CARE OF THE HIGH-RISK NEONATE

THIRD EDITION

Marshall H. Klaus, M.D.

Professor and Chairman
Department of Pediatrics and Human Development
Michigan State University
E. Lansing, Michigan

Avroy A. Fanaroff, M.B. (RAND.), F.R.C.P.E.

Professor of Pediatrics
Vice Chairman, Department of Pediatrics
Case Western Reserve University School of Medicine
Director of Neonatal Nurseries
Rainbow Babies and Childrens Hospital of University Hospitals of Cleveland
Cleveland, Ohio

1986

Ardmore Medical Books, an imprint of
W. B. Saunders Company

Philadelphia / London / Toronto / Mexico City / Rio de Janeiro / Sydney / Tokyo / Hong Kong

W. B. Saunders Company: West Washington Square
                          Philadelphia, PA   19105

Library of Congress Cataloging-in-Publication Data

Main entry under title:

Care of the high-risk neonate.

Includes bibliographies and index.

1. Neonatal intensive care.   2. Infants (Newborn)—
   Diseases.   I. Klaus, Marshall H., 1927–
   II. Fanaroff, Avroy A. [DNLM: 1. Infant Care. 2. Infant,
   Newborn, Diseases—therapy. WS 420 K63c]

RJ253.5.C37 1986   618.92′01   85–19981

ISBN 0–7216–1836–7

Listed here is the latest translated edition of this book together with the language of the translation and the publisher.

German (*1st Edition*)—Gustav Fischer Verlag, Stuttgart, Germany

Japanese (*2nd Edition*)—Igaku Shoin/Saunders Ltd., Tokyo, Japan

Portuguese (*2nd Edition*)—DISCOS CBS Industria E Comercio Ltda., Rio de Janeiro, Brazil

Spanish (*2nd Edition*)—Editorial Medica Panamericana, Buenos Aires, Argentina

Care of the High Risk Neonate   ISBN   0–7216–1836–7

Last digit is the print number: 9   8   7   6   5   4   3   2

This book is dedicated to all students of perinatology, our patients, and their parents—together with Phyllis, Susan, David and Laura, Alisa, Laura, Sarah and grandson Michael (Klaus), and Roslyn, Jonathan, Jodi and Amanda (Fanaroff).

Contributors

Claudine Amiel-Tison, M.D.
Associate Professor of Pediatrics, Medical School Paris V; Staff, Baudelocque Maternity Hospital, Paris, France.

Stephen C. Aronoff, M.D.
Assistant Professor of Pediatrics, Case Western Reserve University School of Medicine; Staff, Division of Pediatric Infectious Diseases, Rainbow Babies and Children's Hospital of University Hospitals of Cleveland, Cleveland, Ohio

June F. Brady, M.B., B.Chir.
Clinical Professor of Pediatrics and Associate Member, Cardiovascular Research Institute, University of California, San Francisco; Director of Nurseries, Children's Hospital of San Francisco, San Francisco, California.

Avroy A. Fanaroff, M.B. (Rand.), F.R.C.P.E.
Professor of Pediatrics and Vice Chairman, Department of Pediatrics, Case Western Reserve University School of Medicine; Director of Neonatal Nurseries, Rainbow Babies and Children's Hospital of University Hospitals of Cleveland, Cleveland, Ohio.

Howard C. Filston, M.D.
Professor of Pediatric Surgery and Pediatrics, Chief, Pediatric Surgery Service, Duke University Medical Center, Durham, North Carolina.

David E. Fisher, M.D.
Associate Professor of Clinical Pediatrics, Pritzker School of Medicine, University of Chicago; Director, Division of Neonatal-Perinatal Medicine, Department of Pediatrics, Michael Reese Hospital and Medical Center, Chicago, Illinois.

Joseph A. Garcia-Prats, M.D.
Associate Professor of Clinical Pediatrics, Baylor College of Medicine; Associate Director of Nurseries and Medical Director, Neonatal Intensive Care Unit of the Winifred Wallace Maternity Center, Jefferson Davis Hospital, Co-Director, Perinatal Outreach Program, Texas Children's Hospital, Houston, Texas.

George A. Gregory, M.D.
Professor of Anesthesia and Pediatrics, University of California, San Francisco, California.

Samuel Gross, M.D.
Professor of Pediatrics, Director of Hematology-Oncology, and Director of Bone Marrow Transplant Unit, University of Florida College of Medicine, Gainesville, Florida.

Warren E. Grupe, M.D.
Associate Professor of Pediatrics, Harvard Medical School; Chief, Division of Nephrology, The Children's Hospital, Boston, Massachusetts.

Maureen Hack, M.B., Ch.B.
Associate Professor of Pediatrics, Case Western Reserve University School of Medicine; Neonatologist University Hospitals (Rainbow Babies and Children's Hospital), Cleveland, Ohio.

Michael A. Heymann, M.D.
Professor of Pediatrics, Physiology and Obstetrics, Gynecology and Reproductive Sciences, University of California, San Francisco; Attending Pediatric Cardiologist, University of California Hospital, San Francisco, California.

Robert J. Izant, Jr., M.D.
Professor of Pediatric Surgery and Professor of Pediatrics, Case Western Reserve University School of Medicine; Director of Pediatric Surgery Division, Department of Surgery, Case Western Reserve University School of Medicine; Director of Pediatric Surgery, Rainbow Babies and Children's Hospital of University Hospitals of Cleveland, Cleveland, Ohio.

John H. Kennell, M.D.
Professor of Pediatrics, Case Western Reserve University School of Medicine; Chief, Division of Child Development, Rainbow Babies and Children's Hospital of University Hospitals of Cleveland, Cleveland, Ohio.

Marshall H. Klaus, M.D.
Professor and Chairman, Department of Pediatrics and Human Development, Michigan State University, East Lansing, Michigan.

Robert M. Kliegman, M.D.
Associate Professor of Pediatrics, Case Western Reserve University School of Medicine; Associate Director of Neonatal Intensive Care Unit, Rainbow Babies and Children's Hospital of University Hospitals of Cleveland, Cleveland, Ohio.

Rowena Korobkin, M.D.
Associate, Pediatric Neurology; Children's Hospital Medical Center, Oakland, California.

Jerome T. Liebman, M.D.
Professor of Pediatrics, Case Western Reserve University School of Medicine, Pediatric Cardiologist, Rainbow Babies and Children's Hospital of University Hospitals of Cleveland, Cleveland, Ohio.

Richard J. Martin, M.B., F.R.A.C.P.
Associate Professor of Pediatrics, Case Western Reserve University School of Medicine; Co-Director, Division of Neonatology, Rainbow Babies and Children's Hospital of University Hospitals of Cleveland, Cleveland, Ohio.

Celeste Martin Marx, Pharm. D.
Assistant Clinical Professor of Pediatrics, Michigan State University College of Human Medicine; Clinical Pharmacy Coordinator, Department of Pharmacy, Edward W. Sparrow Hospital, Lansing, Michigan.

Irwin R. Merkatz, M.D.
Professor and Chairman, Albert Einstein College of Medicine and Affiliated Hospitals, Bronx, New York.

Enrique M. Ostrea, Jr., M.D.
Associate Professor of Pediatrics, Wayne State University School of Medicine; Chief of Pediatrics and Director of Nursery, Hutzel Hospital, Detroit, Michigan.

John B. Paton, M.D.
Associate Professor of Clinical Pediatrics, Pritzker School of Medicine, University of Chicago; Attending Neonatologist, Division of Neonatal-Perinatal Medicine, Department of Pediatrics, Michael Reese Hospital and Medical Center, Chicago, Illinois.

Ronald L. Poland, M.D.
Associate Professor of Pediatrics, Wayne State University School of Medicine; Director of the Neonatal-Perinatal Medicine Division, Children's Hospital of Michigan, Detroit, Michigan.

E. O. R. Reynolds, M.D., F.R.C.P.
Professor of Neonatal Paediatrics, University College of London School of Medicine; Consultant Paediatrician, University College Hospital, London, England.

Arnold J. Rudolph, M.B., B.Ch.
Professor of Pediatrics, Obstetrics and Gynecology, Baylor College of Medicine; Head, Newborn Section, Baylor

College of Medicine, Chief of Neonatology Service, Texas Children's Hospital, Director, Newborn and Premature Service, St. Luke's Episcopal Hospital, Director of Nurseries, Harris County Hospital District, Deputy Chief, Pediatric Service, Methodist Hospital, Chief of Neonatology, The Woman's Hospital of Texas, Houston, Texas.

William T. Speck, M.D.
Professor and Chairman, Department of Pediatrics Case Western Reserve University School of Medicine; Director, Department of Pediatrics, Rainbow Babies and Children's Hospital of University Hospitals of Cleveland, Cleveland, Ohio.

Avron Y. Sweet, M.D.
Professor of Pedatrics, Mount Sinai School of Medicine of The City University of New York; Attending Pediatrician for Neonatology, The Mount Sinai Hospital, New York, New York.

David Teitel, M.D.
Assistant Professor of Pediatrics, University of California, San Francisco, California.

Michael K. Wald, M.D.
Assistant Clinical Professor, Upstate Medical Center—SUNY, Syracuse; Attending Pediatrician, Arnot-Ogden Memorial Hospital and St. Joseph's Hospital, Elmira, New York.

Commenters

Jill E. Baley, M.D.
Assistant Professor of Pediatrics, Case Western Reserve University School of Medicine, Rainbow Babies and Children's Hospital of University Hospitals of Cleveland, Cleveland, Ohio.

Denise Campbell, Ph.D.
Assistant Professor of Medicine, Department of Community Health, University of Calgary, Calgary, Alberta, Canada.

Waldemar A. Carlo, M.D.
Assistant Professor of Pediatrics, Case Western Reserve University School of Medicine, Rainbow Babies and Children's Hospital of University Hospitals of Cleveland, Cleveland, Ohio.

Gabriel Duc, M.D.
Professor of Neonatology, University Women's Clinic, Zurich, Switzerland.

Pamela Fitzhardinge, M.D., F.R.C.P.(C.)
Head of Pediatric Perinatology and Pediatrician in Chief, Mount Sinai Hospital, Toronto, Ontario, Canada.

Emile Gautier, M.D.
Professor, Pediatric Service, University Infants Clinic, Cantonal Hospital, Lausanne, Switzerland.

Maureen Hack, M.B., Ch.B.
Associate Professor of Pediatrics, Case Western Reserve University School of Medicine, Rainbow Babies and Children's Hospital of University Hospitals of Cleveland, Cleveland, Ohio.

David Hull, M.B., Ch.B.
Professor of Child Health, University of Nottingham Medical School, Nottingham, England.

Stanley James, M.D.
Professor of Pediatrics and Obstetrics and Gynecology, Director of Perinatology, Department of Pediatrics, Columbia University College of Physicians and Surgeons, New York, New York.

John Kattwinkel, M.D.
Professor of Pediatrics, University of Virginia School of Medicine, Charlottesville, Virginia.

Lula O. Lubchenco, M.D.
Emeritus Professor of Pediatrics, University of Colorado School of Medicine, Denver, Colorado.

M. Jeffrey Maisels, M.B., B.Ch.(Rand.)
Professor of Pediatrics and Chief of Neonatal Medicine of the Milton S. Hershey Medical Center of Pennsylvania State University, Hershey, Pennsylvania.

George E. McCracken, M.D.
Professor of Pediatrics, University of Texas Health Science Center, Southwestern Medical School; Attending Physician, Parkland Memorial Hospital and Children's Medical Center, Dallas, Texas.

Martha J. Miller, M.D., Ph.D.
Assistant Professor of Pediatrics, Case Western Reserve University School of

Medicine, Rainbow Babies and Children's Hospital of University Hospitals of Cleveland, Cleveland, Ohio.

William Oh, M.D.
Professor of Pediatrics and Obstetrics, Brown University Program in Medicine; Pediatrician-in-Chief, Women and Infants Hospital of Rhode Island, Providence, Rhode Island.

Albert Okken, M.D.
Department of Pediatrics, Division of Neonatology, University Hospital, Groningen, Netherlands.

Frank Oski, M.D.
Professor and Chairman, Department of Pediatrics, Johns Hopkins University, Baltimore, Maryland.

Roberto Paludetto, M.D.
Associate Professor, The University of Naples Faculty of Medicine, Naples, Italy.

Paul Perlstein, M.D.
Professor of Pediatrics, University of Cincinnati College of Medicine, Children's Hospital Research Foundation, Cincinnati, Ohio.

William B. Pittard III, M.D.
Associate Professor of Pediatrics, Medical University of South Carolina, Charleston, South Carolina.

Samuel Prod'hom, M.D.
Professor, Pediatric Service, University Infants Clinic, Cantonal Hospital, Lausanne, Switzerland.

Edward J. Quilligan, M.D.
Professor of Obstetrics and Gynecology, University of California Davis Medical Center, Sacramento, California.

E. O. R. Reynolds, M.D., F.R.C.P.
Professor of Neonatal Paediatrics, University College of London School of Medicine; Consultant Paediatrician, University College Hospital, London, England.

Mildred T. Stahlman, M.D.
Professor of Pediatrics, Vanderbilt University School of Medicine, Nashville, Tennessee.

Leo Stern, M.D.
Professor and Chairman of Pediatrics, Brown University Program in Medicine; Pediatrician-in-Chief, Rhode Island Hospital, Providence, Rhode Island.

John Stork, M.D.
Assistant Professor of Pediatrics, Case Western Reserve University School of Medicine, Rainbow Babies and Children's Hospital of University Hospitals of Cleveland, Cleveland, Ohio.

Norman Talner, M.D.
Professor of Pediatrics, Yale University School of Medicine, New Haven, Connecticut.

Reginald Tsang, M.B.B.S.
Professor of Pediatrics and Obstetrics and Gynecology, Director of Newborn Division, University of Cincinnati College of Medicine and Children's Research Foundation, Cincinnati, Ohio.

Joseph J. Volpe, M.D.
Professor of Pediatrics, Neurology, and Biochemistry, Washington University School of Medicine, St. Louis, Missouri.

William B. Weil, Jr., M.D.
Professor of Pediatrics, Michigan State University, East Lansing, Michigan.

Foreword

During the past four decades, enormous advances have been achieved in the field of neonatal-perinatal medicine. The acquisition of new knowledge through perinatal research and the development of new technology by the combined efforts of scientists and industry are so extensive that they represent somewhat of a "minirevolution" in medicine in general and pediatrics and obstetrics in particular. A few examples are maternal glucocorticoid administration and surfactant replacement therapy for hyaline membrane disease, the use of assisted ventilation and continuous positive airway pressure in the management of infants with respiratory failure, vaccines for the prevention of neonatal hepatitis, and the noninvasive diagnostic technology for such conditions as intraventricular hemorrhage and patent ductus arteriosus. These developments, along with the implementation of perinatal regionalization and firm establishment of neonatal intensive care networks, have accounted for the marked improvement in perinatal mortality and morbidity during the past three to four decades.

The era is also characterized by the publication of several textbooks in neonatology, as well as numerous monographs, symposia, proceedings, and journals dedicated to the field of perinatal medicine. The quality of these publications is, in general, excellent, and they serve as the major reading resources for perinatal health care personnel. The textbook by Marshall Klaus and Avroy Fanaroff, however, stands out as the leader of the pack. The various chapters of this book are written by an impressive group of well-known and well-respected neonatologists and perinatologists assembled by Klaus and Fanaroff. The contents are comprehensive, practical, and clearly written. The editing is superb, and the commentaries by the experts in each field are an excellent addition, representing a real "icing on the cake" to a very fine medical literary product. It is not surprising that this textbook is well read by clinicians and allied health personnel who deal with the care of high-risk neonates. Our sincerest gratitude to both Marshall and Avroy for a job well done.

WILLIAM OH, M.D.

Preface

The field of neonatal-perinatal medicine and specifically neonatal care continues to change, and clinical applications of studies in many disciplines have dramatically improved the outcome of ill neonates.

The past six years have been characterized by refinements in diagnostic and therapeutic techniques as well as new developments, for example, surfactant therapy. Monitoring equipment is now much more sophisticated, provides "trends," and is in many instances software driven so that it should not become outdated. Ultrasonography, CT scan, NMR and PET scans have paved the way for precise and specific diagnoses that were either impossible or delayed until infancy. Malformations are recognized with increased frequency before delivery so that plans can be made for delivery of these high-risk fetuses in tertiary centers, and surgery is now possible for certain lesions formerly regarded as lethal. We continue to strive to sustain life in even smaller, less mature infants. Costs have skyrocketed and there is increased pressure to shorten the duration of hospitalization. Nonetheless, our applications of and understanding of the fundamentals of neonatal physiology remain the cornerstones of neonatal care. It is the attention to detail and fine-tuning that have ultimately been responsible for the continued improvement in outcome. We have, nonetheless, continued to be plagued by iatrogenic disasters and must remain vigilant and cautious about introducing new treatments. The deleterious effects of any new therapeutic regimen should always be carefully considered before the therapy is introduced in the nursery. Detailed and methodical follow-up must be an essential component of all high-risk programs, and evaluations of a new treatment must encompass randomized, controlled studies with not only the immediate and usual side effects but also the equally disastrous late long-term sequelae. Perinatologists must remain the advocates for the newborn.

This third edition attempts to incorporate many of the newer technological and physiologic advances, and in order to accomplish this a larger group of contributors and critical commenters has been gathered to put the current state of the art in perspective. This group includes experts in perinatology from throughout North America and Europe. We are pleased to have several new contributors join us as authors of chapters. Based on practical experience from the first two editions, we have used the same format, presenting new information in the form of text, case problems, or simply questions with descriptive answers that can be explored using an expanded index. There have also been major revisions in all sections. The objective has remained to provide a sound physiologic basis for current perinatal practice.

We would like to thank our many colleagues and the fellows from the past several years for their valuable comments and criticism during the genesis of this, the third edition. We also wish to thank Ellen Rome, Bonnie Siner, Jenny Tucker, and Joseph Alfano who assisted us with proofreading, and Sandra Hartman for coordinating our efforts. In addition, Jennifer Smith, W. B. Saunders Company, has been an extremely valuable copy editor; and, we are most grateful for the continued assistance and encouragement from Al Meier of W. B. Saunders Company.

MARSHALL H. KLAUS
AVROY A. FANAROFF

Contents

1

Antenatal and Intrapartum Care of the High-Risk Infant

IRWIN R. MERKATZ
AVROY A. FANAROFF

Everything ought to be done to ensure that an infant be born at term, well developed, and in a healthy condition. But in spite of every care, infants are born prematurely....

PIERRE BUDIN
THE NURSLING

Parallel to the significant improvements in care of the premature and sick neonate in recent years, there has developed an extensive technology concerned with the evaluation and supervision of the high-risk fetus.[89, 99, 133, 139] Initially stimulated in the 1960s by the pioneering work with amniotic fluid analysis in Rh-isoimmunized pregnancy, this technology has expanded at a rapid rate. Over a mere 15 years, hormonal assessments of fetoplacental function, fetal scalp blood determinations of fetal homeostasis, electronic monitoring of the fetal heart rate during and prior to labor, biochemical estimations of fetal pulmonary maturity, ultrasonographic measurements of fetal head size, fetal growth, and fetal activity, and detailed ultrasonographic evaluation of fetal anatomy have all become commonplace procedures.[2, 13, 124] Visualization of the fetus by fetoscopy, ultrasonic recording of fetal respiration, and sophisticated studies of fetal cardiac function by echocardiography are among newer procedures under current investigation.[49, 119, 140]

The capabilities of accurate diagnosis and treatment of fetal disorders have expanded rapidly.[53–55, 69]

These and other sophisticated approaches may well be routine components of clinical care in the future. However, many of these procedures are expensive and need quality laboratory support, and their results are not always easy to interpret. Advanced training and accreditation for obstetric perinatologists have followed the introduction of new technology, but in this, as in other allied areas, the supply of personnel is limited. Furthermore, epidemiologic studies have indicated that only a small percentage of all pregnant women manifest risk features that necessitate these intensive interventions. Practicalities demand that they be applied in an appropriately effective fashion since underutilized personnel and facilities will not be tolerated by a society increasingly concerned with maximizing cost-benefit ratios and reducing costs.

Nor should overutilization be tolerated. Although perinatal technologies and services are available, their use must be based on a reasonable amount of information about risks, benefits, and alternatives. One of the ill effects of availability of services is to deploy, for instance, neonatal care facilities for all newborns with the result that a large number of infants are admitted to neonatal care units unnecessarily. Health care providers must be vigilant to avoid indiscriminate use of tests and facilities since they may result in more harm than benefits.

D. Campbell

1

Nevertheless, in many centers of excellence, the appropriate utilization of this new technology appears to have contributed to marked reductions of perinatal mortality even among groups of very high-risk patients.[6, 64, 88, 107, 114, 120, 143] It is hoped that wider and more uniform application of these newer concepts of care after controlled studies evaluating their benefits may, in part, offer a solution to the long-standing problem of unacceptably high perinatal mortality and morbidity rates in the United States. Overall, perinatal mortality has fallen dramatically such that most centers are reporting a rate of 12/1000 live births, a decrease of nearly half the rate of the previous decade.[85, 104, 143] Nonetheless, there is an urgent need to tackle the problem of prematurity to reduce these rates further. The recent declines in mortality rates have been attributed to improved neonatal care, with no evidence to date of any impact on the prematurity rate.

Editorial Comment: Neonatologists and perinatologists cannot claim all the credit for reductions in the neonatal mortality rate (NMR). David and Siegel found that 34 per cent of the reduction in NMR in North Carolina in the decade 1968–1977 was attributable to changes in the birth weight and gestational age makeup of the newborn population.

Doing away with poverty would have an even greater effect in reducing the prematurity rate and neonatal mortality.

David, R. J., and Siegel, E.: Decline in neonatal mortality, 1968 to 1977: better babies or better care? Pediatrics 71:531, 1983.

Since many of the determinants of neonatal outcome relate directly to intrauterine and intrapartal events, continued improvement in perinatal care is contingent upon a team approach to high-risk pregnancies. Obstetricians, midwives, nurses, pediatricians, and family physicians collaboratively must develop comprehensive protocols of management that will ensure the best results for the maximum number of mothers and infants.

The team approach to health care delivery has been advocated as an integral part of medical care for the last two decades. Shortages of highly trained professionals may in part serve as an impetus to the development of the team. Caution, however, is necessary since much of the literature on teamwork is mainly anecdotal and has rarely been assessed or evaluated. **D. Campbell**

Maximizing the benefits of the new technology will require regionalization—specifically, the development of a network of providers of perinatal care within a defined geographic area to implement the following objectives: (1) the identification of high-risk pregnancies early in the perinatal period; (2) the further identification of high-risk factors within the intrapartum period; (3) the development of interhospital agreements on criteria for transfer of mothers and infants within the network; (4) the development of support systems of consultation, laboratory services, education, and transportation within a region; and (5) the development of a record-keeping system that will allow adequate monitoring of the performance of the entire program.[123]

IDENTIFYING THE PATIENT AT RISK

Early identification of the high-risk population associated with the largest proportion of untoward perinatal outcome has become a priority for the obstetric care delivery system. Based upon retrospective and prospective studies performed between 1951 and 1965, many of the principal determinants of perinatal morbidity and mortality have been delineated.[56, 74, 75] Included among these are maternal age, race, socioeconomic status, nutrition, past obstetric history, associated medical illness, and current pregnancy problems.

While there is unanimity about the correlation between various sociodemographic characteristics and perinatal morbidity and mortality, nothing has been convincingly established about causality.

Nevertheless, since both prevention of labor and early detection of perinatal morbidity and mortality depend in part on the recognition of sociodemographic variables, various attempts to develop scoring systems for risk of preterm delivery have been made. To date, however, the ability to predict accurately preterm labor or neonatal risk using demographic and other variables has only been modest.[29, 30] Further progress to find better measures to predict outcome is most desirable. **D. Campbell**

Careful analysis indicates that these determinants of morbidity and mortality are composed of historical factors existing prior to pregnancy as well as factors and events associated directly with pregnancy. Together these have provided the basis for the development of several assessment techniques capable of distinguishing most of the high-risk patients from the low-risk patients prior to delivery.

In 1969 Nesbitt and Aubry indicated that 29 per cent of pregnant women could objectively be identified as being at increased risk.[106] The outcome of pregnancy among these women was judged unsatisfactory by the occurrence of premature birth, low birth weight, perinatal mortality, neonatal depression, and respiratory distress syndrome at a rate twice that of the normal population. In Canada, similar results were obtained on more diverse groups of pregnant women by Goodwin, Dunne, and Thomas.[59] Their fetal risk scoring system is now extensively utilized in Nova Scotia. Hobel et al have described a risk assessment system that includes intrapartum as well as prenatal risk factors and have identified four subgroups of patients with ascending rates of perinatal mortality and neonatal morbidity (Table 1–1).[75] In a prospective study of a low socioeconomic population, 18 per cent of pregnant women were categorized as being at high risk both prenatally and intrapartally, and it was from this group that the poorest outcomes were obtained.

In many communities perinatal teams are currently attempting to introduce the concepts of uniform record-keeping and risk identification across broad populations of pregnant women. In this manner it is hoped to better define high-risk indicators among diverse socioeconomic groups. Thus within a defined region all pregnant women will be assessed at the time of the first visit and again in the third trimester, recognizing the possibility of change in risk status upward by intercurrent illness and hopefully downward by preventive intervention. Such risk assessment is repeated early in labor to individualize the technologic interventions appropriately, later in labor to prepare the obstetric and pediatric staffs for delivery, and after birth of the infant to triage potential neonatal difficulties.[92, 93]

Prematurity remains the most significant perinatal problem, accounting for 75 per cent of all perinatal mortality. In the United States, the prematurity rate (about 10%) has remained remarkably constant. Creasy et al[29, 30] in San Francisco, in an effort to identify and intervene in those cases where patients are at greatest risk of delivering prematurely, developed an evaluation (scoring) system which takes into account: (1) the patient's socioeconomic status; (2) her past history; (3) her daily habits; and (4) current pregnancy events. The patients were evaluated at their first office visit and again between 25 and 28 weeks' gestation. Those with a score of 10 were classified as being at high risk for preterm delivery (Table 1–2). Thirty per cent of high-risk patients delivered prematurely in contrast to only 2.5 per cent among the low-risk group.[71] In the second phase of the study those identified as high risk were followed closely and instructed to report immediately any signs or symptoms compatible with early onset of labor. Furthermore, the perinatal staff received inservice education, emphasizing: (1) the need to respond promptly to any subtle signs of preterm labor; (2) the need to admit and observe closely with electronic monitoring those patients with mild signs of early preterm labor or cervical dilatation; (3) the need to attempt tocolysis aggressively when premature labor was present; and (4) an awareness of the contraindications and side effects of tocolysis. Institution of these protocols resulted in a decrease in the prematurity rate from 6.75 per cent to 2.4 per cent. A number of other centers are now testing these protocols in the hope of achieving the same outstanding results.

EVALUATION OF THE FETUS AND SUPERVISION OF ITS CARE[11, 72, 111]

Improved physiologic understanding and multiple technologic advancements now provide the obstetrician with tools for objective evaluation of the fetus. In particular, specific information can now be sought and obtained relative to fetal anatomy, growth, well-being, and functional maturity, and these data are

TABLE 1–1 FETAL RISK ASSESSMENT SYSTEM*

| | Risk Groups | | | | High-Risk Neonate (Morbidity) | | Perinatal (Morbidity) | |
	Prenatal	Intrapartum	N	%	N	% of Group	N	% of Group
I	Low	Low	99	38	5	5.0	0	0.0
II	High	Low	69	27	4	5.8	1	1.4
III	Low	High	43	17	5	11.6	1	2.3
IV	High	High	46	18	8	17.4	2	4.3
			257	100	22	8.6% of 257 births	4	1.5% of 257 births

*From Hobel, C., Hyvarinen, M., Okada, D., et al.: Prenatal and intrapartum high risk screening: Prediction of the high risk neonate. Am J Obstet Gynecol *117*:1, 1973.

TABLE 1–2 SCORING SYSTEM FOR RISK OF PRETERM DELIVERY

Points*	Socioeconomic Status	Past History	Daily Habits	Current Pregnancy
1	Two children at home Low socioeconomic status	One abortion <1 year since last birth	Work outside home	Unusual fatigue
2	Younger than 20 years Older than 40 years Single parent	Two abortions	>10 cigarettes per day	<13 lb gain by 32 weeks Albuminuria Hypertension Bacteriuria
3	Very low socioeconomic status Shorter than 150 cm Lighter than 45 kg	Three abortions	Heavy work Long, tiring trip	Breech at 32 weeks Weight loss of 2 kg Head engaged Febrile illness
4	Younger than 18 years	Pyelonephritis		Metrorrhagia after 12 weeks' gestation Effacement Dilatation Uterine irritability
5		Uterine anomaly Second-trimester abortion Diethylstilbestrol (DES) exposure		Placenta previa Hydramnios
10		Premature delivery Repeated second-trimester abortion		Twins Abdominal surgery

*Score is computed by addition of the number of points given any item. 0–5 = low risk; 6–9 = medium risk; ≥10 = high risk.

Adapted from Creasy, R., Gummer, B., and Liggins, G.: System for predicting spontaneous preterm birth. Obstet Gynecol 55:692, 1980.

utilized to provide a rational approach to clinical management of the high-risk infant prior to birth. For detailed reviews of the many new physical, hormonal, and biochemical approaches to prenatal and fetal assessments, the reader is advised to consult more comprehensive obstetric texts.[9, 11, 69, 133] This section, however, will briefly summarize the clinical applications of the most widely utilized techniques as background for a discussion of practical clinical problems.

Monitoring Fetal Growth

It is important to emphasize that no test or laboratory procedure can serve to supplant the data obtained from a careful history and physical examination. Ultimately the results of all of the newer techniques have to be interpreted in light of the true or presumed gestational age of the fetus. It is therefore essential that the initial pregnancy visit be concerned with a thorough documentation of information relative to the regularity of the patient's menstrual cycles, use of oral contraceptive agents, date of last menstrual period, pregnancy test results, and the like. The initial and subsequent physical examinations are then approached with these facts in mind to ascertain whether the uterine size and growth are consistent with the supposed length of gestation. Similarly, the milestones of quickening (16–18 weeks) and fetal heart tone auscultation by Doppler ultrasound (12–14 weeks) and fetoscope (18–22 weeks) are important and need to be systematically recorded. Although most of this information is gathered early in pregnancy, it may not be used until later in gestation when decisions regarding the appropriateness of fetal size and the timing of delivery are contemplated.

Discrepancies in either direction of size versus dates may suggest the need for an ultrasound evaluation of the uterine contents. Ultrasound is a technique by which short pulses (2 μ sec) of high-frequency (approximately 2.5 m Hz), low-intensity sound waves are transmitted from a piezo-electric crystal (transducer) through the maternal abdomen to the uterus and the fetus.[22, 41, 49, 73, 124, 125] The echo signals reflected back from tissue interfaces provide a two-dimensional picture of the uterine wall, placenta, amniotic fluid, and fetus. Diagnoses of multiple gestation, fetal structural abnormalities, abnormally implanted placentae, and uterine or placental pathologic conditions can be made by this technique. Serial measurements of the fetus can provide a reliable indicator of fetal growth. Furthermore, ultrasound is extensively used to assess fetal well-being and to study fetal physiology. Some indications for ultrasound are contained in Table 1–3. In many instances ultrasound is performed to comply with the mother's request only.

Because of the known susceptibility of the fetus to a multitude of environmental factors, the inherent safety of ultrasound needs to be clearly established. Although a study by Baker and Dalrymple[1] suggests no adverse effects of ultrasound on future child development, some in vitro and animal studies[45, 83] suggest morphologic transformation of embryo cells. The apparently conflicting evidence indicates that more information is needed on the short- and long-term effects of ultrasound.

National Institutes of Health: The use of diagnostic ultrasound imaging in pregnancy. Washington, DC, DHHS Publication, NIH, 1984.

D. Campbell

TABLE 1–3 INDICATIONS FOR ULTRASOUND

Confirmation of pregnancy
Determination of:
  Gestational age
  Fetal number and presentation
  Placental location (vaginal bleeding)
  Fetal anatomy (previous malformations)
Assessment of:
  Size/date discrepancy
  Fetal well-being (biophysical profile—fetal tone,
    movements, and respiration)
  Volume of amniotic fluid (suspected oligo- or
    polyhydramnios)
  Fetal arrhythmias
  Fetal anatomy (abnormal alpha-fetoprotein)
Assist with procedures:
  Amniocentesis
  Intrauterine transfusion

In the first trimester, the gestational age of the fetus is assessed by a crown-to-rump measurement. After the thirteenth week of gestation, measurement of the fetal biparietal diameter (BPD) or cephalometry is the most commonly employed technique (Figure 1–1). Prior to 28 weeks' gestation, this measurement provides a good estimation of gestational age within a range of ± 10 days.[22] After 28 weeks' gestation, the predictability of the measurement is less reliable, so an initial examination should be obtained prior to this stage if a problem pregnancy is anticipated. Follow-up examinations can then be employed to ascertain whether or not fetal growth in utero is proceeding at a normal rate.

When fetal growth is retarded, however, brain sparing may result in an abnormal ratio of growth between the head and the rest of the body. Since the BPD may then remain within normal limits, other measurements are needed to detect the true retardation of growth. Campbell has found that measurement of the ratio between the circumferences of head and abdomen is of particular value under these circumstances.[22] During the second trimester of pregnancy the normal ratio is greater than one in favor of the head, but after 36 weeks' gestation there is a reversal and the abdominal circumference predominates. In many cases of growth retardation this reversal is not seen (Figure 1–2).

Queenan et al (1976) found single biparietal diameter measurements quite unreliable in diagnosing intrauterine growth retardation (IUGR). Only 7 of 16 patients with biparietal diameters below the tenth percentile had IUGR, and of the 16 patients with IUGR, only 9 were diagnosed prenatally—7 with a single low biparietal diameter and 2 with several low values. Thiede, commenting on this paper, stated that in Rochester he had obtained similar results, with only 53 per cent of small-for-gestational-age (SGA) babies having been diagnosed prior to delivery by single or multiple determinations of the fetal biparietal diameter. While it is true that measurement of other fetal parameters such as thoracic or abdominal size may assist in the diagnosis of IUGR, prospective studies like the one cited need to be done to correctly determine the false-positive and false-negative rates.

Queenan, J. T., Kubarych, S. F., Cook, L. N., et al: Diagnostic ultrasound for detection of intrauterine growth retardation. Am J Obstet Gynecol 124:865, 1976.

E. Quilligan

Femur length, which may be less affected by alterations in growth than the head or abdomen, is used to aid in determining gestational age and to identify the fetus with

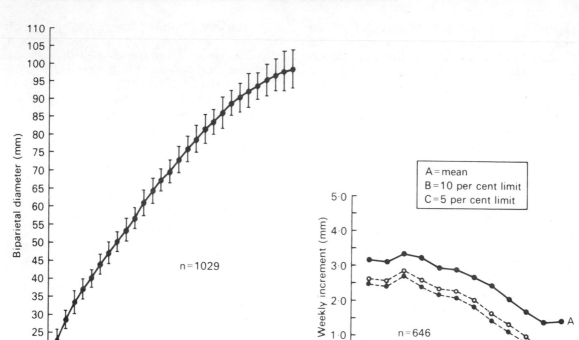

Figure 1–1. *A,* Mean fetal biparietal diameter (mm) ± 2 s.d. for each week of pregnancy from 13 weeks to term. *B,* Mean growth rate of the fetal biparietal diameter with lower tolerance limits related to the size of the biparietal diameter.[22]

abnormal growth. Serial assessment of growth and deviations from normal, including both macrosomia and growth retardation, helps identify the fetus at risk during the perinatal period (see Chapter 4). Nonetheless only about 50 per cent of growth retarded fetuses are identified before delivery.

Editorial Comment: Measurement of total intrauterine volume is also used to identify intrauterine growth retardation.

In prospective studies utilizing antenatal ultrasound,[2, 13] no differences have been noted in neonatal outcome from pregnancies in which ultrasound was not used. Nonetheless, early ultrasound has resulted in more confident establishment of dates, earlier detection of multiple gestation, and earlier diagnosis and more active intervention for infants with intrauterine growth retardation. Furthermore, no adverse short-term effects from ultrasound have been noted. More women who had been screened with ultrasound required antenatal hospitalization.

A clear role for antenatal ultrasound has been established, and it is of extreme value in dating pregnancies, diagnosing multiple

pregnancies, monitoring intrauterine growth, and detecting congenital malformations as well as locating placental site. Additionally ultrasound is invaluable when performing amniocentesis or attempting other invasive procedures such as intrauterine transfusions.

Editorial Comment: Ultrasound may be used during labor to resolve problems related to vaginal bleeding, size/date discrepancies, suspected abnormal presentation, loss of fetal heart tones, delivery of a second twin, attempted version of a breech presentation, and diagnosis of fetal anomalies.

Assessing the Fetal Condition Antepartum

The most widely employed tests to evaluate the function and reserve of the fetoplacental unit and the well-being of the fetus before labor are serial estriol determinations, stress and nonstress monitoring of the fetal heart rate, monitoring of fetal activity, and amnioscopy. Serial measurement of maternal serum alpha-fetoprotein levels and studies of fetal movements and respirations incorporated as part of the multivariable assessment (see the Fetal Biophysical Profile) continue to be evaluated clinically.

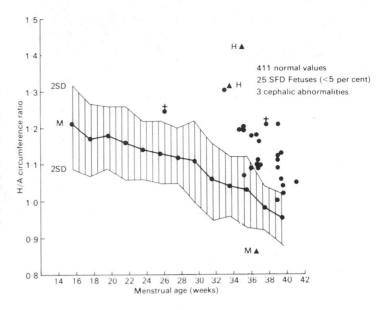

Figure 1–2. The head-to-abdomen circumference ratio (H/A ratio) in small-for-dates fetuses (i.e., below the 5th percentile weight for gestation) and three fetuses with cephalic abnormalities; these are plotted on the normal H/A ratio graph showing the mean, 95th, and 5th percentile confidence limits. Twenty-two of the 25 small-for-dates fetuses had ratios above the 95th percentile limit, and the two fetuses who died (+) had high ratios. Hydrocephalus (H) is associated with very high and microcephaly (M) with very low H/A ratios.[22]

ESTRIOLS

For more than a decade, maternal urine and serum estriol levels were considered the principal tools to evaluate the fetal condition.[78] The fetal adrenal cortex secretes the precursor dehydroepiandrosterone, which is converted by the fetal liver to 16-OH dehydroepiandrosterone sulfate (DHEAS). Placental enzymes readily desulfate 16-OH DHEAS and aromatize Ring A. The product of this conversion is estriol, which, after conjugation in the maternal liver, is excreted in urine. The measurement of estriol in maternal urine or blood thus reflects combined fetoplacental function.[34] Since the placenta has a large reserve in its enzymatic capacity for aromatization, only a marked decrease in availability of fetal precursors will result in decreased estriol production.

Both blood and urinary estriol determinations are available. Serial measurements are necessary because of the daily variation in levels and the problems created by inaccurate or incomplete 24 hour urine collections. Excessive day-to-day fluctuations in urinary estriol levels may be validated by determination of estriol/creatinine ratios.

The testing of estriol has been applied to a wide variety of high-risk pregnancies and has been found most useful in pregnancies complicated by diabetes mellitus, hypertension, preeclampsia, intrauterine growth retardation, prolonged gestation, and previous unexplained fetal loss.[94] Excretion patterns vary, depending upon the pathologic condi-

tion. They may be reassuringly within the normal range and rising, consistently below the normal range and flat, or falling from normal to abnormal, which signifies failing fetoplacental function and impending fetal death. Continuously very low levels are seen in isolated adrenal cortical hypoplasia, placental sulfatase deficiency, or fetal death, in a mother receiving high doses of corticosteroids, or in a mother carrying an anencephalic fetus.[60] Estriols are used less frequently today in following high-risk pregnancies.

ANTEPARTUM FETAL HEART RATE MONITORING

Antepartum electronic monitoring of the fetal heart rate has provided a second useful approach to fetal evaluation. The oxytocin challenge test described by Ray et al[115] records the fetal rate of responsiveness to the stress of induced uterine contractions and thus attempts to assess the functional reserve of the placenta. A negative test (no fetal heart rate decelerations in response to adequate uterine contractions) gives reassurance that the fetus is not in immediate jeopardy.[43, 141] Similar information may be obtained by evaluating the response of the fetal heart rate to spontaneous uterine contractions and perhaps also from the resting heart rate patterns without contractions.[118, 128] Baseline variability of the fetal heart rate and accelerations of the rate with fetal motion have been reported as good indicators of the response to subsequent stress testing and of fetal well-being.[118]

Editorial Comment: During nonstress tests accelerations in fetal heart rate (FHR) $\geq$ 15 beats per minute (bpm) for 15 seconds are indicative of fetal well-being.

The contraction stress test evaluates utero-placental function and was traditionally performed by initiating uterine contractions with oxytocin (Pitocin). Because sophisticated equipment is required together with continuous supervision, attempts have been made to induce uterine contractions with nipple stimulation either by automanipulation or with warm compresses. The nipple stimulation has a variable success rate and, because of inability to regulate the contractions as well as concerns raised by the observation of uterine hyperstimulation accompanied by fetal heart rate changes, has not gained wide acceptance. Nonetheless, breast stimulation provides an alternative, cheap technique for initiating uterine contractions and evaluating placental reserve.[81]

MONITORING FETAL ACTIVITY

Fetal movement has gained increased attention as an expression of fetal well-being in utero. It has been monitored simply by maternal recording of perceived activity or utilizing pressure sensitive electromechanical devices and real time ultrasound. Fetal inactivity is generally defined as less than three movements per hour. Whereas evidence of an active or vigorous fetus is reassuring, an inactive fetus is not necessarily an ominous finding and may merely reflect fetal state (fetal activity is reduced during quiet sleep, by certain drugs including alcohol and barbiturates, and by cigarette smoking). Nonetheless, fetal inactivity requires prompt reassessment including real time ultrasound and electronic fetal heart rate monitoring.

AMNIOSCOPY

Amnioscopy was first introduced as a clinical tool in the early 1960s by Erich Saling.[127] The technique offers a simple, quick, and safe evaluation of the color of the amniotic fluid with the membranes left intact. The principal indications for the procedure are postterm pregnancies and pregnancies complicated by chronic hypertension or preeclampsia. The test can be repeated several times per week, and the visualization of adequate amounts of clear, colorless amniotic fluid is reassuring. Such a finding can be used to support a conservative approach to nonintervention.

If, on the other hand, meconium stained fluid is encountered or an absence of amniotic fluid noted, further evaluation of the metabolic condition of the fetus is indicated before the method of delivery is decided. Several series have demonstrated a significantly increased incidence of fetal acidosis and low Apgar scores among babies with meconium seen at amnioscopy.[133] Therefore, in most instances admission to the hospital, amniotomy, and a fetal blood scalp pH determination would follow the detection of meconium stained fluid in such high-risk patients.

The value of amnioscopy is dubious for two reasons. One is that, not infrequently, meconium may be present and not seen. The second and perhaps more important reason is that the presence or absence of meconium staining of the amniotic fluid gives little information that cannot be obtained more accurately by stress or nonstress fetal monitoring.   E. Quilligan

For these reasons amnioscopy is used sparingly today.

THE FETAL BIOPHYSICAL PROFILE

Antepartum stillbirths (8/1000) account for 66 per cent of all perinatal mortality (Manning et al[89]) and are the result predominantly of chronic asphyxia and congenital malformations. There is an urgent need to detect developing fetal asphyxia accurately in order to intervene and reduce fetal wastage appropriately. A conglomerate of assessments, the biophysical profile, has emerged to address this issue.

Six variables—the nonstress test, fetal movements, fetal breathing movements, fetal tone, amniotic fluid volume, and placental grading—constitute the fetal biophysical profile (Table 1–4). There has been much debate regarding the pros and cons of each component of this evaluation. However, in a prospective evaluation normal tests were highly predictive of a good neonatal outcome. In contrast each abnormal variable was associated with a high false-positive rate. Vintzileos et al[139] noted that the absence of fetal movements was the best predictor of abnormal fetal heart rate patterns in labor (80%); the nonreactive nonstress test best predicted meconium stained amniotic fluid (33%); and

TABLE 1–4 TECHNIQUE OF BIOPHYSICAL PROFILE SCORING

Biophysical Variable	Normal (score = 2)	Abnormal (score = 0)
Fetal breathing movements	At least 1 episode of at least 30 seconds' duration in 30 minutes' observation	Absent or no episode of ≥30 seconds in 30 minutes
Gross body movement	At least 3 discrete body/limb movements in 30 minutes (episodes of active continuous movement considered as a single movement)	Two or fewer episodes of body/limb movements in 30 minutes
Fetal tone	At least 1 episode of active extension with return to flexion of fetal limb(s) or trunk; opening and closing of hand considered normal tone	Either slow extension with return to partial flexion or movement of limb in full extension or absent fetal movement
Reactive fetal heart rate	At least 2 episodes of acceleration of ≥15 bpm and at least 15 seconds' duration associated with fetal movement in 30 minutes	Less than 2 accelerations or acceleration <15 bpm in 30 minutes
Qualitative amniotic fluid volume	At least 1 pocket of amniotic fluid that measures at least 1 cm in 2 perpendicular planes	Either no amniotic fluid pockets or a pocket <1 cm in 2 perpendicular planes

From Manning, F., Morrison, I., Lange, I., et al.: Antepartum determination of fetal health: composite biophysical profile scoring. Clin Perinatol 9:285, 1982.

decreased tone was the best predictor of perinatal death. The biophysical profile was far superior to the contraction stress test in predicting the hypoxic fetus (71 versus 16%). Because the biophysical profile incorporates ultrasonic evaluation of the fetus and may result in the detection of anatomic abnormalities, some investigators have proposed that it should be used as the primary method of fetal surveillance. However, because of its complexity and disagreement about the importance of the various test components, it has not gained wide acceptance.

Early experience with composite biophysical profile scoring has been encouraging, with a reduction in perinatal mortality rate and increased detection of fetal anomalies. A high sensitivity (few fetal asphyxial deaths) and high specificity (minimal inappropriate intervention) are noted from these reports. This contrasts sharply with the high incidence of false-positive tests observed with single assessments such as fetal movements or fetal breathing. A normal fetal biophysical profile appears to indicate intact CNS mechanisms, whereas factors depressing the fetal CNS will reduce or abolish fetal activities. Thus hypoxemia decreases fetal breathing and, with acidemia, reduces body movements. CNS stimulants increase fetal activities. The biophysical profile offers a broader approach to fetal well-being. Perinatologists have become attuned to doing multiple tests in evaluating fetal well-being.

ALPHA-FETOPROTEIN[21, 32, 97]

Alpha-fetoprotein (AFP) is a fetal serum protein genetically and biochemically related to albumin. It has become a valuable marker not only in the prenatal detection of open neural tube defects but also in identifying fetuses likely to have chromosomal abnormalities.

Studies in the United Kingdom documented the correlation of an elevated amniotic fluid AFP level between 16 and 18 weeks' gestation with open neural tube defects. Subsequent testing demonstrated elevated maternal serum AFP levels as well for those fetuses with open defects, and this knowledge has been translated into worldwide screening programs utilizing maternal serum. These programs have been very successful, particularly when it is noted that neural tube defects predominantly occur (95%) in families with no prior history of such defects. The analysis of amniotic fluid has proved to be a reliable, accurate diagnostic test for open neural tube defects, with a 98–99 per cent correlation between amniotic fluid AFP values (plus 3 or more standard deviations from the mean) and affected fetuses. Testing prenatal amniotic fluid AFP levels is indicated under the following circumstances: (1) a previous child with neural tube defect; (2) a parent or close relative with neural tube defect; (3) a previous child with hydrocephalus; (4) elevated maternal serum AFP; or (5) a woman undergoing second trimester amniocentesis for other reasons.

In addition to open neural tube defects an elevated amniotic fluid AFP level may be observed with other fetal anomalies—including abdominal wall defects (gastroschisis and omphalocele), upper gastrointestinal obstruction, congenital nephrosis, and Turner's syndrome—or with fetal demise.

If an elevated AFP level is found in the amniotic fluid, detailed ultrasonography and determination of the amniotic acetylcholinesterase level are indicated.[58] Acetylcholinesterase is an enzyme found in fetal spinal fluid, and its presence is conclusive evidence of fetal CNS malformation.

If an elevated maternal serum AFP level is detected, then the usual protcol followed is to repeat the serum AFP test and perform an ultrasound to establish gestational age and fetal number because both incorrect gestational age and multiple gestations may result in elevated maternal serum AFP. Other causes of elevated maternal serum AFP include the fetal anomalies listed above as well as fetal demise. After the serum AFP and other data have been evaluated, amniocentesis and amniotic AFP measurements may be indicated. Approximately 1–2 per cent of women having serum AFP testing will require amniocentesis.

Recently a new correlation between low maternal serum AFP levels and fetal anomaly has been recognized. First reported by Merkatz et al, this phenomenon has been confirmed in a number of studies.[97] Pregnancies involving fetuses with chromosomal aneuploidy, particularly trisomy 21 but also trisomies 13 and 18, have serum and amniotic fluid AFP significantly below the normal median. Application of this methodology can be of great value in identifying pregnancies at risk, particularly for mothers 34 years old or older.

Assessing Fetal Maturity

The introduction of amniocentesis for study of amniotic fluid in Rh-immunized women paved the way for development of the battery of tests currently available to assess fetal maturity. The initial mcthods developed were based upon amniotic fluid levels of creatinine, bilirubin, and fetal fat cells, and these provided a good correlation with fetal size and gestational age. They were, however, inadequate predictors of fetal pulmonary maturity.[95] For example, the creatinine level rises in amniotic fluid in a linear fashion as pregnancy advances. A concentration greater than 2.0 mg/dl reliably reflects a size consistent with a gestational age of 37 weeks or older.[112, 121] However, in diabetes mellitus with macrosomia, creatinine levels may be prematurely elevated by the increase in muscle mass. Similarly, in toxemia, creatinine levels are greater than normal at corresponding periods of gestation even in the absence of an increase in maternal serum creatinine. This elevation is due to decreased clearance from the fetal compartment.[121] In neither situation does the creatinine level relate to the ability of the infant to adapt to an extrauterine existence.

Since respiratory distress syndrome is a frequent consequence of premature birth and a major component of neonatal morbidity and mortality in many high-risk situations, it was critical that an antenatal assessment of pulmonary status be developed. After it had been found that the pulmonary surface-active materials needed for lung stabilization could be detected in the amniotic fluid and that their concentrations increased with gestational age, it followed logically that amniotic fluid analyses might yield insight into pulmonary maturation. Gluck et al[50, 51] first measured the amniotic fluid lecithin/sphingomyelin (L/S) ratio in the third trimester of pregnancy and demonstrated its clinical application for the prediction of respiratory distress syndrome (Figure 1–3).

Subsequently there has been widespread debate about analytic techniques for testing of the phospholipids and about their specific biochemical nature. There are several advocates of the direct quantitative measurement of lecithin rather than the more qualitative L/S ratio.[17, 105] The introduction of the foam stability test by Clements and coworkers[27] provided a rapid, simple, inexpensive test for surfactant. As with the L/S ratio itself, this test provides two limits of reliable prognostic usefulness and an intermediate zone with more equivocal results. False-positive and false-negative results have been reported with both methods.[35, 138] Investigators have

Figure 1–3. Abnormal elevations of L/S ratio as compared with the curve of progress of the L/S ratio of normal pregnancy. A = Chronic stress, retroplacental bleeding; B = acute stress, membranes ruptured 72–96 hours; C = acute stress, placental infarction; and D = chronic stress, postmaturity.[50]

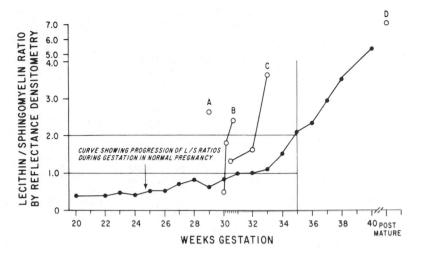

noted that confirmation of the presence of phosphatidyl-glycerol, a component of the more mature surfactant complex, will reduce the incidence of false-positive tests.[67] Nonetheless, in uncomplicated, unstressed situations such as elective repeat cesarean section, any of these techniques are useful, and their utilization should be encouraged, taking into consideration the risk of amniocentesis.

Editorial Comment: The L/S ratio has over the past decade proved to be an excellent predictor of fetal lung maturity. There are suggestions, however, that its use has declined, perhaps concomitant with more precise dating in the first half of pregnancy by means of ultrasound. Furthermore, in the face of fulminant preeclampsia, severe accidental hemorrhage, or acute fetal distress, action is urgent and waiting for the result of an L/S test is not warranted.

Turnbull, A. C.: The lecithin/sphingomyelin ratio in decline. Br J Obstet Gynaecol 90:993, 1983.

However, in many high-risk conditions the developmental biochemical maturation of the fetal lung may be altered, at least as measured by the L/S ratio.[50] Acceleration of mature L/S ratios has been reported in maternal hypertensive states, sickle cell disease, and narcotics addiction, as well as with intrauterine growth retardation and prolonged premature rupture of the membranes.[50] Considerable investigative interest currently centers around the regulatory mechanism leading to such accelerated pulmonary maturation. Experiments in pregnant rabbits and sheep have demonstrated that glucocorticoids can stimulate the appearance of surface-active material in the alveoli of the lungs of the fetuses of these species, presumably by enzyme induction.[103]

Chronic intrauterine stress may initiate earlier lung maturation to permit a premature extrauterine adaptation, but the need persists for careful controlled studies to document this phenomenon in independent high-risk circumstances. In contrast, a delay in the appearance of lung maturation is seen in the infants of some diabetic mothers, particularly where there is macrosomia presumably as the result of poor regulation of maternal blood sugar. The interface between receptors for insulin and cortisone has been implicated in this regard.

Furthermore, studies of patients in whom respiratory distress syndrome occurred in the presence of mature foam stability tests call attention to the separate roles of (1) surfactant deficiency, (2) fetal immaturity, and (3) intrapartum asphyxia in the pathogenesis of this disorder.[138] These assays are useful but there remain many unresolved problems in their clinical interpretation. As with urinary estriols, ultrasound cephalometry, and other tests of fetal condition, each must be employed selectively and properly synthesized into the total assessment of the fetus and the pregnancy management.

Monitoring the Fetus During Labor[26, 79, 100, 144]

Selected high-risk pregnancies should be closely monitored during labor. Forty-seven of 83 term intrapartum fetal deaths reported[95] occurred in mothers who had at least one of the criteria for high risk based on the individual pregnancy history alone.

Careful monitoring with appropriate operative intervention might salvage a significant number of these infants.

The contribution that intrapartum death makes to the stillbirth rate and thus to overall perinatal mortality should not be underestimated. In most series, unexplained peripartum asphyxia (so called) accounts for approximately one third or more of all stillbirths. A very high proportion of these are in turn intrapartum deaths in which the fetus was apparently alive and in good condition at the start of labor but in which fetal death subsequently occurred before labor was completed. It is in this group that monitoring during labor has been shown to be not only efficacious but also highly effective in reducing fetal losses.
L. Stern

Counting the fetal heart rate (FHR) between contractions using a stethoscope is an inadequate method of determining early evidence of fetal distress, since significant rate changes occur early during a contraction and persist for a short time after the contraction is over (Figure 1–4). This is a period when fetal heart tones are least audible with a stethoscope. By continuously monitoring intrauterine pressure and FHR using continuous ultrasound (Doptone) or, when the fetal scalp is accessible, a scalp clip attached to recording electrodes, significant abnormalities can be detected at a time when operative intervention has a greater chance of promoting delivery of a live, neurologically intact newborn infant.

Transient tachycardia with heart rates over 160 beats per minute (Figure 1–4A) may be an isolated finding. It frequently precedes a variable deceleration pattern (Figure 1–4B, C), which may reflect umbilical cord compression, or a late deceleration pattern (Figure 1–5), which is commonly associated with uteroplacental insufficiency. Either of these patterns is compatible with fetal distress (Table 1–5).

Sampling blood from the fetal scalp during labor is another method used for monitoring the fetuses in selected high-risk pregnancies or when fetal distress is suspected. The procedure can be done when membranes are ruptured, the cervix is dilated several centimeters, and the fetal vertex is close to or below the ischial spines.[126, 128] A fetal scalp puncture (only a few millimeters deep) is made under direct visualization, and a sample is collected in a heparinized capillary tube. The values for acid-base parameters on fetal scalp blood correspond to those ob-

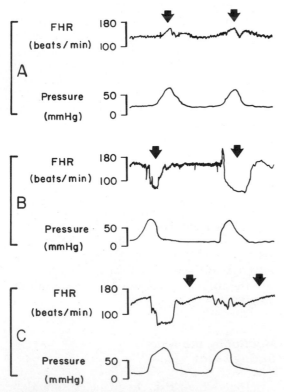

Figure 1–4. Changes in fetal heart rate during uterine contractions as reflection of fetal distress. The arrows indicate transient tachycardia (A), variable deceleration (B), and variable deceleration with slow recovery after uterine relaxation (C), FHR = fetal heart rate. Pressure is uterine pressure. (See text for explanation.)

TABLE 1–5 FHR PATTERNS AND UNDERLYING MECHANISMS

Reflecting Fetal Reserve	
Normal baseline heart rate and FHR	Intact autonomic cardiovascular reflexes
Tachycardia (>160 bpm)	Prematurity, maternal fever, acidosis
Diminished variability (<6 bpm variation)	"Sleep cycle," drug effects, acidosis, congenital anomaly
Bradycardia (<120 bpm)	Normal variant, congenital heart block, cardiac anomaly, maternal hypothermia
Sinusoidal pattern	Anemia, hypoxia, drug effect
Reflecting Acute Environmental Change	
Early deceleration	Head compression
Variable deceleration	Cord compression, acute hemorrhage
Late deceleration	Contraction-induced hypoxia
Acceleration	Intact autonomic response to intrinsic or extrinsic stimuli

Modified from Clark, S. L., and Miller, F. C.: Scalp blood sampling—F.H.R. patterns tell you when to do it. Contemp Ob/Gyn 21:47, 1984.

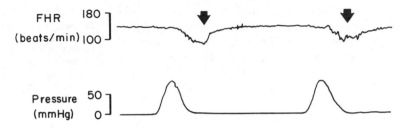

Figure 1–5. Changes in fetal heart rate during uterine relaxation as reflection of fetal distress. The arrows indicate late deceleration pattern with slow recovery after uterine relaxation. FHR = fetal heart rate. Pressure is uterine pressure. (See text for explanation.)

tained from the umbilical cord at cesarean section.[121, 131] The most reliable parameter reflecting the presence of fetal hypoxia and acidosis has been pH.[10] There is a high correlation with fetal distress when the fetal scalp pH is below 7.15 in the presence of normal maternal blood pH. However, a significant number of infants with low pH are born vigorous and with essentially normal acid-base status.[86, 131, 147] At present, continuous fetal heart rate monitoring is the preferred method of identifying fetal distress. Fetal scalp pH is measured when the FHR record is difficult to interpret or in the presence of persistent variable decelerations. Complications of fetal scalp blood sampling and fetal scalp electrode monitoring include significant fetal blood loss and infections in the newborn.

SOME PRINCIPLES RELATED TO FETAL HEART RATE MONITORING (See Table 1–5.)

The normal antepartum fetal heart rate record is characterized by a normal baseline FHR, normal long-term variability, and the presence of accelerations (2/20 minutes, over 15 to 20 bpm) and the absence of decelerations with contractions.

1. Continuous electronic monitoring of fetal heart rate complemented by fetal scalp blood pH best evaluates intrapartum fetal well-being.

2. Whereas a normal fetal heart rate pattern accurately predicts a nondepressed infant (Apgar >7), even with apparently ominous fetal heart rate abnormalities only 50 per cent of the neonates are depressed. Unnecessary interventions based on fetal heart rate abnormalities during labor can be diminished by assessing fetal scalp blood pH. Ninety per cent of infants with a scalp pH of less than 7.2 will be depressed at birth.

3. In the presence of normal fetal heart rate variability infants with late decelerations are unlikely to be acidotic. However if there are late decelerations accompanied by diminished baseline variability together with baseline tachycardia, there is a 60 per cent chance that the fetus is acidotic.

4. Neither baseline bradycardia (FHR<120 bpm) nor tachycardia (FHR>160 bpm) alone is predictive of acidosis.

5. Baseline tachycardia may be due to early asphyxia but is more likely secondary to maternal fever, fetal infection, maternal drugs, or prematurity.

6. Persistent fetal bradycardia with good beat to beat variability is not generally associated with acidosis. It is more likely to be the result of drugs or fetal cardiac anomalies.

7. Variability is a measure of fetal reserve. Both long- and short-term variability should be evaluated. Decreased variability is predictive of fetal acidosis. Normal baseline variability and accelerations occurring spontaneously or after stimulation indicate intact fetal reserves.

8. The occurrence of decelerations except for sporadic mild variable decelerations before labor means antepartum hypoxia. The hypoxia may be mild and may not necessarily compromise the fetus. Persistent or repetitive late and marked atypical variable decelerations before labor are always ominous and require expeditious intervention. Ominous features of variable decelerations include a slow return to baseline, a rising baseline, and a transient smooth rise in baseline following a variable deceleration.

9. If more than a third of contractions are associated with late decelerations or if more than 20 late decelerations are noted during labor, a physiologically depressed baby is likely.

10. Decelerations of less than 15 bpm are considered mild, 15 to 45 moderate, while 45 bpm are considered severe. Gibbs, however, noted that neither the degree of drop of FHR frequency during variable decelerations nor their number was a significant factor in neonatal depression. The duration of the deceleration is most important. Prolonged

decelerations, of 2 minutes or more, are associated with significant fetal asphyxia. They may be induced by uterine hypertonus, local anesthesia, vaginal examination, or an active second stage of labor with the mother bearing down. Since the etiology may be nonrecurrent, a single prolonged deceleration—provided that it is followed by a return to baseline with good beat to beat variability—is not ominous. If there is a recurrence, delivery must be expedited.

11. If there is an increase in fetal heart rate at the time of obtaining a blood gas sample, the gas is usually normal.

Treatment of Fetal Distress (Asphyxia) In Utero

Administration of a high concentration of oxygen to the mother of a distressed fetus is one of the few methods of treating acute fetal asphyxia. Experiments in the rhesus monkey suggest that umbilical blood flow is not adversely affected and that there is an increased amount of oxygen transferred to some hypoxic fetuses.[27]

Although the rise in fetal Po_2 associated with maternal oxygen inhalation is small, this may be reflected in a significant increase in fetal oxygen saturation because of the shift to the left and steep slope of the oxygen hemoglobin dissociation curve for fetal hemoglobin, especially at low Po_2s. **M. Stahlman**

Repositioning the mother in labor occasionally may relieve acute fetal asphyxia caused by mechanical compression of the umbilical cord.[127] Maternal hypotension, secondary to compression of the inferior vena cava, may produce fetal asphyxia by decreasing uterine blood flow and oxygenation. This may be relieved by rotating the mother from a supine to a lateral position.

Prolonged preparation of the mother on the delivery or operating table in a supine position (for instance, during the preparation for cesarean section) may bring about these adverse effects at a time when monitoring is frequently discontinued. **M. Stahlman**

Adequate preparation is desirable for prompt effective resuscitation of the newborn. The pediatrician should be alerted when a decision is being made to intervene operatively for a fetus in distress (Table 1–6).

The tables suggest that meconium staining with a vertex presentation is a factor suggesting fetal distress. In our experience meconium staining with a breech presentation has equal import. Since breech presentations are high-risk deliveries with significant increases in fetal morbidity and mortality, the presence of meconium is more ominous. It used to be thought that, because the baby's buttocks and anus were the presenting parts, meconium was squeezed out of the bowel during delivery. I do not believe that this is the sole mechanism for the appearance of meconium in breech deliveries, but rather that asphyxia, which causes the passage of meconium in the vertex baby and is so very much more frequent in the breech baby, is also the cause of the passage of meconium. **M. Stahlman**

APPLICATIONS OF THE NEW OBSTETRICS

The Diabetic Pregnancy[142]

The diabetic pregnancy may be viewed as an appropriate model for testing the hypothesis that the new technology can result in significantly improved outcomes for defined populations of pregnant women.[110, 120] Major advances in the knowledge of carbohydrate metabolism provide the opportunity for improved screening and identification of the gestational diabetic. Physiologic studies now

TABLE 1–6 OBSTETRIC INDICATIONS FOR PLANNING CARE OF A HIGH-RISK INFANT

Factors Suggesting Fetal Disorders
Meconium staining with vertex presentation
Persistent fetal heart rate >160 bpm
Persistent abnormal fetal heart rate pattern on monitor
Loss of beat-to-beat variation of fetal heart rate on monitor
Fetal acidosis as determined from scalp

Maternal Problems
Toxemia
Intrauterine growth retardation
Diabetes
Erythroblastosis
Abruptio placentae, placenta previa
Dystocia
Elderly primigravida
Prematurity
Gestation >42 weeks
Maternal fever
Premature rupture of membranes >24 hours
Vaginal bleeding other than "show"
Multiple gestation
Abnormal presentation

Other Factors
Polyhydramnios or oligohydramnios
Abnormal stress or nonstress contraction test
Abnormal estriol
Immature L/S ratio
Abnormal labor pattern
General anesthesia
Cesarean section
Difficult delivery

Adapted from Merenstein, G., and Blackmon, L.: *Care of the High Risk Newborn.* San Francisco, Children's Hospital, 1971.

offer a better rationale for management of both the chemical and the overt diabetic pregnant woman and her fetus. Further-more, the increased risks for stillbirth, pre-maturity, and neonatal morbidity associated with diabetes pose a direct challenge to the efficacy of both antenatal surveillance and neonatal intensive care.

Despite insulin, the perinatal mortality among offspring of diabetic mothers has con-tinued to be extraordinarily high. The infant survival rate at the Joslin Clinic from 1922 to 1938 was only 54 per cent. From 1938 to 1958, the survival rate improved to 86 per cent, and from 1958 to 1974 a 90 per cent survival was achieved. Thus, the combined toll from stillbirth and neonatal death may persist at five times the rate of nondiabetics, even at major medical centers. When care is less intensive, perinatal mortality rates for diabetics of 20 to 30 per cent still exist.

Based upon the increased risk of stillbirth during the last month of pregnancy, preterm delivery at 36–37 weeks was the generally ac-cepted recommendation for many years.[48, 66] Möller[102] was one of the first to strive for an avoidance of premature deliveries. In 1970 she reported from Sweden a series of diabetic women carried closer to term when blood sugar regulation comparable to the nondi-abetic pregnancy had been achieved and when evidence of fetal jeopardy or preg-nancy complications such as toxemia did not appear. The perinatal mortality rate in her series of 47 patients was 2.1 per cent as compared with a 21 per cent mortality rate in a prior series from the same obstetric unit.

In recent years, similar favorable results have been reported from other institutions both in Europe and in the United States.[64, 110, 120] Gyves et al[64] have described a reduction in perinatal mortality from 13.5 to 4.1 per cent in a group of 96 diabetic patients in whom the modern technology was applied and preterm delivery was not routinely em-ployed.

For many years good control of maternal blood sugar concentration has been consid-ered important for the well-being of the fetus of the diabetic mother. However, there have been wide differences of opinion as to what constitutes good control. The fasting plasma glucose concentration in pregnancy, both normal and diabetic, has been shown to be lower than in the nongravid state. The con-tinuous siphoning of glucose by the fetus profoundly affects maternal carbohydrate metabolism and, as a result, fasting glucose levels are 15–20 mg/dl lower during preg-nancy than those postpartum. Furthermore, physiologic studies describing diurnal pro-files for blood glucose concentrations in nor-mal pregnancies have shown a remarkable constancy of these concentrations throughout the day. The fetus is thus, in normal circum-stances, provided with a constant glucose environment.

These physiologic principles have provided a rational basis for the care of pregnant diabetic women, and the importance of rigid blood glucose control has been illustrated by several clinical studies. The marked improve-ment in perinatal mortality and morbidity obtained by Möller[102] and Gyves et al[64] was with a mean preprandial blood glucose con-centration kept close to 100 mg/dl, particu-larly during the third trimester. The latter series also described a significant reduction in macrosomia among the infants of such well-controlled diabetic mothers. Karlsson and Kjellmer[77] reported that their perinatal mortality rates could be directly correlated with maternal mean blood glucose concentra-tions. When mean concentrations were above 150 mg/dl, the mortality rate was 23.6 per cent. At concentrations between 100 and 150 mg/dl, the rate declined to 15.3 per cent, and below 100 mg/dl a 3.8 per cent mortality was achieved. The King's College group in Lon-don reported on deliveries in 100 diabetic pregnant women in whom the mean pre-prandial blood glucose concentrations were maintained at approximately 100 mg/dl.[38] There was no perinatal loss in this series.

Since improvements in obstetric and neo-natal management have evolved over the same time span as these studies of intensive blood sugar control, it is difficult to attribute marked improvements in outcome to only one variable. Nevertheless, it appears pru-dent that the therapeutic objective in preg-nant diabetics be an effort at normalization of plasma glucose throughout the day. This approach should apply to the gestational di-abetic as well as to the woman who was diabetic prior to pregnancy.

A critical determinant of the outcome of diabetic pregnancy is the timing of delivery. The risk of intrauterine death increases as term approaches. On the other hand, the infant delivered preterm is exposed to the risks of prematurity, particularly that of res-piratory distress, which may result in neona-tal loss. Over the past 20 years, the feasibility of extending the gestational period and of individualizing delivery timing for the diabetic has been enhanced by the availability of the objective tests for fetal surveillance.

The combined use of daily monitoring by serial urinary estriol measurements and periodic fetal heart rate monitoring provides the best opportunity for following the fetal condition carefully while awaiting the development of functional maturity. Fetal biparietal diameter measurements by ultrasound have proved useful in determining fetal age and growth, particularly when an initial examination is performed early in gestation.[125] This aids in removing some of the uncertainties of pregnancy dating associated with irregular menses in the diabetic woman and late macrosomia in her fetus.

Since the major consequence of premature birth is respiratory distress, fetal pulmonary functional maturity is the most critical objective of current care. Biochemical estimations of this maturity can now be obtained from the amniotic fluid with either the L/S ratio[50] or the foam stability test.[27] These determinations provide an important new dimension in the management of the pregnant diabetic, particularly when maternal blood sugar control has been good and a normal physiologic milieu has been approximated.

Congenital malformations have assumed a major role in diabetic pregnancies. Simpson et al, in a prospective study, documented a 6.6 per cent incidence of major anomalies among offspring of diabetic mothers as compared with 2.4 per cent incidence in control mothers.[132] (Other centers report even higher rates.) Because the anomaly rate in those patients whose diabetes was aggressively managed was similar to that observed by others in patients whose diabetes was less vigorously managed, they hypothesized that abnormal development had occurred before the patients entered the study. There is a major emphasis on carefully managing diabetes before conception and even in the first trimester to reduce the high anomaly rate associated with diabetic pregnancies. This is supported by data generated by Ylinen et al,[145] who measured maternal HbA_{1c} as an indication of maternal hyperglycemia during pregnancy to determine its relationship to fetal malformations. Maternal HbA_{1c} was measured at least once before the end of the fifteenth week of gestation in 139 insulin dependent patients who delivered after 24 weeks' gestation. The mean initial HbA_{1c} was

9.5 per cent of the total hemoglobin concentration in the 17 pregnancies complicated by malformations, which was significantly higher than in pregnancies without malformations (8.0%). Fetal anomalies occurred in 6 of 17 (35%) pregnancies with $HbA_{1c} > 10$ per cent, 8 of 61 (13%) with values initially of 8–9.9 per cent, and only 3 of 63 (5%) in patients who had an initial level below 8 per cent. These data support the notion that there is an increased risk of malformation associated with poor glucose control. Unplanned pregnancies should be avoided in diabetics, and determination of HbA_{1c} prior to conception may assist in planning the optimal time for conception. Whether this will reduce the incidence of malformations has yet to be established.

The application of current technology thus provides the clinical team with the means of minimizing both fetal death in utero and preventable neonatal morbidity and mortality from the hazards of prematurity. Together with intensive control of maternal blood glucose, the technology of fetal surveillance offers the possibility of normalizing perinatal outcomes in large numbers of diabetic pregnancies.

Obstetric Management of the Low-Birth-Weight Infant

Low birth weight is the key determinant of perinatal outcome.[40] Major obstetric complications resulting in delivery of very low-birth-weight infants include premature rupture of membranes or PROM (75%), premature labor (45%), multiple gestation (16%), amnionitis (14%), and premature separation of the placenta (7%). The rationale for a group of specific obstetric interventions directed at optimizing the outcome of low-birth-weight infants now exists and will be illustrated in the following section. The following basic principles apply:

1. Prevent prematurity through maximal antenatal care, avoidance of unnecessary iatrogenic interventions, and conservative management of pregnancy problems whenever feasible.

2. Inhibit premature labor pharmacologically when favorable conditions permit.

3. Avoid asphyxia and expedite delivery when the intrauterine environment becomes too unfavorable for allowing further fetal maturation.

4. Avoid excessive medications or the inappropriate use of anesthetic agents that may depress the low-birth-weight infant.

5. Maintain a controlled delivery of the low-birth-weight infant—this is critical in avoiding birth trauma and injury. A more liberal use of cesarean section is favored over arduous inductions of labor or extensive vaginal manipulations.

6. Anticipate problems and communicate management plans to pediatric and nursing colleagues. The team approach furthers a continuity of care between the delivery room and the nursery.

7. Promote healthy maternal-infant attachments by avoidance of separations, maintenance of an air of optimism, and a positive, supportive approach to the emotional needs of both parents.

Pharmacologic Inhibition of Premature Labor

For properly selected patients, the option to inhibit uterine contractions must be available when premature onset of labor cannot be prevented. When such treatment is contraindicated or unsuccessful, optimal obstetric management and expert neonatal care need to be in readiness to maximize the outcome for the very small premature infant. After exclusion of cases in which arrest of labor is either contraindicated or doomed to failure, a group of patients remains for whom a program of pharmacologic control of labor can materially improve the perinatal outcome (approximately 25 per cent of patients delivering premature infants).[149]

Pharmacologic inhibition of threatened premature labor is generally contraindicated under these conditions: (1) active vaginal bleeding, (2) ruptured membranes, (3) advanced dilatation of the cervix (>4–5 cm), (4) coexisting medical problems such as diabetes mellitus or cardiovascular disease, (5) premature separation of the placenta, and (6) evidence of intrauterine growth failure or chronic fetal distress.

Time-honored approaches to therapy have included the use of bed rest, intravenous fluids, tranquilizers, sedatives, and narcotics. Since it remains difficult to distinguish those patients in true early labor from those in false labor, each of these approaches has at times been credited with some degree of success by obstetricians. However, it is agreed that their actual therapeutic influence on inhibiting the myometrium is minimal, and the groups of drugs employed have the potential for depressing the very small premature infant. The use and dosage of such drugs should be carefully considered when there is threatened delivery of a small premature infant, and they should be discontinued completely when delivery appears inevitable. Castrén et al[24] have emphasized the therapeutic value derived from placebos when the mother is assigned to bed rest and reassured that she is being treated.

It is in light of such background that the evaluation and introduction of newer pharmacologic agents for the control of premature labor have posed particular difficulties. Patient selection, criteria for premature labor, and suitable controls are the areas of greatest controversy.

Following experimental evidence that ethanol inhibits the release of both vasopressin and oxytocin, the first large clinical trial with intravenous ethanol demonstrated a 65 per cent success rate in postponing delivery for at least 72 hours.[46] It was criticized for lack of suitable controls. The firmest evidence for effectiveness of ethanol was later provided by Zlatnik and Fuchs,[149] utilizing sequential analysis of a randomized controlled study. It required only 42 patients to prove statistically the efficacy of the ethanol compared with a solution of glucose and water.

The other commonly used method for clinical suppression of premature labor has been treatment with beta-adrenergic stimulators, an approach in use since the early 1960s. Stimulation of myometrial beta-receptors inhibits activity as it does in smooth muscles. The myocardium responds with increased activity when its beta-receptors are stimulated.

Isoxsuprine was one of the first synthetic beta-mimetic agents to be employed clinically for labor suppression.[18, 70] Although various studies demonstrated an inhibition of labor in as many as 50 per cent of patients treated, a randomized controlled trial was not performed. The significant cardiovascular side effects of isoxsuprine have limited the drug's clinical effectiveness in control of premature labor.

A series of other beta-mimetic agents with fewer cardiovascular side effects studied in various parts of the world have been shown to have considerable therapeutic value in the prevention of premature delivery. These drugs include ritodrine, metaproterenol, fenoterol, salbutamol, and terbutaline.

Aminophylline, salicylates, indomethacin and other nonsteroidal antiinflammatory agents, ethanol, magnesium sulfate, isoxsuprine, and terbutaline all have their clinical proponents. Most of these agents are in widespread use in centers throughout the United States because, in contrast to ritodrine, they have been readily available for other nonpregnancy or pregnancy indications without restriction. Not only are these agents not approved to date for use in treating preterm labor but they, like ritodrine, have their unique side effects and potential risks to mother and baby.

Ritodrine hydrochloride was the first of the agents to undergo rigorous clinical investigation in the United States. Whereas ritodrine was specifically synthesized for its predominant B_2 effect, by which uterine relaxation is achieved, there is invariably a degree of B_1 stimulation resulting in tachycardia, widened pulse pressure, tremor, and restlessness. (Additionally, ritodrine causes fluid retention, a short-lived elevation in blood glucose, and a fall in hematocrit and potassium.) In an initial study involving three perinatal centers, the effectiveness of ritodrine was compared with that of ethanol.[81] One hundred and thirty-five patients considered to be in premature labor were randomly divided into two treatment groups. The results are summarized in Table 1–7. In a larger multicenter series of randomized prospective double blind studies, ritodrine was compared with either ethanol or placebo in the treatment of idiopathic preterm labor. When compared with controls, offspring of ritodrine-treated mothers experienced a significantly reduced incidence of neonatal death and respiratory distress syndrome; also a significantly higher proportion of these infants achieved a gestation of greater than 36 weeks or a birth weight of more than 2500 gm, or both. There was thus a significant improvement in gestational age at delivery as a result of more days gained in utero among

ritodrine-treated patients. These results coupled with the generally acceptable side effects resulted in ritodrine becoming the first drug approved for the treatment of preterm labor in the United States.[5, 23, 98]

It has nonetheless been difficult to assess the efficacy of various treatment modalities of preterm labor. First, because the exact mechanisms that trigger the onset of either term or preterm labor remain incompletely understood, efficacy can only be assessed in terms of subsequent clinical events rather than precise or discriminating biochemical or physiologic parameters. Furthermore, there is a significant margin of error attendant to an accurate diagnosis of preterm labor made early enough for the interventions to work effectively. Criteria establishing premature labor vary among physicians and institutions. Those centers with a positive attitude to arresting premature labor pharmacologically tend to intervene earlier, with a greater chance for success but also the likelihood of overtreating patients in false labor. On the other hand, those less enamored of the available agents who await clear evidence of progressive labor are risking excessive delays. By the time unquestionable changes in cervical effacement and dilatation can be documented it is often too late for effective inhibition of uterine activity.

Table 1–8 summarizes the analysis of a number of controlled studies with ritodrine. In patients who do not tolerate tachycardia or tremor associated with ritodrine or in those with diabetes or hyperthyroidism, magnesium sulfate may be used for tocolysis.

It has been suggested that agents that block the synthesis of prostaglandins from arachidonic acid might have a role in labor inhibition. Aspirin and indomethacin, especially in high doses, have been documented as having prevented labor in some circumstances.[82, 150] Because of their general availability, there was some tendency to employ these drugs as therapeutic agents without prior controlled study, until evidence appeared that prostaglandin inhibition might result in premature closure of the ductus arteriosus and perhaps fetal death.

INTRAUTERINE GROWTH RETARDATION

Intrauterine growth retardation (IUGR) is associated with both significantly increased rates of perinatal mortality and long-term

TABLE 1–7 PROLONGATION OF PREGNANCY: MEAN TIME GAINED (DAYS)[80]

	Singletons (120)	Twins (15)	Combined* (135)
Ethanol	26.6 ± 3.4	30.7 ± 9.2	27.6 ± 3.1
Ritodrine	46.2 ± 4.1	22.0 ± 6.0	44.0 ± 3.9

*p <.001

TABLE 1–8 CONTROLLED TRIALS—PREMATURE LABOR*

Efficacy Criterion	Ritodrine (%)	Analysis of Cases Control (%)	Significance
Neonatal death	5	13	p<.05
Neonatal RDS†	11	20	p<.05
Attaining >36 weeks' gestation	52	38	p<.05
Weeks' gestation at delivery	35.5	34.5	p<.05
Mean days gained	32.6	21.3	p<.001
Birth weight >2500 gm	58	43	p<.05

*Phase III controlled studies. (See Merkatz et al.[98])
†RDS = respiratory distress syndrome.

morbidity.[36, 42, 61, 62, 86] Unfortunately, prior to the widespread use of ultrasound, most studies revealed that only a small percentage of intrauterine growth-retarded infants were actually detected before birth. Improved perinatal outcome depends upon early identification, which requires an awareness of developing signs of uterine growth lag. Confirmation of diagnosis, based upon continued lack of clinical growth or serial ultrasonography, still requires a delay, often of several weeks, following initial suspicions. On the other hand, even when an awareness of the problem exists and a high index of suspicion is maintained, a significant number of false-positive diagnoses will result, especially when there is coincident ambiguity about pregnancy dating. Beard and Roberts[9] reported that in 35 per cent of their suspected cases the infants turned out not to be growth retarded. In our own studies, 50 per cent of patients with suspected IUGR of the fetus eventually delivered an infant whose weight was appropriate for gestational age, although conservative management and prolonged bed rest may well have been ameliorating in some instances.

Once the identification of possible growth retardation has been made, hospitalization is recommended. Bed rest, nutritional support, and when appropriate, control of maternal blood pressure constitute the therapeutic approach for both mother and baby. Placental perfusion, however, must not be compromised by overly aggressive treatment of maternal hypertension.

Fetal growth and well-being are evaluated by regular clinical measurements of fundal height and ultrasonographic measurements of fetal diameters, daily 24 hour maternal urinary estriol determinations, and serial external cardiotachography. The decision regarding appropriate timing of delivery rests on whether the fetus will continue to benefit from its environment in utero or whether it will profit more from premature delivery. Aggressive intervention increases the risk of fetal immaturity, particularly when the diagnosis of IUGR has not been fully substantiated. Expectant management, on the other hand, may result in intrauterine death or irreversible damage to a surviving neonate.

To date, none of the current laboratory estimations of fetal well-being have been able to provide supportive data adequate to formulate a clear decision.[94, 95] As a result, one commonly advocated approach is to deliver the growth-retarded baby soon after it has been diagnosed, or following earliest evidence of pulmonary maturity by amniotic fluid analysis. However, amniocentesis in severe cases of IUGR, particularly those identified prior to 35 weeks, is often complicated by the presence of oligohydramnios and by difficulty in obtaining the amniotic fluid specimen. Traumatic taps may force unplanned interventions and at times may further compromise fetal homeostasis.

In our hands, the use of antepartum cardiotachography without oxytocin (spontaneous contraction stress test [SCST]) on a daily or alternate-day basis has proved to be an aid in individualizing the timing of delivery in such situations involving suspected IUGR. Delivery is expedited at any time beyond 28 weeks' gestation if repetitive fetal heart rate decelerations are observed in response to spontaneous uterine contractions. Otherwise, expectant management is advocated, and prolongation of the time in utero is sought. The ominous significance of a positive SCST was described initially by Fairbrother et al,[39] who observed the presence of late deceleration fetal heart rate patterns in response to Braxton-Hicks contractions in four infants who were severely growth retarded and born prior to 35 weeks' gestation. Two infants were delivered by immediate cesarean section and did well, whereas the other two were not delivered immediately

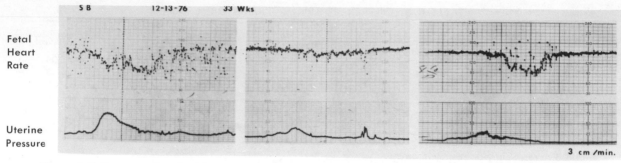

Figure 1–6. Recurrent late fetal heart rate decelerations following spontaneous uterine contractions in a patient with hypertension, delivered by cesarean section of an SGA infant.

and died within days of the observation. Emmen et al[37] described five patients in whom late decelerations of the fetal heart rate were seen in response to nonlabor spontaneous contractions shortly prior to intrauterine fetal demise. After these five stillbirths, this fetal heart rate pattern was interpreted as a "terminal state" and was thereafter managed by immediate cesarean section.

The data from MacDonald House confirm and extend these two studies from abroad. In a series of 26 patients with suspected IUGR whose supervision included frequent nonstressed monitoring, no stillbirth occurred. Immediate cesarean sections were performed in nine instances in which late deceleration fetal heart rate patterns were noted after Braxton-Hicks contractions (Figure 1–6). Eight of the nine infants demonstrated severe IUGR, and the ninth weighed less than the twenty-fifth percentile. In contrast, only 5 of the 17 patients who did not develop a positive SCST eventually delivered small-for-gestational-age (SGA) infants, and all of these babies tolerated labor well. The biophysical profile (see the foregoing section) is an added dimension in monitoring these pregnancies.

EXPECTANT MANAGEMENT FOR PREMATURE RUPTURE OF FETAL MEMBRANES

Depending upon definitions employed, the reported incidences for pregnancies complicated by premature rupture of fetal membranes generally vary from 7 to 20 per cent.[63, 122, 136] The incidence of low-birth-weight infants associated with premature rupture of membranes (PROM) has been shown to approximate 20 per cent, or twice that of the usual occurrence.[63] Furthermore, perinatal mortality rates among premature infants are markedly increased when there has been coexisting premature rupture of membranes. In the 10 year retrospective study from the University of California, Los Angeles, 16 per cent of all perinatal deaths were associated with PROM.[63] The vast majority of these deaths were among low-birth-weight infants.

The obstetric management of this major complication remains controversial, and there is considerable polarization of opinion.[15, 16, 33, 47, 90, 116] There has been strong advocation of an aggressive or dynamic management that favors early delivery of the fetus by induction of labor or cesarean section. There has been equally strong advocation, particularly when the fetus is premature, of an approach predicated on a hands-off policy of expectant management. This latter approach has as its objective the continued growth and maturation of the fetus in utero, unless the onset of labor or infection otherwise dictates.

At term, approximately 80 to 90 per cent of women who experience ruptured membranes will be in spontaneous labor within 24 hours, so any controversy regarding management at term pertains principally to a small minority of patients.[122] However, when preterm pregnancies are considered, only 35 to 50 per cent of women will be in labor within 24 hours, and the probability of an infant not being delivered within 72 hours after premature rupture of membranes is reported to be about 30 per cent.[63] In general, the earlier in gestation that rupture occurs, the greater the likelihood of a delay in onset of labor. Some patients will experience delays of 14 days or more, and such an extension of gestation for the small premature infant can be critical.

The interval between occurrence of membrane rupture and onset of regular uterine contractions resulting in progressive cervical dilatation is defined as the *latent period*. The longer the latent period, the greater the risk of the eventual development of amnionitis. Therefore the expectant management of PROM in the preterm gestation represents a balancing of the risks of low-birth-weight delivery versus the risk of infection. The likelihood of infection in turn is directly related to the number and frequency of vaginal examinations. It can be argued that such examinations serve little useful purpose and that in most instances they can be avoided entirely to minimize infection. Since the most frequent cause of perinatal mortality in the low-birth-weight group with PROM is prematurity itself, in our institution expectant management is advocated.

Delivery of a patient with a small premature infant and premature rupture of membranes is generally avoided until labor ensues. In those instances when early clinical manifestations of amnionitis such as low-grade fever, leukocytosis, or uterine tenderness appear, the strategy is reversed, and delivery is expedited within a few hours.

If one is going to manage premature rupture of the membranes conservatively, it is important to look for signs of infection. In addition to monitoring for fetal tachycardia, maternal temperature should be taken frequently. Examination of the amniotic fluid for bacteria is helpful, but the presence of white cells in the amniotic fluid does not correlate well with subsequent maternal infection. If signs of infection develop, antibiotics should be given and the fetus delivered.   **E. Quilligan**

Our experience at MacDonald House has been consistent with that of the Denver group,[136] whose data first demonstrated that less than 2 per cent of infants of mothers with premature rupture of membranes who are conservatively managed develop neonatal sepsis and that the perinatal mortality for low-birth-weight infants is not increased by this conservative approach. Furthermore, in contrast to other reports, our experience indicates that such management can be appropriate for patients from poor socioeconomic environments as well as for the more advantaged patient.

Garite et al followed 251 patients with PROM prospectively to evaluate the maternal and neonatal effects of chorioamnionitis.[47] The period of gestation ranged from 28 to 34 weeks at time of rupture. Nineteen per cent developed intrauterine infection prior to delivery. Fetal tachycardia, maternal leukocytosis, and uterine contractions were not predictive of intrauterine infection in afebrile patients; however, amniocentesis positive for bacteria either with Gram stain or with subsequent positive culture correlated with antenatal maternal fever. Postpartum endometritis was the only major maternal complication associated with chorioamnionitis. Neonatal outcome—as evidenced by an increased perinatal mortality rate and a higher incidence of neonatal infection and respiratory distress syndrome—was adversely affected in the presence of maternal infection. In patients with chorioamnionitis the duration of labor did not affect neonatal outcome, but the presence of maternal fever prior to the onset of labor was prognostically an ominous sign for the fetus.

Patients with premature rupture of membranes are admitted to the hospital and placed at bed rest. Careful abdominal examination is performed to evaluate the fetal size, presentation, and estimated station. In many instances, the diagnosis of PROM can be confirmed by history and perineal inspection without requiring vaginal examination.[44] The continued leakage of amniotic fluid from the vagina is often obvious, and Nitrazine testing or the collection of fluid for ferning can be performed at the introitus. The vagina is examined by sterile speculum under aseptic conditions only when the diagnosis remains questionable and visualization of the cervix or posterior vaginal pool is necessary for confirmation. Digital examinations are contraindicated since they may add markedly to the risk of infection and usually add little to either diagnosis or management. Particularly when on Leopold's maneuvers the presenting part has been found to be high and floating free from the pelvis, it should not come as a surprise that the examining fingers find only a "long and closed" cervix.

A period of electronic monitoring of the fetal heart rate and uterine activity is routinely initiated by external cardiotachography. The absence of progressive labor with or without occasional mild contractions is documented. Fetal tachycardia may be an early indicator of incipient amnionitis, and its finding should be considered significant. Furthermore, variable decelerations of fetal heart rate in response to even minimal uterine activity are indicative of occult umbilical cord prolapse. We have used this finding to diagnose early cord complications for the premature infant even in the presence of a closed cervix and have therefore been reassured as to the wisdom of avoiding even the single vaginal examination (Figure 1–7). Actually, cord prolapse is not a common complication of prematurely ruptured membranes.[19, 63] In early gestations complicated by PROM, the incidence has been reported to be as low as 0.7 to 3.0 per cent—only slightly higher than in the general population.

It is the complications of prematurity per se, notably respiratory distress syndrome, which are the principal threats to the very low-birth-weight infant with associated premature rupture of membranes. There are contradictory reports as to whether PROM decreases the chance of respiratory distress syndrome. Yoon and Harper first suggested that rupture of membranes more than 24 hours prior to delivery protected against the development of respiratory distress syndrome.[146] Other investigators reporting similar findings suggested acceleration of fetal lung maturation by endogenous corticosteroids.[7, 117] However, more recent studies focusing retrospectively on the incidence of respiratory distress syndrome with premature rupture of membranes found no such protective influence.[14, 76]

The role of exogenous corticosteroids in preventing respiratory distress syndrome (RDS) has been the focus of much attention lately in many reports including the large collaborative study.[3, 4, 28, 108, 135] Glucocorticoids play a major role in development of the fetal lung and are stimulators of surfactant synthesis. In a double-blind controlled study of premature labor, Liggins[84] demonstrated a more favorable outcome in a betamethasone-treated group as compared with a control group. There were reduced incidences of RDS, pneumonia, intraventricular hemorrhage, and perinatal mortality recorded in the betamethasone-treated group. Infants born less than 1 day or more than 7 days after steroid therapy and those above 34 weeks' gestation demonstrated no benefit from treatment. Furthermore, the use of steroid therapy to enhance surfactant maturation may present hazards. In addition to an increased risk of fetal death in pregnancies complicated by hypertension and an increased occurrence of maternal infections, adverse effects of betamethasone therapy could arise as a consequence of accelerated maturation of organs other than lungs. Potentially long-term adverse effects of glucocorticoids on brain development are being evaluated.

Editorial Comment: Surprisingly, gut maturation is apparently also enhanced by corticosteroids, and the incidence of necrotizing enterocolitis was reduced in the steroid group.

Bauer, C. R., Morrison, J. C., Poole, W. K., et al: A decreased incidence of necrotizing enterocolitis after prenatal glucocorticoid therapy. Pediatrics 73:682, 1984.

CESAREAN SECTION FOR THE PREMATURE BREECH DELIVERY

Premature deliveries of very low-birth-weight infants are associated with a greatly increased incidence of breech presentations.[20] When compared with cephalic presentations, breech births, with or without associated prematurity, demonstrate increased perinatal mortality and morbidity stemming from associated birth trauma, growth retardation, prolapse of the umbilical cord, placental accidents, fetal anomalies, and multiple gestation. Whereas the overall incidence of breech presentation is only 3 to 4 per cent of deliveries, for infants weighing less than 1500 gm at birth the incidence may be 30 per cent or greater.[57] An analysis of over 30,000 deliveries at MacDonald House revealed that more than one quarter of all breech births occurred at or prior to 34 weeks' gestation.[57]

How should the preterm breech delivery be managed? At most centers, there is an increasing tendency to use cesarean section as the mode of delivery for all but the most uncomplicated of breech presentations.[113] Because vaginal delivery of a fetus in breech presentation entails delivery of successively larger fetal parts, most complications have to be anticipated in advance. With a premature fetus, the size of the head is even greater in relation to that of the buttocks than with a term fetus, and the chance for entrapment is markedly increased. Trauma to the fetus, cord complications, or a period of hypoxia may prove particularly disastrous for a tiny infant, for whom there is a much narrower margin for error. Cesarean section as a preferable method of delivery would certainly appear at least as rational for this group as for any other category of breeches.

A rise in perinatal mortality in breech delivery has been shown to correlate with birth

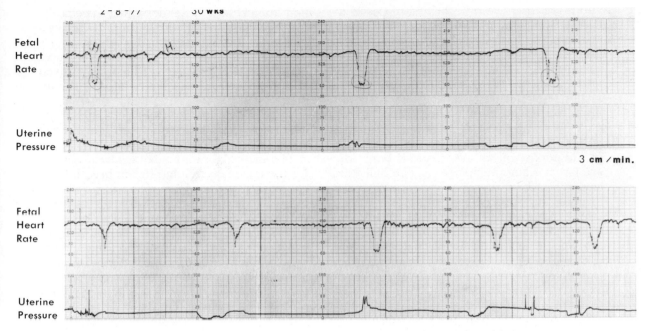

Figure 1–7. External electronic monitoring tracing from a patient at 30 weeks' gestation with premature rupture of the membranes. Cesarean section was performed because of the abnormal fetal heart rate patterns.

weights in amounts decreasing from 2500 gm.[101] One study has contrasted a perinatal mortality rate of 51 per 1000 in breech deliveries of term fetuses for primigravidas with a rate of 310 per 1000 in breech deliveries of premature fetuses weighing between 1000 and 2499 gm.[109] Goldenberg and Nelson[57] found that during labor the premature fetus in breech presentation was 16 times more likely to die than the premature fetus in vertex presentation. Although the corrected perinatal mortality rate for breech deliveries in their study was greater than that for vertex deliveries in every weight category, the difference was greatest and statistically significant between 750 and 1500 gm.

A study at MacDonald House demonstrated that, at each stage of gestation, the incidence of intrapartum stillbirths, neonatal deaths, and low Apgar scores increased for breech as compared with nonbreech deliveries.[20] Furthermore, from as early as 32 weeks' gestation onward, vaginal delivery could be shown to result in higher rates of perinatal loss and lower Apgar scores than did delivery by cesarean section. In fact, it was in the gestational period of 32 to 35 weeks that the most measurable advantage could be ascribed to delivery of the fetus in breech presentation by cesarean section rather than by the vaginal route. The time period covered by this study preceded many of the recent advances in

neonatal care that have resulted in improved survival expectations for the tiny infant weighing 1000 to 1500 gm. Few cesarean sections were performed prior to 32 weeks, and as a consequence there were no data available to evaluate the potential benefits of cesarean section for breeches in the gestational period of 28 to 31 weeks. One may presume, however, that today these benefits would be quite substantial.

It is the opinion of many obstetric perinatologists therefore that modern management of premature, low-birth-weight fetuses in breech presentation includes the widespread use of cesarean section. Depending upon the supporting neonatal services available within an institution, opinions may vary as to whether such an approach should be initiated after 28 or after 32 weeks' gestation. From 1973 at MacDonald House, we have advocated cesarean section when delivery must be accomplished for an apparently healthy premature fetus in breech presentation of 1000 gm estimated weight and/or 28 weeks' gestation.[40]

More recently, with improved outcome for smaller, less mature infants, these criteria have been expanded. The lower limits of expected weight and gestational age remain fuzzy. It must be acknowledged, however, that several problems with the premature fetus in breech presentation remain unsolved and merit discussion. In the first place, cesarean section cannot be utilized for all circumstances. Many breech deliveries of very small, potentially viable infants occur after rapid, unanticipated labors in which there may be little opportunity to prepare for cesarean section. Furthermore, having to set a lower limit for fetal weight and gestational age, particularly in view of the known maternal risks of cesarean section, means that errors in judgment will always occur. Infants who are larger than anticipated may be delivered vaginally when there is a desire to avoid unnecessary procedures on women who might deliver previable infants. Ultrasound cephalometry may be helpful in this regard but only when there is adequate time and accessibility to the labor suite for an accurate examination. For the most part, the decision in such circumstances will need to be based on clinical parameters, and it must be understood that these are subject to error.

A second problem with the more liberal use of cesarean sections for the premature fetus in breech presentation stems from the high incidence of associated congenital anomalies. Most series on premature breeches provide "corrected perinatal mortality rates" eliminating both the high incidence of stillbirths prior to labor and the serious anomalies. Congenital abnormalities are more frequent in infants of breech deliveries as compared with infants of nonbreech deliveries at all durations of gestation.[20] The MacDonald House data demonstrated that the percentage of congenital anomalies in infants of breech deliveries peaks at about 35 weeks and that in the period between 30 and 35 weeks the anomaly rate for infants delivered in breech presentation is 10 to 15 per cent.

Chervenak et al raised the question of whether routine cesarean section is necessary for vertex-breech or vertex-transverse twin gestations.[25] Analysis of a 5 year experience at Yale University documented first the high proportion (97%) of twins confirmed before labor. Seventy-eight per cent of the vertex-breech and 53 per cent of vertex-transverse twins were delivered vaginally by breech extraction for a total of 76 second twins. Infants with birth weights <1500 gm had low 5 minute Apgar scores (67%) and accounted for the six neonatal deaths. These data support the concept of cesarean section delivery for infants <1500 gm with abnormal presentations.

Extending the indications for cesarean section to include those described specifically for the very low-birth-weight infant creates a new set of experiences for the contemporary obstetrician. The traditional transverse lower uterine segment incision, which has proved so successful for delivery of most term infants, may not always be ideal for cesarean section done prior to 34 weeks' gestation. This is particularly true with very small breech or twin premature fetuses.

The principal rationale of cesarean section for the low-birth-weight fetus in breech presentation is that the fetus tolerates poorly the trauma associated with delivery per vaginum. If this trauma is to be avoided with cesarean section, the uterine incision must at least be adequate. A low vertical incision has the advantage of permitting upward extension as needed, and this can prove critical when the extremities of the breech fetus are not readily accessible or clearly identifiable.

The same concept applies at least as well to the abdominal delivery of premature twins, particularly when one or both of the infants must be extracted in breech presentation. Furthermore, with small twins an additional complication may develop. The volume of amniotic fluid may be disproportionately large compared with the total uterine contents. Following rupture of the membranes and delivery of twin A, there is the potential for twin B to be displaced high in the contractile portion of the fundus and to become trapped. In such circumstances, a vertical incision that can be extended can avoid both excessive trauma and delay in the delivery of the trapped fetus and the alternative need for a second uterine incision.

It is with these factors in mind that we have advocated consideration of the low vertical cesarean section for the abdominal delivery of infants of very low birth weight. It is recommended that, once the abdomen is opened, the uterine size and morphology be examined and the position of the presenting part of the fetus be assessed. At times a transverse uterine incision will be considered appropriate, but if doubt exists about reaching the fetus easily, the vertical incision should be strongly considered.

Questions

How safe are diagnostic x-rays for the fetus and newborn?

Much of our knowledge of the changes caused by x-radiation comes from the more immediately apparent results of large doses such as those from radiation therapy, radiation accidents, and atomic bomb explosions. To estimate the longer-term effects of the much lower doses derived from diagnostic radiation, we can make theoretical extrapolations from the effects of large doses or employ epidemiologic methods.

The latter approach was applied to offspring of mothers who had received diagnostic x-rays for purposes of pelvic measurement during the latter part of pregnancy. We know that radiation may damage the embryo even prior to its implantation in the uterus. Also, during embryogenesis in early pregnancy, relatively high levels of radiation have been shown to cause anomalies in experimental animals.

Is it possible to induce leukemia by diagnostic x-rays? Are premature infants at greater risk?

In this regard, there is evidence that mothers of leukemic children had been radiographed more frequently during the relevant pregnancy than those of normal children. The studies that showed this increased risk for leukemia, which may be as much as two-fold, have been challenged by some because of unavoidable statistical bias.

It is quite true that the premature infant can be considered to be a fetus in a chronologic sense, and some organ systems may be immature. It is doubtful, however, that the risk of induction of malignancies per unit of absorbed dose differs significantly in the fetus from that of adults who have also had whole-body exposures. Moreover, most of the radiographic exposures of newborn infants concentrate on specific regions of the body, most often the chest, rather than the enire body. Consequently, fewer of the critical blood-forming areas of the newborn are exposed than would be the case during intrauterine life. Incidentally, the characteristics of scattered radiation are such that exposure of a carefully composed radiograph will result in negligible radiation of a neighboring patient.

While it can be stated that there is an increased risk of inducing malignancy by radiation, even at very low levels, this risk is small when compared with the probability of cancer occurring naturally. The risk becomes more acceptable when it is appreciated in terms of the increased morbidity or mortality that would result from the withdrawal of diagnostic x-rays from critically ill infants. Theoretically, during a lifetime, nearly 2000 chest radiographs would be necessary to cause any appreciable increase in probability of occurrence of a fatal malignancy over the natural incidence.

It has been only in recent years that large numbers of premature babies have survived. The more immediate effects of the various medical advances necessary for this increased survival are now becoming known. However, the latency period between delivery and effect of low-dose diagnostic radiation is measured in years and decades. Although we can be very optimistic, we can only guess the eventual outcome. In the meantime, it is up to the many concerned neonatologists, radiologists, and technicians to improve radiographic techniques, to substitute less invasive methods whenever possible, and to exercise care and judgment in the use of diagnostic radiation for this fragile portion of the human population.

Bross, I., and Natarajan, N.: Genetic damage from diagnostic radiation. JAMA 237:2399, 1977.

Gregg, E.: Radiation risks with diagnostic x-rays. Radiology 123:447, 1977.

Harvey, E. B., Boice, J. D., Honeyman, J., et al.: Prenatal x-ray exposure and childhood cancer in twins. N Engl J Med 312:541, 1985.

Margulis, A.: The lessons of radiobiology for diagnostic radiology. Am J Roentgenol 117:741, 1973.

Mazzi, E., Herrera, A., and Herbert, L.: Neonatal intensive care and radiation. Johns Hopkins Med J 142:15, 1978.

Pochin, E.: Radiology now. Malignancies following low radiation exposures in man. Br J Radiol 49:577, 1976.

Above questions and references provided by B. Fletcher.

True or False

Ultrasonography may produce major anatomic malformations in the fetus.

Diagnostic ultrasonography is now performed 1.4 million times annually in the United States for fetal visualization and gestational aging. The Food and Drug Administration issued a report (82:8190) expressing concerns about ultrasonography. While acute dramatic effects are unlikely, less obvious long-term or cumulative effects remain unexplored. Studies on mouse tissue reveal changes when exposed to pulsed ultrasound of the same intensity used in obstetrics. Whether the results apply to human tissue cells is unknown. The statement is false.

Diminished amniotic fluid has a serious implication for the fetus.

Reduced amniotic fluid is defined by ultrasound when no vertical pool measures 30 mm.[31] The association between oligohydramnios and renal anomalies has long been recognized. Mercer et al[91] reviewed ultrasound for detection of diminished amniotic fluid and eliminated those cases secondary to rupture of membranes. A 7 per cent malformation rate was noted, and if diminished amniotic fluid was present before 27 weeks, outcome was poorer. Crowley et al[31] noted more meconium staining, fetal distress, and growth retardation in pregnancies with decreased amniotic fluid. The statement is true.

Amniocentesis should be a routine part of the management of patients with PROM.

Some investigators would support this notion because knowledge of the L/S ratio, Gram stains, and quantitative colony counts would dictate further management policies. Thus if the L/S ratio is mature or the Gram stain shows evidence of bacteria, irrespective of gestational age, delivery is expedited. Not everyone would agree that amniocentesis should be routine even with ultrasound guidance. The statement is false.

Amniocentesis and determination of alpha-fetoprotein should be performed in pregnancies subsequent to one that produced an infant with neural tube defect.

Open neural tube defects have an increased recurrence rate of 1 in 20 with a previously affected child, and this risk is even greater when two previous children have been affected. Routine antenatal screening of amniotic fluid alpha-fetoprotein concentration together with careful ultrasonographic study of the fetus is thus recommended in such pregnancies.[95] The statement is true.

Gestational diabetics may contribute significantly more to perinatal mortality than do insulin-dependent diabetics.

Since the incidence of gestational diabetes far exceeds that of the overt form, its potential impact on perinatal outcome for a defined population may be more significant. It has been estimated that many pregnancies in the United States have resulted in perinatal death from undiagnosed or untreated gestational diabetes. Therefore the importance of screening for abnormal glucose tolerance during pregnancy must be reemphasized.[120]

In identification of the gestational diabetic, clinical features suggestive of potential gestational diabetes include a family history of diabetes, a prior delivery of a baby weighing over 4000 gm, maternal obesity, a prior unexplained stillbirth, neonatal death, or major fetal anomaly. Glucose in a second fasting urine specimen and clinical hydramnios are additional factors that raise the index of suspicion during pregnancy.[134] The statement is true.

The presence of blood and/or meconium in the amniotic fluid does not affect the L/S ratio.

Serum contains an L/S ratio of approximately 1.31 to 1.46; therefore its addition lowers high L/S ratios and raises low L/S ratios. The addition of meconium to amniotic fluid increases the L/S ratio. Therefore the statement is false.

REFERENCES

1. Baker, M. L., and Dalrymple, G. V.: Biological effects of diagnostic ultrasound: a review. Radiology 126:479, 1978.
2. Bakketeig, L. S., Jacobsen, G., Brodtkorb, C. J., et al: Randomized controlled trial of ultrasonographic screening in pregnancy. Lancet 2:207, 1984.
3. Ballard, P.: Corticosteroids and respiratory distress syndrome: status, 1979. Pediatrics 63:163, 1979.
4. Ballard, R., Ballard, P., Granberg, J., et al: Prenatal administration of betamethasone for prevention of respiratory distress syndrome. J Pediatr 94:97, 1979.
5. Barden, T. P., Peter, J. B., and Merkatz, I. R.: Ritodrine hydrochloride: a betamimetic agent for use in preterm labor. I. Pharmacology, clinical history, administration, side effects, and safety. Obstet Gynecol 56:1, 1980.
6. Barrett, J. M., Boehm, F. H., and Vaughn, W. K.: The effect of type of delivery on neonatal outcome in singleton infants of birth weight of 1,000 g or less. JAMA 250:625, 1983.
7. Bauer, C., Stern, L., and Colle, E.: Prolonged rupture of membranes associated with a decreased incidence of respiratory distress syndrome. Pediatrics 53:7, 1974.
8. Beard, R., and Nathanielsz, P.: *Fetal Physiology and Medicine: The Basis of Perinatology.* Philadelphia, W. B. Saunders Co., 1976.
9. Beard, R., and Roberts, G.: A prospective approach to the diagnosis of intrauterine growth retardation. Proc R Soc Med 63:501, 1970.
10. Beard, R., Morris, E., and Clayton, S.: pH of foetal capillary blood as an indicator of the condition of the foetus. J Obstet Gynaecol Br Cwlth 74:812, 1967.
11. Beard, R. W., and Nathanielsz, P. W.: *Fetal Physiology and Medicine.* New York, Marcel Dekker, 1984.
12. Behrman, R., Peterson, E., and deLannoy, C.: The supply of O_2 to the primate fetus with two different O_2 tensions and anesthetics. Resp Physiol 6:271, 1969.
13. Bennett, M. J., Little, G., Dewhurst, Sir J., et al: Predictive value of ultrasound measurement in early pregnancy: a randomized controlled trial. Br J Obstet Gynaecol 89:338, 1982.
14. Berkowitz, R., Bonta, B., and Warshaw, J.: The relationship between premature rupture of the membranes and the respiratory distress syndrome. Am J Obstet Gynecol 124:712, 1976.
15. Berkowitz, R. L., Hoder, E. L., Freedman, R. M., et al: Results of a management protocol for premature rupture of the membranes. Obstet Gynecol 60:271, 1982.
16. Berkowitz, R. L., Kantor, R. D., Beck, G. J., et al: The relationship between premature rupture of the membranes and the respiratory distress syndrome. Am J Obstet Gynecol 131:503, 1978.
17. Bhagwanani, S., Fahmy, D., and Turnbull, A.: Prediction of neonatal respiratory distress by estimation of amniotic-fluid lecithin. Lancet 1:159, 1972.
18. Bishop, E., and Wouterez, T.: Isoxsuprine, a myometrial relaxant. Obstet Gynecol 17:442, 1961.
19. Breese, M.: Spontaneous premature rupture of the membranes. Am J Obstet Gynecol 81:1086, 1961.
20. Brenner, W., Bruce, R., and Hendricks, C.: The characteristics and perils of breech presentation. Am J Obstet Gynecol 118:700, 1974.

21. Brock, D. J. H.: Impact of maternal serum alpha-fetoprotein screening on antenatal diagnosis. Br Med J 258:365, 1982.
22. Campbell, S.: Fetal Growth. In Beard, R., and Nathanielsz, P. (eds.): Fetal Physiology and Medicine: The Basis of Perinatology. Philadelphia, W. B. Saunders Co., 1976.
23. Caritis, S. N., Edelstone, D. I., and Mueller-Heubach, E.: Pharmacologic inhibition of preterm labor. Am J Obstet Gynecol 133:557, 1979.
24. Castrén, O., Gummerus, M., and Saarikoski, S.: Treatment of imminent premature labor. Acta Obstet Gynecol Scand 54:95, 1975.
25. Chervenak, F., Johnson, R., Berkositz, R., et al: Is routine Cesarean section necessary for vertex breech and vertex transverse twin gestations? Am J Obstet Gynecol 148:1, 1984.
26. Clark, S. L., Gimovsky, M. L., and Miller, P. C.: Fetal heart rate response to scalp blood sampling. Am J Obstet Gynecol 144:706, 1982.
27. Clements, J., Platzker, A., Tierney, D., et al: Assessment of the risk of the respiratory distress syndrome by a rapid test for surfactant in amniotic fluid. N Engl J Med 286:1077, 1972.
28. Collaborative Group of Antenatal Steroid Therapy: Effect of antenatal dexamethasone administration on the prevention of respiratory distress syndrome. Am J Obstet Gynecol 141:276, 1981.
29. Creasy, R., and Herron, M.: Prevention of preterm birth. Semin Perinatol 5:295, 1981.
30. Creasy, R., Gummei, B., and Liggins, G.: System for predicting spontaneous preterm birth. Obstet Gynecol 55:692, 1980.
31. Crowley, P., O'Herlihy, C., Boylan, P., et al: The value of ultrasound measurement of amniotic fluid volume in the management of prolonged pregnancies. Br J Obstet Gynaecol 91:444, 1984.
32. Cuckle, H. S., Wald, N. J., and Lindenbaum, R. H.: Maternal serum alpha-fetoprotein measurement: a screening test for Down Syndrome. Lancet 1:926, 1984.
33. Daikoku, N. H., Kaltreider, D. R., Johnson, T. R. B., et al: Premature rupture of membranes and preterm labor: neonatal infection and perinatal mortality risks. Obstet Gynecol 58:417, 1981.
34. Diczfalusy, E.: Endocrine function of the human feto-placental unit. Fed Proc 23:791, 1964.
35. Donald, I., Freeman, R., Goebelsmann, U., et al: Clinical experience with the amniotic fluid lecithin-sphingomyelin ratio. Am J Obstet Gynecol 115:547, 1973.
36. Drillien, C.: The small-for-dates infant: etiology and prognosis. Pediatr Clin North Am 17:9, 1970.
37. Emmen, L., Huisjes, H., Aarnoudse, J., et al: Antepartum diagnosis of the "terminal" fetal state by cardiotocography. Br. J Obstet Gynaecol 82:535, 1975.
38. Essex, N., Pyke, D., Watkins, P., et al: Diabetic pregnancy. Br Med J 4:89, 1973.
39. Fairbrother, P., VanCoeverden De Groot, H., Coetzee, E., et al: The significance of prelabour type II deceleration of fetal heart rate in relation to Braxton-Hicks contractions. S Afr Med J 48:2391, 1974.
40. Fanaroff, A., and Merkatz, I.: Modern obstetrical management of the low birth weight infant. Clin Perinatol 4:215, 1977.
41. Filly, R. A., Golbus, M. S., Carey, J. C., et al: Short-limbed dwarfism: Ultrasonographic diagnosis by mensuration of fetal femoral length. Radiology 138:653, 1981.
42. Fitzhardinge, P., and Steven, E.: The small for date infant. II. Neurologic and intellectual sequelae. Pediatrics 50:50, 1972.
43. Freeman, R.: The clinical value of antepartum fetal heart rate monitoring. In Gluck, L. (ed.): Modern Perinatal Medicine. Chicago, Year Book Medical Publishers, Inc., 1974.
44. Friedman, M., and McElin, T.: Diagnosis of ruptured fetal membranes. Am J Obstet Gynecol 104:544, 1969.
45. Frost, H. M., and Stratmeyer, M. E.: In-vivo effects of diagnostic ultrasound. Lancet 1:999, 1977.
46. Fuchs, F., Fuchs, A., Poblete, V., Jr., et al: Effect of alcohol on threatened premature labor. Am J Obstet Gynecol 99:627, 1967.
47. Garite, T. J., Freeman, R. K., Linzey, E. M., et al: Prospective randomized study of corticosteroids in the management of premature rupture of the membranes and premature gestation. Am J Obstet Gynecol 141:508, 1981.
48. Gellis, S., and Hsia, D.: The infant of the diabetic mother. Am J Dis Child 97:1, 1959.
49. Gluck, L.: Modern Perinatal Medicine. Chicago, Year Book Medical Publishers, Inc., 1974.
50. Gluck, L., and Kulovich, M.: Lecithin-sphingomyelin ratios in amniotic fluid in normal and abnormal pregnancy. Am J Obstet Gynecol 115:539, 1973.
51. Gluck, L., Kulovich, M., Borer, R., et al: Diagnosis of RDS by amniocentesis. Am J Obstet Gynecol 109:440, 1971.
52. Goebelsmann, U., Freeman, R., Mestman, J., et al: Estriol in pregnancy. II. Daily urinary estriol assays in the management of the pregnant diabetic woman. Am J Obstet Gynecol 115:795, 1973.
53. Golbus, M. S.: Antenatal diagnosis of hemoglobinopathies, hemophilia and hemolytic anemias. Clin Obstet Gynecol 24:1055, 1981.
54. Golbus, M. S.: The current scope of antenatal diagnosis. Hosp Pract 17:179, 1982.
55. Golbus, M. S., Loughman, W. D., Epstein, C. J., et al: Prenatal genetic diagnosis in 3,000 amniocenteses. N Engl J Med 300:157, 1979.
56. Gold, E.: Identification of the high-risk fetus. Clin Obstet Gynecol 11:1069, 1968.
57. Goldenberg, R., and Nelson, K.: The premature breech. Am J Obstet Gynecol 127:240, 1977.
58. Goldfine, G., Miller, W. A., and Haddow, J. E.: Amniotic fluid gel cholinesterase density ratios in fetal open defects of the neural tube and ventral wall. Br J Obstet Gynaecol 90:238, 1983.
59. Goodwin, J., Dunne, J., and Thomas, B.: Antepartum identification of the fetus at risk. Can Med Assoc J 101:458, 1969.
60. Greene, J., Jr., and Touchstone, J.: Urinary estriol as an index of placental function. Am J Obstet Gynecol 85:1, 1963.
61. Gruenwald, P.: Infants of low birth weight among 5,000 deliveries. Pediatrics 34:157, 1964.
62. Gruenwald, P.: Growth and maturation of the foetus and its relationship to perinatal mortality, perinatal problems. In Butler, N., and Alberman, E. (eds.): The Second Report of the 1958 British Perinatal Mortality Survey. Edinburgh and London, E & S Livingstone Ltd., 1969, pp. 141–162.
63. Gunn, G., Mishell, D., and Morton, D.: Premature rupture of the fetal membranes. Am J Obstet Gynecol 106:469, 1970.

64. Gyves, M., Rodman, H., Little, A., et al: A modern approach to management of pregnant diabetics: a two-year analysis of perinatal outcomes. Am J Obstet Gynecol 128:606, 1977.

65. Hack, M., Fanaroff, A., Klaus, M., et al: Neonatal respiratory distress following elective delivery—A preventable disease? Am J Obstet Gynecol 126:43, 1976.

66. Hagbard, L.: Pregnancy and diabetes mellitus. In Hamblen, E. (ed.): American Lecture Series (No. 449). Springfield, Ill., Charles C Thomas, 1961.

67. Hallman, M., Feldman, B., Kirkpatrick, E., et al: Absence of phosphatidyl glycerol in respiratory distress syndrome in the newborn: study of the minor surfactant phospholipids in newborns. Pediatr Res 11:714, 1977.

68. Harrison, M. R., Filly, R. A., Golbus, M. S., et al: Fetal treatment. N Engl J Med 307:1651, 1982.

69. Harrison, M. R., Golbus, M. S., and Filly, R. A.: The Unborn Patient. Prenatal Diagnosis and Treatment. New York, Grune & Stratton, 1984.

70. Hendricks, C., Cibils, L., Pose, S., et al: The pharmacologic control of excessive uterine activity with isoxsuprine. Am J Obstet Gynecol 83:1064, 1961.

71. Herron, M., Katz, M., and Creasy, R.: Evaluation of a preterm birth prevention program: preliminary report. Obstet Gynecol 59:452, 1982.

72. Hobbins, J. C. (ed.): Prenatal diagnosis and treatment. Semin Perinatol 9:8, 1983.

73. Hobbins, J. C., and Winsberg, F.: Ultrasonography in Obstetrics and Gynecology. Baltimore, Williams and Wilkins Co., 1977.

74. Hobel, C.: Recognition of the high-risk pregnant woman. In Spellacy, W. (ed.): Management of the High-Risk Pregnancy. Baltimore, University Park Press, 1975, pp. 1–28.

75. Hobel, C., Hyvarinen, M., Okada, D., et al: Prenatal and intrapartum high risk screening: prediction of the high risk neonate. Am J Obstet Gynecol 117:1, 1973.

76. Jones, M., Jr., Burd, L., Bowes, W., Jr., et al: Failure of association of premature rupture of membranes with respiratory distress syndrome. N Engl J Med 292:1253, 1975.

77. Karlsson, K., and Kjellmer, I.: The outcome of diabetic pregnancies in relation to the mother's blood sugar level. Am J Obstet Gynecol 112:213, 1972.

78. Klopper, A.: The assessment of placental function in clinical practice. In Klopper, A., and Dicztalusy, E.: Foetus and Placenta. Oxford, Blackwell Scientific Publications, 1969, pp. 471–555.

79. Krebs, H. B., Petres, R. E., Dunn, L. J., et al: Intrapartum fetal heart rate monitoring. I. Classification and prognosis of fetal heart rate patterns. Am J Obstet Gynecol 133:762, 1979.

80. Lauersen, N., Merkatz, I., Tejani, N., et al: Inhibition of premature labor: a multicenter comparison of ritodrine and ethanol. Am J Obstet Gynecol 127:837, 1977.

81. Lenke, R. R.: Use of nipple stimulation to obtain contraction stress test. Obstet Gynecol 63:345, 1984.

82. Lewis, R., and Schulman, J.: Influence of acetylsalicylic acid, an inhibitor of prostaglandin synthesis, on the duration of human gestation and labour. Lancet 2:1159, 1973.

83. Liebeskind, D., Bases, R., Elequin, F., et al: Diagnostic ultrasound: effects on the DNA and growth patterns of animal cells. Radiology 131:177, 1979.

84. Liggins, G.: Prenatal glucocorticoid treatment: Prevention of respiratory distress syndrome. In Moore, T.: Report of 70th Ross Conference on Pediatric Research. Columbus, Ohio, Ross Laboratories, 1976, p. 97.

85. Lilien, A.: Term intrapartum fetal death. Am J Obstet Gynecol 107:595, 1970.

86. Low, J., and Galbraith, R.: Pregnancy characteristics of intrauterine growth retardation. Obstet Gynecol 44:122, 1974.

87. Low, J. A., Cox, M. J., Karchmar, E. J., et al: The prediction of intrapartum fetal metabolic acidosis by fetal heart rate monitoring. Am J Obstet Gynecol 135:299, 1981.

88. Main, D. M., Main, E. K., and Maurer, M. M.: Cesarean section versus vaginal delivery for the breech fetus weighing less than 1,500 grams. Am J Obstet Gynecol 146:580, 1983.

89. Manning, F., A., Morrison, I., Lange, I. R., et al: Antepartum determination of fetal health: composite biophysical profile scoring. Clin Perinatol 9:285, 1982.

90. Mead, P. B.: Management of the patient with premature rupture of the membranes. Clin Perinatol 7:243, 1980.

91. Mercer, L. J., Brown, L. G., Petres, R. E., et al: A survey of pregnancies complicated by decreased amniotic fluid. Am J Obstet Gynecol 149:355, 1984.

92. Merkatz, I. R., and Fanaroff, A.: The regional perinatal network. In Sweeney, W., and Caplan, R.: Advances in Obstetrics and Gynecology. Vol. II. Baltimore, Williams and Wilkins Co., 1978, pp. 1–12.

93. Merkatz, I. R., and Johnson, K.: Regionalization of perinatal care for the United States. Clin Perinatol 3:271, 1976.

94. Merkatz, I. R., and Solomon, S.: The fetoplacental unit. Clin Obstet Gynecol 13:665, 1970.

95. Merkatz, I. R., Aladjem, S., and Little, B.: The value of biochemical estimations on amniotic fluid in management of the high-risk pregnancy. Clin Perinatol 1:301, 1974.

96. Merkatz, I. R., Goldfarb, J. M., Gyves, M. T., et al: Diagnosis and management of the suspected growth retarded fetus. In Rathi, M., and Kumar, S. (eds.): Perinatal Medicine—Clinical and Biochemical Aspects. Vol. II. Washington, D.C., Hemisphere Publishing Corp., 1982.

97. Merkatz, I. R., Nitowsky, H. M., Macri, J. N., et al: An association between low maternal serum alpha-fetoprotein and fetal chromosome abnormalities. Am J Obstet Gynecol 148:886, 1984.

98. Merkatz, I. R., Peter, J. N., and Barden, T. P.: Ritodrine hydrochloride: a betamimetic agent for use in preterm labor. II. Evidence of efficacy. Obstet Gynecol 56:7, 1980.

99. Milunsky, A.: Symposium on the management of the high-risk pregnancy. Clin Perinatol 1:2, 1974.

100. Modanlou, H. D., and Freeman, R. K.: Sinusoidal fetal heart rate pattern: its definition and clinical significance. Am J Obstet Gynecol 142:1033, 1982.

101. Moir, J., and Meyerscough, P.: *Kerr's Operative Obstetrics*. 8th ed. London, Bailliere, Tindall and Cassell, 1971.

102. Möller, E.: *Studies in Diabetic Pregnancy*. Lund, Student Literature, 1970.

103. Moore, T.: Lung maturation and the prevention of hyaline membrane disease. *In:* Report of 70th Ross Conference on Pediatric Research. Columbus, Ohio, Ross Laboratories, 1976.

104. Morrison, I.: Annual perinatal mortality reports. College of Physicians and Surgeons of Manitoba, 1980.

105. Nelson, G.: Relationship between amniotic fluid lecithin concentration and respiratory distress syndrome. Am J Obstet Gynecol *112*:827, 1972.

106. Nesbitt, R., Jr., and Aubry, R.: High-risk obstetrics. II. Value of semi-objective grading system in identifying the vulnerable group. Am J Obstet Gynecol *103*:972, 1969.

107. O'Driscoll, K., and Foley, M.: Correlation of decrease in perinatal mortality and increase in cesarean section rates. Obstet Gynecol *61*:1, 1983.

108. Papageorgiou, A., Desgranges, M., Masson, M., et al: The antenatal use of betamethasone in the prevention of respiratory distress syndrome: a controlled double-blind study. Pediatrics *63*:73, 1979.

109. Patterson, S., Mulliniks, R., Jr., and Schrier, P.: Breech presentation in the primigravida. Am J Obstet Gynecol *98*:404, 1967.

110. Pedersen, J.: *The Pregnant Diabetic and Her Newborn: Problems and Management*. Baltimore, Williams and Wilkins Co., 1967.

111. Petrie, R. (ed.): Fetal monitoring. Clin Perinatol *9*:231, 1982.

112. Pitkin, R., and Zwirek, S.: Amniotic fluid creatinine. Am J Obstet Gynecol *98*:1135, 1967.

113. Pritchard, J., and MacDonald, P.: *Williams Obstetrics*. 15th ed. New York, Appleton-Century-Crofts, 1976.

114. Quilligan, E., Paul, R., and Sacks, D.: Results of fetal and neonatal intensive care. *In* Gluck, L.: *Modern Perinatal Medicine*. Chicago, Year Book Medical Publishers, Inc., 1974, pp. 425–430.

115. Ray, M., Freeman, R., Pine, S., et al: Clinical experience with the oxytocin challenge test. Am J Obstet Gynecol *114*:1, 1972.

116. Reid, D., and Christian, C.: *Controversy in Obstetrics and Gynecology II*. Philadelphia, W. B. Saunders Co., 1974.

117. Richardson, C., Pomerance, J., Cunningham, M., et al: Acceleration of fetal lung maturation following prolonged rupture of the membranes. Am J Obstet Gynecol *118*:1115, 1974.

118. Rochard, F., Schifrin, B., Goupil, F., et al: Nonstressed fetal heart rate monitoring in the antepartum period. Am J Obstet Gynecol *126*:699, 1976.

119. Rodeck, C. H.: Fetoscopy and the prenatal diagnosis of inherited conditions. J Genet Hum *28*:41, 1980.

120. Rodman, H., Gyves, M., Fanaroff, A., et al: The diabetic pregnancy as a model for modern perinatal care. *In* New, M., and Fiser, R., Jr. (eds.): *Diabetes and Other Endocrine Disorders During Pregnancy and in the Newborn. Progress in Clinical and Biological Research*. Vol. 10. New York, Alan R. Liss, 1976, pp. 13–32.

121. Roopnarinesingh, S.: Amniotic fluid creatinine in normal and abnormal pregnancies. J Obstet Gynaecol Br Cwlth *77*:785, 1970.

122. Rovinsky, J., and Shapiro, W.: Management of premature rupture of membranes. I. Near term. Obstet Gynecol *32*:855, 1968.

123. Ryan, G.: Toward improving the outcome of pregnancy: recommendations for the regional development of perinatal health services. Obstet Gynecol *46*:375, 1975.

124. Sabbagha, R. E., Tamura, R. K., and Dal Compo, S.: Obstetric ultrasonograph in perspective. Perinatol Neonatol *9*:53, 1982.

125. Sabbagher, R., Twiner, H., Rockette, H., et al: Sonar biparietal diameter and fetal age. Obstet Gynecol *43*:7, 1974.

126. Saling, E.: A new method of safe-guarding the life of the foetus before and during labor. J Int Fed Gynecol Obstet *3*:100, 1965.

127. Saling, E.: Amnioscopy and fetal blood sampling. *In* Adamsons, K. (ed.): *Diagnosis and Treatment of Fetal Disorders*. New York, Springer Verlag, Inc., 1968.

128. Schifrin, B., Lapidus, M., Doctor, G., et al: Contraction stress test for antepartum fetal evaluation. Obstet Gynecol *45*:433, 1975.

129. Schwarz, R., Fields, G., and Kyle, G.: Timing of delivery in the pregnant diabetic patient. Obstet Gynecol *34*:787, 1969.

130. Seeds, A.: Adverse effects on the fetus of acute events in labor. Pediatr Clin North Am *17*:811, 1971.

131. Seeds, A., and Behrman, R.: Acid-base monitoring of the fetus during labor with blood obtained from the scalp. J Pediatr *74*:804, 1969.

132. Simpson, J. L., Elias, S., Martin, A. O., et al: Diabetes in pregnancy. Northwestern University series (1977–1981). I. Prospective study of anomalies in offspring of mothers with diabetes mellitus. Am J Obstet Gynecol *146*:263, 1983.

133. Spellacy, W.: *Management of the High-Risk Pregnancy*. Baltimore, University Park Press, 1975.

134. Sutherland, H., and Stowers, J.: The detection of chemical diabetes during pregnancy using the intravenous glucose tolerance test. *In* Sutherland, H., and Stowers, J. (eds.): *Carbohydrate Metabolism in Pregnancy and the Newborn*. Edinburgh, Churchill Livingstone, 1975, p. 153.

135. Taeusch, H., Jr., Frigoletto, F., Kitzmiller, J., et al: Risk of respiratory distress syndrome after prenatal dexamethasone treatment. Pediatrics *63*:64, 1979.

136. Taylor, E., Morgan, R., Bruns, P., et al: Spontaneous premature rupture of the fetal membranes. Am J Obstet Gynecol *82*:1341, 1961.

137. Taylor, K.: Current status of toxicity investigation. J Clin Ultrasound *2*:149, 1974.

138. Thibeault, D., and Hobel, C.: The interrelationship of the foam stability test, immaturity, and intrapartum complications in the respiratory distress syndrome. Am J Obstet Gynecol *118*:56, 1974.

139. Vintzileos, A., Campbell, W., Ingardia, C., et al: The fetal biophysical profile and its predictive value. Obstet Gynecol *62*:271, 1983.

140. Warshaw, J. B., and Hobbins, J. C. (eds.): *Principles and Practice of Perinatal Medicine: Maternal, Fetal, and Newborn Care*. Menlo Park, California, Addison-Wesley, 1983.

141. Weingold, A., DeJesus, T., and O'Keife, J.: Oxytocin challenge test. Am J Obstet Gynecol 123:466, 1975.
142. White, P.: Diabetes mellitus in pregnancy. Clin Perinatol 1:331, 1974.
143. Williams, R. L., and Chen, P. M.: Identifying the sources of the recent decline in perinatal mortality rates in California. N Engl J Med 306:4, 1982.
144. Yeh, S., Bruce, S. L., and Thornton, Y. S.: Intrapartum monitoring and management of the postdate fetus. Clin Perinatol 9:381, 1982.
145. Ylinen, K., Aula, P., Stenman, U. H., et al: Risk of minor and major fetal malformations in diabetics with high hemoglobin A_{1C}. Values in early pregnancy. Br Med J 289:345, 1984.
146. Yoon, J., and Harper, R.: Observations on the relationship between duration of rupture of the membranes and the development of idiopathic respiratory distress syndrome. Pediatrics 52:161, 1973.
147. Zanini, B., Paul, R. H., and Huey, J. R.: Intrapartum fetal heart rate correlation with scalp pH in the preterm fetus. Am J Obstet Gynecol 134:43, 1980.
148. Zlatnik, F.: The applicability of labor inhibition to the problem of prematurity. Am J Obstet Gynecol 113:704, 1972.
149. Zlatnik, F., and Fuchs, F.: A controlled study of ethanol in threatened premature labor. Am J Obstet Gynecol 112:610, 1972.
150. Zuckerman, H., Reiss, U., and Rubinstein, I.: Inhibition of human premature labor by indomethacin. Obstet Gynecol 44:787, 1974.

2

Resuscitation of the Newborn Infant

DAVID E. FISHER
JOHN B. PATON

If the child does not breathe immediately upon Delivery, which sometimes it will not, especially it has taken Air in the Womb; wipe its Mouth, and press your Mouth to the Child's, at the same time pinching the Nose with your Thumb and Finger, to prevent the Air escaping; inflate the Lungs; rubbing it before the Fire; by which Method I have saved many.

BENJAMIN PUGH (1754)

Although mouth-to-mouth resuscitation has been known since antiquity and isolated mention of positive-pressure ventilation appeared in the literature of the seventeenth, eighteenth, and nineteenth centuries,[17] it was not until the second quarter of the twentieth century that a basis for resuscitation of the newborn infant emerged. The use of positive-pressure ventilation with an endotracheal tube was described in 1928,[31] as was a positive-pressure device with a pressure regulator,[49] which, with modifications,[48] is still in use today. With the knowledge available in 1928 one would have expected that an orderly, progressive development of resuscitation techniques would have taken place, but this was not the case.

Until the last two decades, methods of resuscitation were based on empirical observations in the human infant without animal experimentation under controlled conditions. Since many infants were resuscitated during primary apnea (Figure 2–I), methods

now discarded seemed to work, including the Bloxsom positive-pressure oxygen-air lock,[9] body rocking,[5, 28, 55] intragastric oxygen,[44] hyperbaric oxygen,[11] analeptic drugs,[19] and electrical stimulation of the phrenic nerve.[15]

This chapter presents an approach to the resuscitation of the asphyxiated human new-

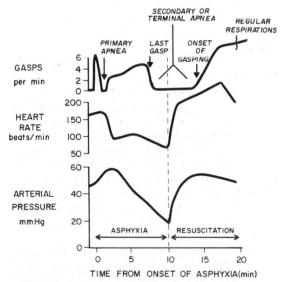

Figure 2–1. Changes in physiologic parameters during asphyxiation and resuscitation of the rhesus monkey fetus at birth. Rhesus monkeys were asphyxiated at birth by tying the umbilical cords while their heads were in saline-filled rubber bags. Resuscitation was by positive-pressure ventilation. (Adapted from Dawes[21] and Adamsons et al.[3])

31

born infant. Anticipation is the key to good care; an understanding of the obstetric events preceding delivery (see Chapter 1) is an important component in planning rational neonatal management, of which resuscitation is the critical initial intervention. After reviewing pertinent background information, the sequential steps necessary to resuscitate the asphyxiated neonate are presented. In addition, special problems associated with very low birth weight, meconium aspiration, acute blood loss, and progressive distress after birth are discussed.

PATHOPHYSIOLOGY OF ASPHYXIA

An understanding of the pathophysiology of asphyxia is preliminary to considering the approach to resuscitation of an asphyxiated human newborn infant. A significant amount of information is, of necessity, based on animal experiments, and there is great variability among different species in their response to asphyxia when measured in terms of the time to last gasp or survival time, which are commonly used end points.[21] These species differences may be very important factors influencing the course and effect of asphyxia. Furthermore, there are significant differences in degrees of maturation at birth and subsequent rates of development in the diverse species used to study asphyxia, such as the rat, guinea pig, rabbit, cat, sheep, and monkey. Therefore, caution must be exercised when extrapolating such data to the human newborn infant.

The events associated with asphyxia in the human fetus are probably closely analogous to those described for the rhesus monkey. A useful example is the observation of the natural history of total asphyxia at birth in the rhesus monkey fetus delivered by cesarean section, in which, prior to delivery, catheters were placed in fetal vessels and the head was covered with a saline-filled rubber bag to prevent air breathing during gasping. At delivery, the umbilical cord was immediately tied. (Figure 2–1 illustrates the course of selected physiologic parameters during 10 minutes of total asphyxia and subsequent resuscitation.) Rapid gasps occurred shortly after the onset of asphyxia, accompanied by muscular effort producing thrashing movements of the extremities. This ceased after a little more than a minute and heralded the onset of primary apnea (during which spontaneous respirations can still be induced by appropriate sensory stimuli), which lasted almost a minute. The heart rate dropped considerably but was still approximately 100 beats per minute. (Normal is 180 to 220 beats per minute in an infant monkey.) A series of spontaneous deep gasps then followed for 4 to 5 minutes, gradually becoming weaker and terminating at the last gasp after approximately 8 minutes of total asphyxia. Secondary apnea (during which spontaneous respirations cannot be induced by sensory stimuli) begins after the last gasp, and death occurs if secondary apnea is not reversed within several minutes. The longer the delay in initiating adequate resuscitation measures (artificial ventilation) after the last gasp, the longer the time to the first gasp after resuscitation: for every 1-minute delay, the time to first gasp is increased by about 2 minutes, and the time to onset of rhythmic breathing is delayed, on the average, by over 4 minutes[3] (Table 2–1).

During total asphyxia, dramatic changes occurred in acid-base parameters: pH dropped from 7.3 just prior to asphyxia to 6.8 at 10 minutes; PCO_2 rose from 45 mm Hg prior to asphyxia to 150 mm Hg at 10 minutes; and PO_2 fell from 25 mm Hg prior to asphyxia to virtually zero at 10 minutes.[21] Concomitantly, the levels of blood lactate, reflecting anaerobic metabolism and accumulation of excess acid, rose rapidly with asphyxia. The concentration of blood lactate fell slowly when positive-pressure oxygen ventilation was initiated.

Clinically, fetal hypoxia is usually incomplete and intermittent. The effects of this pattern of fetal hypoxia on fetal mortality have been described in a rabbit model.[66] Fetal survival decreased significantly at lower maternal inspired O_2 concentrations used to produce hypoxia, longer durations of hypoxia, and shorter recovery intervals between hypoxic episodes.

TABLE 2–1 EFFECT OF DELAYING RESUSCITATION IN NEWBORN MONKEYS*

Duration of Asphyxia (min)	Minutes of Assisted Ventilation Before:	
	Gasping	Breathing
10.0	2.3	9.7
12.5	9.4	20.5
15.0	13.6	30.0

*Adapted from James.[43]

The human fetus and newborn may be less mature and may tolerate greater amounts of asphyxia than the rhesus monkey without developing brain damage, and the time to last gasp is probably longer than in the rhesus monkey.[21] The frequency distribution of duration of primary apnea and time to last gasp studied in newborn rabbits shows a reasonably wide range.[11] This variability may also occur in the human infant, with the possibility of a marked prolongation of primary apnea and/or time to last gasp. This means that in the individual newborn patient the actual time course of asphyxia and the possibility of subsequent manifestations of anoxic brain damage cannot be easily estimated. When an apneic newborn is encountered in the delivery room, it is extremely difficult to determine whether primary or secondary (terminal) apnea is present. The latter must be assumed and resuscitative measures started at once. Retrospectively, on the basis of the infant's response, it may be possible to estimate the severity of the asphyxial episode.

Circulatory Changes During Asphyxia

During the course of total asphyxia in the rhesus monkey (Figure 2–1) the blood pressure, after an initial rise, fell steadily. At the same time, the skin became successively blue, blotchy, and then white as the infant responded to the circulatory failure with generalized peripheral vasoconstriction. A study of the effects of hypoxia on the rhesus monkey in utero indicated that concomitant with the decrease in cardiac output was a redistribution of the available cardiac output in an attempt to provide oxygenated blood to vital organs—brain, heart, and adrenal glands.[7] This was done at the expense of kidneys, spleen, lungs, and carcass. In this study, mild to moderate asphyxia, as indicated by oxygen uptake and acid-base studies, was induced by a gradual reduction in maternal arterial oxygen tension. Umbilical blood flow decreased by 50 per cent, as did fetal oxygen consumption. The oxygenated blood returning to the heart from the ductus venosus contributed a proportionately larger volume to the blood perfusing the brain and heart in control and hypoxic fetuses than did blood from the superior or inferior vena cava. In addition, during hypoxia there was increased shunting of superior vena caval blood across the foramen ovale, temporarily maintaining the absolute volume of blood perfusing the heart and brain on a per gram of tissue basis in the face of a falling cardiac output.

Five minutes of total asphyxia in the newborn monkey[30] during the first week of life produced similar alterations in the distribution of cardiac output. With a decrease in cardiac output of 80 per cent, the percentage of cardiac output going to the heart, adrenal glands, and paleoencephalon (midbrain, brainstem, and cerebellum) increased significantly, although not enough to preserve the organ flow per gram of tissue.

The observation of an alteration in the distribution of the circulation during periods of oxygen deprivation is not new. Reflex circulatory adjustments occur in diving seals, with profound bradycardia, decrease in oxygen consumption, decrease in body temperature, and accumulation of lactic acid in muscle but not in the blood.[72] Central blood pressure is usually maintained, and arterial blood contains oxygen whereas peripheral blood does not. When the seal surfaces, the predive state resumes, and after air breathing starts, the lactic acid is taken away from the muscle by the blood stream and delivered to the liver for metabolism.

It has been postulated that such circulatory adjustments occur in the human infant to protect vital organs from the hypoxia occurring at the time of delivery. This is based in part on the observation that the blood lactate level in the newborn increases shortly after the onset of respiration, with higher levels noted in the severely depressed newborn.[42] However, there is a fundamental difference in the stress to the human infant. In the diving mammal, which may remain submerged for 25 minutes, the circulatory changes are not overwhelmed under the conditions of a normal dive; in the asphyxiated primate, however, the circulatory changes are in response to life-threatening pathologic conditions, and the protective effects are quickly overwhelmed after short periods of asphyxia as noted above. Calculations reveal that these circulatory adjustments will account for only a small portion of the increased length of time that the newborn can survive asphyxia. Survivors of sublethal asphyxia often show evidence of organ damage, particularly acute renal failure, feeding intolerance, seizures, and myocardial ischemia.

Biochemical Changes During Asphyxia

The most important biochemical event during asphyxia is the conversion from aerobic oxidation of glucose to anaerobic glycolysis in response to hypoxia, with the accumulation of lactate and the development of a metabolic acidosis. Lactate is metabolized by oxidation predominantly in the neonatal liver. There is an increase in lactic acid dehydrogenase (LDH) activity in the liver immediately after birth; this activity is further increased in response to hypoxia. In addition to the development of severe metabolic acidosis secondary to hypoxia, there is an immediate, rapid elevation of PCO_2 during asphyxia. This respiratory acidosis generally occurs first when there is cord compression of the fetus, acute placental insufficiency (placental respiratory acidosis), or obstruction of the airway in a newborn infant. The profound drop in pH is thus a result of a mixed acidosis that is coincident with the hypoxia.

Respiratory acidosis in the immediate newborn period also may be secondary to drug depression of the infant. Use in the mother of drugs that are known respiratory depressants, such as barbiturates and meperidine in repeated or large doses, and use of general inhalation anesthetics such as cyclopropane may induce apnea in the newborn. **M. Stahlman**

Free fatty acids and glycerol, both products of neutral fat hydrolysis, increase in blood in response to hypoxia. It has been postulated that a decrease in transfer of glucose across the placenta secondary to hypoxia may mobilize free fatty acids by release of epinephrine and norepinephrine.[79]

Hepatic glycogen is mobilized immediately after birth to provide a continuing source of glucose to the brain when the maternal blood glucose supply is terminated. At the time of delivery, maternal blood glucose is usually elevated secondary to sympathetic stimulation, and the neonate has a parallel elevation, although the levels are lower in fetal than in maternal blood.

Animal studies indicate that adenosine triphosphate (ATP) levels initially are maintained at the expense of phosphocreatine.[86] As the level of high-energy phosphate falls, cell processes begin to fail, including resynthesis of acetylcholine and the "sodium pump," which results in cell losses of potassium and amino acids.[69] The cell accumulates carbon dioxide, inorganic phosphate, ammonia, and γ-aminobutyric acid (GABA), which is a neuroinhibitory substance.[69] These changes take considerably longer to occur in the newborn infant with immature nervous tissue than in the adult animal.

Several studies[18, 32, 38, 39, 51, 73, 75] suggest that brain tissue can utilize glycerol, ketone bodies (β-hydroxybutyrate, acetoacetate), and lactate as metabolic substrates; however, the oxygen requirements are high, and it is unlikely that this pathway is utilized under conditions of hypoxia and glycogen depletion.

ABILITY OF THE NEWBORN TO SURVIVE ASPHYXIA

There are several factors that enable the newborn infant to survive asphyxia better than the adult.[53] The lower metabolic rate of particular tissues is probably most important. The relatively immature brain of the newborn animal has a resting metabolic rate less than that observed in the adult. The state of activity of a given tissue, as well as the temperature, is also significant. For example, the metabolic requirements of the myocardium are probably initially increased during asphyxia. Environmental temperatures outside the neutral thermal range may also increase metabolic requirements.

Hypothermia[56] has been recommended for resuscitation of the asphyxiated human newborn on the basis of findings in very small newborn mammals cooled to 15° C, in which all metabolic processes and therefore, presumably, oxygen consumption were slowed. A significant benefit from cooling was not noted in the rhesus monkey asphyxiated at birth.[20] In the human neonate with much greater mass it is unrealistic to expect to achieve a core temperature considered "therapeutic hypothermia"; partial cooling represents an additional stress to the asphyxiated newborn, with an increased metabolic rate and oxygen requirement.

Another major factor enabling the newborn to survive asphyxia is the availability of substrate for anaerobic degradation. The substrate may be locally stored, as with myocardial glycogen, or mobilized via the circulation to supply the brain with carbohydrate from liver glycogen. The mobilization of hepatic glycogen during hypoxia makes the finding of hypoglycemia extremely unusual in the infant being resuscitated because of asphyxia, and administration of a hypertonic glucose solution under such circumstances is probably of little value in the term or large preterm infant.

An intact circulation is of major importance in the ability to survive asphyxia, and it was shown as early as 1812 by Le Gallois (cited by Dawes[21]) that rabbits asphyxiated by immersion in water or opening of the thorax gasped significantly longer than those from which the heart was removed. An intact circulation is able to redistribute lactate and hydrogen ion to tissues still being perfused (that may have a lower hydrogen ion production) and thus may provide a means of buffering cerebral cells during asphyxia.[1, 21] It is as an adjunct to this that sodium bicarbonate, administered during asphyxia, may exert a beneficial effect if CO_2 gas is being removed.

Although a beneficial effect (prolongation of last gasp) from the infusion of alkali and glucose has been reported in the rhesus monkey asphyxiated at birth,[2, 22] the glucose levels were not low even in the control group, and the effect may be related to improvement in the circulating vascular volume. Data in fetal and newborn lambs suggest that the hypertonicity of the infused solution (glucose, saline, or sodium bicarbonate), independent of the effect of pH, may be responsible for increasing pulmonary blood flow and cardiac output.[46] In the human this benefit must be weighed against the risk of precipitating intracerebral hemorrhage in poorly supported vascular areas, particularly in the low-birth-weight infant.

In summary, as shown in the rat brain,[45] immature brain tissue with a lower rate of energy metabolism can possibly increase the rate of anaerobic glycolysis and use the available energy more efficiently, so that the biochemical ultrastructure is maintained within recoverable limits in response to hypoxia. Unfortunately, severe sustained hypoxia overcomes these protective mechanisms, and brain damage or death then occurs.

AN APPROACH TO RESUSCITATION OF THE NEWBORN

In this section the rationale is provided for the various components of the resuscitation technique presented later.

Many early methods depended on uncomfortable stimuli to initiate the onset of respirations, including gentle, intermittent traction on the tongue, spanking the feet or buttocks, dilation of the anal sphincter, and alternately immersing the infant in hot and cold water.[77] There is little experimental basis for these methods, and they should be avoided, since injury may be produced and they waste time that can be used more effectively.

Current resuscitation methods, based on the previous discussion of asphyxia and clinical assessment of the neonate utilizing the Apgar score (Table 2–2), are directed to providing oxygen and removing carbon dioxide by positive-pressure ventilation, maintaining the circulation by external cardiac massage (described in 1962[61]), using a volume expander to combat shock, and infrequently, using a cardiotonic agent and providing alkali for buffering the excess acid produced during anaerobic metabolism.

The asphyxiated newborn should be placed in a neutral thermal environment for resuscitation. At the present time an overhead radiant heat source is most effective and should be used in every delivery room. It has been demonstrated that the naked, wet, term neonate placed on an open table in the delivery room with an ambient temperature of 25° C will lose 4° C in skin temperature in 5 minutes and 2° C in core temperature in 20 minutes.[16]

TABLE 2–2 APGAR SCORE*

Sign	Score		
	0	1	2
Heart rate	Absent	Below 100	Over 100
Respiratory effort	Absent	Weak, irregular	Good; crying
Muscle tone	Flaccid	Some flexion of extremities	Well flexed
Reflex irritability (Catheter in nose or slap sole of foot)	No response	Grimace	Cry
Color	Pale	Blue	Completely pink

*Adapted from data of Apgar.[4]

A dried infant under a radiant heat source loses almost no heat over the same time. The need to keep an infant warm during the resuscitation procedure cannot be overemphasized.

Adequate ventilatory support is the cornerstone of neonatal resuscitation since hypoxic cardiorespiratory depression is the underlying problem in the presence of otherwise normal tissues. Prompt reversal of respiratory insufficiency results in cardiocirculatory and metabolic function being stabilized. This may be partially a result of maintaining circulatory autoregulation and avoiding progressive shock. Hyperventilation is relatively common during resuscitation in the presence of normal pulmonary compliance and will tend to abort the progress of, and partially compensate for, metabolic acidosis without the obligate use of pharmacologic support, except in situations of the most severe compromise. Moderately asphyxiated infants (Apgar scores of 3–6) will usually respond to pharyngeal suctioning or respiratory stimulation (resuscitation bag and mask or tube) with spontaneous respiratory efforts. Severely asphyxiated infants (Apgar scores of 0–2) usually need positive-pressure ventilation, which may initially require greater pressure (>20–30 cm H_2O) to achieve lung expansion, similar to pressures described for the initial breaths after birth.[47, 58]

Prolonged, unnecessary exposure to high concentrations of oxygen in the delivery room should be avoided, especially in the small, preterm infant susceptible to retrolental fibroplasia. Arterial Po_2 values in excess of 400 mm Hg by 15 minutes of age have been demonstrated[41] in the normal term infant breathing 75 per cent O_2; comparable data are not available for the premature infant.

Maintaining an adequate circulation is an essential component of resuscitation if the progressive effects of hypoxia are to be avoided. In the majority of infants this is a spontaneous consequence of adequate ventilation and oxygenation, and recovery should be documented as promptly as possible after birth by clinical evaluation and blood pressure measurement. In the absence of response to initial resuscitation efforts, cardiocirculatory failure with shock may be the most important factor, and volume expansion may be more important than drugs. Circulation should be maintained by external cardiac massage in the infant unexpectedly born without heart rate or in whom heart rate falls below or fails to rise above 80 beats per minute in response to ventilation. Cardiac stimulants, therefore, have little role in neonatal resuscitation other than to allow additional time for further evaluation and definitive intervention in the infant who fails to respond.

When a potential problem is anticipated at the time of delivery, based on the identification of a high-risk pregnancy or evidence of fetal distress (asphyxia) during labor, the physician on call for the delivery room should be alerted (see Table 1–6). The need for sophisticated assessment and educated intervention beyond the initial resuscitation efforts requires the provision of a specifically identified resuscitation area within the delivery suite, preferably in close proximity to the special care nursery, which can be quickly staffed by trained personnel to provide appropriate monitoring, diagnostic, and therapeutic supports for extended resuscitation based on specific infant needs.

Volume depletion can represent either acute blood loss around the time of delivery—as in fetomaternal transfusion, placenta previa, or abruptio placentae—or passive vascular compartment expansion, as occurs following asphyxia or with infection. Under such circumstances, volume replacement becomes the logical treatment of choice. When blood loss seems the likely diagnosis, replacement, which includes red cells for oxygen transport, may be an essential component of successful resuscitation. Umbilical vessels provide the easiest route for intravascular access. The umbilical vein is easier to catheterize and in addition provides the most direct vascular access for cardiac stimulants, despite the qualification that insertion be limited to approximately 5 cm to avoid the risk of mechanical or pharmacologic injury to liver parenchyma. Umbilical artery catheterization is technically more difficult to perform, and in the absence of radiographic localization the catheter is as likely to be positioned in an area of increased risk for complications as the umbilical vein catheter (see Appendix I–2).

Blood is the best agent for volume expansion, and if an infant in shock is anticipated prior to delivery (because of severe fetal distress, severe Rh disease, actively bleeding placenta previa, or abruptio placentae), low antibody titer O-negative blood that has been cross-matched against the mother's blood should be available at the time of delivery.

The placenta, containing the infant's own blood, is theoretically the ideal replacement source. However, placental blood should only be used in immediately life-threatening situations because of the risk of bacterial contamination and possible infusion of blood clots or red blood cell microaggregates. Risks can be minimized by using a small priming volume blood filter between the syringe and infusion line. Placental blood may be drawn aseptically at the time of delivery from the umbilical vein or its major tributaries on the surface of the placenta into a plastic syringe rinsed with heparin solution (1000 units/ml). Usually 20–30 ml (occasionally up to 50 ml) may be collected and administered immediately or may accompany the infant to the nursery for use in the first 1 to 2 hours of life.

If blood is not available or if acute blood loss is not considered the most likely diagnosis, then normal saline or a plasma preparation is an alternative volume expander.

The use of a plasma preparation (colloid) for volume expansion is associated with prompt increase in colloid osmotic pressure, whereas use of normal saline (crystalloid) is associated with a decrease in colloid osmotic pressure.[76, 87] In moderate quantities sufficient to bring about cardiocirculatory homeostasis, either choice will be effective, although duration of effect on colloid osmotic pressure may vary with the specific solution. In the neonate, in whom volume deficits usually reflect real or functional whole blood loss and the colloid osmotic pressure is normally low (relative to the older child), the use of both colloid and crystalloid is frequently necessary when several increments of volume replacement are needed.

Initial volume expansion should be 10–20 ml/kg, and additional increments of 10 ml/kg can be given depending on the response observed. Every effort should be made to initiate objective serial measurements of response (blood pressure, venous pressure, hematocrit, blood gases) as promptly as possible. The volume of fluid required for correction is variable but may be over half the infant's total blood volume (85 ml/kg).

Infrequently an infant fails to respond to adequate ventilation, external cardiac massage, and volume expansion. When this occurs the infant may be presumed to be acidotic, hypoxic (tissue), and volume depleted, necessitating intervention with both epinephrine and sodium bicarbonate. Under such

TABLE 2–3 ESTABLISHING EFFECTIVE VENTILATION

What Is Required	What Can Interfere
Responsive respiratory center	Immaturity, asphyxia, trauma, drugs
Adequate neural transmission	Spinal cord injury, phrenic nerve injury
Normal musculoskeletal effector	Diaphragmatic hernia, chest deformity
Patent airways and normal lung parenchyma	Airway obstruction, lack of surfactant, meconium, blood, or exudate filling air spaces

circumstances sodium bicarbonate will serve a volume expanding role as well as provide alkalinization (partial) to improve the effectiveness of epinephrine. Epinephrine can be given via an umbilical vessel catheter; an alternative route is via endotracheal tube,[27, 35, 71] which, although not yet validated by more than a case report in the human neonate,[36, 70] would seem preferable to transmyocardial administration. Direct cardiac puncture should be avoided unless all else has failed.

Table 2–3 is helpful as an outline in approaching infants who do not establish effective ventilation.

Resuscitation Techniques

Resuscitation of the newborn infant is one of the major pediatric emergencies. There is no substitute for adequate training and periodic review of the techniques required. The physician should arrive early enough to set out the necessary equipment and see that it is functioning properly. The procedure is facilitated when the supplies are identified and organized in a prearranged manner on a resuscitation cart or attached to a wall board.[13] Another major advantage of arriving before the delivery is that useful information obtained from the obstetrician concerning the pregnancy and labor makes it possible to anticipate problems that may be present at birth. Transmitting this information to personnel in the nursery will enable special preparations to be made for anticipated problems. The pediatrician who arrives after the delivery is obviously at a disadvantage with respect to organizing equipment and obtaining the relevant history. In addition, it may be difficult to assess accurately the time sequence of events following delivery of the infant.

The physician should be familiar with both the premature (size 0) and the infant (size 1) Miller laryngoscope blades (Figure 2–2). The infant size is more flexible, in that the length is adequate for all newborns even if somewhat cumbersome. The premature blade is not long enough to permit adequate visualization of the larynx in the newborn weighing over 2500 gm. The straight endotracheal tube (Murphy) may be passed either orally or nasally, but care is needed to avoid insertion into the right main-stem bronchus. Some currently available tubes are marked with a circumferential black ring 3 cm proximal from the tip to facilitate proper placement by direct visualization (Figure 2–2). An alternative may be the Cole tube, which has a flare to prevent passage of the tube beyond the tracheal bifurcation. In either case, the tube size (2.5 to 3.5 mm) should be the largest that will allow an air leak and avoid pressure injury to subglottic structures.

The brightness of the light on the laryngoscope blade should be tested. Endotracheal tube obturators (Figure 2–2) should be available to facilitate oral intubation. The resuscitation bag should be checked for proper function, and adapters should be available to connect the bag to the face mask and endotracheal tube. This connection is preferably separated by a T-piece, which allows interposition of an aneroid manometer to estimate inflation pressure. The oxygen flowmeter and wall suction equipment, when used, should be checked for proper function. Oxygen should be warmed and humidified and compressed air available to adjust the oxygen concentration administered. Syringes, DeLee mucus trap, needles, umbilical vessel catheters, drugs (1 mEq/ml of sodium bicarbonate and epinephrine 1:10,000), and sterile water for injection should all be available. All resuscitation efforts should be carried out under a radiant heat unit.

The current approach to resuscitation of the newborn infant closely follows guidelines recommended by the American Heart Association.[78]

The severity of depression of the newborn infant must be evaluated to determine the course of immediate management. The most practical emergency guideline is based on the Apgar scoring chart (Table 2–2).

The infant with an Apgar score above 7 will rarely need any resuscitation unless the Apgar score drops suddenly several minutes after birth. If this occurs, then management is as described below. It is important to avoid prolonged vigorous nasopharyngeal suctioning of these infants, since it may cause reflex bradycardia and apnea.[14]

The infant with an Apgar score of 3 to 6 when first seen has probably had mild to moderate asphyxia. If apnea is present it is usually primary, and gasping respiratory efforts can be anticipated. In such situations, brief suctioning of the airway followed by ventilation by positive-pressure mask and bag often will result in rapid improvement. In the rare infant who becomes worse over several minutes and whose Apgar score drops into the range of the severely asphyxiated infant (a score of 0 to 2), subsequent management should proceed as for severe asphyxia.

An infant with an Apgar score of 0 to 2 is

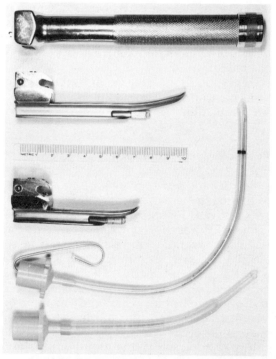

Figure 2–2. Equipment for intubation of the newborn. Note in particular the difference in length between the size 1 (term infant) and size 0 (premature infant) blades. The size 0 blade will not be long enough for adequate visualization of the larynx in the near-term infant. Note the short distal segment of the Cole endotracheal tube (without obturator) that passes between the vocal cords and the proximal wider portion that prevents the tube from being advanced too far. The straight endotracheal tube (Murphy), shown with obturator, has a black ring proximal to the tip to aid placement in the trachea (ring is located at entrance to larynx by direct visualization) and to avoid passage down the right main stem bronchus.

considered severely asphyxiated until proven otherwise. The assistance of another skilled person should be requested immediately to help with this infant's resuscitation. Very brief (15 second) suctioning should be done initially to clear the airway, preferably under direct laryngoscopic visualization. An endotracheal tube should be inserted (Figures 2–3 and 2–4). Adequate ventilation with oxygen should be provided by positive pressure established by bag to tube inflation of the lungs at the rate of approximately 50 times per minute; the inspiratory phase should be slightly less than half the time of a ventilation cycle. Approximately 20–25 cm H_2O pressure is needed to inflate the lungs of a normal newborn infant, but pressure twice as high may be necessary initially.[47, 58] The adequacy of ventilation can be determined best by observing the chest wall excursion or by listening to the chest with a stethoscope. If too much pressure is generated, the procedure may be complicated by the development of a pneumomediastinum and/or pneumothorax (see Respiratory Problems, Chapter 8). If the initial heart rate is over 100 beats per minute, primary apnea is more likely, and optionally a brief 15–20 second attempt to resuscitate can be made, using a tight-fitting face mask and positive-pressure oxygen by bag. If there is no immediate response, indicated by an increase in heart rate, endotracheal intubation should be performed.

Bag and mask resuscitation frequently works for moderately to severely depressed infants who are delivered per vaginam and apparently acts by stimulating the stretch receptors in the trachea, causing the infants to inspire. It sometimes has the effect of causing frothing of fluid in the trachea, particularly in those infants delivered by cesarean section. The pressure is insufficient to expand the alveoli, and the frothy fluid pours out of the trachea into the back of the pharynx at such a rate that it is almost impossible to view the larynx when intubation has to be resorted to.

As a generalization the trend to employ the bag and mask as a "more simple technique" for resuscitation is not in the best interest of the infant because the pressures applied are distributed not only to the lungs but also to the stomach, which fills with gas. It is by no means as effective as intubation and direct line expansion.

S. James

The infant with primary apnea or gasping at the time resuscitation is started will usually respond promptly to suction or the administration of oxygen by face mask with an increase in heart rate, spontaneous increased gasping, improved color, and some spontaneous movement. For infants who do not respond promptly (within 30 seconds) to effective ventilation with oxygen with an increase in heart rate to over 100 beats per minute, further deterioration can be anticipated. External cardiac compression should be started if the heart rate falls below 80.

External cardiac massage is performed by placing the hands around the neonate's chest with both thumbs over the midsternum; the fingers are used to support the back.[85] The

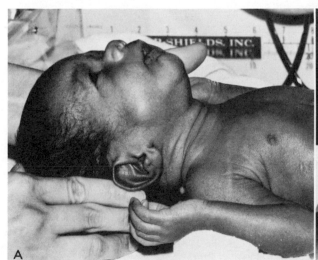

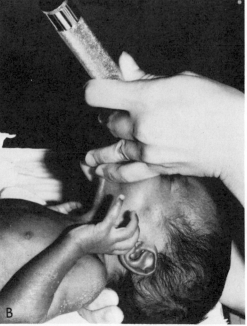

Figure 2–3. Note the positioning of the hand for intubation with chin up and shoulders slightly elevated. The laryngoscope is held in the left hand, and the fourth and fifth fingers can help control the position of the head. When held properly, the blade should be easy to control and soft tissue injury avoided.

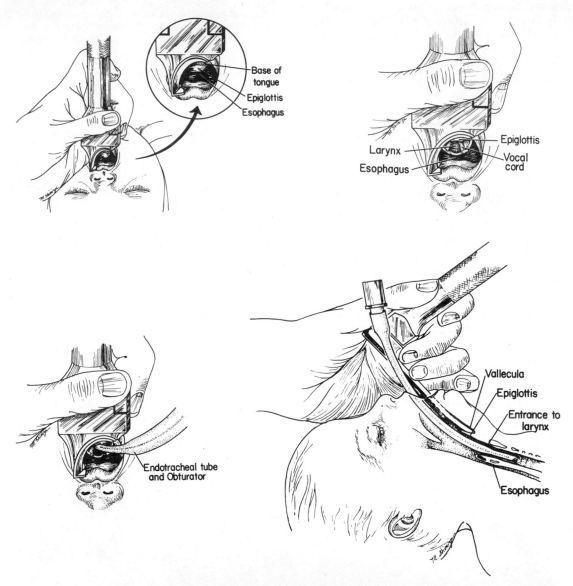

Figure 2–4. Technique of endotracheal intubation. The Miller blade should be inserted near the midline and moved to the left side of the mouth, gently deflecting the tongue. As it is advanced, the base of the tongue and epiglottis are visualized. The blade should be advanced in the same plane of movement into the vallecula (as at lower right); as the blade is gently raised, the epiglottis swings anteriorly, revealing the opening of the larynx. If secretions or meconium is noted, gentle suctioning should be done before insertion of the endotracheal tube. On certain occasions when the epiglottis is not adequately raised, the blade tip may be placed posterior to the epiglottis, which can then be gently raised to expose the vocal cords. The endotracheal tube is advanced from the right corner of the mouth and inserted while maintaining direct visualization. Pitfalls include inadequate visualization of structures and inability to control the direction of the tip of the endotracheal tube. Repeat suctioning or depression of the larynx by the fourth or fifth finger of the left hand may help the physician to visualize the vocal cords; the endotracheal tube should be kept clear of the line of vision of the laryngoscope blade when inserted. A counterclockwise, semicircular movement of the tube in the right hand prevents contact with the alveolar ridge of the maxilla and enables the tube to enter the airway easily. An obturator may be helpful in maintaining the appropriate curve of the tube. After intubation the laryngoscope blade is carefully withdrawn while the position of the tube is maintained by the right hand on the infant's face. Note the tip of the blade in the vallecula.

sternum is then compressed 1–1.5 cm at a rate of 100–120 times/minute. The chest compression should be synchronized with ventilation at a ratio of three to four chest compressions for every breath. The effectiveness of cardiac massage can be assessed by monitoring heart rate, femoral pulses, and status of the peripheral circulation. Observation of pupil reactivity may be helpful.

If the heart rate does not improve or progressively worsens, then a significant metabolic acidosis can be presumed as well as a need for myocardial stimulation by epinephrine in a dose of 0.1 ml/kg of 1:10,000 solution administered via an umbilical vessel catheter. Administration of sodium bicarbonate (2 mEq/kg as a 0.5 mEq/ml solution) may partially correct the metabolic acidosis and improve the effectiveness of the epinephrine dose, which can be repeated.

In the presence of severe shock or apparent asystole or if an umbilical vessel catheter has not yet been placed, epinephrine absorption may be facilitated by the endotracheal route of administration. The same dose as for intravenous administration is utilized and diluted with sterile water to a volume of 1 ml; instillation directly into the endotracheal tube or into the trachea is followed by five rapid ventilations to deliver the medication to distal airways where rapid absorption occurs. Blood levels persist for a much longer period of time by this route,[27] and a second dose should only follow evidence of efficacy succeeded by clinical deterioration. Administration of epinephrine by external cardiac puncture should only be used as a last resort.

We rarely, if ever, use cardiac stimulants in the delivery room. Good ventilation and the restoration of oxygenation seem to be the most important procedures.

S. James

After successful resuscitation of the newborn infant, a feeding tube should be passed into the stomach and any secretions or air removed by gentle suction.

Special Problems

VERY LOW-BIRTH-WEIGHT NEONATE

The need for effective resuscitation of the very low-birth-weight infant occurs with greater frequency and assumes greater importance as survival rates increase. An even better outcome for the very low-birth-weight infant can be predicted for the next decade; there will probably be few factors as significant as the condition at birth and the initial care provided at that time. The very low-birth-weight infant tolerates labor and delivery less well and is less likely to have a normal neonatal transition. On the other hand, neonatal depression may be overestimated when the Apgar score criteria, based on the term neonate, are rigidly applied, since reflex activity and muscle tone are less well developed. Prompt, effective resuscitation and avoidance of unnecessary instability during transition are most important.

Airway stabilization with the provision of continuous positive airway pressure (CPAP) and elective endotracheal intubation by a skilled operator has been suggested to avoid unnecessary hypoxia.[26] Although this is routine practice in some nurseries, the controlled data that validate the concept are meager; no comparison is available that includes the use of CPAP by nasal prongs to minimize the risks associated with endotracheal intubation of the very low-birth-weight infant by other than a skilled operator. The benefits of such intervention must be weighed against the risk of prolonging asphyxia or interfering with spontaneous respiratory effort during intubation attempts by a less skilled operator; spontaneous respiratory effort when sustained is probably more effective in increasing tidal volume and establishing the functional residual capacity associated with mechanical stabilization of the lung.[9]

The anticipation of impending vascular collapse or frank hypotension and the early provision of appropriate fluids may avoid the need for rapid changes in intravascular volume or the use of vasoactive agents, which predispose to intracranial hemorrhage—a frequent cause of secondary mortality or long-term morbidity. These are thorny problems, particularly if there is loss of autoregulation of cerebral blood flow in the presence of mild or severe asphyxia, as has been proposed.[52, 57] Systemic hypotension may be associated with cerebral ischemia, which is difficult to document shortly after birth; a new imaging method utilizing phosphorus nuclear magnetic resonance may eventually make this assessment possible.[23] Aggressive correction of hypotension with excessive amounts of fluid may result in systemic hypertension and exposure of the cerebral capillary blood vessels to high pressure, leading to rupture with periventricular and/or intraventricular hemorrhage,[33, 34] now easily documented by portable ultrasound examination.[74]

The tendency to administer fluid for hypotension has in recent years been greatly overdone. Administration of fluid to restore blood pressure should only be done when there is definite evidence of acute blood loss. Restoration of oxygenation is the most effective means of restoring cardiac output and blood pressure. We are very conservative with fluid administration in both the small immature infants and the larger severely asphyxiated infants. For the latter we basically restrict fluids until we know the state of the kidneys and the amount of urine output. Until that is ascertained fluids are only given sufficient to replace insensible water loss.   **S. James**

Editorial Comment: Moscoso reported a rather dramatic upward trend in blood pressure occurring spontaneously within the first hours of life in infants weighing less than 1.25 kg. Many infants, hypotensive on standard charts at 2 hours, became normotensive by 7 hours of age. The use of volume expansion to correct hypotension in the absence of acute blood loss should be approached cautiously. In many preterm infants who are mildly hypotensive but clinically stable, a conservative expectant approach may prevent unnecessary treatment. This approach is supported by an increasing body of evidence that, as a result of poor autoregulation, rapid volume expansion may increase cerebral blood flow and possibly cause or aggravate intracranial hemorrhage in very low-birth-weight infants.

Moscoso, P., Goldberg, R. N., Jamieson, J., et al: Spontaneous elevation in arterial blood pressure during the first hours of life in the very-low-birth-weight infant. J Pediatr *103*:114, 1983.

Following the initial resuscitation, an intravenous glucose infusion of approximately 5 mg/kg/min is necessary to avoid hypoglycemia in the preterm infant with poor glycogen stores.

MECONIUM ASPIRATION

The presence of fresh meconium in amniotic fluid prior to delivery should initiate concern about possible meconium aspiration in the newborn. Frequently there is a history of prenatal stress. At the time of delivery the obstetrician should carefully suction the hypopharynx before delivery of the shoulders; this may be the most important factor in preventing severe meconium aspiration syndrome.[12] If meconium is present around the face or in the mouth of the infant, direct visualization of the larynx should be done with removal by suction of any meconium seen. This should be done even if respirations have been initiated, since tenacious meconium may still be removable. When thick meconium is seen within the larynx, endotracheal intubation should be done and direct suctioning of the trachea accomplished through a gauze pad or paper face mask. This procedure reduces the incidence of significant morbidity and mortality (see Respiratory Problems, Chapter 8).[37, 84]

PROGRESSIVE DISTRESS AFTER BIRTH

Infrequently an infant born without significant evidence of perinatal asphyxia will rapidly develop progressive distress and a low 5 minute Apgar score despite appropriate management. A diagnosis must be established as promptly as possible; initial management may need to be based on clinical suspicion confirmed as promptly as possible by appropriate diagnostic studies. An infant with a diaphragmatic hernia will benefit from early intubation and insertion of a nasogastric tube to prevent further inflation of the gastrointestinal tract during bag and mask ventilation. Identification of a scaphoid abdomen, progressive respiratory distress, shift in cardiac apex, and asymmetric breath sounds may be noted. Progressive tension pneumothorax may require aspiration by intravenous catheter or the equivalent shortly after birth, based on sudden deterioration and auscultatory findings of a marked shift in the cardiac apex and significant decrease in breath sounds on the affected side. Infants with these problems can rapidly progress to develop clinical shock since impaired lung function and elevated intrathoracic pressures are associated with decreased venous return through the vena cava and low cardiac output. Emergency chest x-ray will establish a definitive diagnosis. Transillumination of the chest may identify a pneumothorax more quickly; this is particularly useful in the preterm infant with less body fat and a relatively thinner chest wall. Bilateral choanal atresia, a very rare condition, will benefit from orotracheal intubation, which will immediately establish normal ventilation. Infants with severe micrognathia and respiratory distress will benefit from an endotracheal tube placed in the hypopharynx via the nose, which breaks the seal to the upper airway produced by a posteriorly displaced tongue.

Rarely, an infant may be depressed secondary to narcotic sedation of the mother and may improve after administration of a narcotic antagonist, naloxone (0.01 mg/kg, given by umbilical vein). However, an airway should be established first and adequate ventilation initiated before this diagnosis is considered. This problem can be expected to be of greater significance when associated with perinatal asphyxia or prematurity.

An infant with a severe congenital abnormality such as severe pulmonary hypoplasia associated with a diaphragmatic hernia may not respond to any resuscitative interventions.

BRAIN DAMAGE FOLLOWING ASPHYXIA AND RESUSCITATION

By appropriate intervention with adequate resuscitative measures the severely asphyxiated infant can be saved and brain damage prevented or minimized. Brain injury occurs when prolonged hypoxia overwhelms the compensatory mechanisms previously described. The damage may be severe and manifested early in the form of a seizure disorder, cerebral palsy, or profound developmental retardation. Damage also may be reflected by very subtle neurologic findings in early childhood or as a learning disorder at school age. Current efforts to minimize damage are directed at managing or preventing problems of inadequate cerebral blood flow, cerebral edema, and intracerebral hemorrhage. The usefulness of phenobarbital administration immediately after birth—to prevent seizures and cerebral edema and to decrease cerebral oxygen consumption and the incidence of hemorrhage by minimizing the fluctuations of blood pressure related to activity—remains uncertain.[24, 40, 60, 82] A new drug that is reported to stabilize the capillary vessel wall and increase platelet adhesiveness has been shown in a preliminary study to decrease the frequency and severity of periventricular hemorrhage without altering mortality[59]; more studies are indicated. Measurement of intracranial pressure across the anterior fontanelle has been done and cerebral perfusion pressure estimated—mortality and morbidity in this small series were associated with markedly decreased cerebral perfusion pressure.[67] No generally accepted approach to manage cerebral edema in the neonate is available. Hyperventilation is frequently used, sometimes in conjunction with hyperosmotic agents or diuretics, although the effectiveness of any of these treatments is not well documented.

In the future, monitoring of anterior cerebral blood flow by ultrasound may provide a way of assessing the effectiveness of altering physiologic parameters of cerebral blood flow.

Behavioral abnormalities have been described in experimental animals following various periods of asphyxiation and resuscitation.[6, 68] Similarly, characteristic pathologic changes in the brain have been described in the nonhuman primate[10] and in the human fetus and newborn.[50, 64]

The Apgar scoring system has shown a significant relationship between 1 minute and 5 minute scores and neonatal mortality and morbidity.[25] The initial assessment (1 minute score) identifies the neonatal infant needing immediate attention (Apgar score of 0 to 6) and helps estimate the degree of asphyxia likely to be present. The 5 minute Apgar score is more closely correlated with neonatal mortality and morbidity. Based on the information already presented, infants with prolonged hypoxia, which mimics the secondary apnea described for the nonhuman primate, will be more depressed and take longer to resuscitate, resulting in a low Apgar score at 5 minutes of age. Of those infants with a 5 minute score of 0 or 1, 44 per cent did not survive the second day of life, and 49 per cent did not survive the neonatal period (to 28 days).[25] Follow-up of infants with a 5 minute Apgar score of 0 to 3 compared with a score of 7 to 10 indicated that, at 1 year of age, neurologic abnormality appeared in over 3 times as many infants with a 0 to 3 score[25]; for infants surviving to age 7 years, cerebral palsy was 21 times more likely in those with an Apgar score of 0 to 3 compared with a 7 to 10 score.[63] Eighty-seven per cent of infants with an Apgar score of 0 to 3 at 20 minutes of age died by the end of the first year, and 38 per cent of known survivors had cerebral palsy at age 7 years.[63] Similar neurologic disadvantage for the term infant in this 0 to 3 Apgar score group has been noted more recently, particularly associated with the onset of seizures before 24 hours of age.[29] If the original data[25] are rearranged, either on a weight basis or by individual Apgar scores, the higher the score, the lower the associated mortality and long-term morbidity.

Follow-up of infants born in the decade of the 1970s has generally suggested that improved mortality statistics have not been at the expense of increased morbidity, particularly in the very low-birth-weight groups.[81]

The association of an increased risk of dying in the presence of perinatal asphyxia has been noted to be greater at the higher gestational ages and greatest at term.[53]

It can be concluded that every effort should be made to identify potential obstetric pathologic conditions, to manage the pregnancy as optimally as possible, and to be prepared to resuscitate an asphyxiated newborn skillfully when necessary. The goal is to present each mother with a healthy newborn infant who has maximal potential for growth and development.

Unsuccessful Resuscitation

Since there appears to be a wide range of tolerance of asphyxia by individual infants, it is difficult to know when to discontinue resuscitative efforts. The infant should be given the benefit of any doubts. Such a decision is rarely an emergency and can be deferred to the intensive care nursery or equivalent stabilization unit with the advantages of monitoring equipment, biochemical data, radiographic assistance, and consultation as appropriate. Continuation of resuscitative efforts past the point at which a neurologically intact infant may be reasonably expected is usually not in the best interests of the neonate or parents. The only firm guideline that can be extrapolated from previous reports[80, 83] would indicate that infants who have not had spontaneous respirations during the first hour of life have a uniformly poor neurologic prognosis if they survive; discontinuation of resuscitation seems reasonable under such circumstances. In our opinion initiation of ventilator support should be reserved for infants judged to be "successfully" resuscitated.

When to stop resuscitation. Because the heart rate continues after the infant has stopped gasping and indeed continues during the period when brain damage is occurring, we approach the resuscitation of an infant born with no audible heart beat as follows: Lungs are ventilated and expanded two or three times with a high oxygen mixture. If there is no heart beat at that point, cardiac massage is instituted vigorously for approximately six to ten compressions. The lungs are again ventilated two or three times, and then a second period of cardiac massage is instituted. Those infants with a reflex cardiac arrest will usually respond to this. Possibly a third period of ventilation and cardiac massage will be necessary. If no heart beat can be heard after the third attempt at ventilation and cardiac massage, we do not recommend further resuscitation. I do not believe that any normal infants will be lost by adhering to these principles. Indeed by adhering to them we have salvaged a number of severely damaged infants. We certainly need better methods of assessing antenatal asphyxia and predicting those infants who will survive with minimal or no deficits.

S. James

PRACTICAL HINTS

1. All newborn infants have some degree of respiratory acidosis and hypoxia at birth.

2. The asphyxiated newborn infant has more profound hypoxia and respiratory acidosis as well as metabolic acidosis if asphyxia has been present for a long time. The low-birth-weight and particularly the very low-birth-weight infant will be at increased risk from asphyxia. Hypothermia may further aggravate these problems and is to be avoided.

3. The resuscitation of the asphyxiated newborn must include ventilatory (P_{CO_2}, P_{O_2}, and mechanical effect of inflation of the lung), circulatory (external cardiac massage and blood volume correction), and metabolic (sodium bicarbonate) correction as appropriate.

4. Hypotension and hypovolemia are often difficult to diagnose clinically immediately after delivery; any infant being observed following perinatal asphyxia should have serial determinations of blood pressure and microhematocrit done in anticipation of these problems.

5. Acidosis cannot be diagnosed clinically and must be suspected in any infant with a history of asphyxia.

6. Newborn infants may have cardiorespiratory problems because of asphyxia, maternal drugs (anesthetics, reserpine, etc.), intrathoracic disease (pneumothorax, diaphragmatic hernia, paralysis, etc.), anemia, hypotension, hypoglycemia, etc. The reason should be sought.

7. Rarely, a clinical trial of naloxone may be warranted for suspected narcotic overdose after establishment of adequate ventilation. Use of nonspecific central nervous system stimulants (caffeine, etc.) has no place in the treatment of asphyxia.

8. Meconium aspiration syndrome is usually a preventable disease, provided that prompt and appropriate resuscitation is performed.

CASE PROBLEMS

The clinical relevance of the foregoing information can be best understood by the following case examples and the questions they raise. The answer to each question follows immediately after the question, but we encourage readers to think out their own answers before reading the ones provided.

Case One

E. A., an 1800 gm male infant, was delivered after a 38 week gestation. The fetal heart rate varied widely (40 to 110 beats per minute) 30 minutes prior to delivery. The amniotic fluid was heavily meconium stained. At the age of 1 minute, the infant was noted to be limp and cyanotic, with a pulse rate of 84 per minute. He made no spontaneous effort to breathe and was unresponsive to stimuli. The 1 minute Apgar score was 1. At the age of 2 minutes, the pulse was 40 per minute, with no respirations.

How would you proceed to establish respiration?

The condition of this infant is urgent indication for resuscitation as follows: (1) Clear the upper airway by a short period of gentle suction with direct vision of the pharynx and larynx. (2) Establish adequate ventilation with oxygen by positive pressure, either with mask and bag or preferably with endotracheal tube. If there is no immediate response to mask and bag ventilation, then an endotracheal tube should be passed and positive-pressure ventilation carried out in this manner. (3) Because the heart rate is only 40 beats per minute, after ventilating the lungs a few times begin closed chest cardiac massage. (4) If there is no response as evidenced by prompt increase in heart rate, then administer over a 1 minute period 1–2 mEq/kg of sodium bicarbonate, diluted with equal parts of sterile water, and 0.1 ml/kg (1:10,000) of epinephrine. The initial dose of epinephrine, in the absence of an umbilical vessel catheter, can be given via the endotracheal tube. (5) If a response occurs with increase in heart rate, then volume expansion with 10–20 ml/kg of blood or plasma would be appropriate. (6) To minimize heat loss during resuscitation, keep the infant warm and dry. Attempt to maintain the skin temperature between 36 and 36.5° C. Once respiration has been restored, the infant can be further assessed.

With a birth weight of 1800 gm at 38 weeks, this infant is small for gestational age (SGA). (The antenatal diagnosis might have been made by the finding of a lag in fundal growth by ultrasound and by a fall in estriols.) Under these circumstances, prolonged labor, difficult delivery, or excessive sedation must be avoided, since SGA infants are particularly prone to perinatal asphyxia. Because there was fetal distress, evidenced by both a fall in fetal heart rate and the passage of meconium prior to delivery, the problem should have been anticipated, and a person skilled in resuscitation of the newborn should have been present at the delivery. Fetal scalp sampling might also have indicated this problem. Low Apgar scores are correlated with metabolic acidosis, which requires early correction. The SGA infant is likely to develop hypoglycemia, and the blood sugar should be monitored. Blood gas determinations, an x-ray of the chest, and a hematocrit are necessary in the further management of this infant.

Was this infant in "primary" or "secondary" apnea?

In attempting to determine whether the infant was in primary or secondary apnea, the history of whether the infant cried or breathed before becoming apneic is obviously important. If either crying or breathing took place, it is primary apnea. In this case, there is no indication of these having taken place, and it is the events during the recovery that will aid in arriving at the diagnosis. If the color is restored before the onset of breathing, then the infant is usually in secondary apnea. On the other hand, if gasping commences quickly before the onset of improvement in color, then the infant is in primary apnea. A number of infants in primary apnea will commence gasping while preparation is being made to start the resuscitation with the initial handling, suction, or oxygen blowing over their faces. In primary apnea, the heart rate and blood pressure are maintained, and there is some muscle tone present. Although the vast majority of infants who require resuscitation will be in primary apnea, this infant was probably in secondary apnea.

What is the relationship between the duration of asphyxia and reestablishment of spontaneous respiration?

The duration of asphyxia prior to artificial ventilation appears to influence the reestablishment of gasping and spontaneous ventilation. It is presumed, based on data obtained in the nonhuman primate, that for each minute after the last gasp that ventilation is delayed, there is a further delay of 2 minutes before gasping begins again and 4 minutes before rhythmic breathing is established. Thus, the longer artificial ventilation is delayed during secondary apnea, the longer it will take to resuscitate the infant (see Table 2–1).

What factors prolong the interval until the last gasp?

There are a number of factors purported to prolong the interval until the last gasp, including the maintenance of pH, hypothermia, administration of analgesic or anesthetic agents, and the maintenance of cerebral blood flow. Cooling alone does not reinitiate gasping in secondary apnea, nor does it produce a significant difference in time to the last gasp in the experimental animal unless the cooling is initiated prior to the asphyxia.

What are the effects of alkali infusion?

The beneficial effects of correcting pH, in addition to protecting against cerebral damage, include (1) increased myocardial responsiveness to sympathetic amines, (2) a fall in pulmonary vascular resistance with increased pulmonary blood flow, (3) volume expansion as a function of the hyperosmotic solution, and (4) correction, by the administration of sodium bicarbonate, of the shift in the oxygen dissociation curve to the right with acidosis.

These apparent benefits must be weighed against the risk of an increased incidence of intracranial hemorrhage, which has been associated with rapid volume expansion, particularly in the very low-birth-weight infant.

What are some of the sequelae that may be anticipated after asphyxia?

1. Lungs—respiratory distress syndrome and meconium aspiration.
2. Heart—cardiomegaly, heart failure, and persistent fetal circulation.
3. Kidneys—anuria, hematuria, and proteinuria.
4. Brain—cerebral edema, seizures, cerebral hemorrhage, tremulousness, irritability, and intraventricular hemorrhage, particularly in premature infants, often 48 hours after a severe asphyxial episode.
5. The onset of disseminated intravascular coagulation.
6. Following severe asphyxia with any cellular damage there will be a rise in serum potassium. The serum sodium may be influenced by the renal status as well as the amount of sodium administered in the form of bicarbonate. The blood sugar rises during a period of asphyxia and may be followed by hypoglycemia in infants with poor glycogen stores, particularly very low-birth-weight and SGA neonates.
7. Traumatic purpura—the distribution will depend on the type of delivery; thus, there may be extensive purpura, bruising of the legs after breech delivery, or facial purpura if the umbilical cord was tight around the neck.
8. Edema.
9. Necrotizing enterocolitis.

What prognostic significance does the onset of convulsions at the age of 12 hours have in an asphyxiated infant?

The etiology of the convulsions must be known to give a meaningful answer. A number of infants will have seizures following a severe asphyxial episode as a result of the ensuing cerebral edema. Provided that at the time of discharge from the hospital there are no neurologic deficits detectable, the prognosis for normal development is excellent, irrespective of the symptomatology in the early neonatal period.

Case Two

A repeat cesarean section was performed on a well-controlled white diabetic woman at 38 weeks' gestation. The mother's blood sugar just before delivery was 140 mg/dl. The male infant, B. W., weighed 3900 gm and at 1 minute was found to be hypotonic, making gasping respirations. His pulse rate was 120 per minute, and he was slightly cyanotic. The 1 minute Apgar score was 5. There was some improvement when the airways were cleared and oxygen was administered. The heart rate remained 100 per minute, and the respiratory rate at 5 minutes was 40 per minute. He remained slightly hypotonic and had slightly pale color. At age 15 minutes, respirations were noted to be 60 per minute. He had gasping movements with the use of accessory muscles of respiration, and his mouth opened with each respiration. The rectal temperature was 35° C. He had good air entry, with no cyanosis.

What investigations should be carried out immediately?

Factors predisposing to asphyxia in this case are diabetes and cesarean section. There is no information as to the type of anesthesia used for the cesarean section; the anesthetic may be a contributing factor. The Apgar score is in the 4 to 7 range, so this infant is in no immediate danger. Significantly, his color is poor, and he is using the accessory muscles of respiration with an open mouth, which indicates air hunger. The poor color may reflect poor peripheral circulation or may be genuine pallor due to anemia. Air hunger may be due to airway obstruction, but there is good air entry and no cyanosis at 15 minutes, so this is unlikely; it may be a result of lack of oxygen-carrying capacity. The urgent investigations required, therefore, comprise hematocrit, blood pressure, and blood gases, including pH, P_{O_2}, P_{CO_2}, and bicarbonate. A blood sugar test is not necessarily indicated at this stage, since it is extremely unlikely that hypoglycemia is the cause of the symptomatology. However, estimation of the blood sugar by Dextrostix or bG Chemstrip will be a useful baseline in the further management of the infant. Chest x-ray is also required. In this infant, a diagnosis of anemia and hypotension was established. The hematocrit was 32 per cent, and the blood pressure was 45/25 mm Hg by indirect measurement. (Note: the blood pressure may be falsely high with acidosis. When this is corrected vasodilation occurs, and the pressure can fall precipitously.)

The anemia was partially corrected by the administration of whole blood, 10 to 15 ml/kg at 30 minutes. While the blood was being collected, the circulation was supported with an infusion of 0.9 per cent saline, 10 ml/kg.

It is not uncommon for anemia to occur following cesarean section. Blood loss from the infant may occur if the placenta is incised. In addition, the infant does not get the full placental transfusion, because the normal gravitational effect is lost and the cord is often clamped before the first breath, before the transfusion from placenta to baby. Fetomaternal bleeding is not rare, and the mother's blood should be evaluated for the quantitative presence of fetal red cells to establish the diagnosis. Other features to be searched for in a full-term anemic infant include concealed hemorrhage, such as a ruptured viscus (e.g., liver and/or spleen). (See Chapter 15, Hematologic Problems.)

Is gastric aspiration essential immediately after delivery by cesarean section?

Although it has been established that the gastric contents are greater following cesarean section than vaginal delivery, it is not essential to aspirate the stomach immediately. It is important that the procedure be delayed until normal ventilation has been established; otherwise, apnea, bradycardia, and even cardiac arrest may be induced when an attempt is made to aspirate the stomach.

Case Three

A 2900 gm, 42 weeks' gestation male infant, covered with "pea soup" meconium, is delivered.

How should he be managed?

The initial responsibility for managing this infant belongs to the obstetrician, who should carefully suction the hypopharynx using a DeLee trap immediately after delivery of the head. Following complete delivery of the infant, the larynx is directly visualized with a laryngoscope. If meconium is seen at the level of the larynx or below, then direct endotracheal suctioning is indicated.[12] The suctioning is best performed by covering the tube connector with gauze or directly suctioning by mouth through a face mask as the endotracheal tube is withdrawn. Repeated intubation and suctioning may be necessary to clear the trachea completely. A chest x-ray should be obtained once the child is stable.

Shortly after birth, chest x-ray reveals infiltrates in both lower lung fields consistent with meconium aspiration. At 3 hours of age the infant suddenly deteriorates.

Considering the previous history, what is the most likely diagnosis?

A meconium-stained infant who suddenly deteriorates should immediately raise suspicion of air-leak syndrome (e.g, pneumothorax, a pneumomediastinum, or pneumopericardium). In this situation, aspirated meconium functions as a foreign body creating a ball-valve obstruction that can lead to overdistension and eventual rupture of alveoli.

What clinical findings support the diagnosis of pneumothorax?

The findings would include shift of the apical impulse, liver down 2 cm from the previous examination, hypotension, and asymmetric transillumination of the chest. As air accumulates in the pleural space, tension builds, resulting in a shift of mediastinal structures. In addition, descent of the diaphragm on the affected side would lead to downward displacement of the liver or spleen. Since an air-filled structure transmits light very well, a high intensity fiberoptic light may be used to demonstrate asymmetric transillumination of the chest when a pneumothorax is present. This is most effective in the low-birth-weight infant with less body fat and a thinner chest wall. (X-ray shows left pneumothorax.)

Case Four

A 780 gm female infant is delivered vaginally after the spontaneous onset of labor at 26 weeks' gestation, 12 hours following premature rupture of the amniotic sac and subsequent leaking of amniotic fluid. You had been notified of this high-risk delivery in advance and are present with an associate, all of the necessary equipment is ready for use. Spontaneous respiratory efforts are noted at completion of the delivery, and you receive this small infant noted to have extensive facial bruising, spontaneous irregular respirations, spontaneous but weak movement of extremities, duskiness, and a heart rate of 150 beats per minute.

What is your initial assessment and management?

The prompt onset of spontaneous respirations and movement along with a normal heart rate suggests that severe asphyxia is not present; relatively poor tone and absence of a grimace response may reflect immaturity more than underlying pathology. On the other hand, facial bruising is of some concern here, since delivery probably occurred through an incompletely dilated cervix with greater possibility of injury to fragile intracranial contents. In addition the risks associated with hyperbilirubinemia may be heightened.

Immediate attention is directed toward maintaining body temperature utilizing a radiant heat source and gently drying the skin. Because of a lack of subcutaneous tissue and relatively greater surface area to body weight when compared with a term infant, this baby is at great risk for hypothermia. The airway is briefly suctioned with a DeLee mucus trap. Since respirations are irregular and the infant is dusky, prompt endotracheal intubation is indicated, and bag to tube ventilation is initiated utilizing an oxygen-enriched gas mixture until CPAP or positive-pressure ventilation (if needed) can be initiated. With this intervention the Apgar score at the end of 2 minutes was 5. If regular respirations, pink color, and more vigorous movement had been present in the first minute of life, then endotracheal intubation would probably not be needed, although prompt use of nasal CPAP would be appropriate.

What information would you need as promptly as possible to manage this infant further?

Since mild to moderate asphyxia is present based on the Apgar score and an oxygen-enriched environment has been provided, blood gas and pH determinations are needed on blood preferably obtained from a promptly placed umbilical artery catheter (see Appendix I–2). Hyperoxia in the very low-birth-weight infant at risk for retrolental fibroplasia should be avoided; inspired oxygen concentration can be reduced initially based on clinical response, followed as promptly as possible by laboratory confirmation aimed at maintaining arterial Po_2 between 50 and 80 torr. Since very low-birth-weight infants are frequently hypotensive, blood pressure determination should be made—directly, utilizing the umbilical artery catheter and pressure transducer, or indirectly, by oscillometric or Doppler methods. Serial microhematocrit and glucose (bG Chemstrip or Dextrostix) determinations are initiated. With the insertion of the umbilical catheter, an intravenous infusion of glucose in water at a rate of 5 mg/kg/dl is begun.

The initial laboratory values (at 20 minutes of age) show a blood pH of 7.23, Pco_2 of 42 mm Hg, Po_2 of 70 mm Hg with Fi_{o_2} of 0.45, base deficit (BD) of 11.5, microhematocrit of 48 per cent, and glucose by bG Chemstrip of over 40 mg/dl. Blood pressure by transducer was 28/18 mm Hg.

How do you interpret these data?

The most important finding is the low blood pressure along with a borderline hematocrit value. In addition the acidosis, mostly metabolic, might be aggravated in the presence of poor peripheral perfusion. Volume expansion may improve all of these parameters, and fresh whole blood would be preferred; plasma and packed cells would be an alternative. Close monitoring should be done to avoid producing hypervolemia and hypertension and thereby increasing the risk for intracerebral hemorrhage.

At 2 days of age a cerebral ultrasound reveals periventricular hemorrhage on the right side without extension into the ventricle (grade I). The infant has periodic apneic episodes that are abolished by minimal ventilator support. (IMV = 5, PIP = 18 cm H_2O, CPAP = 3 cm H_2O, and Fi_{o_2} = 0.25.)

What is this infant's prognosis?

The short-term prognosis will depend on whether intercurrent life-threatening complications develop, including respiratory distress syndrome, pneumothorax, sepsis, feeding intolerance and nutritional problems, necrotizing enterocolitis, extensive bilateral intraventricular hemorrhage, etc. The long-term prognosis depends on the successful resolution of many problems associated with very low-birth-weight infants (see subsequent chapters). For the baby presented here, if there is no further extension of the intracerebral bleeding, then the prognosis would generally be good, and normal growth and development could be anticipated.[65]

REFERENCES

1. Adamsons, K., Jr.: Brain damage in the fetus and newborn from hypoxia or asphyxia. *In* James, L., Myers, R., and Gaull, G. (eds.): *Report of the 57th Ross Conference on Pediatric Research.* Columbus, Ohio, Ross Laboratories, 1967, p. 75.
2. Adamsons, K., Jr., Behrman, R., Dawes, G., et al: The treatment of acidosis with alkali and glucose during asphyxia in foetal rhesus monkeys. J Physiol *169*:679, 1963.
3. Adamsons, K., Jr., Behrman, R., Dawes, G., et al: Resuscitation by positive pressure ventilation and tris-hydroxy-methyl-aminomethane of rhesus monkeys asphyxiated at birth. J Pediatr *65*:807, 1964.
4. Apgar, V.: A proposal for a new method of evaluation of the newborn infant. Anesth Analg *32*:260, 1953.
5. Avery, M., and O'Doherty, N.: Effects of bodytilting on the resting and end-respiratory position of newborn infants. Pediatrics *29*:255, 1962.
6. Becker, R.: Learning ability after asphyxiation at birth, especially as it concerns the guinea pig. *In* Windle, W., Hinman, E., and Bailey, P. (eds.): *Neurological and Psychological Deficits of Asphyxia Neonato-*

rum. Springfield, Ill., Charles C Thomas, 1958, p. 44.
7. Behrman, R., Lees, M., Peterson, E., et al: Distribution of the circulation in the normal and asphyxiated fetal primate. Am J Obstet Gynecol *108*:956, 1970.
8. Bloxsom, A.: Resuscitation of the newborn infant. J Pediatr *37*:311, 1950.
9. Boon, A., Milner, A., and Hopkin, I.: Lung expansion, tidal volume and formation of the functional residual capacity during resuscitation of asphyxiated neonates. J Pediatr *95*:1031, 1979.
10. Brann, A., and Myers, R.: Central nervous system findings in the newborn monkey following severe in utero partial asphyxia. Neurology *25*:327, 1975.
11. Campbell, A., Cross, K., Dawes, G., et al: A comparison of air and O_2 in a hyperbaric chamber or by positive pressure ventilation, in the resuscitation of newborn rabbits. J Pediatr *68*:153, 1966.
12. Carson, B., Losey, R., Bowes, W., et al: Combined obstetric and pediatric approach to prevent meconium aspiration syndrome. Am J Obstet Gynecol *126*:712, 1976.

13. Clark, J., Brown, Z., and Jung, A.: Resuscitation equipment board for nurseries and delivery rooms. JAMA 236:2427, 1976.
14. Cordero, L., Jr., and Hon, E.: Neonatal bradycardia following nasopharyngeal stimulation. J Pediatr 78:441, 1971.
15. Cross, K., and Roberts, P.: Asphyxia neonatorum treated by electrical stimulation of the phrenic nerve. Br Med J 1:1043, 1951.
16. Dahm, L., and James, L.: Newborn temperature and calculated heat loss in the delivery room. Pediatrics 49:504, 1972.
17. Daily, W., and Northway, W., Jr.: Perspectives in mechanical ventilation of the newborn. Adv Pediatr 18:253, 1971.
18. Daniel, P., Love, E., Moorehouse, L., et al: Factors influencing utilization of ketone-bodies by brain in normal rats and rats with keto acidosis. Lancet 2:637, 1971.
19. Daniel, S., Dawes, G., James, L., et al: Analeptics and the resuscitation of asphyxiated monkeys. Br Med J 2:562, 1966.
20. Daniel, S., Dawes, G., James, L., et al: Hypothermia and the resuscitation of asphyxiated monkeys. J Pediatr 68:45, 1966.
21. Dawes, G.: Foetal and Neonatal Physiology. Chicago, Year Book Medical Publishers, 1968.
22. Dawes, G., Hibbard, E., and Windle, W.: The effect of alkali and glucose infusion on permanent brain damage in rhesus monkeys asphyxiated at birth. J Pediatr 65:801, 1964.
23. Delpy, D., Gordon, R., Hope, P., et al: Noninvasive investigation of cerebral ischemia by phosphorus nuclear magnetic resonance. Pediatrics 70:310, 1982.
24. Donn, S., Roloff, D., and Goldstein, G.: Prevention of intraventricular hemorrhage in preterm infants by phenobarbitone: a controlled trial. Lancet 2:215, 1981.
25. Drage, J., and Berendes, H.: Apgar scores and outcome of the newborn. Pediatr Clin North Am 13:635, 1966.
26. Drew, J.: Immediate intubation at birth of the very-low-birth-weight infant. Am J Dis Child 136:207, 1982.
27. Elam, J.: The intrapulmonary route for CPR drugs. In Safar, P., and Elam, J. (eds.): Advances in Cardiopulmonary Resuscitation. New York, Springer-Verlag, 1977, p. 132.
28. Eve, F.: Artificial circulation produced by rocking. Br Med J 2:295, 1947.
29. Finer, N., Robertson, C., Richards, R., et al: Hypoxic-ischemic encephalopathy in term neonates: perinatal factors and outcome. J Pediatr 98:112, 1981.
30. Fisher, D. E., Paton, J. B., and Behrman, R. E.: The effect of phenobarbital on asphyxia in the newborn monkey. Pediatr Res 9:181, 1975.
31. Flagg, P.: Treatment of asphyxia in the newborn. JAMA 91:788, 1928.
32. Gardiner, R.: The effects of hypoglycemia on cerebral blood flow and metabolism in the newborn calf. J Physiol 298:37, 1980.
33. Goddard, J., Lewis, R., Armstrong, D., et al: Moderate rapidly induced hypertension as a cause of intraventricular hemorrhage in the newborn beagle model. J Pediatr 96:1057, 1980.
34. Goldberg, R., Chung, D., Goldman, S., et al: The association of rapid volume expansion and intraventricular hemorrhage in the preterm infant. J Pediatr 96:1060, 1980.

35. Greenberg, M., Roberts, J., Baskin, S., et al: The use of endotracheal medication for cardiac arrest. Topics Emerg Med 1:29, 1979.
36. Greenberg, M., Roberts, J., and Baskin, S.: Use of endotracheally administered epinephrine in a pediatric patient. Am J Dis Child 135:767, 1981.
37. Gregory, G., Gooding, C., Phibbs, R., et al: Meconium aspiration in infants—a prospective study. J Pediatr 85:848, 1974.
38. Hawkins, R., Williamson, D., and Krebs, H.: Ketone-body utilization by adult and suckling rat brain in vivo. Biochem J 122:13, 1971.
39. Hellmann, J., Vannucci, R., and Nardis, E.: Blood-brain barrier permeability to lactic acid in the newborn dog: lactate as a cerebral metabolic fuel. Pediatr Res 16:40, 1982.
40. Hope, P., Stewart, A., Thorburn, R., et al: Failure of phenobarbitone to prevent intraventricular hemorrhage in small preterm infants. Lancet 1:444, 1982.
41. Huch, A., Huch, R., and Gosta, R.: Monitoring the intravascular pO$_2$ in newborn infants. J Perinat Med 1:53, 1973.
42. James, L.: Biochemical aspects of asphyxia at birth in adaptation to extrauterine life. Report of the 31st Ross Conference on Pediatric Research. Columbus, Ohio, Ross Laboratories, 1959, p. 66.
43. James, L.: Onset of breathing and resuscitation. J Pediatr 65:807, 1964.
44. James, L., Apgar, V., Burnard, E., et al: Intragastric oxygen and resuscitation of the newborn. Acta Paediatr Scand 52:245, 1963.
45. Jilek, L., Travnickova, E., and Projan, S.: Characteristic metabolic and functional responses to oxygen deficiency in the central nervous system. In Stave, U. (Ed.): Physiology of the Perinatal Period. New York, Appleton-Century-Crofts, 1970.
46. Johnson, G., Kirschbaum, T., Brinkman, C., III, et al: Effects of acid base and hypertonicity on fetal and neonatal cardiovascular hemodynamics. Am J Physiol 220:1798, 1971.
47. Karlberg, P., Cherry, R., Escardo, F., et al: Pulmonary ventilation and mechanics of breathing in the first minutes of life, including the onset of respiration. Acta Paediatr Scand 51:121, 1962.
48. Kreiselman, J.: An improved apparatus for treating asphyxia of the newborn infant. Am J Obstet Gynecol 39:888, 1940.
49. Kreiselman, J., Kane, H., and Swope, R.: A new apparatus for resuscitation of asphyxiated newborn babies. Am J Obstet Gynecol 15:552, 1928.
50. Larroche, J.: Developmental Pathology of the Neonate. Amsterdam, Excerpta Medica, 1977.
51. Levitsky, L., Fisher, D., Paton, J., et al: Fasting plasma levels of glucose, acetoacetate, D-β-hydroxybutyrate, glycerol, and lactate in the baboon infant: correlation with cerebral uptake of substrates and oxygen. Pediatr Res 11:298, 1977.
52. Lou, H., Lassen, N., and Friis-Hansen, B.: Impaired autoregulation of cerebral blood flow in the distressed newborn infant. J Pediatr 94:118, 1979.
53. MacDonald, H., Mulligan, J., Allen, A., et al: Neonatal asphyxia. I. Relationship of obstetric and neonatal complications to neonatal mortality in 38,405 consecutive deliveries. J Pediatr 96:898, 1980.
54. Merenstein, G., and Blackmon, L.: Care of the High Risk Newborn. San Francisco, Children's Hospital, 1971.
55. Millen, R., Rowson, A., and Mayberger, H.: Prevention of neonatal asphyxia with the use of a rocking respirator. Am J Obstet Gynecol 70:1087, 1955.

56. Miller, J.: New approaches to preventing brain damage during asphyxia. Am J Obstet Gynecol 110:1125, 1971.
57. Milligan, D.: Failure of autoregulation and intraventricular hemorrhage in preterm infants. Lancet 1:896, 1980.
58. Milner, A., and Vyas, H.: Lung expansion at birth. J Pediatr 101:879, 1982.
59. Morgan, M., Benson, J., and Cooke, R.: Ethamsylate reduces the incidence of periventricular haemorrhage in very low birth-weight babies. Lancet 2:830, 1981.
60. Morgan, M., Massey, R., and Cooke, R.: Does phenobarbitone prevent periventricular hemorrhage in very low-birth-weight babies? A controlled trial. Pediatrics 70:186, 1982.
61. Moya, F., James, L., Burnard, E., et al: Cardiac massage in the newborn infant through the intact chest. Am J Obstet Gynecol 84:798, 1962.
62. Mulligan, J., Painter, M., O'Donoghue, P., et al: Neonatal asphyxia. II. Neonatal mortality and long-term sequelae. J Pediatr 96:903, 1980.
63. Nelson, K., and Ellenberg, J.: Neonatal signs as predictors of cerebral palsy. Pediatrics 64:225, 1979.
64. Pape, K., and Wigglesworth, J.: *Haemorrhage, Ischemia and the Perinatal Brain.* Clinics in Developmental Medicine, Nos. 69/70. London, S.I.M.P. with Heinemann; Philadelphia, Lippincott, 1979.
65. Papile, L. A., Burstein, J., Burstein, R., et al: Incidence and evolution of subependymal and intraventricular hemorrhage: a study of infants with birth weights less than 1500 gm. J Pediatr 92:529, 1978.
66. Power, G., Bennett, T., and Longo, L.: Survival in the fetal rabbit exposed to intermittent hypoxia. Am J Obstet Gynecol 127:428, 1977.
67. Raju, T., Vidyasagar, D., and Papazafiratou, C.: Cerebral perfusion pressure and abnormal intracranial pressure wave forms: their relation to outcome in birth asphyxia. Crit Care Med 9:449, 1981.
68. Ranck, J., Jr., and Windle, W.: Brain damage in the monkey, Macaca mulatta, by asphyxia neonatorum. Exp Neurol 1:130, 1959.
69. Richter, D.: Brain damage in the fetus and newborn from hypoxia or asphyxia. *In* James, L., Myers, R., and Gaull, G. (Eds.): *Report of the 57th Ross Conference on Pediatric Research.* Columbus, Ohio, Ross Laboratories, 1967, p. 56.
70. Roberts, J., Greenberg, M., and Baskin, S.: Endotracheal epinephrine in cardiorespiratory collapse. JACEP 8:515, 1979.
71. Roberts, J., Greenberg, M., Knaub, M., et al: Blood levels following intravenous and endotracheal epinephrine administration. JACEP 8:53, 1979.
72. Scholander, P.: The master switch of life. Sci Am 209:92, 1963.
73. Shambaugh, G., Mrozak, S., and Freinkel, N.: Fetal fuels. I. Utilization of ketones by isolated tissues at various stages of maturation and maternal nutrition during late gestation. Metabolism 26:623, 1977.
74. Silverboard, G., Horder, M., Ahmann, P., et al: Reliability of ultrasound in diagnosis of intracerebral hemorrhage and posthemorrhagic hydrocephalus: comparison with computerized tomography. Pediatrics 66:507, 1980.
75. Sloviter, H., Shimkin, P., and Suhara, K.: Glycerol as a substrate for brain metabolism. Nature 210:1334, 1966.
76. Sola, A., and Gregory, G.: Colloid osmotic pressure of normal newborns and premature infants. Crit Care Med 9:568, 1981.
77. Special Committee on Infant Mortality of the Medical Society of The County of New York: Resuscitation of newborn infants. Obstet Gynecol 8:336, 1956.
78. Standards and Guidelines for cardiopulmonary resuscitation (CPR) and emergency cardiac care (ECC). V. Advanced cardiac life support for neonates. JAMA 244:453, 1980.
79. Stave, U., and Wolf, H.: Metabolic effects in hypoxia neonatorum. *In* Stave, U. (Ed.): Physiology of the Perinatal Period. New York, Appleton-Century-Crofts, 1970.
80. Steiner, H., and Neligan, G.: Perinatal cardiac arrest. Arch Dis Child 50:696, 1975.
81. Stewart, A., Reynolds, E., and Lipscomb, A.: Outcome for infants of very low birth weight: survey of world literature. Lancet 1:1038, 1981.
82. Svenningsen, N., Blennow, G., Lindroth, M., et al: Brain-orientated intensive care treatment in severe neonatal asphyxia. Effects of phenobarbitone protection. Arch Dis Child 57:176, 1982.
83. Thomson, A., Searle, M., and Russell, G.: Quality of survival after severe birth asphyxia. Arch Dis Child 52:620, 1977.
84. Ting, P., and Brady, J.: Tracheal suction in meconium aspiration. Am J Obstet Gynecol: 122:767, 1975.
85. Todres, I., and Rogers, M.: Methods of external cardiac massage in the newborn infant. J Pediatr 86:781, 1975.
86. Vannucci, R., Nardis, E., Vannucci, S., et al: Tolerance of the perinatal brain to graded hypoxemia. Neurology 30:443, 1980.
87. Wu, P.: Colloid oncotic pressure: current status and clinical applications in neonatal medicine. Clin Perinatol 9:645, 1982.

3

Anticipation, Recognition, and Transitional Care of the High-Risk Infant

ARNOLD J. RUDOLPH
JOSEPH A. GARCIA-PRATS

Appraisal of the newborn infant, just as of older children, requires a knowledge of the history of the infant. It must be remembered that he *does* have a past history, for he is not really "new" but only newly born. One cannot stress sufficiently the importance of this past history (that is, the maternal history prior to conception and throughout the pregnancy, the course of labor and delivery, and any signs of fetal distress), because the infant will, on examination, reflect the sum total of his genetic and environmental past and the minor or major insults to which he has been subjected.

Normal development of the fetus is threatened by a myriad of factors, both singly and in combination. Maternal complications (obstetric factors) play a threatening role, but of greater importance are the environmental factors (unfavorable social conditions, nutritional deficits, etc.). An interaction between many of these factors occurs and adversely affects the perinatal mortality rate and the quality of survivors. Such factors have resulted in the identification of high-risk pregnancies and high-risk infants.[2, 18, 19, 22]

A *high-risk pregnancy* is one in which the fetus has a significantly increased chance of dying, either before or after birth, or of being disabled. Some fetuses may be damaged early, others late; many infants will be born prematurely or will be unusually small for their gestational age. A few will be too large or will have remained in utero too long. Each situation has its special hazards. The high-risk infant is thus one, regardless of gestational age or birth weight, whose extrauterine existence is compromised by a number of factors (prenatal, natal, or postnatal) and who is in need of special medical care.

ANTICIPATION AND RECOGNITION OF HIGH-RISK FACTORS

The list of medical and obstetric problems of pregnancy, labor, and delivery known to affect the infant and of problems in the infant per se making him at high risk is lengthy (see Chapter 1).

A patient may make her first prenatal visit soon after she misses a period. It is becoming increasingly apparent, however, that by the time pregnancy is confirmed the fetus has already passed the most critical period in its development. If anything is to be done to influence the events in the pre- or periconceptional period—probably the most dangerous time in any individual's lifetime—it must be done before rather than after a woman thinks she is pregnant. Under these circumstances, it becomes advisable to have patients see their doctor before they expect to start a pregnancy.

Preconceptional Visit

The physician has an excellent opportunity in a preconceptional visit for discussion and for counseling the aspiring parents. The mother has certain intrinsic attributes, such as age, stature, nutritional status, immunologic make-up (Rh and ABO factors), and past obstetric history. These usually are unchangeable and may to some extent be influenced by the extrinsic features of her socioeconomic level. The interaction of all of these factors has a definite influence on the course of pregnancy, labor, and delivery. The father should also be interviewed.

Past illnesses can be discussed, and the physician can become aware of unfavorable factors in the family history, such as diabetes or congenital abnormalities. Occasionally, abnormalities that could influence the course of a pregnancy will make further investigation desirable. It is usually better to carry out such investigations before rather than after conception has taken place. The physician should check both mother and father for immunizations and previous illnesses, such as rubella and syphilis.

The prospective mother should be given advice about the importance of an adequate diet and the effects of smoking (pregnant women who smoke give birth to smaller babies) and alcohol consumption (fetal alcohol syndrome). There are no conclusive reports on the effect of chronic malnutrition in the mother as a single factor on the fetus, but it is known that malnutrition in the fetus does have an effect on tissue replication and growth, especially that of brain tissue. Furthermore, adequate folate intake significantly decreases the incidence of neural tube defects.

The hazardous effects on the fetus of medicines that the mother might take should be discussed. All drugs may be teratogenic, and there seems to be no satisfactory way of determining which ones are safe; therefore obstetricians have retreated into a position approaching therapeutic nihilism. Such a policy may indeed be a wise one, since in several reported studies the average woman takes between four and ten different drugs during pregnancy, with the consequence that now the fetus is potentially at greater risk from medications taken with good intentions than from the vicissitudes of pregnancy and delivery.[23]

The noxious effects of therapeutic drugs taken during pregnancy range from fetal death to various types of malformations involving different organ systems with varying degrees of severity (Table 3–1). Many of these drugs may influence profoundly the developmental processes in the fetus.[1, 5, 7, 9, 10, 23–25, 27, 30]

The newborn infant's response to drugs may not only be a quantitative difference but also a profound qualitative difference. These differences are even more striking when one considers the developing embryo. During the first weeks of embryonic development, characterized by a period of rapid cell division and differentiation of organ systems, drugs such as thalidomide, aminopterin, and others may result in complete disruption of the embryo or a nonlethal aberration producing a congenital defect. These agents may be relatively benign in their effects on the older fetus. The variability in response of the fetus to maternal drug exposure during pregnancy can be explained by the dosage of the drug, gestational age of the fetus, timing of the exposure, organ system predilection of the drug, and species differences in response to specific drugs.

Other factors to be considered in the effects of maternal medication on the fetus and newborn are the *distribution, metabolism, and excretion of the drug*. Permeability of the blood-brain barrier to pharmacologic agents is generally greater in the neonate than in the adult. For example, the neonate has an increased sensitivity to morphine, which readily traverses the immature blood-brain barrier and attains concentrations three to four times greater than those in adults given comparable doses. Barbiturates penetrate the unmyelinated white matter of the neonatal brain more rapidly than they penetrate the gray matter and produce much longer sleeping times in newly born than in adult animals given equal doses per unit of body weight.

At birth, there is significant limitation of the activity of drug-metabolizing enzymes (located primarily in the liver), which convert drugs into products that are generally less active or toxic than the parent compounds. Studies have also shown impaired capacity in infants for conjugation of chloramphenicol, acetylation of sulfonamides, and other effects. Excretion regulates the actual removal

Text continued on page 56

TABLE 3–1 POSSIBLE EFFECTS OF MATERNAL MEDICATION ON THE FETUS OR NEWBORN*

Name of Drug	Effect on the Fetus or Newborn
Inhalation anesthetics (Cross placenta rapidly; neonatal depression directly related to depth and duration of anesthesia):	
Ether	Depresses infant by direct narcotic effect
Cyclopropane	
Nitrous oxide	No significant depression if oxygen concentration administered to mother is adequate (20% or more)
Trichloroethylene (Trilene)	No significant depression unless mother deeply anesthetized
Methoxyflurane (Penthrane)	
Halothane (Fluothane)	No significant depression if drug given to mother for short duration; danger of maternal hypotension with possible fetal hypoxia
Local anesthetics:	
Lidocaine (Xylocaine)	Indirect effect of maternal hypotension with possible fetal hypoxia
Mepivacaine (Carbocaine)	
Procaine (Novocain)	Direct injection into fetus produces intoxication
Tetracaine (Pontocaine)	
Narcotics (Dose and time interval between administration and delivery important in neonatal depression):	
Morphine	Depression of fetal respirations, bradycardia, hypothermia; decreased responsiveness of newborn
Meperidine (Demerol)	
Heroin	Babies born to narcotics addicts develop withdrawal symptoms of hyperirritability, shrill cry, vomiting; can be fatal
Methadone (Dolophine)	
Alphaprodine (Nisentil)	
Levorphanol (Levo-Dromoran)	
Dihydrocodeine	
Narcotic antagonists:	May in themselves have respiratory depressant action
Nalorphine (Nalline)	
Levallorphine (Lorfan)	
Naloxone (Narcan)	No evidence of effects on the fetus or neonate
Sedatives:	
Barbiturates†	
Phenobarbital	All barbiturates and thiobarbiturates cross the placenta; in usual clinical doses they cause minimal fetal depression
Amobarbital (Amytal)	
Secobarbital (Seconal)	Larger doses cause apnea, depression, depressed EEG
Pentobarbital (Nembutal)	Neonatal bleeding
Thiopental (Pentothal sodium)	Increase rate of fetal or neonatal drug metabolism/withdrawal symptoms
Thiamylal (Surital)	Decreased responsiveness and poor sucking ability in early neonatal period
Chloral hydrate	Incomplete evidence of effects on fetus or neonate
Ethchlorvynol (Placidyl)	Withdrawal reported
Paraldehyde	If given in large doses to mother, may cause respiratory depression or drowsiness of infant
Thalidomide	Congenital anomalies, especially extremity anomalies (phocomelia)
Ethyl alcohol	May decrease uterine contractions
	Babies born to chronic alcoholic mothers may have fetal alcohol syndrome and/or withdrawal symptoms of twitching, hyperirritability, sweating, and fever
	Neonatal depression can occur
*Tranquilizers:**	
Chlorpromazine (Thorazine)	No appreciable depressant action on fetus or neonate
Promethazine (Phenergan)	All tranquilizers may cause alterations of postnatal clinical behavior (withdrawal syndrome); these appear during neonatal period and during early infancy and last for months; extrapyramidal signs sometimes noted
Prochlorperazine (Compazine)	
Hydroxyzine (Atarax, Vistaril)	
Meprobamate (Equanil, Miltown)	
Benzodiazepines (Librium, Valium)	May produce loss of beat-to-beat variation in fetal heart rate pattern
Reserpine	Nasal congestion with respiratory distress, excessive secretions, lethargy, decreased activity, bradycardia, hypothermia

Table continued on following page

TABLE 3–1 POSSIBLE EFFECTS OF MATERNAL MEDICATION ON THE FETUS OR NEWBORN* *Continued*

Name of Drug	Effect on the Fetus or Newborn
Skeletal muscle relaxants (Neuromuscular blocking agents):	
Curare	In usual clinical doses, these drugs do not cross placenta in amounts
Gallamine thiethiodide (Flaxedil)	that cause any noticeable effect on fetus
Succinylcholine chloride (Anectine)	
Decamethonium iodide (Syncurine)	
Pancuronium bromide (Pavulon)	
Steroids:	
Cortisone	Possible relation to cleft palate in animals only
Hydrocortisone	
Prednisone	Mild growth retardation
Prednisolone	
Dexamethasone (Decadron)	Placental insufficiency syndrome, fetal distress during labor—not fully substantiated; leukopenia and leucocytosis
Progestin	Masculinization of female fetus (nonadrenal pseudohermaphroditism of
Testosterone	the female)
Diethylstilbestrol	Adenocarcinoma of lower genital tract reported in female offspring years later (14–25 years)
Thyroid compounds:	
Desiccated thyroid extract	Crosses the placenta slowly but not known whether untoward effect
Triiodothyronine (Cytomel)	occurs in fetus
Antithyroid drugs:	
Propylthiouracil	All antithyroid drugs cross the placenta and can result in fetal goiters
Methimazole (Tapazole)	and hypothyroidism
Potassium iodide	Iodine compounds in excessive amounts (for control of asthma, expectorants) cause fetal nontoxic goiter
I^{131}	When administered to the pregnant woman, even in the first trimester of pregnancy, may be disastrous for the fetus (athyrotic cretin)
Antidiabetic drugs:	
Insulin	No proven untoward effect
Chlorpropamide (Diabinese)	Respiratory distress and neonatal hypoglycemia; teratogenic effects suggested but not proved
	Treated diabetic mothers have 3 times the incidence of fetal death in utero as compared with diabetic gravidas on insulin and diet alone
Tolbutamide (Orinase)	Teratogenic effects suggested but never proved
Anticoagulants:	
Heparin	No untoward effect
Coumarins (Warfarin, Dicumarol)	Risk of fetal hemorrhage and death in utero; hemorrhagic manifestations in newborn; mental retardation, deafness, optic atrophy reported with second trimester use
	Fetal Warfarin syndrome (hypoplastic nasal cartilage, stippled epiphyses)
Anticonvulsant drugs:	
Hydantoin (Dilantin)	Fetal hydantoin syndrome (digit and nail anomalies, unusual facies; growth and mental deficiency)
	Neonatal hemorrhage, ↓ clotting factors
Antihistamines and antiemetics:	
Dimenhydrinate (Dramamine)	No evidence of adverse effect in human beings
Cyclizine (Marezine)	
Meclizine (Bonine)	
	Reports of multiple congenital malformation (gastroschisis, limb malformations, spinal deformities) in infants of mothers on dicyclomine hydrochloride and doxylamine succinate (Debendex)
Antimicrobial agents:	
Cephalothin (Keflin)	No untoward effect demonstrated
Chloramphenicol (Chloromycetin)	"Gray syndrome" (gastrointestinal irritability, circulatory collapse, death) in newborns treated with this drug (never proved to occur in newborn if drug given only to mother)

Table continued on opposite page

TABLE 3–1 POSSIBLE EFFECTS OF MATERNAL MEDICATION ON THE FETUS OR NEWBORN* *Continued*

Name of Drug	Effect on the Fetus or Newborn
Erythromycin	No untoward effects demonstrated
Kanamycin	Ototoxicity suspected but never proved in infants born to mothers treated for prolonged periods
Novobiocin	Increase in hyperbilirubinemia if newborn treated, but not proved to occur if drug given only to mother
Penicillin	No untoward effect
Ampicillin	No untoward effect
Streptomycin	Hearing loss (very rare) in infants whose mothers have been treated for prolonged periods in early pregnancy
Tetracycline (Achromycin) Chlortetracycline (Aureomycin) Oxytetracycline (Terramycin) Demethylchlortetracycline (Declomycin)	Staining of deciduous teeth; inconclusive association with congenital cataracts; potential for bone growth retardation but not proved to occur in utero
Sulfonamides: Short-acting Sulfadiazine Sulfisoxazole (Gantrisin)	Fetal and maternal levels equilibrate in 2 to 3 hours; competes with bilirubin for binding sites on albumin
Long-acting Sulfamethoxypyridazine (Kynex)	Present in fetal blood in 2 hours; newborn serum levels present for 5–6 days
Sulfadimethoxine (Madribon)	Sulfonamides compete with bilirubin for binding sites on albumin, but no untoward effect on newborn proved if only mother received drug
Metronidazole (Flagyl)	No untoward effect
Griseofulvin	No untoward effect
Isoniazid (INH)	Unconfirmed, retrospective, circumstantial evidence of psychomotor retardation
Quinine, quinidine	Early reports of ototoxicity and congenital malformations unsubstantiated by extensive experience of many authors; danger of fetal damage probably minimal; thrombocytopenia has been reported
Nitrofurantoin (Furadantin)	Megaloblastic anemia in fetus with glucose-6-phosphate dehydrogenase deficiency
Cancer chemotherapeutic agents: Aminopterin Amethopterin (Methotrexate)	Fetal death and multiple malformations; congenital anomalies
Miscellaneous: Hexamethonium	Paralytic ileus
Ammonium chloride	Acidosis
Thiazides	Neonatal thrombocytopenia
Salicylates (Aspirin)	No untoward effect in usual amounts Death in utero; hemorrhagic manifestations in newborn; congenital salicylate poisoning reported in mother who took overdose
Indomethacin (Indocin)	Prostaglandin synthetase inhibitor; may affect developing cardiopulmonary system of the fetus (constriction of ductus arteriosus and pulmonary arterioles)
Propranolol (Inderal)	Hypoglycemia and postnatal bradycardia; placental transfer of unchanged drug; side effects in fetus include blockade of reflex tachycardia and of hypoxia-induced hypertension; delayed onset of respiration at delivery; in neonate, respiratory depression at birth
Vitamin K and analogues: Menadione sodium bisulfite (Hykinone) Phytonadione (AquaMEPHYTON)	Hyperbilirubinemia, kernicterus
Vitamin D_2 (irradiated ergosterol)	Large quantities administered to pregnant mother may cause congenital cardiac malformation

Table continued on following page

TABLE 3–1 POSSIBLE EFFECTS OF MATERNAL MEDICATION ON THE FETUS OR NEWBORN* *Continued*

Name of Drug	Effect on the Fetus or Newborn
Intravenous fluids	Electrolyte imbalance, usually hyponatremia (lethargy, poor muscle tone, poor color)
Smoking	Intrauterine growth retardation
Radiation	Fetal death in utero or congenital anomalies (microcephaly, etc.)
	Actual teratogenic dose of ionizing radiation in humans not yet determined: I rad to fetus may probably be harmless; up to 10 rads may be potentially dangerous; 10 rads or more probably harmful (numerous individuals receiving 2.5 rads had normal infants)
Heavy metals (Environmental pollution):	
Lead	Abortion; growth retardation; congenital anomalies
Mercury	Mental retardation
Hallucinogens:	
Lysergic acid diethylamide (LSD), mescaline, etc.	"Fractured chromosomes" anomalies (?)

*Adaped from Bowes, W., Jr., Brackbill, Y., Conway, E., et al.: The effects of obstetrical medication on fetus and infant. Monogr Soc Res Child Dev, Serial No. 137, Vol. 35, No. 4, June 1970.
†Barbiturates and some tranquilizers may potentiate the effects of inhalation agents and narcotics.

REFERENCES

1. Forfar, J., Nelson, M.: Epidemiology of drugs taken by pregnant women—drugs that may affect the fetus adversely. Clin Pharmacol Ther *14*:632, 1973.
2. Mirkin, B.: Maternal and fetal distribution of drugs in pregnancy. Clin Pharmacol Ther *14*:643, 1973.
3. Chez, R., Fleischman, A.: Fetal therapeutics—challenge and responsibilities. Clin Pharmacol Ther *14*:754, 1973.
4. Eriksson, M., Catz, C., and Yaffe, S.: Drugs and pregnancy. Clin Obstet Gynecol *16*:199, 1973.
5. Anderson, P.: Drugs and breast feeding: a review. Drug Intelligence and Clinical Pharmacy *2*:208, 1977.
6. Briggs, G., Bodendorfer, P. W., Freeman, R. K., et al.: *Drugs in Pregnancy.* Baltimore, William & Wilkins, 1983.
7. Stern, L.: *Drug Use in Pregnancy.* Balgowlah, Australia, ADIS Press, 1984.
8. Kalter, H., and Warkany, J.: Congenital malformation. N Engl J Med *308*:424, 1983.

of an unchanged drug and its metabolites from the body, mainly in urine and feces. Since the glomerular filtration rate of the immature newborn is 30 to 40 per cent of that in the adult, drugs and their metabolites are removed more slowly and can achieve higher tissue levels (see Chapter 14).

This limited excretory function has significant clinical implications. In newborns less than 48 hours of age, tetracycline, streptomycin, kanamycin, chloramphenicol, ampicillin, penicillin, methicillin, gentamicin, colistin, and cephaloridine have extremely long plasma half-lives and may readily accumulate to toxic levels if dosage regimens are not altered. The limited excretory function can also serve as a positive therapeutic function. For example, small doses of penicillin G, the least toxic of the penicillins, can be given every 12 hours to the newborn and will provide drug levels that are effective in combating infection.

The prepregnancy visit provides an opportunity to inquire into the patient's drug usage, regular or sporadic, and to advise discontinuing all but the essential drugs. While much has been written about the teratogenic effects of many drugs, until recently little attention has been paid to fetal hazards from environmental pollution with certain nonessential trace elements, such as mercury and lead. Minamata disease is an example of a condition produced by mercury contamination in which pregnant women who ingest mercury compounds give birth to infants with severe congenital neurologic problems. Another example of environmental pollution is the increased incidence of congenital malformations in the offspring of operating room personnel, probably due to their constant exposure to waste anesthetic gases.

Prenatal Care

During the course of prenatal examination, the first warning signs of fetal danger invariably can be discovered. Complications of pregnancy known to be associated with fetal risk can be identified in prenatal visits. During pregnancy, the mother may suffer from acute medical illnesses (infections, toxemia, drug addiction) and obstetric problems (acute bleeding, premature labor) that may affect the fetus.

Infections known to influence the fetus and newborn are rubella (German measles), syphilis, gonorrhea, toxoplasmosis, cytomegaloviral disease, genital herpes, and others (see Chapter 12).[3, 6, 17, 26]

The chronically ill mother presents other problems. Chronic kidney disease, for example, is associated with vascular insufficiency and hence inadequate uterine arterial blood flow, and the mother may give birth to an infant with intrauterine growth retardation. The mother with congenital heart disease may present similar problems. Maternal diabetes, which subjects the fetus to an abnormal metabolic environment, also creates problems for the fetus.

Fetal factors require consideration. These include the undesirable effects of multiple births, including twin-to-twin (fetofetal) transfusion syndrome and discrepancy in the size of twins, abnormalities in presentation, and cord anomalies.

Lack of prenatal care has been shown to be the single most important factor predisposing to serious illness in low-birth-weight infants during the first 9 months of life. Hence, lack of prenatal care would appear to continue to affect the infant following labor and delivery.

It has been shown that intensive inpatient prenatal care applied to high-risk cases pays good dividends. Efficiently organized prenatal care remains the mainstay of successful reproduction. During the last 15 years it has been supplemented by a more direct approach, in selected cases, to what has come to be known as the *fetomaternal unit,* by which is meant the placenta, the amniotic fluid, and the fetus. The emphasis in medical care of the newborn has been on instituting aggressive action at the birth of the infant. The events preceding the delivery are equally important. In fact, the product delivered—the infant—is probably more influenced by factors present during its in utero development than by those during delivery. The pediatrician, no matter how proficient, can make only limited progress in further reducing perinatal loss unless presented with a healthier infant.

Many techniques have been developed to assess placental and fetal function. Sudden falls in serial urinary estriol levels indicate fetal distress. The use of stress testing and monitoring of the fetal electrocardiogram and amniotic fluid studies for evidence of lung maturity and ultrasound diagnosis have all increased the armamentarium of the obstetrician (see Chapter 1).

TRANSITION

Birth is an obligatory change of environments, and with the dynamic changes occurring during this transition, the signs of disease are frequently difficult to differentiate from the rapidly changing signs that accompany these physiologic adjustments. Every infant, whether sick or well, mature or immature, must successfully complete the transition to extrauterine life at delivery if he is to survive and develop. If neonatal morbidity and mortality are to be decreased, the focus must be on early detection of those infants whose transition is in jeopardy.

Transition to extrauterine life is a complex process. It encompasses, first, *changes in function* of organ systems (onset of respiration, changeover of fetal to neonatal circulation with a change in cardiovascular hemodynamics, alterations of hepatic and renal functions, and clearance of meconium from the bowel). Secondly, there is a *reorganization of metabolic processes* to achieve a new steady state or postnatal homeostasis. For most infants, transition is so smooth as to appear superficially uneventful; for some, transition is delayed or complicated; and for a small percentage of infants, transition is never achieved.

Change is essential for survival once birth takes place and the cord is clamped. The cardiovascular system of the fetus functions completely differently from that of the neonate, but the transition at birth normally is instantaneous.[29] (See Chapter 13.)

Since respiratory movement occurs in utero it is probably incorrect to state that "breathing" begins at birth; however, the birth process stimulates a sequence of events that quickly transforms the fluid-filled lung to an organ for gas exchange. Multiple factors, such as cutaneous stimulation, cold, mild acidosis, and removal from an aquatic medium, are in part responsible for the initiation of vigorous gasping respiration. This is augmented by chemoreceptors in the large airways (Head's paradoxic reflex). Considerable fluid is removed in the first few breaths by the thoracic squeeze, the lymphatics, or the pulmonary blood vessels. This is so effective that after only a few breaths the functional residual capacity is nearly normal. If transition is to occur satisfactorily, adequate stores of surface-active materials must be present to reduce the surface tension created by the establishment of the air-fluid interface on the alveolar surface of the lungs.

Fetal thermal homeostasis is provided entirely by the environment. A 0.5° to 1.0° C gradient between fetus and mother exists to dissipate heat across the placenta. Although the initial cold stress caused by being born soaking wet into a cold environment may help establish adequate ventilation, it is well known that stress from heat and cold diminishes the likelihood of survival. (See Chapter 5.)

Reaction of the Infant to Delivery

As labor progresses, the biochemical milieu undergoes progressive change, and sensory input to the fetus increases (e.g., amniotomy, oxytocic stimulation of labor, forceps application, fundal pressure, varying methods of delivery, hyperventilation, and various agents administered to the mother, such as drugs, anesthetics, and glucose).

The stimuli of labor are reinforced by the avalanche of new stimuli encountered immediately upon emergence of the infant from an intrauterine existence (dark, warm, and watery, where there was minimal sensory stimulation, and respiration and nutrition were provided by the maternal organism) into a new environment in which the medium is air, temperatures are unstable, sensory stimuli are increased and constant, and the physiologic functions of respiration and nutrition must be performed by the infant. The sum of the stimuli causes a massive sympathetic reaction.

These changes are reflected in the changes in fetal and neonatal heart rate at the time of delivery. In vigorous high Apgar score term infants at the end of labor, the fetal heart rate fluctuates around a baseline rate with a rapid return to this baseline after either tachycardia or bradycardia. These wide swings mirror the intensity of the input reaching the fetus at the end of labor and the rapidity of response to these stimuli. Following delivery there is an abrupt increase in heart rate. For a short time oscillations

occur around a higher baseline, then the rate begins to fall irregularly.

In infants with a suboptimal response to delivery and low 1 minute Apgar scores, the heart rates may remain at an extremely low or extremely high level and do not return promptly to baseline levels after the wide oscillations. The inability to return to baseline rate constitutes an autonomic imbalance.

On delivery, if the infant is vigorous and reactive to the experience of being born, a characteristic series of changes in vital signs and clinical appearance takes place. These changes include a first period of reactivity, a relatively unresponsive interval or sleep period, and a second period of reactivity (Figure 3–1).

During the first 15 to 30 minutes after birth (*first period of reactivity*) the normal infant with an Apgar score of 7 to 10 will be very vigorous and highly responsive because of the numerous stimuli he has been subjected to during the labor and delivery process. During the first 60 minutes of life, he spends up to 40 minutes in a quiet, alert state in which he is unusually responsive. This is often the longest period of this state during the first 4 days! In this state, he can turn his head to sound, follow a face, and be taught to mimic (see Chapter 16).

The infant exhibits changes that are at first predominantly sympathetic, including tachycardia (mean peak heart rate of 180 beats per minute occurs at 3 minutes of age), with some lability of the heart rate. An active cry initiates filling and expansion of the lungs. The lung fluid remaining after the "squeeze" coming through the birth canal is rapidly reabsorbed. As a result, rapid and irregular respiration (ranging from 60 to 90 per minute), transient rales, grunting, flaring of alae nasi, and retraction of the chest give evidence of the establishment of pulmonary respiration in the neonate. There is a falling body temperature with increased activity, increased muscle tone, and alerting exploratory behavior. Characteristic reactions and responses with alerting exploratory behavior include nasal flaring or "sniffing" unrelated to respiratory activity; movements of the head from side to side; spontaneous startles and the Moro reflex; grimacing; sucking; chewing and swallowing; pursing and smacking of the lips; tremors of the extremities and mandible; opening and closing of the eyelids; short, rapid, jerky movements of the eyeballs; and outcries and sudden onset and

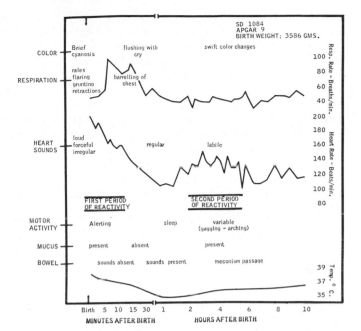

Figure 3–1. A summary of the physical findings in normal transition (the first 10 hours of extrauterine life in a representative high–Apgar-score infant delivered under spinal anesthesia without premedication).[14]

cessation of crying. Bowel sounds become evident as the parasympathetic nervous system activates peristaltic activity in the intestine, and the bowel begins to inflate as the baby swallows air. Saliva production is also increased by parasympathetic stimulation, resulting in increased mucus in the mouth. Brief periods of apnea and sternal retraction are not unusual during this period. This massive reaction dissipates rapidly, and after this first period of reactivity (usually between 10 and 60 minutes of age), heart and respiratory rates decline. The diffuse, apparently purposeless motor activity reaches a peak and then diminishes, and the infant passes into an *unresponsive* or *sleep period.*

With return of tonus to normal and diminished responsiveness, color should be excellent. A fast respiration rate without dyspnea should not be alarming at this time. An increase in the anteroposterior diameter (barrelling) of the chest may be noted accompanying the periods of shallow, rapid respiration. The chest, however, is not fixed in this position; the barrelling disappears promptly with any change in respiratory pattern if the infant is handled or begins to cry spontaneously. It recurs with resumption of rapid, shallow, synchronous breathing. The abdomen should be rounded and bowel sounds audible.

Peristaltic waves beginning in the left upper quadrant of the abdomen and moving from left to right (gastric peristalsis) may

occasionally be visible during periods of quiet activity or sleep. Small amounts of watery mucus may be visible at the lips. General responsiveness declines, and the infant sleeps. Heart rate at this time (average 120 to 140 beats per minute) is relatively unresponsive. During this sleep period spontaneous jerks and twitches are common, but the infant quickly returns to rest.

After this sleep period, the infant enters a *second period of reactivity* (between 2 and 6 hours of age). Responsiveness returns and may become exaggerated. This is not unlike the reactivity of a patient following anesthesia. The infant again exhibits tachycardia, brief periods of rapid respiration, and abrupt changes in tonus, color, and bowel sounds. Oral mucus may again become prominent, and gagging and vomiting are not unusual; the infant becomes more responsive to exogenous and endogenous stimuli, and heart rate becomes labile. The bowel is cleared of meconium. In some infants, the secondary reactivity period results in waves of heightened autonomic activity. Wide swings in heart rate (bradycardia to tachycardia) occur, along with the passage of meconium stools and the clearing of mucus, vasomotor instability, and irregular respiration with apneic pauses. The second period of reactivity may be brief or may last over a period of several hours. As it diminishes, the infant appears to be relatively stable and ready for feeding.

The sequence of clinical behavior just described is common to *all* newborns after birth, regardless of gestational age or route of delivery. The time sequence of changes is altered, however, in infants who are immature or who have demonstrated difficulty in establishing respiration promptly on delivery (low Apgar score infants). The length of time these periods last is also affected by the length and difficulty of labor, the amount of stress to the fetus during labor, maternal medication and anesthesia, and other factors. All the events occurring during labor and delivery need to be carefully monitored and recorded, since they may profoundly influence the immediate as well as the long-term outcome of the newborn.

Complicated Transition[11, 12, 14, 15]

Complicated transition or neonatal morbidity occurs when the process of transition is disturbed by the addition of one or more adverse factors. For example, administration of anesthesia, barbiturates, or narcotics to the mother near or during delivery often causes marked depression of the neonate. Respiratory effort and rate are affected; the infant will be slow to cry initially, and full expansion of the lungs will be inhibited by shallow respirations. It is common for the depressed infant to be floppy immediately after birth, with the poor muscle tone afterward becoming hypertonic in an exaggerated or rebound response. The infant may require occasional ventilatory support with bagging and external stimulation to assist him to ventilate his lungs adequately. In general there is delay of the whole transition period.

The infant born to a diabetic mother may present with additional problems such as hypoglycemia (twitching, jitteriness, weak cry, convulsions, etc.) that interfere with and complicate transition (see Chapter 10).

There are, therefore, many additional factors to be considered when caring for an infant experiencing a delayed or altered period of transition. Although patterns of postnatal events are altered, these events still occur, since every infant must pass through the transition process before truly becoming an extrauterine independent being.

PHYSICAL EXAMINATION OF THE NEWBORN

Serial evaluation of the infant is more valuable than a single examination at any particular age. *Optimum evaluation would include a delivery room examination, a natal day examination, and a more detailed examination after the infant is 24 hours old.* With such serial evaluation, it is possible to determine the infant's progress in making the transition and to detect problems that are interfering with transition. The detailed examination after 24 hours of age provides a good basis for judging the infant's future growth and development.

Editorial Comment: Early discharges (<24 hours after delivery) make multiple examinations difficult. The importance of the initial examination together with careful review of the history is therefore exaggerated.

Delivery Room Examination

The Apgar score, which consists of an evaluation of five factors (heart rate, respiratory effort, muscle tone, responsiveness, and color) at 1 minute after delivery, gives an immediate appraisal of the infant's condition. This "instant physical" assesses the cardiopulmonary and neurologic function. The results are reproducible and significantly related to neonatal mortality. Perhaps the greatest value of the score lies in the clarity of the picture of the infant's clinical condition, which the number representing the total and component score conveys to those accustomed to its use (see Table 2–2).

A second scoring at 5 minutes after delivery gives added information concerning the infant's ability to recover from the stress of birth and to adapt to the extrauterine environment. Statistically, mortality and the clinical course of survivors have been related to both 1 and 5 minute Apgar scores.

In addition to the Apgar score, the infant is checked for cyanosis or pallor (anemia), congenital anomalies, state of maturity, and evidence of neonatal disease.

Following this immediate appraisal or "instant physical" in the delivery room, there has been a supervisory limbo of the infant's first hours when he is "nobody's baby" until seen by the pediatrician. Thus the early detection of problems not apparent in the delivery room frequently becomes the reponsibility of nursery personnel. Our concern at Jefferson Davis Hospital, Houston, about this limbo period instigated the concept of the transitional care nursery.

A thorough understanding of the transition period is necessary in order to identify delays or abnormalities in transition.

Natal Day Examination

Ideally, the examination of a newborn should be gentle, rapid, and sufficiently thorough to obtain the desired information. Since much of the examination is based on observation, the first portion may be performed while the infant is still in the incubator.

Postnatal Day Examination

Examination of the infant performed 24 hours after birth is of great value as a basis for following the infant's growth and development in future years. After 24 hours, the infant has largely recovered from the intense sensory experiences accompanying labor and delivery; thus a complete examination at this time is advantageous. During the first hours postdelivery, excessive handling of the infant, particularly the premature infant, may be followed by clinical deterioration. The infant is still under the influence of maternal anesthesia and analgesia, and body temperature may be low. Reexamination after the infant is 24 hours old may reveal new findings, since many neonatal problems may not be evident during the first day. These include cephalhematoma, bleeding into tissues, fat necrosis, jaundice, apneic episodes, seizures, intestinal obstruction, genitourinary disorders, and other conditions.

Guidelines for the Physical Examination of the Newborn Infant

GENERAL APPEARANCE. General inspection of the infant is the first and most important step in the examination, and this will tell much in a short time.

- Gross anomalies such as anencephaly, omphalocele, and phocomelia are immediately obvious and should be recorded in as much detail as possible.
- State of maturity. If the infant seems mature, no description is required, but if there is evidence of immaturity or malnutrition, this should be described. Assess gestational age (see Chapter 4). In postmature (placental insufficiency) infants, note evidence of acute or chronic weight loss, eye movements, "old man" appearance, dryness of skin, desquamation, long fingernails and toenails, etc.
- State of nutrition—e.g., loss of subcutaneous tissue in postmature infants or plethoric infants.
- Activity. Note whether activity of the infant is excessive or whether it is lethargic.
- Cry. The cry is described—if it is high-pitched or hoarse or if the child is slow to respond by crying when stimulated.
- Color. Presence or absence of cyanosis, jaundice, pallor, and plethora should be noted. Also note evidence of mottling or vasomotor instability, such as harlequin color change.
- Edema should be noted as to location and degree.
- Evidence of respiratory difficulty as manifested by tachypnea, flaring of alae nasi, expiratory grunt, xiphoid and intercostal retraction, etc.
- Posture. The newborn infant tends to retain a posture reflecting his recent intrauterine position. We call this "position of comfort" because attempts to change it produce resistance and often crying. If unusual, it should be described; e.g., posture in breech presentations is usually quite characteristic—the legs are not bowed but straight, and in a frank breech, they are markedly abducted and externally rotated. In face or brow presentations the head is usually extended in a position of opisthotonos, and the neck appears long.
- Measurements. The head and chest circumferences and the length of the infant are measured and recorded. The head at birth should be 2 to 3 cm larger than the chest in the term infant and more than 3 cm larger in the premature infant. If there is any question about hydrocephalus developing, measurements should be repeated at daily intervals. In low-birth-weight infants do head measurements routinely every week. Ultrasound of the head for ventricular size is a noninvasive approach to establish the diagnosis.

SKIN. Note the skin color, consistency and hydration, and any evidence of tumors, injuries, rashes, etc.

- Color.
  (1) Cyanosis. Note whether generalized or localized and whether persistent or variable.
  (2) Pallor—e.g., due to blood loss or hemolysis of red cells.
  (3) Red color—e.g., as seen in infants of diabetic mothers or in polycythemia.
  (4) Jaundice.

(5) Meconium staining of skin, umbilical cord, or nails.

(6) Vasomotor changes—e.g., harlequin color change, cutis marmorata (dappled or marblelike appearance, especially seen in premature infants).

- Vernix caseosa. Note whether present and if discolored; virtually absent after 40 weeks' gestation.
- Consistency and hydration. Dehydration immediately after birth may indicate malnutrition or placental insufficiency.

Generalized edema is common in premature infants and infants of diabetic mothers, especially if the infant has respiratory distress. Localized edema may be noted in a presenting part, e.g., genitalia in a breech delivery.

Generalized hardness of the skin (sclerema) occurs with overcooling of the infant and also occurs in debilitated infants. Isolated scleroderma-like indurated areas (subcutaneous fat necrosis) may occur in the skin, especially at forceps pressure areas, and on the back, buttocks, and pectoral areas. There is overlying erythema.

- Excessive dryness of the skin with desquamation is noted, especially in malnutrition or placental insufficiency.
- Congenital skin anomalies and tumors are common and should be described (including size and location).
  (1) Mongolian spots are almost universally present over the sacrogluteal area in black infants and also occur in about 10 per cent of white infants. In addition to the sacrogluteal area, they may occur over the back and extensor surfaces. They are caused by pigment cells in the deep layers of the skin and become less and less conspicuous as the overlying epidermal pigment becomes more intense.
  (2) Telangiectatic nevi are commonly found at the back of the neck and often over the forehead, the upper eyelids, the wings of the nose, and the upper lip. These tend to become less and less conspicuous with increasing age.
  (3) Vascular nevi, pigmented nevi, lymphangiomata, branchial clefts or cysts, dermal sinuses, etc., should be noted.
- Trauma as a result of delivery or application of forceps should be recorded. Abrasions, petechiae, and ecchymoses are frequently seen. However, petechiae and ecchymoses in the newborn can be caused by sepsis, erythroblastosis fetalis, and blood diseases.
- Rashes are very common and should be described in detail—e.g., milia, heat rash, and erythema toxicum.
- Nails. Note the length of nails (short in premature infants and unusually long in postmature infants). Also note any defects of nails or any staining from meconium.

HEAD. The head, being the usual presenting part, seldom fails to show evidence of molding and some degree of "physiologic" trauma. Note is made of the following.
- Size. Measure head, chest, and abdominal circumference, and note if the head is larger or smaller than expected.
- Molding and shape of head. Immediately after birth, the fontanelles may appear to be very small or entirely closed, and the suture lines will be represented by hard ridges caused by overriding. Within a few days the distortion caused by molding disappears, and one can estimate better the shape of the head, the fontanelles, and the suture lines. Failure of normal expansion may be the earliest sign of microcephaly or craniostenosis.
- Fontanelles and suture lines. Note is made of the shape and size of the fontanelles. A tense fontanelle any time after birth indicates increased intracranial pressure. A depressed fontanelle may be normal or may be early evidence of dehydration in the newborn infant. Describe the sutures' location and size.
- Caput succedaneum is an example of "physiologic" trauma to the area of the head that presents at the cervical os. The position and extent of caput should be noted. It is seen on examination as a soft, ill-defined swelling with pitting edema and a bruised-looking scalp and is not limited by the margins of the cranial bones.
- Cephalhematoma is frequently not present at birth but appears on the first or second day. It is a fluctuant tumor from a subperiosteal hemorrhage and has a well-defined outline confined within the margins of a cranial bone (usually the parietal on one or the other side). It begins to calcify in the first few days of life, and a ridge, giving the impression of a depressed fracture, can be felt at the limits of the tumor.
- Craniotabes is especially noted in the parietal region where, as a result of areas of

thinness in the bone, it gives under pressure like a Ping-Pong ball.

EYES. These are difficult to examine since they are often swollen and edematous as a result of prophylactic use of silver nitrate. If conjunctivitis persists or is thought to be purulent, do a bacteriologic study. Note is made of the following.
- Conjunctival or scleral hemorrhage and edema.
- Size of the eyeball. Exophthalmos is rare but may occur with buphthalmos and congenital glaucoma. Enophthalmos usually is due to Horner's syndrome (ptosis and constricted pupil).
- Cornea and lens. Note any haziness or cloudiness of these.
- Pupil. May be constricted for about 3 weeks or may respond to light at birth by contracting.
- Retina is examined for hemorrhage, etc., and a red reflex is obtained.

EARS. The canals are usually filled with vernix so that the drums may not be visualized at birth, but after a few days they are usually easily visualized.

Abnormalities and/or abnormally positioned ears are noted.

NOSE. Patency of the nasal canals may be tested by closing the infant's mouth and listening to breathing through the nostrils. Also note presence of nasal discharge.

MOUTH. Cleft lip and cleft palate are noted. The gums should be checked carefully for epidermal patches, inclusion cysts, or tooth buds. The palate should be checked for completeness, Epstein's pearls, Bednar's aphthae, and high arching.

Excessive mucus should be noted, and esophageal atresia should be excluded.

NECK. The neck is checked for mobility and masses. It should be flexed to examine the posterior portion and then extended to examine the anterior portion, since many infants' necks are physiologically short at birth in cephalic presentations.
- Mobility. Normal flexion and extension should be obtained. Resistance is rare but may indicate meningeal irritation. Poor mobility also occurs with the Klippel-Feil syndrome.
- Masses. Small cystic masses in the upper part of the sternocleidomastoid may be branchial cleft cysts. A mass in the lower part is usually due to a hematoma and causes a torticollis, but this does not usually become evident for several weeks.

A midline mass may be a thyroglossal duct cyst or a congenital goiter, and a soft mass over the clavicle that transilluminates may be a cystic hygroma. Always palpate the clavicles carefully for evidence of fracture.

THORAX. The following are noted.
- Shape. Normally the chest of the newborn is almost circular, but sometimes there are peculiarities of shape such as flattening of the lateral aspects due to compression by the arms in utero or to the presence of funnel chest or pigeon breast deformities. Occasionally an enlarged heart will cause a bulging of the thorax on the left.
- Breast hypertrophy or abnormality.
- Evidence of respiratory distress.

LUNGS. Note the following.
- Rate and character of respiration.
- Retraction—xyphoid, subcostal, and intercostal.
- Grunting and flaring of the alae nasi.
- Percussion, to be of any value, must be very light, since the chest wall is thin. Make certain that the infant lies so that the head and neck are not turned, because increased or decreased areas of dullness may occur simply because of the position of the infant.
- Auscultation requires patience since breathing may be so shallow that vesicular sounds can scarcely be heard, but if one waits long enough, the infant will take a succession of deep inspirations from which conclusions can be drawn.

Remember that in the first day of life, fine crepitant rales are very often normal.

HEART
- The heart size is percussed and the apical impulse palpated, but heart size is difficult to evaluate clinically (and even radiologically) because of its great variability in the neonatal period.
- Heart rate and rhythm are noted. The heart rate at birth varies from 100–200, but stabilizes shortly after birth at 120–140. The rhythm is usually regular. Any arrhythmia or tachycardia should be considered abnormal. Poor or distant heart sounds occur with pneumothorax, pneu-

momediastinum, pneumopericardium, hypovolemia, and cardiac failure.
- Murmurs should be described as to loudness, location, and intensity but at this age can be misleading. If present, they are usually heard at the third or fourth interspace along the left sternal border or over the base of the heart.
- Palpate femoral and brachial pulses.
- Check blood pressure.

ABDOMEN
- General inspection. Abdominal examination should include an overall evaluation of the size of the abdomen—its roundness, distension, or concavity. If the abdomen is distended, one should consider intestinal obstruction, a ruptured viscus, enlargement of abdominal organs, ascites, and tumors. If the abdomen is flat or scaphoid, consider a diaphragmatic hernia or esophageal atresia without a fistula.

  Diastasis recti is a normal finding. Visible peristalsis indicates intestinal obstruction, but remember that it may be seen in otherwise normal infants, especially shortly after birth.
- Palpation of the abdomen is easy in the normal newborn if the infant is not crying.

  The liver is normally palpated as much as 2 cm below the right costal margin. The spleen is usually not palpable, but sometimes the tip is felt in normal infants. The lower pole of the right kidney and the left kidney can usually be palpated. The bladder can be palpated or percussed 1–4 cm above the symphysis.

  Any other masses palpable in the abdomen must be identified and described.
- The umbilical cord is inspected and the following noted.
  (1) Abnormal staining of the cord as with meconium.
  (2) Whether it is excessively large and jellylike or excessively small.
  (3) Any oozing of blood from the stump.
  (4) Redness around the cord or a fetid odor, since these usually signify the presence of omphalitis.
  (5) Pulsations of the cord.
  (6) Number of vessels. The presence of a single umbilical artery has been associated with an increase in congenital anomalies. However, prospective studies on newborns with a single umbilical artery as the only abnormal finding have demonstrated no increase in anomalies.[16]

- Examination for inguinal and umbilical hernia.

  GENITALIA. Any abnormalities of the male or female genitalia should be described.
- Male. Physiologic phimosis is the rule in newborn males, but in some, the foreskin may be retracted sufficiently to reveal the urethral meatus. The testes, whether in the canal or scrotum, should be palpated. The scrotum is often edematous, especially following breech delivery, and note should be made of the amount of pigmentation. Also note the presence of a hydrocele.
- Female. Note the presence of any discharge from the vagina, and describe this, since it may be blood-tinged or frankly bloody (withdrawal bleeding). Also note the size of the clitoris—e.g., an unusually large clitoris is found in pseudohermaphroditism. Hymenal tags are not uncommon. The labia, especially the labia minora, are relatively large in the newborn. Normal labia may be confused with a bifid scrotum. The genitalia, as in the male, may be edematous, especially following breech delivery.

  ANUS. The anus should be inspected for hemorrhoidal tags and patency. Routine rectal examination in the neonatal period is superfluous and, because it is traumatic, is unwise. It should, however, be done if there is any question about the free passage of meconium, or if the nurse has had difficulty in passing a thermometer.

  TRUNK AND SPINE. Note any obvious deformity of the trunk or spine, and check the end of the coccyx for a pilonidal sinus or dimple.

  EXTREMITIES. Check extremities for any congenital abnormalities such as polydactyly and syndactyly. Fractures, paralysis, and dislocations are looked for. The hips are examined for dislocation by flexing the knees and then abducting the thighs. Intrauterine posture is responsible for some deformities of the extremities, especially of the feet. In nearly every newborn, the feet are markedly dorsiflexed, and the dorsum of the foot can be made to lie against the anterior aspect of the tibia without effort. This is talipes or pes calcaneus, which corrects itself. There is often pronation of one or both feet, and a metatarsus varus is also fairly common.

Editorial Comment: Hip dislocation or subluxation can be confirmed by ultrasound.

NEUROMUSCULAR STATUS

- Reflexes. The nervous system of the neonate is still immature, and this is demonstrated in evaluation of reflexes. The following reflexes should be observed.
  (1) Moro's reflex—record whether this is complete or incomplete and if a unilateral response is obtained.
  (2) The grasp reflex as elicited in the hands and feet.
  (3) The plantar reflex, which may give a positive (Babinski) response in the newborn.
  (4) Chvostek's sign, which is frequently normally present.
  (5) Patellar reflex.
  (6) Rooting and sucking reflexes—if these are absent then check the gag and swallow reflexes.
- Tone should be checked.
- Tremulousness, jitteriness, etc., should be noted.

Editorial Comment: The importance of the states of consciousness and alertness of the infant must be noted during the examination, since they markedly alter the responses during the neuromuscular examination (see Chapter 16).

OTHER CHARACTERISTICS

- Passing of meconium is to be checked for. Normally, in the majority of infants, the passage of the first meconium stool is seldom delayed longer than 12 hours. If delayed, then check patency of anus and also check for intestinal obstruction. Presence of bright red blood in the meconium is usually due to the infant ingesting mother's blood and can be checked by the Apt test (see Appendix G–5).
- Voiding of urine. Urine is usually passed soon after birth, but may be unnoticed. If, however, there is no voiding of urine by 24 hours of age, it is highly suggestive of urinary tract obstruction, etc., and requires further investigation.

RECOMMENDATIONS FOR CARE OF THE NEWBORN*

1. Newborn infants should be regarded as recovering patients (few surgical procedures stress the patient more than the birth process) and kept under close surveillance during the first few hours after birth.

2. Assign a specific person (physician or nurse) to each delivery. This person is responsible for obtaining a pertinent history of pregnancy, labor, and delivery.

3. On delivery, place the infant in a prewarmed incubator or infant warmer. The infant should be dried immediately in a towel, and the mouth and nose should be very gently suctioned. The Apgar score is checked at 1 and 5 minutes (or, if low, until a good score is reached), and appropriate care is given. Every attempt should be made to facilitate and encourage maternal-infant interaction.

4. Transfer the infant to the transitional care (recovery) nursery or, if brief physical examination is normal, allow the infant to remain with the mother. In either case, trained personnel aware of the changes to be expected during the transitional state should observe the infant frequently and intensively until a smooth transition has been achieved. Vital signs, first recorded in the delivery room, are noted on a check sheet until the infant's condition is stable. In this manner, departures from the orderly progress of transition may be noted at their earliest appearance.

Editorial Comment: For the majority of infants, a short, thorough examination (by either nurse or doctor) during the first 5 to 10 minutes of life will show whether the infant is normal. Normal infants should then have a private time to meet their parents. This special time can be interrupted every 20 minutes to palpate the mother's uterus, take her blood pressure, and glance at the infant.

5. Infants who prove to be normal, as evidenced by a smooth transition, or infants with transient difficulties should be transferred to regular nurseries or remain with the mother. If transition is complicated, appropriate measures should be taken in the management of the infant.

6. If the infant requires continued monitoring, it is recommended that he be transferred to the intensive care area. The length of stay of the infant in the transitional care nursery should be determined by the physician.

In conclusion, the course of the individual infant during the natal day is unpredictable and variable. Optimal care of the neonatal patient should be prospective and anticipatory.

---

*Standards and Recommendations for Hospital Care of Newborn Infants, 6th edition, American Academy of Pediatrics, 1977, and Guidelines for Perinatal Care, American Academy of Pediatrics and American College of Obstetricians and Gynecologists, 1983.

Questions

True or False

Withdrawal symptoms are seen in neonates delivered to narcotics addicts but not in infants of chronic alcoholic mothers.

There have been several reports of a withdrawal syndrome in infants of alcoholic mothers. The clinical picture is much like that of delirium tremens seen in the adult. The infants often become hypoglycemic also. The fetal alcohol syndrome (small for gestational age, microcephaly, postnatal growth deficiency, developmental delay, and characteristic facies) is seen in many of these infants. Therefore the statement is false.

The fetal lungs are collapsed, and pulmonary blood flow is negligible.

The lungs in utero are not collapsed but are filled with fluid. This fluid is removed rapidly with the onset of air breathing. The pulmonary artery receives about 10 per cent of the cardiac output in the fetus. Although low, this blood flow seems to be very important in the development of the pulmonary vascular bed. Both parts of this statement are false.

Blood perfusing the brain in utero has the same oxygen saturation as that perfusing the kidney.

Oxygenated blood returns to the fetal heart via the umbilical vein and inferior vena cava. A portion of this is shunted across the foramen ovale and ultimately supplies the upper half of the body. Since blood supplying the lower half of the body is composed of a mixture of superior and inferior vena caval blood return, the oxygen saturation is lower. Hence the statement is false.

A good Apgar score at 1 minute suggests that the effect of maternal medications is minimal.

Birth is a tremendously stimulating process for the infant; thus the effect of depressant medications can be temporarily overcome. Therefore a 5 minute score that is less than the 1 minute score might suggest a medication-related problem. Therefore the statement is false.

Barrelling (increased AP diameter) of the chest is frequently seen in normal infants.

During normal transition in the unresponsive period between the first and second periods of reactivity, increase in the anteroposterior diameter of the chest may be noted to accompany the periods of shallow rapid respiration. The chest is not fixed in this position, since, if the infant cries or is handled, the barrelling disappears promptly only to return with resumption of rapid, shallow breathing. The same pattern may be seen in infants affected by maternal medication. Therefore the statement is true.

Gastric peristalsis (peristalsis from left to right) is usually indicative of bowel obstruction.

Gastric peristalsis is often noted during the transition period, especially in the relatively unresponsive interval between the first and second periods of reactivity. Therefore the statement is false.

A scaphoid abdomen is diagnostic of an esophageal atresia or diaphragmatic hernia.

Although the diagnosis of esophageal atresia without a fistula or diaphragmatic hernia should always be considered, a scaphoid abdomen is noted frequently during transition in infants with low Apgar scores or infants depressed by maternal medication. Therefore the statment is false.

Seizures (unless terminal) seldom occur in the severely depressed neonate.

In the majority of infants with convulsions, it has been noted that when they are severely depressed they seldom convulse. As their condition improves with increased responsiveness, spontaneous activity, and improved color, the brain becomes more irritable, and the seizure threshold is lowered. Similarly, transplacental sedation will raise the seizure threshold. Therefore the statement is true.

The clinical behavior during transition of the small-for-dates infant follows the course of that of an immature infant of comparable weight.

The more mature infant of low birth weight reacts like a larger infant of comparable gestational age. Small-for-dates infants have neurologic hyperexcitability and a lowered threshold for seizure activity. Therefore the statement is false.

Match

Match the following clinical findings in the neonate with the most likely maternal medication.
   A. Hypoglycemia
   B. Neonatal goiter
   C. Congenital malformations
   D. Floppiness
   E. Thrombocytopenia

   1. Thiazides
   2. Diazepam
   3. Aminopterin
   4. Potassium iodide
   5. Propranolol

A–5, B–4, C–3, D–2, E–1.

Match the following findings in the infant with the most likely maternal infection.

A. Meningoencephalomyocarditis
B. Intracranial calcification
C. Granulomatosis infantiseptica
D. "Celery stick" appearance of long bones
E. Conjunctivitis and pneumonia
F. Periostitis

1. Listeriosis
2. Syphilis
3. Coxsackievirus infection
4. Cytomegalovirus infection
5. Chlamydia
6. Rubella

A–3, B–4, C–1, D–6, E–5, F–2.

CASE PROBLEMS

Case One

B. A., a 21 year old gravida II para I mother, was admitted in labor with no history of prenatal care. Her blood pressure was 150/100, and she had 3+ proteinuria. She was treated with magnesium sulfate and thiazides. Two hours later she delivered a 3000 gm male infant under caudal analgesia with mepivacaine. The infant was flaccid at birth, with an Apgar score of 3 at 1 minute, but resuscitation was successful.

Describe the possible effects of the maternal medication.

Mepivacaine, when used for caudal analgesia, has caused intoxication and death of the fetus if accidentally injected into the fetal scalp. Magnesium sulfate administered to the mother in large doses may cause severe neonatal depression. Thiazides have been reported to cause thrombocytopenia.

Describe the pattern of transition expected in this infant.

Transition would be complicated, and the infant would manifest a combination of the changes seen during transition in low Apgar score infants and those depressed by maternal medications (see Table 3–1).

What complications could be expected during recovery?

During recovery, the infant may possibly require ventilatory assistance and parenteral fluids, since respiration and sucking and swallowing responses are often poor. The infant will require close observation for onset of hypoglycemia, apneic attacks, and seizures.

Case Two

G. S., a 20 year old gravida II para I, had an uncomplicated pregnancy and delivered a 2700 gm male infant under spinal anesthesia. The infant had an Apgar score of 8 at 1 minute, and his initial physical examination was described as normal. At 8 hours of age, the infant began to cry constantly, became extremely hyperactive and tremulous, and had vasomotor instability. Apart from the above findings, physical examination was again unremarkable. The hematocrit was 54, blood glucose was 100 mg/dl, and calcium was 9 mg/dl.

What would be the first approach in establishing a diagnosis?

Obtain a detailed history from the mother, especially in regard to medications. Of prime concern in this infant is a "withdrawal syndrome." One will repeatedly find that a personal interview with the mother is critical in delineating problems in a neonate. The infant was normal at birth and had no metabolic problems. The mother was a narcotics addict.

Is the fact that transition was apparently normal surprising?

Transition may be normal, since the infant has adapted to his abnormal intrauterine environment, and it is only when withdrawal effects occur that he becomes symptomatic. Withdrawal effects occurring during the course of transition will alter the pattern, but if they occur after transition is achieved, the clinical behavior during transition can be normal.

Having established a diagnosis, how would you manage the infant?

Management of these infants consists in giving specific therapy and supportive care. Withdrawal effects may be relieved by the administration of paregoric, starting with 1 to 2 drops/kg every 4 to 6 hours. If necessary, this dose may be increased once symptoms are under control. Paregoric is gradually withdrawn by reducing the dose about 10 per cent daily. It may be necessary to continue therapy for several weeks. Chlorpromazine and diazepam have been used with good results. Swaddling of the infant is of great value and will decrease the amount of medication required. These infants may require supportive therapy for diarrhea, vomiting, and dehydration.

REFERENCES

1. Adamsons, K., Jr., and Joelsson, I.: The effects of pharmacologic agents upon the fetus and newborn. Am J Obstet Gynecol 96:437, 1966.
2. Anderson, J.: High-risk groups—Definitions and identifications. N Engl J Med 273:308, 1965.
3. Babson, S., Benson, R., Pernoll, M., et al.: *Management of High-Risk Pregnancy and Intensive Care of the Neonate.* 4th ed. St. Louis, C. V. Mosby Co., 1979.
4. Baker, C., and Barrett, F.: Transmission of group B streptococci among parturient women and their neonates. J Pediatr 83:919, 1973.
5. Baker, J.: The effects of drugs on the fetus. Pharmacol Rev 12:37, 1960.
6. Barrett-Connor, E.: Infections and pregnancy: a review. Southern Med J 62:2715, 1969.
7. Brackbill, Y.: Long-term effects of obstetrical anesthesia on infant autonomic function. Dev Psychobiol 10:529, 1977.
8. Clark, C. E., Clyman, R. T., Roth, R. S., et al: Risk factor analysis of intraventricular hemorrhage in low birth weight infants. J Pediatr 99:625, 1981.
9. Cohlan, S.: Fetal and neonatal hazards from drugs administered during pregnancy. NY J Med 64:493, 1964.
10. Corke, B.: Neurobehavioural responses of the newborn. The effect of different forms of maternal analgesia. Anaesthesia 32:539, 1977.
11. Desmond, M., and Rudolph, A.: Progressive evaluation of the newborn. Postgrad Med 37:207, 1965.
12. Desmond, M., and Rudolph, A.: The clinical evaluation of the low-birth weight infant with regard to head trauma. *In* Angle, C., and Bering, E., Jr., (Eds.): *Physical Trauma as an Etiologic Agent in Mental Retardation. Proceedings of a Conference on the Etiology of Mental Retardation.* Omaha, Nebraska, October 13–16, 1968, p. 241.
13. Desmond, M., Franklin, R., Blattner, R., et al: The relation of maternal disease to fetal and neonatal morbidity and mortality. Pediatr Clin North Am 8:421, 1961.
14. Desmond, M., Franklin, R., Vallbona, C., et al: The clinical behavior of the newly born. I. The term baby. J Pediatr 62:307, 1965.
15. Desmond, M., Rudolph, A., and Phitaksphraiwan, P.: The transitional care nursery. Pediatr Clin North Am 13:651, 1966.
16. Froehlich, L. A., and Fujikura, T. Follow-up of infants with single umbilical artery. Pediatrics 52:6, 1973.
17. Fulginiti, V.: Bacterial infections in the newborn infant. J Pediatr 76:646, 1970.
18. Glass, L., Kolka, N., and Evans, H.: Factors influencing predisposition to serious illness in low birth weight infants. Pediatrics 48:368, 1971.
19. Gold, E.: Identification of the high risk fetus. Clin Obstet Gynecol 11:1069, 1968.
20. Gold, E.: Interconceptional nutrition. J Am Diet Assoc 55:27, 1969.
21. Harris, T. R., Isaman, J., and Giles, H. R.: Improved neonatal survival through maternal transport. Obstet Gynecol 52(3):294, 1978.
22. Hendricks, C.: Delivery patterns and reproductive efficiency among groups of differing socioeconomic status and ethnic origins. Am J Obstet Gynecol 97:608, 1967.
23. Hill, R., Craig, J., Chaney, M., et al: Utilization of over-the-counter drugs during pregnancy. Clin Obstet Gynecol 20:381, 1977.
24. Moya, F., and Thorndike, V.: Passage of drugs across the placenta. Am J Obstet Gynecol 84:1778, 1962.
25. Nora, J., Nora, A., Sommerville, R., et al: Maternal exposure to potential teratogens. JAMA 202:1065, 1967.
26. Overall, J., Jr., and Glasgow, L.: Virus infections of the fetus and newborn infant. J Pediatr 77:315, 1970.
27. Palmisano, P., and Polhill, B.: Fetal pharmacology. Pediatr Clin North Am 19:3, 1972.
28. Redwine, F., and Petres, R. E.: Fetal surgery—past, present, and future. Clin Perinatol 10:399, 1983.
29. Rudolph, A.: *Congenital Diseases of the Heart.* Chicago, Year Book Medical Publishers, Inc., 1974, chaps. 1–3.
30. Scanlon, J., Brown, W., Jr., Weiss, J., and Alper, M.: Neurobehavioral responses of newborn infant after maternal epidural anesthesia. Anesthesiology 40:121, 1974.

4

Classification of the Low-Birth-Weight Infant

AVRON Y. SWEET

... there are tiny, puny infants with great vitality. Their movements are untiring and their crying lusty, for their organs are quite capable of performing their allotted functions. These infants will live, for although their weight is inferior ... their sojourn in the womb was longer.

PIERRE BUDIN
THE NURSLING

In the past, newborn infants weighing 2500 gm or less were arbitrarily identified as premature, while those weighing more were designated full term. When it became widely accepted that not all neonates of 2500 gm or less at birth were prematurely born (<38 weeks' gestation), the designation low birth weight was applied to them instead. Accordingly, low birth weight now refers to all infants whose weight at birth is ≤ 2500 gm, irrespective of the cause and without regard to the duration of gestation.

The concept that small neonates do not constitute a homogeneous group and that babies of low birth weight are often undergrown full-term infants did not gain wide acceptance and attention until after the meticulous studies of investigators such as Gruenwald[46] demonstrated fetal malnutrition, or chronic fetal distress, as he termed it. The idea of intrauterine growth retardation (IUGR) had been proposed earlier,[22, 120] but Gruenwald's work and the wide support of his concepts did much to curtail the use of birth weight alone as a measure of matu-

rity of newborn infants. The importance of birth weight was not diminished, but the necessity for relating it to the duration of gestation was established.

Almost simultaneously, Lubchenco et al[69] presented standards of intrauterine growth of white infants in which birth weight was related to gestational age. The graphic display of the relationship provides a useful and simple method for determining the appropriateness of weight with respect to gestational age in a given infant. The reliability of weight measurement and the determination of gestational age are critical. Unfortunately, the accuracy of the determination of the duration of gestation from obstetric information is sometimes difficult, whether based on menstrual history or obstetric milestones such as quickening, appearance of fetal heart sounds, and fundal height. Serial studies of the fetus by ultrasound are often helpful in estimating gestational age (see Chapter 1); however, occasionally they, too, may be misleading. A reliable assessment of gestational age, based on direct examination of the infant, has been derived from neurodevelopmental criteria[5, 58, 98] and a variety of external physical characteristics[37, 38, 116] that change as pregnancy progresses. Although the techniques have faults, it is possible to assess each neonate with reasonable accuracy. By these means, newborn infants can now be categorized as *appropriate for gestational age* (in weight) (AGA), *small for gestational age* (SGA) (also referred to as *small for dates*), or *large for gestational age* (LGA). At the same time, they may be identified as *preterm* (<38 weeks' gestation), *term* (38–42 weeks' gestation), or *postterm,* also referred to as *postmature* (>42 weeks' gestation) (Figure 4–1).

One major "adaptation" in this chart is the change in the dividing line between preterm and term from 38 to 37 weeks. The reason for this change probably is related to the World Health Organization's use of 37 weeks as a definition of preterm. The dividing line is, at best, arbitrary. One might ask what factors support one or the other choice. There seems to be a practical need, especially for underdeveloped countries, to select the smallest number of the newborn population (those at highest risk of neonatal morbidity) for observation. In some countries, only infants with birth weights ≤2000 gm are given special attention. It is understandable that infants with the highest chance of illness and death will be selected for observation in understaffed obstetric and newborn services, but it is a mistake to equate these practices with optimum care. Infants with gestational ages of 37 to 38 weeks have a higher neonatal mortality and morbidity rate than do infants with gestational ages ≥ 38 weeks, and also they have a higher long-term morbidity for growth and development.

Approximately 80 per cent of births in the United States occur at gestational ages of 38 to 42 weeks or ± 2 weeks around the peak gestational age of 40 weeks; thus there is a division at 38 and 42 weeks. Why choose 3 weeks on one side of the peak incidence and 2 weeks on the other side, unless to avoid observation of moderate-risk infants? Nine per cent of our institution's population are neonates of 37 weeks' gestation.

L. Lubchenco

When infants of low birth weight are properly classified, about one third are found to be small for gestational age, while two thirds are appropriate for gestational age and preterm (gestational age <38 weeks).

Based on this classification, the clinician can now anticipate clinical problems peculiar to the category to which the patient belongs. Furthermore, one is able to prognosticate better with respect to growth and development and to seek out inapparent congenital abnormalities intelligently.

This chapter presents procedures for classifying young neonates, the physical differences between immature and small for gestational age infants, and the clinical significance of these differences. (Antenatal evaluation of fetal maturity is considered in Chapter 1.)

BASIC CONSIDERATIONS

An understanding of the dimensional changes that occur in normally or abnormally grown fetuses has resulted from the application of techniques that permit the determination of cell number and cell size. These techniques are based on the assumption that the proteins of any organ are contained within the cells and that the amount of DNA within the diploid nucleus of all cells of a given species is constant (k). Accordingly, the measurement of the DNA and total protein content of an organ permits the estimation

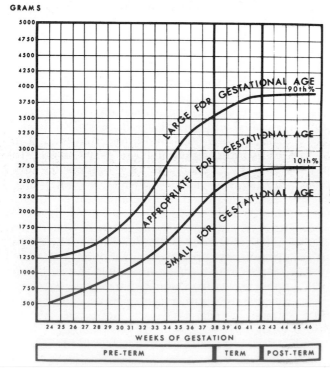

Figure 4–1. The birth weights of live-born singleton white infants at gestational ages from 24 to 42 weeks. (From Battaglia and Lubchenco.[13])

of cell size (protein/DNA) and number (DNA/k). These techniques have been used in valuable studies of animals with and without growth retardation and in studies of normal and malnourished human infants.

During early fetal life, virtually all growth is due to increases in cell number (*hyperplasia*). Increases in cell size (*hypertrophy*) become dominant during the latter part of gestation. It is not clear how long the increase in cell number continues or what variations occur in different organs.

Interference with the growth of the fetus during the period of hyperplasia results in organs that contain fewer cells than normal but cells of normal size. If the insult occurs during the period of hypertrophy, the cells will be normal in number but small in size. An intrauterine insult throughout the periods of both hyperplastic and hypertrophic growth will result in fewer and smaller cells. The classic example of this is the infant with the rubella syndrome.

Brain cell numbers continue to increase after birth. However, there is some disagreement as to when cell number no longer increases. Estimates vary between 8 and 15 months beyond 40 weeks' gestation. Thus, until more is known, malnutrition at any time during the 2 years following conception should be regarded as a potential hazard to brain development.

Total brain DNA content is directly and linearly related to head circumference, if no abnormal accumulation of intracranial fluid is present. Postmortem studies of marasmic infants have shown brain weight and protein to be reduced proportionate to head circumference. These findings support the use of changes in head circumference as a measure of postnatal brain growth. It should be pointed out that short-term reduction in rate of increase of head circumference has been associated with catching up in growth among very small preterm infants and some small for dates infants whose mothers had toxemia.

Every organ can be affected by intrauterine growth retardation. When the onset occurs toward the end of pregnancy, brain and skeletal growth, together with that of the heart and lungs, appears to be the least affected, while the adrenals, liver, spleen, and thymus often are severely reduced in size.[78]

ETIOLOGY

There are multiple causes of intrauterine growth retardation, and their effects upon

TABLE 4–1 SUGGESTED DISTRIBUTION OF CAUSES OF SMALL-FOR-DATES BABIES IN THE UNITED KINGDOM[30]

Cause	Percentage
Normal variation	10
Chromosomal and other congenital anomalies	10
Infections (maternal and fetal)	5 (? <5)
Poor uterus	1
Placenta and cord defects	2
Vascular disease in mother (including diabetes and heart disease)	35
Drugs, medicaments, and smoking	5
Other	32

the fetus vary according to the mode and duration of their action and the stage of fetal development during which they take place.

The etiologic factors are protean and difficult to categorize even in such broad terms as shown in Table 4–1.

The Placenta

In view of the importance of the placenta to the fetus in such matters as nutrition and respiration, when the question of fetal deprivation arises, the placenta must be suspect. Benirschke and Driscoll[14] suggest that large infarcts early in pregnancy may compromise placental function and impair fetal growth, while Rolschau[97] found small infarcts in 17 per cent of normal pregnancies and concluded that they played no role in fetal growth retardation. Abnormal insertions of the cord play a minor role,[99] and it is common knowledge that vascular tumors of the placenta, which occur infrequently, are usually associated with fetal stunting.[57] From the standpoint of discernible pathology, it is apparent that gross anatomic lesions are of little importance as causes of fetal growth impairment. Minute lesions, on the other hand, may be of importance. Among some placentas of growth-retarded infants of normotensive and toxemic mothers, atheromatous changes have been demonstrated in the decidual spiral arteries that are due to fibrin deposition and lipid-laden cells in the vessel walls.[102] It has been pointed out that the physiologic dilatation of the spiral arteries of the placental bed occurs in association with preeclampsia.[45] In any event, identifiable placental pathology is not a major etiologic factor.[46, 99]

Finally, eight pregnant women with growth-retarded fetuses studied between the thirty-second and thirty-ninth weeks of gestation were found to have uteroplacental blood flow one third of that demonstrated in women with normal fetal growth.[70]

Malnutrition

Nutritional inadequacy was the accepted cause of prematurity when the term referred to all infants weighing ≤2500 gm at birth. It is evident that many such infants were the products of women from areas of urban poverty. Naeye et al[81] found that women considered to be poor (as determined by weekly income and family size) more often delivered stillborn infants or liveborn infants who died within 48 hours of age and were smaller than comparable infants of more affluent mothers. Having removed from consideration infants with growth retardation from other known causes, they assumed that intrauterine growth was retarded because of poor maternal nutrition.

In an attempt to evaluate the effects of maternal nutritional deprivation upon the fetus, Smith[106] reviewed the hospital records in Rotterdam before, during, and after the "hunger winter" in northwestern Holland toward the end of World War II. During that winter (1944–1945), there was a paucity of food to the point of near (sometimes actual) starvation. Women who were pregnant during that period gave birth to infants who tended to be about 200 gm below expected weight when compared with mean birth weights of infants born before and after the episode. It appears that no significant undergrowth of infants in utero occurred during the hunger winter if food supplies were restored before the last weeks of pregnancy. If, however, the last weeks of pregnancy occurred during the time of severe food shortage, the infants were somewhat underweight. A similar trend was noted in Japan, where food became scarce toward the end of the war in the Pacific.[48]

Winick's studies favoring nutritional inadequacy as a cause of growth retardation in humans impressively demonstrate poor placental growth in nutritionally deprived pregnant women.[123] Less direct studies suggest impaired brain growth in the intrauterine-growth-retarded infants of poorly nourished mothers.

The work of Ferguson et al[40] supports the importance of nutrition as a factor in intrauterine growth retardation. A comparison of rosette-forming lymphocytes in the blood of AGA and SGA infants of equal gestational age revealed the undergrown infants to have a lower percentage of rosettes.[40] A similar decrease has been demonstrated in protein-calorie–malnourished infants. Other investigators have found similarities of abnormal energy metabolism of leukocytes between protein-calorie–malnourished and intrauterine-growth-retarded infants.[125] The evidence that supports a role for nutritional factors in human fetal growth retardation offers no clue as to whether the problem results from inadequate caloric intake or specific deficiencies of nutritional elements, such as certain fats, proteins, vitamins, etc.

Mothers with jejunoileal bypass have a high frequency of small-for-dates infants, including those who had AGA children born prior to surgery.[2] The basis of the growth retardation is not clear, for these women have several metabolic problems in addition to the nutritional consequences of the intestinal shunt.

Although it has been demonstrated that nutritional inadequacy causes intrauterine growth retardation in a variety of laboratory animals, there is no comparable evidence in the human. This difference may well be explained by the comparatively slow growth of the human fetus relative to the size of its mother. A nutritional problem of even short duration might prove catastrophic to the fast-growing rat fetus; however, since the rate of growth of the human is not nearly so demanding, a protracted and severe nutritional insult is required to produce an effect.

Infection

Certain intrauterine infections are known to cause diminished fetal growth. Newborn infants with overt cytomegalic inclusion disease may be small for gestational age. On the other hand, the disease most commonly occurs without growth retardation or other clinical signs among infants of young primiparous mothers.

Similarly, congenital rubella is associated with infants who are undergrown, particularly if they demonstrate the "expanded" rubella syndrome. In a study of 58 infants with congenital rubella who were born in New York City during the 1964 outbreak, 60 per cent fell below the tenth percentile for weight, and 90 per cent fell below the fiftieth percentile.[24] Studies of cord blood immunoglobulins have failed to implicate infections as a major cause of intrauterine growth retardation in human infants.[6, 72, 91, 111] In addition, viral cultures of stool, urine, and saliva of SGA infants during the first 3 days of life have failed to identify viral agents as a cause of prenatal growth failure.[6] At present it appears that only rubella and cytomegalic inclusion disease are known to cause a disparity in weight and gestational age in humans.

Although congenital syphilis has been identifed as a cause of prematurity, Naeye[79] found no evidence of intrauterine growth retardation from the examination of body weight, organ size, and cell number in organs of infected infants.

Intrauterine toxoplasmosis causes preterm birth. From the only study in which intrauterine growth retardation is mentioned, it was found in two of ten infants, but there was no evidence that toxoplasmosis was the cause.[95]

Bacterial infections are known to occur in utero, but they are not associated with growth retardation. These primarily occur during or just prior to labor (possibly causing premature labor), so that there is insufficient time for them to cause growth difficulties.

Inherited Factors

A woman who has produced a small for dates infant has a 20 per cent chance of doing so in subsequent pregnancies.[9] There are families in which infants are SGA without associated abnormalities, except for mental retardation. A family has been reported by Warkany et al[120] in which four generations contained several members who were below the expected weight at birth, and virtually all grew to be of normal size. Infants whose parents are small tend to be small at birth, sometimes sufficiently so to be classified as SGA.

Inherited abnormalities not associated with evident peculiarity of chromosome structure occur in association with intrauterine growth retardation. This is obvious, for example, in diastrophic dwarfs, achondroplastic dwarfs, and the like; it is also true of disorders in which mass is diminished for reasons other than diminutive or missing anatomic parts such as arms or legs—for example, Bloom's

syndrome, Smith-Lemli-Opitz syndrome, and Cornelia de Lange's syndrome.

It is characteristic of infants with excessive autosomal chromosomal material to be small for gestational age. This is true with regard to trisomy 13 and trisomy 18 and in the uncommon trisomy 8 mosaicism. It appears to be less common in infants with trisomy 21, who as a rule weigh 10 to 15 per cent less than normal at birth; half weigh less than 2700 gm.[105]

Inadequacy of sex chromosomal material, as exemplified by Turner's syndrome (45/XO), is known to be associated with fetal growth retardation. Reisman[94] suggests that material on the short arm of the X chromosome is important for intrauterine as well as postnatal growth and that a homologous locus is present on the Y chromosome. Individuals with excessive numbers of sex chromosomes, such as 47/XXY (Klinefelter's syndrome), may or may not exhibit growth retardation at birth. Barlow[12] found a regular and linear fall in birth weight with an increase of sex chromosomes, especially chromosome X. For each chromosome added, weight decreased about 300–400 gm.

Infants with chromosome anomalies characterized by simple deletions usually are SGA. Although the cri-du-chat syndrome, in which there is deletion of the short arm of No. 5 (5p−), serves as the most common example, growth retardation is most marked in infants with deletion of No. 4 (4p−).[89]

Toxemia and Hypertension

In the past, it was widely believed that toxemia was a cause of prematurity. It is now apparent that mothers with hypertension, who may or may not have toxemia, give birth to a higher than expected percentage of infants who are preterm, small for dates, or both. The basis for this association is not clear; however, with toxemia, numerous placental infarcts, atheromatous changes in the decidual spiral arteries, or failure of the normal physiologic dilatation of the placental spiral arteries may be sufficient to decrease perfusion of the placenta below what is adequate to meet the needs of the fetus. This is particularly likely toward the latter part of the third trimester. Probably more important is the finding that umbilical arteries of infants born to preeclamptic women produce prostacyclin (PGI_2) in much lower quantity than do those of infants whose mothers are normal.[28] This, together with an increasing volume of related research, strongly suggests that decreased prostacyclin synthesis may play a significant role in causing inadequate placental perfusion and its resultant effect upon the fetus. Along these lines, it has been found that the earlier the onset of preeclampsia, the worse the prognosis for intrauterine growth.[65] The incidence of SGA infants among pregnant women with hypertension is about 10 per cent. The weight deficiency is from 5 to 30 per cent below normal and can be manifested at any time after the twenty-fourth week of gestation. From Table 4–1, it can be seen that almost a third of SGA infants result from maternal problems of circulation (hypertension, toxemia, heart disease, class C or other insulin-dependent diabetes), of which hypertension and toxemia are the most common.

Other Factors

A wide variety of miscellaneous circumstances are associated with aberrations of intrauterine growth.

As a rule, products of *multiple births* are small for dates. This is usually apparent only if birth occurs after 35 weeks of gestation,[67] presumably because the placenta becomes inadequate to meet the needs of more than one fetus.

At *high altitudes,* infants tend to be light in weight for the duration of pregnancy, although linear growth is unaffected.[67] The reason for this phenomenon is not known, but it is known that intrauterine growth retardation occurs at high altitudes if the mother has hypoventilation, hypoxemia, or anemia.[76]

Mothers who smoke *cigarettes* during pregnancy produce infants who are small for dates.[1, 15, 29, 75, 92] At high altitudes, smoking has a two- to threefold greater unfavorable effect on birth weight than at sea level.[76] Moderate smokers have double the incidence of small for dates infants that nonsmokers do, while among heavy smokers it is threefold. The cause of this is not known. It is assumed by some to be a result of the vascular effects of smoking, while others attribute it to the hypoxemia in the mother and fetus that results from elevated levels of carboxyhemoglobin. No effects occur if smoking is stopped before pregnancy or in the face of smoking if extra food is provided during gestation.[87] Decreased fetal breathing activity, as demonstrated by sonography, was shown when women in the thirty-second to thirty-eighth week of pregnancy smoked two cigarettes in succession.[71] It is assumed that regular breathing movements reflect normalcy. Although cigarette smoking is not considered to be teratogenic, it does cause an increase in fetal wastage.[96]

Suspicion that maternal smoking during pregnancy is associated with an adverse outcome, such as growth retardation, perinatal mortality, and complications of pregnancy, is well established in the medical literature. Implicit in this literature is the assumption that smoking seems to be, at least in part, a causal factor. However, it should be recognized that it is difficult to assess the independent effect of smoking, since this variable is likely to be linked with low socioeconomic status, overcrowding, stressful situations, and excess in coffee and alcohol consumption.

Because of the dearth of studies that statistically control for lifestyle factors, the causal relationship of cigarette smoking remains to be established by further studies of smoking withdrawal. Nevertheless, even though all the scientific questions have not been answered, the cumulative evidence warrants the conclusion that it is better for infants if the mother does not smoke.

D. Campbell

Maternal *chronic alcoholism* has a marked retarding effect upon fetal growth. Ulleland,[112] while admitting the difficulty of identifying alcoholics, discovered 12 alcoholic mothers who gave birth to 10 SGA infants (83 per cent), while only 2.3 per cent of 1582 infants of nonalcoholic mothers from the same population were SGA. The birth weight of infants of historical alcoholics is about 250 gm below nonalcoholic controls, while offspring of active alcoholics weigh about 235 gm less than those of historical alcoholics and more than 500 gm below nonalcoholic controls.[64] Intrauterine growth retardation was found in 32 per cent of chronic alcoholics in a collaborative study of the National Institute of Neurological Disease and Stroke.[56] It has been reported that, among susceptibles, for each 10 gm of alcohol ingested daily, intrauterine growth is retarded about one per cent.[90]

It must be kept in mind that the spectrum of risks described above relates specifically to heavy alcohol consumption. The issue of any effect in human pregnancy of alcohol consumption that is moderate or minimal is unresolved. The fact that a variety of adverse outcomes are reported at levels of alcohol consumption deemed to be socially acceptable is puzzling and raises important concerns about the extent of the effects within the general population. **D. Campbell**

The long-term effects of maternal alcoholism on her offspring are disheartening. The growth retardation persists, and mental deficiency is common, presumably due to the lack of brain cells.[17]

Aside from the intrauterine growth retardation, infants of alcoholic mothers have a pattern of dysmorphogenesis that includes cardiocirculatory, limb, craniofacial, and genital (in females) abnormalities.[85] Two thirds of the infants involved are female.[93] The mechanisms underlying the aberrations of intrauterine growth and development and altered sex ratio are not clear. The basis is probably enzymatic. It is known, however, that the retardation is not due to a deficiency of growth-promoting hormones.[17]

Insulin is an important growth hormone for the fetus, according to clinical and experimental evidence. The prolonged hyperinsulinemia of the fetuses of diabetic women results in large overall size and macrosomia in these offspring. Conversely, when there is an absence of the pancreas (and its islets of Langerhans), intrauterine growth is well below standard.[62] Transient neonatal diabetes (hyperglycemia without ketoacidosis) in SGA neonates was first described by Gentz and Cornblath[44] and has since been ascribed to insufficient production of insulin or inactivation of it.[27] Streptozotocin ablation of the endocrine pancreas of fetal lambs results in significantly lower insulin content of the pancreas compared with controls and appreciable intrauterine growth retardation.[16]

Certain *noxious agents* have an unfavorable effect upon the growth (and often the development) of the fetus.

X-irradiation causes intrauterine growth retardation and microcephaly. *Aminopterin and other antimetabolites* given to the mother during pregnancy result in growth impairment and malformations of the brain and cranial vault as well as other anomalies, depending on the stage of gestation when the drug is taken.

Certain anticonvulsants administered during pregnancy result in fetal growth retardation. This is especially true of the *hydantoins (phenytoin, mephenytoin, ethotoin)*, which also have been incriminated in the causation of microcephaly, postnatal growth retardation, and craniofacial and limb abnormalities.[50] Less frequently, *trimethadione* intake has been associated with intrauterine growth retardation, mental retardation, dental irregularities, and ear abnormalities in infants.[126]

Infants born to mothers who are addicted to *narcotics* are often small for gestational age. Methadone has an effect but not as great as that of opiates.[108] Women with *hyperalaninemia* produce small babies also.

It has been accepted by most that infants born into families of *low socioeconomic level* tend to be small for gestational age. A study in Great Britain has shown that mothers from that class have SGA babies because of maternal height, youth, smoking, and hypertension. When these factors are corrected for, there is a marked decrease in the frequency of growth-retarded infants produced by those women.[83]

Several observers have noted intrauterine-growth-retarded offspring among women who develop *high hematocrit* values or *high hemoglobin* concentrations during the latter half of pregnancy.[35, 59, 73, 109] These mothers have abnormally high blood viscosity and decreased erythrocyte deformity.[109] The implication of these associations is that the hyperviscosity impedes uterine and placental perfusion with the result that the fetus is poorly supported and undergrown. Meberg[73] pointed out that decreased estriol and intrauterine growth retardation are related and that estriol production permits decreased restriction of red cell production, which results in greater than usual hematocrit values and hemoglobin concentrations.

Finally, *first-born infants* are usually smaller than their siblings, and sometimes they are sufficiently undergrown to be designated SGA. Usually there is no identifiable cause for the problem.

CLINICAL PRINCIPLES

Assessment of Gestational Age

Clinical decisions often require the knowledge of whether neonates are small, appropriate, or large for gestational age. The clinical course, outcome, and problems are quite different for each group of infants. Hypoglycemia, congenital malformations, and pulmonary aspiration are far more common among infants who are SGA, while hyaline membrane disease, spells of apnea, hyperbilirubinemia, etc., are more common among preterm, immature AGA infants. The need for precision in the estimation of gestational age cannot be overemphasized. If there is an incorrect estimation of gestational age (see Figure 4–1) by 4 weeks, an AGA infant weighing 2000 gm at 35 weeks who is incorrectly assessed as having a gestational age of

39 weeks will be labeled as a small for gestational age term infant.

This accuracy, however, may be difficult to obtain. X-rays of bone epiphyseal centers are unreliable in establishing gestational age because of the wide range of fetal age when the centers appear normally. Furthermore, when bone growth is impaired, fibular length is diminished, and there is a delay in the time of appearance of the distal and proximal tibial epiphyses.[122]

Although the mother's dates are useful, they are sometimes confusing because of irregular menstrual periods, bleeding in the first trimester, and the irregular or abnormal growth of the fetus. To avoid dependence on maternal information, several methods based upon the physical characteristics of infants have been developed. Three techniques most commonly used to determine gestational age are (1) the assessment of external physical characteristics, (2) the neurologic evaluation, and (3) scoring systems that combine the external physical characteristics and the neurologic evaluation.

ASSESSMENT OF GESTATIONAL AGE ACCORDING TO EXTERNAL CHARACTERISTICS. Farr and her associates[37, 38] and Usher and his coworkers[116] have defined certain external physical characteristics of newborn infants that progress in an orderly fashion during gestation. A wide variety of physical characteristics are available for evaluation (Table 4–2), such as sole creases (Figure 4–2) and the form and rigidity of the external ears (Figure 4–3).

ASSESSMENT OF GESTATIONAL AGE BY NEUROLOGIC EXAMINATION. Unlike the assessment of gestational age by physical criteria, which can be performed immediately after birth, neurologic evaluation requires the infant to be in a quiet, rested state. Uncompromised normal infants and some appropriate-for-gestational-age preterm infants without other problems can be accurately examined during the first hour or so after birth; however, this can be accomplished in others only during the latter part of the first day of life, and for many it cannot be done until the second or third day. In addition, "depressed," asphyxiated, neurologically damaged, or otherwise sick infants are difficult to assess. It is unfortunate that the neurologic assessment as a means of judging gestational age is not always practical at the time it is needed most.

Judgment of gestational age according to posture, passive range of motion of certain parts, active tone, righting reactions, and a variety of reflexes has been beautifully described by Amiel-Tison.[5]

SCORING SYSTEM FOR ASSESSING GESTATIONAL AGE FROM PHYSICAL AND NEUROLOGIC FINDINGS. Dubowitz and colleagues[34]

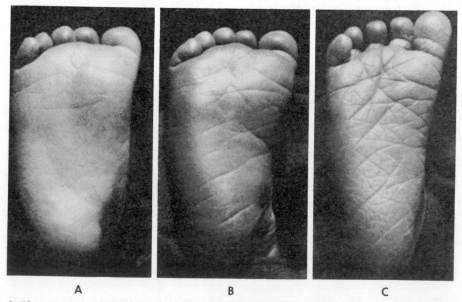

A   B   C

Figure 4–2. Plantar aspect of the foot of infants of varying gestational ages. *A*, Thirty-six weeks' gestation. Note the transverse creases on the anterior third only. *B*, Thirty-eight weeks' gestation. Note transverse creases extending to heel. *C*, Forty weeks' gestation. Note transverse creases over entirely of the sole and additional wrinkling. (From Usher et al.[116])

TABLE 4–2 SCORING SYSTEM OF EXTERNAL PHYSICAL CHARACTERISTICS*

External Sign	Score†				
	0	**1**	**2**	**3**	**4**
Edema	Obvious edema of hands and feet; pitting over tibia	No obvious edema of hands and feet; pitting over tibia	No edema		
Skin texture	Very thin, gelatinous	Thin and smooth	Smooth; medium thickness; rash or superficial peeling	Slight thickening; superficial cracking and peeling, especially of hands and feet	Thick and parchment-like; superficial or deep cracking
Skin color	Dark red	Uniformly pink	Pale pink; variable over body	Pale; only pink over ears, lips, palms, or soles	
Skin opacity (trunk)	Numerous veins and venules clearly seen, especially over abdomen	Veins and tributaries seen	A few large vessels clearly seen over abdomen	A few large vessels seen indistinctly over abdomen	No blood vessels seen
Lanugo (over back)	No lanugo	Abundant; long and thick over whole back	Hair thinning, especially over lower back	Small amount of lanugo and bald areas	At least half of back devoid of lanugo
Plantar creases (Figure 4–2)	No skin creases	Faint red marks over anterior half of sole	Definite red marks over > anterior half; indentations over < anterior third	Indentations over > anterior third	Definite deep indentations over > anterior third
Nipple formation	Nipple barely visible; no areola	Nipple well defined; areola smooth and flat, diameter < 0.75 cm	Areola stippled, edge not raised, diameter < 0.75 cm	Areola stippled, edge raised, diameter > 0.75 cm	
Breast size	No breast tissue palpable	Breast tissue on one or both sides, < 0.5 cm diameter	Breast tissue on both sides, one or both 0.5 to 1.0 cm	Breast tissue on both sides, one or both > 1 cm	
Ear form	Pinna flat and shapeless, little or no incurving of edge	Incurving of part of edge of pinna	Partial incurving of whole of upper pinna	Well-defined incurving of whole of upper pinna	
Ear firmness	Pinna soft, easily folded, no recoil	Pinna soft, easily folded, slow recoil	Cartilage to edge of pinna but soft in places, ready recoil	Pinna firm, cartilage to edge, instant recoil	
Genitals: Male	Neither testis in scrotum	At least one testis high in scrotum	At least one testis right down		
Genitals: Female (with hips half abducted)	Labia majora widely separated, labia minora protruding	Labia majora almost cover labia minora	Labia majora completely cover labia minora		

*Adapted by Dubowitz et al[34] from Farr et al.[38] To be used in conjunction with Figures 4–4 and 4–5.
†If score differs on two sides, take the mean.

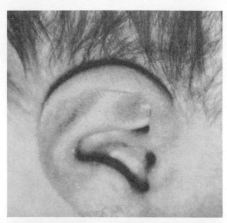

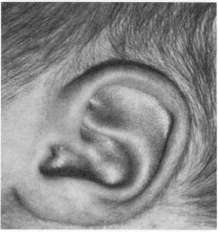

Figure 4–3. *Top,* This ear, an infant's of 36 weeks' gestation, characteristically demonstrates a rolled margin only superiorly, appears thin and shapeless, contains little cartilage, and has only a moderate tendency to spring back to its original contour when it is manually deformed. *Bottom,* The ear of an infant of 40 weeks' gestation, with a rolled margin everywhere but inferiorly and good cartilaginous support providing rigidity and a vigorous return to normal shape when it is deformed. (From Usher et al.[116])

devised a scoring system combining neurologic findings similar to those of Amiel-Tison[5] and physical characteristics described by Farr et al.[38] The changes in external physical characteristics are weighted according to their appearance as pregnancy progresses (Table 4–2). Table 4–3 and Figure 4–4 describe and depict the procedures for the neurologic evaluation.

Dubowitz et al have given us the most reliable method of assessing gestational age. Two of the most helpful neurologic findings are really not neurologically determined. These are wrist and ankle flexion patterns. They are not related to muscle tone and, in fact, as maturity and tone progress they "mature" in the opposite direction. They are related more to mobility of the joints rather than to muscle tone. The exact mechanism has not been worked out, but it parallels mobility of pelvic joints of the mother during the last trimester. Supporting this observation is the finding of Amiel-Tison that joint mobility in preterm infants does not progress postnatally, as it does in utero, and that preterm infants grown to 40 weeks tend to walk on their toes, rather than on the whole sole as do infants born at term.

There are physical characteristics that are altered with intrauterine growth retardation, and these patterns are helpful in accurately identifying the small for gestational age infant. The small for gestational age infant usually has lost his vernix, has more skin desquamation, and has more sole creases than expected. At the same time, there is less breast tissue and ear cartilage than is present at the normal gestation. **L. Lubchenco**

The scores obtained from the assessment of each of the 10 neurologic signs (Figure 4–5) are totaled and added to the scores of each of the 11 external signs (Table 4–2). The gestational age is then found by using the graph in Figure 4–5.

Ballard et al[10] have produced an abbreviated version of the system of Dubowitz et al (Figure 4–6) in which certain neurologic criteria are retained that do not require the infant to be alert and vigorous.

Every infant should be evaluated physically and neurologically as soon as possible after birth. In following published directions for evaluation, it is important to adhere closely to the directions of the original author and to use the same method in following the neurologic development. Only by repetition can one obtain proficiency, reliability, and reproducibility. Under the best circumstances, physical and neurologic examinations are only accurate to within plus or minus 2 weeks, so history and all other factors must be taken into consideration when determining gestational age.

Many abbreviations of the assessment of gestational age are appearing, with valid reasons. This comes in response to the need to know gestational age immediately after birth, since management is based on the clinical assessment, and also to minimize handling of the infant in the transition period. The complete neurologic score requires more handling and exposure than are recommended in the first hour after birth. **L. Lubchenco**

The weight, length, and head circumference of all newborn infants should be compared with a set of normal standards (Figure 4–7 and Appendices G–1, 2, and 3). In this way, a number of SGA and LGA infants who would not otherwise be recognized will be identified.

ESTIMATION OF GESTATIONAL AGE BY EXAMINATION OF THE ANTERIOR VASCULAR CAPSULE OF THE LENS. Careful studies have demonstrated changes in the vessels of the anterior vascular capsule of the lens as pregnancy progresses (Figure 4–8).[54] There is an excellent correlation of the vascular changes and the gestational age as determined by the method of Dubowitz et al,[34] but only from the twenty-seventh through the thirty-fourth week of pregnancy. The relationship is unaffected by size at birth.[53]

INTRAUTERINE GROWTH CURVES. It should be apparent that impaired growth may vary in duration and cause and that small-for-dates infants are not a homogeneous group. Without a comparison with expected norms, proper classification of infants cannot be made. The most commonly used normal values are those compiled in Denver, which have been used to construct smoothed curves as shown in Figure 4–1.[68] As with all such data, they are compiled from records that are deemed to contain reliable obstetric data and to exclude infants with obvious problems known to cause abnormal birth weight–gestational duration relationships such as hydrocephalus, anencephaly, and maternal diabetes. Unfortunately, the data are from singleton white infants born at high altitude. Similar data of singleton white infants born at sea level are shown in Appendix G–4.[115] Similar data concerning monochorionic and dichorionic twins have also been used in constructing curves.[80]

The curves alluded to above are constructed from values of birth weights attained by infants born at specific weeks of gestation by history. The lowest 10 per cent of values in each week of gestation represents the tenth percentile, etc. An infant whose birth weight is on or below the tenth percentile curve is considered to be small for gestational age, while a large-for-gestational-age infant has a birth weight on or above the ninetieth percentile curve.

Since the curves considered to represent normal intrauterine growth for any particular segment of the population are constructed from values obtained from a large number of pregnancies exclusive of those with vague or obviously erroneous histories and malformed products, inapparent errors tend to be few and therefore fail to skew the data because of the overwhelming volume of correct information.

The weight/length ratio or ponderal index (100 × weight in gm/length in cm³), when plotted against the duration of gestation in weeks (Figure 4–7), allows for an assessment of concordance or the degree of discordance in growth of the two parameters. Weight/length ratios between the tenth and ninetieth percentiles at any gestational age indicate symmetry of growth regardless of the presence or absence of growth retardation. Ratios at or below the tenth percentile indicate that ponderal growth is appreciably below linear growth at any gestational age. Using the weight/length ratio, one can further categorize SGA infants as symmetrically or asymmetrically growth retarded, a differentiation whose importance is discussed below.

Small-for-Gestational-Age Infants

APPEARANCE AT BIRTH

The majority of small-for-dates infants are born at or near term. In fact, of all infants who weigh less than 2500 gm at birth, about one third are full term.[22, 47]

Although infants who are small for dates represent a heterogeneous group, there are no definitions or descriptions of the subgroups contained within that population. Some appear simply to be dwarfed (symmetrically undergrown), while others are designated *dysmature* or said to show evidence of the *placental insufficiency syndrome*. These are undefined terms, but they imply nutritional inadequacy late in pregnancy, and in clinical appearance the infants so designated seem to differ little from the wasted infant born after 42 weeks' gestation (the *postmaturity syndrome*).

Dysmature SGA infants are asymmetrically growth retarded, being primarily underweight, and therefore appear thin and wasted. The skin is loose, often dry, and frequently scaling. Meconium staining of the skin, nails, and umbilical cord is common. There is little subcutaneous tissue. The face is not full, nor do the trunk and extremities seem to have as much musculature as expected. While weight is low, quite often length is not affected, and head size is usually normal. This disparity between length and/or head size and weight has led to the designation of these infants as asymmetrically growth retarded. A study of pregnancies in Yugoslavia identified 80 per cent of SGA infants to be asymmetrically growth retarded.[61] Hair on the head tends to be sparse. These babies are usually alert and active and seem hungry, although not necessarily from the first minutes of life. Often they do not urinate in the first hours after birth and may not for 24 hours or more if fluids are not provided early. The cord dries rapidly.

The spectrum of small-for-dates infants

TABLE 4–3 TECHNIQUES OF NEUROLOGIC ASSESSMENT*

Posture

With the infant supine and quiet, score as follows:

Arms and legs extended	= 0
Slight or moderate flexion of hips and knees	= 1
Moderate to strong flexion of hips and knees	= 2
Legs flexed and abducted, arms slightly flexed	= 3
Full flexion of arms and legs	= 4

Square Window

Flex the hand at the wrist. Exert pressure sufficient to get as much flexion as possible. The angle between the hypothenar eminence and the anterior aspect of the forearm is measured and scored according to Figure 4–4. Do not rotate the wrist.

Ankle Dorsiflexion

Flex the foot at the ankle with sufficient pressure to get maximum change. The angle between the dorsum of the foot and the anterior aspect of the leg is measured and scored as in Figure 4–4.

Arm Recoil

With the infant supine, fully flex the forearm for 5 seconds, then fully extend by pulling the hands and release. Score the reaction as follows:

Remain extended or random movements	= 0
Incomplete or partial flexion	= 1
Brisk return to full flexion	= 2

Leg Recoil

With the infant supine, the hips and knees are fully flexed for 5 seconds, then extended by traction on the feet and released. Score the reaction as follows:

No response or slight flexion	= 0
Partial flexion	= 1
Full flexion (less than 90° at knees and hips)	= 2

Popliteal Angle

With the infant supine and the pelvis flat on the examining surface, the leg is flexed on the thigh and the thigh fully flexed with the use of one hand. With the other hand the leg is then extended and the angle attained scored as in Figure 4–4.

Heel-to-Ear Maneuver

With the infant supine, hold the infant's foot with one hand and move it as near to the head as possible without forcing it. Keep the pelvis flat on the examining surface. Score as in Figure 4–4.

Scarf Sign

With the infant supine, take the infant's hand and draw it across the neck and as far across the opposite shoulder as possible. Assistance to the elbow is permissible by lifting it across the body. Score according to the location of the elbow:

Elbow reaches the opposite anterior axillary line	= 0
Elbow between opposite anterior axillary line and midline of thorax	= 1
Elbow at midline of thorax	= 2
Elbow does not reach midline of thorax	= 3

Head Lag

With the infant supine, grasp each forearm just proximal to the wrist and pull gently to bring the infant to a sitting position. Score according to the relationship of the head to the trunk during the maneuver:

No evidence of head support	= 0
Some evidence of head support	= 1
Maintains head in the same antero-posterior plane as the body	= 2
Tends to hold the head forward	= 3

Ventral Suspension

With the infant prone and the chest resting on the examiner's palm, lift the infant off the examining surface and score according to the posture shown in Figure 4–4.

*According to Dubowitz et al[34] from Amiel-Tison.[5] To be used in conjunction with Figures 4–4 and 4–5.

includes a group who are proportionately small (dwarfed) without wasting, meconium staining, etc. They are referred to as symmetrically growth retarded. These neonates seem to have been undergrown for a long time and appear old for their size. It is in them that anomalies tend to occur. Aside from the evident problems of the rubella syndrome and the various trisomies, congenital heart disease, genitourinary malformations, and alimentary tract abnormalities are encountered. The presence of a unilateral or bilateral single palmar crease, single umbilical artery, and peculiarities of the ears may serve as additional clues that hidden problems exist.

The clinical problems encountered among SGA infants are different from those seen among AGA, preterm infants. Some of these are given in Table 4–4 and considered below.

CLINICAL PROBLEMS

There is a considerable amount of literature dealing with clinical problems of SGA infants. Unfortunately the infants are rarely identified as symmetrically or asymmetrically growth retarded. Accordingly, proper and useful interpretation of the findings has been unusual, and much dogma concerning small-for-dates infants is true only for an unspecified segment of that population.

As many as 65 per cent of SGA infants are likely to present in the delivery room with one or more severe and often life-threatening problems.[84] In the main, these include as-

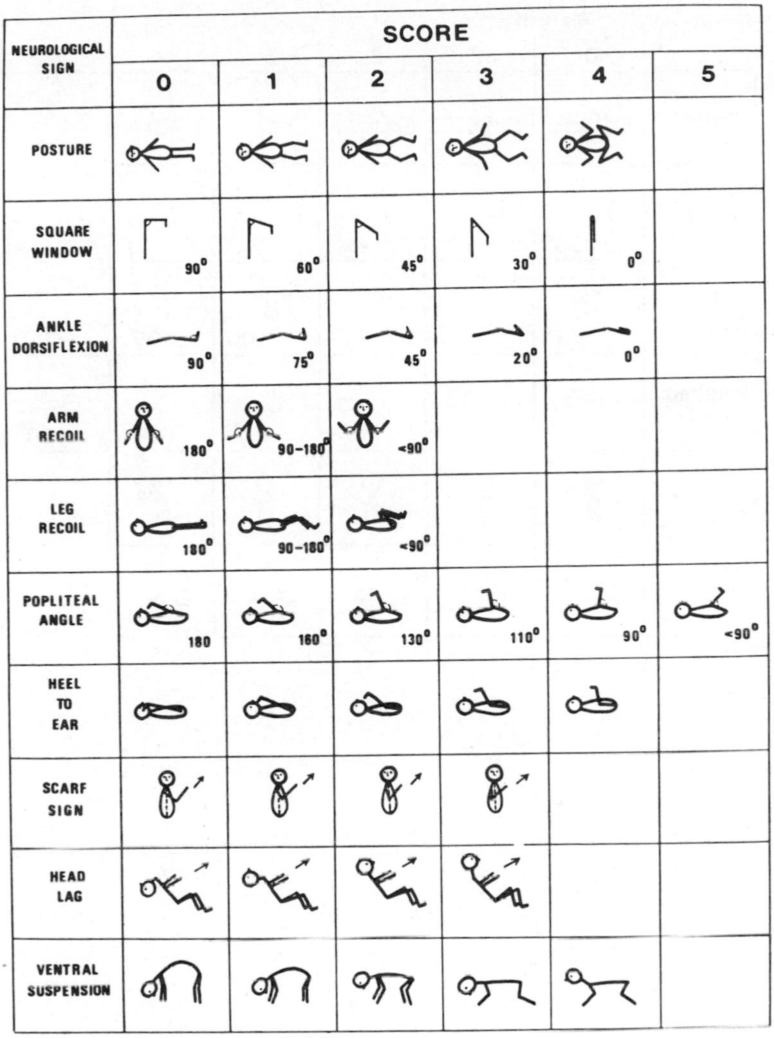

NEUROLOGICAL SIGN	SCORE					
	0	1	2	3	4	5
POSTURE						
SQUARE WINDOW	90°	60°	45°	30°	0°	
ANKLE DORSIFLEXION	90°	75°	45°	20°	0°	
ARM RECOIL	180°	90–180°	<90°			
LEG RECOIL	180°	90–180°	<90°			
POPLITEAL ANGLE	180	160°	130°	110°	90°	<90°
HEEL TO EAR						
SCARF SIGN						
HEAD LAG						
VENTRAL SUSPENSION						

Figure 4–4. The scoring of neurologic findings according to Dubowitz et al[34] from Amiel-Tison.[5] (To be used in conjunction with Table 4–3.)

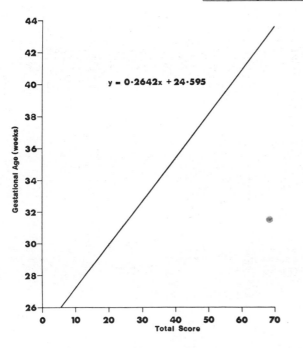

$$y = 0{\cdot}2642x + 24{\cdot}595$$

Figure 4–5. Graph for ascertaining gestational age from the total score of physical and neurologic development according to Dubowitz et al.[34]

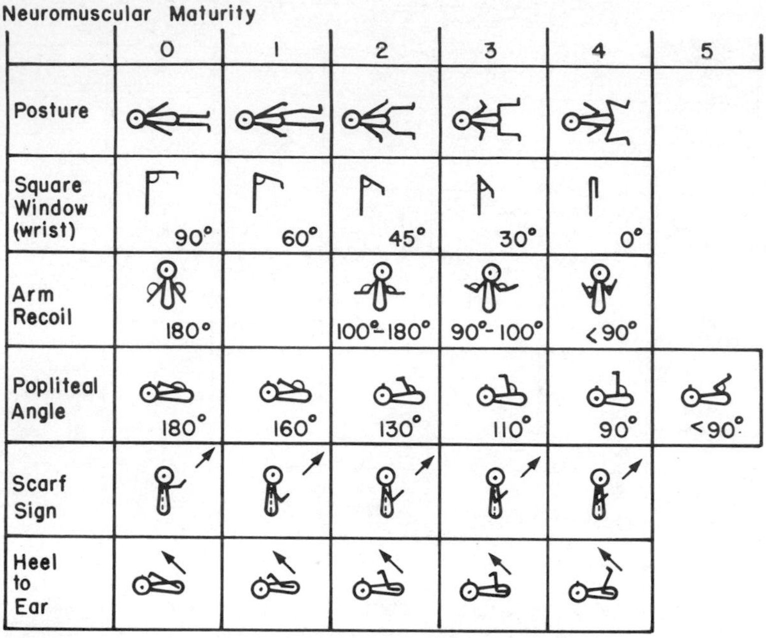

Neuromuscular Maturity

	0	1	2	3	4	5
Posture						
Square Window (wrist)	90°	60°	45°	30°	0°	
Arm Recoil	180°		100°–180°	90°–100°	<90°	
Popliteal Angle	180°	160°	130°	110°	90°	<90°
Scarf Sign						
Heel to Ear						

Apgars _____ 1 min _____ 5 min

Age at Exam _____ hrs

Race _____ Sex _____

B.D. _____

LMP _____

EDC _____

Gest. age by Dates _____ wks

Gest. age by Exam _____ wks

B.W. _____ gm. _____ %ile

Length _____ cm. _____ %ile

Head Circum. _____ cm. ____ %ile

Clin. Dist. None _____ Mild _____

Mod. _____ Severe ____

PHYSICAL MATURITY

Skin	gelatinous red, transparent	smooth pink, visible veins	superficial peeling &/or rash few veins	cracking pale area rare veins	parchment deep cracking no vessels	leathery cracked wrinkled
Lanugo	none	abundant	thinning	bald areas	mostly bald	
Plantar Creases	no crease	faint red marks	anterior transverse crease only	creases ant. 2/3	creases cover entire sole	
Breast	barely percept.	flat areola no bud	stippled areola 1–2 mm bud	raised areola 3–4 mm bud	full areola 5–10 mm bud	
Ear	pinna flat, stays folded	sl. curved pinna; soft with slow recoil	well-curv. pinna; soft but ready recoil	formed & firm with instant recoil	thick cartilage ear stiff	
Genitals ♂	scrotum empty no rugae		testes descending, few rugae	testes down good rugae	testes pendulous deep rugae	
Genitals ♀	prominent clitoris & labia minora		majora & minora equally prominent	majora large minora small	clitoris & minora completely covered	

MATURITY RATING

Score	Wks
5	26
10	28
15	30
20	32
25	34
30	36
35	38
40	40
45	42
50	44

Figure 4–6. Assessment of gestational age. (Modified from Ballard et al.[10])

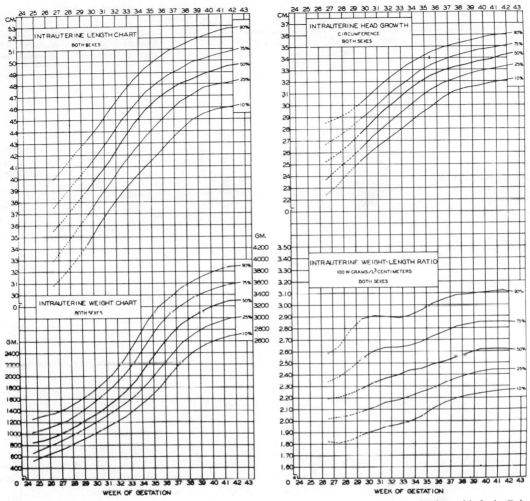

Figure 4–7. Intrauterine growth curves for length, head circumference, and weight for singleton births in Colorado. (From Lubchenco et al.[68])

phyxia, hypoglycemia, polycythemia, and hypothermia; they occur most commonly among term SGA infants who have a low ponderal index.[119] Because of these and other important problems, undergrown infants frequently require prompt attention in the de-livery room. Accordingly, persons skilled in resuscitation of newborn infants and knowledgeable of their physiologic and clinical peculiarities should be present at the delivery of infants who have intrauterine growth retardation.

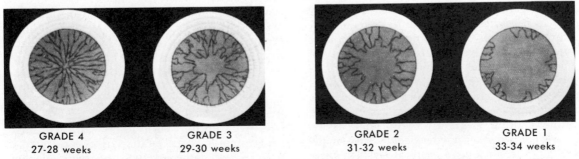

GRADE 4	GRADE 3	GRADE 2	GRADE 1
27-28 weeks	29-30 weeks	31-32 weeks	33-34 weeks

Figure 4–8. Assessment of gestational age from examination of the anterior vascular capsule. (From Hittner et al.[53])

Table 4–4 COMPARISON OF PROBLEMS OF SMALL-FOR-GESTATIONAL-AGE AND IMMATURE NEWBORN INFANTS

	Immature AGA	Immature SGA	Mature SGA (Symmetric)	Mature SGA (Asymmetric)
Early weight change	5–10% loss, then slow gain	5–10% loss, then slow gain	5–10% loss, then slow gain	≤5% loss, then rapid gain
Congenital infection	+	+ +	+ +	±
Respiratory problems	Hyaline membrane disease	Hyaline membrane disease	Unusual	Aspiration syndrome Pneumomediastinum Pneumothorax
Persistent fetal circulation	+	+	0	+ +
Apneic spells	+ + + +	+ + + +	0	0
Polycythemia	0	0	±	+ +
Hyperbilirubinemia	+ + + +	+ + + +	+	+ +
Hypoglycemia	+	+	+	+ + +
Hypocalcemia	+	+	±	+
Congenital malformation	±	+	+ +	±
Intracranial hemorrhage	+ + +	+ + +	±	+
Asphyxia	+ +	+ +	±	+ +
Growth (linear)	Normal	Subnormal (rare catch-up)	Subnormal (rare catch-up)	Normal
Neurobehavioral residua	+ + (mostly in very low birth weight infant)	+ + +	+ + +	+ (more if asphyxia is severe)

ASPHYXIA. Neonatal asphyxia tends to be more common and profound among small-for-dates infants, especially the ones who are underweight for their length.[63, 66, 119] Because these infants do not enjoy adequate placental support toward the end of their intrauterine stay, they are deprived of the usual glucose input from the mother, have low carbohydrate reserves, and are often marginally oxygenated. Therefore, severe hypoxemia is common, and acidemia appears rapidly. Prior to the advent of reliable continuous fetal heart rate monitoring, these infants would be born dead or near dead to the surprise of everyone attending the delivery. Now such occurrences are unusual—or should be. Resuscitation must be prompt and vigorous and carried out according to the techniques described in Chapter 2.

RESPIRATORY DIFFICULTIES. Term or near-term asymmetrically undergrown SGA infants are prone to aspiration of amniotic fluid. This is a result of the antenatal asphyxia that causes the fetus to gasp. In response to the asphyxia, often meconium is passed, and although it is very viscid material, it spreads throughout the volume of the amniotic fluid. Evidently then, when asymmetrically growth-retarded, near-term, small-for-dates infants have respiratory difficulty, as a rule it is due to aspiration of amniotic fluid. The infants present one or more of the usual signs of respiratory distress: grunting, flaring of the anterior nares, subcostal and/or intercostal retractions, tachypnea, and cyanosis. The severity of the illness is related to the quantity of material aspirated. Although those who aspirate uncontaminated amniotic fluid may be very ill at the outset, their respiratory difficulty abates rapidly, within 48 hours. If fresh meconium is aspirated with the amniotic fluid, the problem is more severe, more prolonged (commonly 10 days or more), and likely to be complicated by pneumomediastinum or pneumothorax (see Chapter 8). Occasionally pulmonary hemorrhage occurs as a manifestation of asphyxia- or hypothermia-induced disseminated intravascular coagulation.

Very prematurely born SGA babies are usually symmetrically growth retarded, and their respiratory problems are usually due to hyaline membrane disease, just as those of their preterm AGA peers are.

PERSISTENT FETAL CIRCULATION. No infant at or near term is immune from persistent fetal circulation, which is a frightening, life-threatening functional abnormality whose major manifestation is cyanosis. Initially it was believed that the basis of the disease was the persistence of the pulmonary hypertension of the fetus, causing shunting of unoxygenated blood from the pulmonary circuit to the aorta via the ductus arteriosus. Recently it has been demonstrated that in some infants the shunting is not through the ductus arteriosus but through the foramen ovale instead. In addition, some functional problems of the cardiac musculature may be present also.

Persistent fetal circulation occurs most frequently among asymmetrically undergrown SGA (dysmature/postmature) infants, particularly if asphyxia has occurred. Polycythemia has not been a concomitant finding, but the aspiration of amniotic fluid, often containing meconium, is commonly associated. It is not only asymmetric SGA newborns who are vulnerable to persistent fetal circulation but also infants of diabetic mothers. It may be noteworthy that both are associated with abnormal placentae.

HYPOGLYCEMIA. This condition is encountered most frequently during the neonatal period among infants of diabetic mothers, small-for-dates infants (including the smaller of discordant twins), and stressed, small, preterm infants. Neonatal symptomatic hypoglycemia (blood glucose concentration < 20 mg/dl) is more common among males and, predominantly, SGA infants.[25] It is seen most frequently (50 per cent) among the SGA infants who are markedly wasted (asymmetrically growth retarded), with weights below the third percentile for gestational age.[113, 119] Hypoglycemia is most likely to occur during the first 12 hours of life but may appear as late as 48 hours. Accordingly, blood sugar concentration of SGA infants should be monitored carefully and, if necessary, treatment begun promptly. As with most conditions of neonates in which hypoglycemia occurs, hypocalcemia is frequently a concomitant problem.[110] (For the clinical manifestations and management of symptomatic hypoglycemia, see Chapter 10.)

It is generally accepted that hypoglycemia results from the high metabolic rate of SGA infants together with their already low and rapidly depleted glycogen stores. Shelley,[101] in a study of human tissues, found SGA infants to have low carbohydrate content in heart, liver, and skeletal muscles, often one tenth or less of the amount expected normally.

Gluconeogenesis in infants with intrauterine growth retardation is seen to be impaired when compared with that of adults and AGA infants. The response of SGA infants to oral or intravenous administration of the glucogenic amino acid alanine during the first 24 hours of life is minimal with respect to blood glucose and insulin concentrations.[121] This failure of gluconeogenesis in response to alanine is more pronounced in hypoglycemic SGA infants than in those who are normoglycemic.[74] Furthermore, hypoglycemic SGA infants have increased plasma concentrations of the glycogenic amino acid precursors (alanine, glycine, proline, and valine),[74] implying that there is an appropriate response in the production and outflow from their peripheral pool. However, the marked hyperaminoacidemia suggests that hepatic gluconeogenesis is impaired.

The hypoglycemia of SGA infants may reflect an additional burden on the meager carbohydrate stores imposed by poor fat stores and inadequate functioning of enzyme systems involved in fat metabolism.

THERMAL REGULATION. It is not surprising that SGA infants have difficulties in thermal regulation in view of their metabolic fuel problems. This is especially true of the asymmetrically undergrown infants.[119] Carbohydrates are in short supply,[101] there is a lack of response to glucogenic amino acids,[74, 121] fat insulation is poor, and lipid metabolism is impaired.[7, 31, 82] To these abnormalities is added a decrease in stores of brown fat,[3] a special heat-producing tissue of the body.

In view of these metabolic deficiencies and problems of body composition, the usual tables (based on weight) for ascertaining the neutral thermal environment and critical temperature do not apply to SGA infants. Incubator settings should be determined by closely monitoring the temperature of each infant with a view to maintaining abdominal skin temperature between 36.0 and 36.5° C.

POLYCYTHEMIA. Central hematocrit values ≥ 65 per cent occur in 15 to 39 per cent of small-for-dates infants at or near term who have sustained asymmetric intrauterine growth retardation.[45, 52, 55, 119] In addition, infants with intrauterine growth retardation have been found to have increased red blood cell volume[114] and elevated erythropoietin levels.[41, 42]

The cause of the polycythemia among SGA infants is unknown. It is of interest that SGA infants have higher ratios of fetal to adult hemoglobin than their gestational age peers.[11] Usually, as pregnancy progresses, there is a decrease in the proportion of fetal to adult hemoglobin. This is not true among SGA infants, supporting Gruenwald's hypothesis that intrauterine hypoxemia is an important factor in growth retardation,[46] since, in vitro, a decrease of oxygen tension or glucose in the environment results in an increase of fetal hemoglobin synthesis as compared with adult hemoglobin production.[4]

It is noteworthy that among newborns who are large for gestational age, infants of diabetic mothers often have polycythemia.

Polycythemic infants are usually asymptomatic, but some manifest one or more clinical abnormalities. Symptoms may be related to increased viscosity, which rises precipitously as hematocrit values reach 70 per cent. These symptoms include tachypnea, intercostal retraction, grunting, nasal flaring, tachycardia with or without cardiac failure, pleural effusion, scrotal edema, priapism, and convulsions. Hyperbilirubinemia is not uncommon.

Treatment is usually provided to infants whose venous hematocrit reaches 65 per cent or more and consists of an exchange transfusion, in which plasma is used to replace the blood withdrawn. A large volume is not necessary, since a small decrease in hematocrit results in a large decrease in blood viscosity and improvement in symptoms. The amount of blood removed is calculated as:

$$\text{estimated blood volume (ml)} \times \frac{\text{actual} - \text{desired hematocrit}}{\text{actual hematocrit}}$$

The desired hematocrit should be 50 to 60 per cent.

CONGENITAL MALFORMATIONS. With the separation of the true premature (< 38 weeks) from the small-for-dates infant, it became apparent that congenital malformations occur more frequently among undergrown infants. More recently it has become evident that, among SGA infants, structural anomalies appear most commonly when growth retardation is symmetric. Usher[113] found congenital malformations to occur 10 to 20 times more frequently among SGA infants than among AGA infants. Van den Berg and Yerushalmy[117] reviewed the records of 469 liveborn infants whose birth weights were between 1501 and 2500 gm and found that SGA infants with the longest gestation had the highest incidence (18 per cent) of severe malformations. Drillien[32, 33] also found the

frequency of congenital malformations to increase as the duration of gestation increased. The more severe, prolonged, and symmetric the intrauterine growth retardation, the more likely the chance of malformation.

Most infants with anomalies tend to have problems that are immediately evident upon physical examination at birth or that manifest themselves in the first few days of life. Because urinary tract abnormalities may be silent, it is often questioned whether excretory urograms and other diagnostic studies are necessary to demonstrate abnormalities in SGA infants who appear to be normal otherwise. We do not study these patients unless there are physical findings suggestive of abnormalities, such as enlargement of one or both kidneys, ear abnormalities, or the presence of a single palmar crease together with a single umbilical artery.

Usher et al[116] found that 6 per cent of the SGA infants they studied had congenital heart disease.

The majority of congenital anomalies in SGA infants are not associated with demonstrable chromosomal peculiarities, nor is there a specific pattern of abnormalities identified with SGA neonates.

Although the presence of congenital anomalies is commonly associated with intrauterine growth retardation, there are certain notorious exceptions. Infants with transposition of the great vessels tend to be large for gestational age. Infants of diabetic mothers, well known for their increased frequency of malformations, are very commonly large for dates.

IMMUNE STATUS. For many years clinicians have been aware of the increased susceptibility to infection of undernourished children. Only recently has that possibility been raised with regard to infants who were undernourished in utero.

Serum immunoglobulin G (IgG) values of SGA infants are appreciably lower than those of AGA infants of the same gestational age (Figure 4–9).[6, 86, 100, 111, 124] The longer the time in utero, the lower the serum IgG value.[86] It has been postulated that the low IgG value reflects poor placental perfusion or poor placental function.[86] In addition, Shapiro et al,[100] studying the complement system of newborn infants, found C3 values to be significantly lower among SGA infants when compared with AGA controls. There were no differences in C4 values or classical pathway and alternate pathway function. The

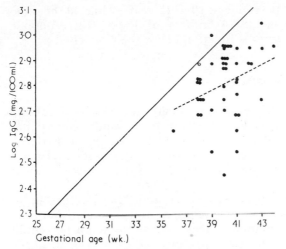

Figure 4–9. A comparison of the log of serum IgG values at various gestational ages among AGA infants (———) and SGA infants (--------). Each circle (●) represents an SGA infant. (From Papadatos et al.[86])

reduced opsonic function of the plasma of SGA infants was attributed, in part at least, to the decreased C3 levels.[18]

The number of peripheral T lymphocytes is decreased in SGA infants, as are the rosetting T lymphocytes and the lymphocyte proliferation. Cell-mediated immunity in growth-retarded infants is significantly impaired at birth in comparison with term newborns.[18–20] It has been suggested that the low serum thymic hormone activity associated with the impaired cell-mediated immunity in SGA infants indicates the possibility that thymic hypofunction contributes causally to the immunodeficiency. Compared with term infants, SGA newborns have polymorphonuclear leukocytes whose function is impaired with regard to chemotaxis and bactericidal capacity, although the phagocytosis of organisms is not different.

Following birth there tends to be persistence of the immunologic weakness of growth-retarded infants. Chandra[20] found decreased cell-mediated immunity and serum thymic hormone activity to persist for 12 months, and Ferguson[39] demonstrated impairment of cellular immunity in 5 year old children who were SGA at birth.

There are no reports of increased numbers of infections among infants and children who were small for dates; however, there is no indication that studies have been done. At 3 months of age, SGA infants have demonstrated antibody response to tetanus toxoid and *Salmonella typhi* comparable to healthy term infants at that age, but the growth-retarded infants had impaired antibody response to poliovirus vaccine.[18] Polymorphonuclear leukocyte killing of bacteria and chemotaxis were still abnormal.

TWIN TRANSFUSION (PARABIOSIS) SYNDROME. The occurrence of monochorionic twins with grossly disparate size in association with vascular communications in the placenta may produce a type of malnutrition in the small twin. This is referred to as the *twin transfusion* or *parabiosis syndrome*. Aside from differences in weight, length, and head size, there is comparable discrepancy in the size of all organs. The smaller (donor) infant is anemic, while the large (recipient) infant is polycythemic. Naeye[77] found that the anemic member is always on the arterial side of the placental shunt; the plethoric recipient is on the venous side. Often the smaller twin is dead and may present as a fetus papyraceus. The smaller of the pair is small for dates. Peculiarly, hypoglycemia is not prominent among the smaller of these twins—in the usual circumstances in which there is discordance, the smaller tends to be hypoglycemic. Hyperbilirubinemia, probably as a consequence of polycythemia, is common in the recipient twin, who also is prone to develop cardiac failure because of hypervolemia. Hyaline membrane disease is not uncommon and may be found in either twin. In the common occurrence of discordance, the twins are of rather good size (1500 gm or more), whereas with the parabiosis syndrome, the infants tend to be very small and are usually immature. In Shanklin's group of seven such sets of twins, both members of five sets were 815 gm or less; one pair weighed 1270 and 1125 gm, respectively; and one pair weighed 2960 and 2100 gm.[99]

POSTNATAL GROWTH. Among SGA infants, postnatal growth varies according to the duration of the intrauterine problem that caused the stunting. Of all categories of infants, those who are very small and symmetrically growth retarded have the lowest growth velocity at all times during the first year of life.[26]

So-called dysmature or asymmetric SGA infants tend not to lose weight in the first days of life, nor do they gain. After a period of weight stability inversely related to their gestational age, they gain weight rather rapidly, and most of them are not different from their appropriately grown gestational age peers at 3 months.[118] On the other hand, symmetric SGA infants who are undergrown with respect to height, weight, and head circumference tend not to catch up in any parameter. In one large study, 92 per cent of such infants were in the fiftieth percentile or below in all parameters at 4 to 6 years.[43] If catching up has not occurred by 3 years of age, the child will remain small.[33, 43] It is noteworthy that the SGA infants who fail to catch up tend to have serious congenital anomalies.[122]

INTELLIGENCE. The possibility of permanent impairment of brain function has been suggested, since head growth retardation is associated with poor brain development and there is often subsequent failure to catch up postnatally. This concept is supported by studies that relate low IQ not only to SGA infants with known syndromes of malformations but also to a large percentage of low-birth-weight infants of 37 weeks' or more gestation.[21, 107] In New South Wales nearly 15 per cent of 1345 mentally retarded patients with intelligence quotients of 50 or below were small for gestational age at birth.[21]

On the other hand, a careful long-term study of girls who at birth were small in height, weight, and head circumference failed to indicate a significant handicap in mental development, regardless of whether or not head catch-up growth had occurred.[8]

The failure to characterize the intrauterine growth retardation of study subjects has caused otherwise carefully done follow-up investigations to yield confusing and conflicting results. From properly done reports, it appears that fetal growth retardation with head involvement (symmetric type) results in neurologic deficits whose severity is inversely related to the duration of pregnancy prior to the onset of abnormal head growth—that is, the earlier the appearance of head growth retardation, the greater the neurobehavioral problem.[36, 51, 88]

The long-term morbidity includes problems in the areas of cognition, language, hearing, motor function, attention, and behavior. A careful 2 year prospective study of 71 preterm small-for-dates infants indicates the severity of neurodevelopmental handicap to be related to the asphyxia suffered rather than to the degree of intrauterine growth retardation.[23]

Finally, Drillien[32] has shown that SGA infants born into high socioeconomic group families do as well as or better than their peers at age 10 to 12 years, while, at the same age, SGA infants of lower socioeconomic groups function below their matched peers.

MORTALITY

The risk of death for newborn infants according to their birth weight–gestational age relationship is shown in Figure 4–10. In general, the mortality rate for any given gestational age group increases as birth weight decreases. This is most evident among infants between 26 and 32 weeks' gestation. Beyond 36 weeks, mortality is related only to the infant's being below the tenth percentile in weight.

The causes of death among SGA infants are related to the type of growth retardation. Asymmetric SGA infants die mainly of asphyxia, aspiration pneumonia and its complications, and persistent fetal circulation. Early onset (symmetrically) growth-retarded infants die of malformations and, because so often they are born early in the third trimester, problems of immaturity.

PRACTICAL HINTS

1. If at all possible, the diagnosis of growth retardation should be anticipated, and delivery should take place at a center with a special high-risk nursery (see Chapter 1).

2. Every neonate requires an immediate

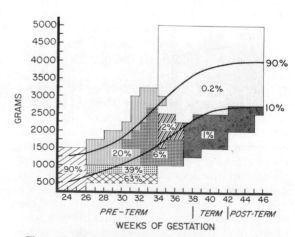

Figure 4–10. Mortality risk according to birth weight–gestational age relationship. Based on 14,413 live births at University of Colorado Health Sciences Center (1974–1980).

assessment for early recognition of any problem. The first step in this process is to classify the baby as mature, immature, or postmature and small for gestational age, appropriate for gestational age, or large for gestational age. From the weight/length ratio (ponderal index), SGA infants should be classified as symmetrically or asymmetrically undergrown.

3. The gestational age calculated from an adequate maternal history of menstrual periods should not be downgraded. Estimates calculated in this fashion should be seriously considered when caring for neonates.

4. A scoring sheet for assessment of gestational age should be part of every newborn infant's record.

5. Infants of the same weight but of various gestational ages may have different obstetric complications and problems in the neonatal period and, as a result, different prognoses.

6. Neonatal asphyxia tends to be more common and accentuated among small-for-dates infants; this is particularly true among underweight infants of normal length at or near term. The problem of poor growth in utero may be recognized by serial measurements of fundal height, fetal biparietal diameter by ultrasound, and maternal urinary estriols. Personnel skilled in resuscitation should be present at the delivery of infants who have recognized intrauterine growth retardation.

7. Symmetrically growth-retarded infants are at greater risk of having a major congenital anomaly than appropriately grown infants and should be followed closely for the detection of hidden genitourinary or cardiovascular anomalies.

8. Neonatal symptomatic hypoglycemia is commonly found (15 per cent) among infants who are asymmetrically small for gestational age. Blood sugar should be closely monitored in these infants (see Chapter 10).

9. Polycythemia is a common finding among asymmetrically undergrown small-for-dates infants. Although usually asymptomatic, they may present with tachypnea, intercostal retractions, grunting, nasal flaring, tachycardia with or without failure, pleural effusion, scrotal edema, and convulsions—all of which can be relieved by reducing the hematocrit. Central hematocrit should be checked and appropriate therapy instituted promptly.

Questions

True or False

The brain is the most severely stunted organ in infants with intrauterine growth retardation secondary to malnutrition.

The brain is usually the least affected organ. Therefore the statement is false.

The intrauterine twin transfusion (parabiosis) syndrome results in twins of unequal size, and the larger will usually be polycythemic. Neither twin is prone to hypoglycemia.

In other instances of twin discordance the smaller twin is often hypoglycemic. The above statement, however, is true.

Although an infant has suffered intrauterine growth retardation secondary to malnutrition, there is no increased risk of developing problems during labor.

Small-for-dates infants of appropriate length for gestational age usually have low levels of liver and cardiac glycogen and are not prepared for the rigors of labor. Although mild to moderate degrees of asphyxia are noted in every infant at birth, it appears to be accentuated in these small for-dates babies. Therefore the statement is false.

Twin pregnancies are unlikely to yield small-for-dates infants if delivery occurs at 30 to 34 weeks' gestation.

There is usually a relative reduction in weight only if the infants are delivered after 35 weeks' gestation. The statement is therefore true.

Neurologic assessment of gestational age of every neonate while still in the delivery room might well afford an opportunity to identify high-risk infants more accurately.

Neurologic assessment is not highly reliable in the first hour of life. The statement is therefore false. The state of wakefulness, hunger, irritability, or effects of maternal sedation may all affect the neurologic examination. When discordance is found between gestational and neurologic age, repeat the examination—further studies may be required.

Small-for dates infants have a higher mortality rate than preterm infants of the same weight who are appropriate in weight for gestational age.

According to Koops et al,[60] at each gestational age SGA infants do less well than AGA infants (Figure 4–10). This phenomenon is more pronounced at less than 34 weeks' gestation.

Small-for-dates infants often have an alert appearance not found in other newborns.

Asymmetrically undergrown small-for-dates infants do appear alert as compared with infants of the same weight or gestational age. Therefore the statement is true.

Small-for-dates infants have low fat stores but a normal amount of brown fat.

Brown fat is also reduced. Therefore these infants have a decreased ability to control their body temperature in a cool environment. The statement is false.

Carbohydrate stores of small-for-dates infants are low, and their oxygen consumption per unit weight is higher than that of AGA preterm infants.

The carbohydrate content of several organs, including the heart, liver, and skeletal muscles, is quite low in SGA infants. In addition, based on their body weight, infants who are small for gestational age have a high oxygen consumption. Therefore the statement is true.[104]

The ratio of fetal to adult hemoglobin synthesis is greater in small-for-dates infants than in normally grown infants.

Usually, as pregnancy progresses, there is a decrease in normal infants in the proportion of fetal to adult hemoglobin. This is not true in small-for-dates infants. The existence of this decrease supports Gruenwald's hypothesis that intrauterine hypoxemia is an important cause of growth retardation,[46] since, in vitro, decreased oxygen tension or glucose concentration results in increased fetal hemoglobin synthesis as compared with adult hemoglobin synthesis.[11] Therefore the statement is true.

Large parents tend to have large babies.

Infants of large parents do tend to be large at birth, and they contribute significantly to the category of large-for-gestational-age neonates. The statement is therefore true.

Gross placental lesions frequently are found in association with growth-retarded infants.

While minute lesions may be of importance, in only a small number of instances do gross lesions of the placenta provide an explanation for the inappropriate growth. Identifiable placental pathologic conditions are not a major etiologic factor. Therefore the statement is false.

Women who smoke cigarettes have a greater than expected frequency of SGA infants. That disadvantage disappears if smoking is discontinued throughout pregnancy.

It is assumed that the effects upon the fetus are due to diminished perfusion, which apparently occurs at the time of cigarette smoking. The statement is true.

Editorial Comment: Cigarette smoking accounts for 21–39 per cent of low-birth-weight infants (< 2500 gm) according to a review reporting in excess of 100,000 deliveries in the U.S., Canada, and Wales. It is perhaps the single most powerful determinant of poor fetal growth in the developed world. The term *fetal tobacco syndrome* has been coined to identify undergrown infants whose mothers smoked > 5 cigarettes per day throughout pregnancy and had no evidence of hypertension or preeclampsia. The fetus has symmetric growth retardation at term, for which there is no other obvious cause.

Nieberg, P., Marks, J. S., McLaren, N. M., et al.: The fetal tobacco syndrome. JAMA *253*:2998, 1985.

SGA infants should be fed early to prevent hypoglycemia.

Because SGA infants usually do not have good hepatic carbohydrate stores, it seems reasonable that the provision of sugar and gluconeogenic amino acids by feedings would be helpful, but this is not always so. Although the sugar is valuable, amino acids do not yield effective gluconeogenesis in all SGA babies. Monitor blood sugar carefully, and treat with intravenous glucose as well as oral feedings. The statement is true.

If SGA infants are going to catch up in growth, it will happen by the end of 6 months after birth.

True, and beware of the ones who remain small—they may have a significant hidden anomaly.

It is important to differentiate between low-birth-weight infants who are small for gestational age and those who are appropriate for gestational age. Check the following statements, marking those that are correct.
  A. *Estimation of bone development by x-ray is a precise measure of gestational age.*
  B. *Maturity of organs correlates better with birth weight than with gestational age.*
  C. *With intrauterine growth retardation, the earlier the onset, the greater the chance of neurobehavioral handicap.*
  D. *Hyperbilirubinemia is a major problem in small-for-gestational-age infants.*

A. Although organ maturation parallels gestational age, delay in the appearance of ossification centers makes radiologic investigation unreliable for estimating gestational age. Therefore the statement is false.
B. Organ maturity correlates best with gestational age. The statement is therefore false.
C. True. Early impairment of growth causes a decrease in production of cells (hyperplastic

growth), an insult that the brain withstands poorly and cannot compensate for. Late onset growth retardation tends to spare the brain.

D. Liver function in SGA infants is similar to that of term infants; thus, hyperbilirubinemia is not a major problem in the absence of blood-group incompatibility or polycythemia. Therefore the statement is false.

Around 8 per cent of all infants with birth weights greater than 2500 gm have gestational ages less than 37 weeks and masquerade as full-term infants.

This statement is true, and these infants should definitely be identified. Often their poor sucking reflex, limpness, and poor temperature control incorrectly suggest to the parents and the physician that they are ill. They are subject to problems of immaturity (hyaline membrane disease, hyperbilirubinemia, poor ability to maintain body temperature, etc.) and must be observed closely in the early hours and days after birth.

CASE PROBLEMS

Case One

A 1600 gm male infant presents with no problems in the delivery room, is 48 cm in length, and has a head circumference of 33 cm and no evidence of physical abnormality. Assessment of gestational age from menstrual history and neurologic examination indicates he was born at 38 weeks' gestation.

The most likely complication in the next 12 hours is (check one):
  A. Hypoglycemia.
  B. Hypocalcemia.
  C. Septicemia.
  D. Apneic episodes.

This patient is small for dates and asymmetrically so; therefore hypoglycemia (blood glucose concentration less than 20 mg/dl) is the most likely complication of those listed to appear in the first 12 hours of life. Therefore the answer is A. Although hypocalcemia might occur, it is very much less likely than hypoglycemia. Septicemia is not a specific problem for small-for-dates infants. Apneic episodes are generally observed in very immature infants.

It is likely that he will (check any that are appropriate):
  A. Lose little if any weight in the first 24 hours of life.
  B. Not reach birth weight for 5 to 10 days after an initial fall in weight.
  C. Gain more slowly than an AGA infant of the same birth weight.
  D. Gain more rapidly than an AGA infant of the same birth weight.

It is likely he will lose little if any weight in the first 24 hours and will gain more rapidly than an AGA infant of the same birth weight. This is true for the first few weeks of life; thereafter the rate of gain most likely will decrease. The answers are A and D.

He has a greater chance than an AGA infant of the same weight of having (check any that are appropriate):
  A. A central hematocrit > 65 per cent.
  B. A serum bilirubin greater than 12 mg/dl.
  C. A congenital anomaly.
  D. Mental retardation evident later in life.

He has a greater chance than an AGA infant of the same weight of having polycythemia and, because of that, of developing hyperbilirubinemia. Congenital malformations, including those of the brain, are problems more likely to occur among symmetrically undergrown SGA infants. Since this infant was asymmetrically growth retarded and asphyxia was not evident at birth, there is no more likelihood for this infant of having mental retardation in later life than for an AGA infant of the same weight. Therefore the answers are A and B.

Case Two

A 1600 gm female infant 47.5 cm long is delivered of a preeclamptic primipara. The infant is cyanotic and poorly responsive to stimuli and ventilates poorly. She is meconium stained and at examination is deemed to be of 37 weeks' gestation. Resuscitation is successful, but grunting respiration, flaring of the alae nasi, intercostal retractions, hyperinflation of the chest, and dusky skin color in room air are present.

The most likely cause of the problem is (check one):
  A. Hyaline membrane disease.
  B. Massive aspiration of meconium.
  C. Hypoglycemia.
  D. Intraventricular hemorrhage.

Among dysmature (asymmetrically undergrown) small-for-dates infants, this clinical picture is usually due to massive aspiration of meconium. Hyaline membrane disease may occur in an infant of 37 weeks' gestation, but it is not the most likely cause of these symptoms. Therefore the answer is B.

It is appropriate to add that this complication has decreased markedly, since the introduction of treatment of aspiration of meconium with deep nasopharyngeal suction while the head is on the perineum, before the infant takes the first breath (see Chapter 8).

L. Lubchenco

The most likely complications are (check any that are appropriate):
  A. Pneumonitis.
  B. Pneumothorax.
  C. Hemorrhagic disease of the newborn.

D. Seizures.
E. Apneic episodes.
F. Jaundice.

The most likely complications are pneumonitis from meconium aspirated with the amniotic fluid and pneumothorax. (Pneumothorax is a common occurrence in infants with meconium aspiration.) Therefore the answers are A and B.

It is necessary immediately to (check any that are appropriate):
A. Obtain an x-ray of the chest.
B. Obtain an x-ray of the skull.

C. Perform a lumbar puncture.
D. Give oxygen.
E. Give glucose.

Every cyanotic, poorly responsive infant requires oxygen. An x-ray of the chest is necessary to verify the lung disease, evaluate its extent, and note the presence or absence of complications. X-ray studies of the skull and examination of cerebrospinal fluid are inappropriate to the problem. Although there is nothing to be gained by the immediate administration of glucose, it is important to make frequent assessment of the blood glucose concentration. Therefore the answers are A and D.

REFERENCES

1. Abernathy, J., Greenberg, B., Wells, H., et al: Smoking as an independent variable in a multiple regression analysis upon birth weight and gestation. Am J Public Health 56:626, 1966.
2. Abramovici, H., Brandes, J. M., and Schramek, A.: Small for gestational age infants in pregnancies following jejunoileal bypass. Int Surg 65:135, 1980.
3. Aherne, W., and Hull, D.: Brown adipose tissue and heat production in the newborn infant. J Pathol Bacteriol 91:223, 1966.
4. Allen, D., and Jandl, J.: Factors influencing relative rates of synthesis of adult and fetal hemoglobin in vitro. J Clin Invest 39:1107, 1960.
5. Amiel-Tison, C.: Neurological evaluation of the maturity of newborn infants. Arch Dis Child 43:89, 1968.
6. Andréasson, B., Svenningsen, N. W., and Nordenfelt, E.: Screening for viral infections in infants with poor intrauterine growth. Acta Paediatr Scand 70:673, 1981.
7. Andrew, G., Chan, G., and Shiff, D.: Lipid metabolism in the neonate. I. The effects of intralipid infusion on plasma triglyceride and free fatty acid concentrations in the neonate. J Pediatr 88:273, 1976.
8. Babson, S., and Henderson, N.: Fetal undergrowth: relation of head growth to later intellectual performance. Pediatrics 53:890, 1974.
9. Bakketeig, L. S., Hoffman, H. J., and Harley, E. E.: The tendency to repeat gestational age and birth weight in successive births. Am J Obstet Gynecol 135:1086, 1979.
10. Ballard, J. L., Novak, K. K., and Driver, M.: A simplified score for assessment of fetal maturation of newly born infants. J Pediatr 95:769, 1979.
11. Bard, H., Makowski, E., Meschia, E., et al: The relative rates of synthesis of hemoglobins A and F in immature red cells of newborn infants. Pediatrics 45:766, 1970.
12. Barlow, P.: The influence of inactive chromosomes on human development. Anomalous sex chromosome complements and the phenotype. Humangenetik 17:105, 1973.
13. Battaglia, F., and Lubchenco, L.: A practical classification of newborn infants by weight and gestational age. J Pediatr 71:159, 1967.
14. Benirschke, K., and Driscoll, S.: *The Pathology of the Human Placenta.* New York, Springer-Verlag New York, Inc., 1967.
15. Bosley, A. R., Sebert, J. R. and Newcombe, R. G.: The effects of maternal smoking on fetal growth and nutrition. Arch Dis Child 56:727, 1981.
16. Brinsmead, M. W., and Thorburn, G. D.: Effect of streptozotocin on fetal lambs in mid-pregnancy. Aust J Biol Sci 35:517, 1982.
17. Castells, S., Mark, E., Abaci, F., et al: Growth retardation in fetal alcohol syndrome. Unresponsiveness to growth-promoting hormones. Dev Pharmacol Ther 3:232, 1982.
18. Chandra, R. K.: Fetal malnutrition and postnatal immunocompetence. Am J Dis Child 129:450, 1975.
19. Chandra, R. K.: Impairment of immunity in children with intrauterine growth retardation. J Pediatr 95:157, 1979.
20. Chandra, R. K.: Serum thymic hormone activity and cell-mediated immunity in healthy neonates, preterm infants and small-for-gestational-age infants. Pediatrics 67:407, 1981.
21. Collins, E., and Turner, G.: The importance of the "small-for-dates" baby to the problem of mental retardation. Med J Aust 2:313, 1971.
22. Colman, H., and Rienzo, J.: The small term baby. Obstet Gynecol 19:87, 1962.
23. Commey, J. O. O., and Fitzhardinge, P. M.: Handicap in the preterm small-for-gestational-age infant. J Pediatr 94:779, 1979.
24. Cooper, L., Green, R., Krugman, S., et al: Neonatal thrombocytopenic purpura and other manifestations of rubella contracted in utero. Am J Dis Child 110:416, 1965.
25. Cornblath, M., Wybregt, S., Baens, G., et al: Symptomatic neonatal hypoglycemia. Studies of carbohydrate metabolism in the newborn infant. VIII. Pediatrics 33:388, 1964.
26. Cruise, M.: A longitudinal study of the growth of low birth weight infants. I. Velocity and distance growth, birth to three years. Pediatrics 51:620, 1973.
27. Dacou-Voutetakis, C., Anagnostakis, D., and Xanthou, M.: Macroglossia, transient neonatal diabetes mellitus and intrauterine growth failure: a new distinct entity? Pediatrics 55:127, 1975.
28. Dadak, C., Kefalides, A., Sinzeringer, H., et al: Reduced umbilical artery prostacycline formation in complicated pregnancies. Am J Obstet Gynecol 144:792, 1982.
29. Davies, D., Gray, O., Ellwood, P., et al: Cigarette

smoking in pregnancy: associations with maternal weight gain and fetal growth. Lancet *1*:385, 1976.

30. Dawes, G.: *Size at Birth*. Ciba Foundation Symposium 27. Amsterdam, Associated Scientific Publishers, 1974, p. 393.

31. De Leeuw, R., and de Vries, I.: Hypoglycemia in small-for-dates newborn infants. Pediatrics *58*:18, 1976.

32. Drillien, C.: Intellectual sequelae of "fetal malnutrition." *In* Waisman, H., and Kerr, G. (eds.): *Fetal Growth and Development*. New York, McGraw-Hill, 1970.

33. Drillien, C.: The small-for-dates infant: etiology and prognosis. Pediatr Clin North Am *17*:9, 1970.

34. Dubowitz, L., Dubowitz, V., and Goldberg, C.: Clinical assessment of gestational age in the newborn infant. J Pediatr *77*:1, 1970.

35. Dunlap, W., Furness, S. C., and Hill, L. M.: Maternal haemoglobin concentration, haematocrit and renal handling of urate in pregnancies ending in the birth of small-for-dates infants. Br J Obstet Gynaecol *85*:938, 1978.

36. Fancourt, R., Campbell, S., Harvey, D. R., et al: Follow-up study of small-for-dates babies. Br Med J *1*:1435, 1976.

37. Farr, V., Kerridge, D., and Mitchell, R.: The value of some external characteristics in the assessment of gestational age at birth. Dev Med Child Neurol *8*:657, 1966.

38. Farr, V., Mitchell, R., Neligan, G., et al.: The definition of some external characteristics used in the assessment of gestational age of the newborn infant. Dev Med Child Neurol *8*:507, 1966.

39. Ferguson, A. C.: Prolonged impairment of cellular immunity in children with intrauterine growth retardation. J Pediatr *93*:52, 1978.

40. Ferguson, A. C., Lawlor, G. J., Jr., Neumann, C. G., et al: Decreased rosette-forming lymphocytes in malnutrition and intrauterine growth retardation. J Pediatr *85*:717, 1974.

41. Finne, P.: Erythropoietin levels in cord blood as an indicator of intrauterine hypoxia. Acta Paediatr Scand *55*:478, 1966.

42. Finne, P.: Erythropoietin production in fetal hypoxia and in anemic uremic patients. Ann NY Acad Sci *149*:497, 1968.

43. Fitzhardinge, P., and Steven, E.: The small-for-date infant. I. Later growth patterns. Pediatrics *49*:671, 1972.

44. Gentz, J. C. H., and Cornblath, M.: Transient diabetes of the newborn. Adv Pediatr *16*:345, 1969.

45. Gerretsen, G., Huisjes, H. J., and Elema, J. D.: Morphological changes of the spiral arteries in the placental bed in relation to pre-eclampsia and fetal growth retardation. Br J Obstet Gynaecol *88*:876, 1981.

46. Gruenwald, P.: Chronic fetal distress and placental insufficiency. Biol Neonate *5*:215, 1963.

47. Gruenwald, P.: Infants of low birth weight among 5,000 deliveries. Pediatrics *34*:157, 1964.

48. Gruenwald, P., Funakawa, H., Mitani, S., et al: Influence of environmental factors in foetal growth in man. Lancet *1*:1026, 1967.

49. Hakanson, D. O., and Oh, W.: Hyperviscosity in the small-for-gestational-age infant. Biol Neonate *37*:109, 1980.

50. Hanson, J., and Smith, D.: The fetal hydantoin syndrome. J Pediatr *87*:285, 1975.

51. Harvey, D., Prince, J., Bunton, J., et al: Abilities of children who were small-for-gestational-age babies. Pediatrics *69*:296, 1982.

52. Haworth, J., Dilling, L., and Younsoszai, M.: Relation of blood glucose to hematocrit, birth weight, and other body measurements in normal and growth-retarded newborn infants. Lancet *2*:901, 1967.

53. Hittner, H. M., Gorman, W. A., and Rudolph, A. J.: Examination of the anterior vascular capsule of the lens. II. Assessment of gestational age in infants small for gestational age. J Pediatr Ophthalmol Strabismus *18*:(Mar-Apr)52, 1981.

54. Hittner, H. M., Hirsch, N. J., and Rudolph, A. J.: Assessment of gestational age by examination of the anterior vascular capsule of the lens. J Pediatr *91*:455, 1977.

55. Humbert, J. R., Abelson, H., Hathway, W. E., et al: Polycythemia in small for gestational age infants. J Pediatr *75*:812, 1969.

56. Jones, K., and Smith, D.: The fetal alcohol syndrome. Teratology *12*:1, 1975.

57. King, C. R., and Lovrien, E. W.: Chorioangioma of the placenta and intrauterine growth failure. J Pediatr *93*:1027, 1978.

58. Koeningsberger, M.: Judgment of fetal age. I. Neurologic evaluation. Pediatr Clin North Am *13*:823, 1966.

59. Koller, O., Sagen, N., Ulstein, M., et al: Fetal growth retardation associated with inadequate hemodilution in otherwise uncomplicated pregnancy. Acta Obstet Gynecol Scand *58*:9, 1979.

60. Koops, B. L., Morgan, L. J., and Battaglia, F. C.: Neonatal mortality risk in relation to birth weight and gestational age: Update. J Pediatr *101*:969, 1982.

61. Kurjak, A., Latin, J., and Polak, J.: Ultrasonic recognition of two types of growth retardation by measurement of four fetal dimensions. J Perinat Med *6*:102, 1978.

62. Lemons, J. A., Ridenour, R., and Orsini, E. N.: Congenital absence of the pancreas and intrauterine growth retardation. Pediatrics *64*:255, 1979.

63. Lin, C. C., Moawad, A. H., Rosenow, P. J., et al: Acid-base characteristics of fetuses with intrauterine growth retardation during labor and delivery. Am J Obstet Gynecol *137*:553, 1980.

64. Little, R. E., Streissguth, A. P., Barr, H. M., et al: Decreased birth weight in infants of alcoholic women who abstained during pregnancy. J Pediatr *96*:974, 1980.

65. Long, P. A., Abell, D. A., and Beischer, N. A.: Fetal growth retardation and pre-eclampsia. Br J Obstet Gynaecol *87*:13, 1980.

66. Low, J., Boston, R., and Pancham, S.: Fetal asphyxia during the intrapartum period in intrauterine growth-retarded infants. Am J Obstet Gynecol *113*:351, 1972.

67. Lubchenco, L., Hansman, C., and Bäckström, L.: Factors influencing fetal growth. *In* Jonxis, J., Visser, H., and Troelstra, J. (eds.): *Nutricia Symposium: Aspects of Prematurity and Dysmaturity*. Springfield, Ill., Charles C Thomas, 1968.

68. Lubchenco, L., Hansman, C., and Boyd, E.: Intrauterine growth in length and head circumference as estimated from live births at gestational ages from 26 to 42 weeks. Pediatrics *37*:403, 1966.

69. Lubchenco, L., Hansman, C., Dressler, M., et al al: Intrauterine growth as estimated from liveborn birth weight data at 24 to 42 weeks of gestation. Pediatrics *32*:793, 1963.

70. Lunell, N. O., Sarby, B., Lewonder, R., et al: Comparison of utero-placental blood flow in normal and in intrauterine growth retarded preg-

nancy. Measurements with indium-113 m and a computer-linked gammacamera. Gynecol Obstet Invest *10*:106, 1980.

71. Manning, F., Wyn Pugh, E., and Boddy, K.: Effect of cigarette smoking on fetal breathing movements in normal pregnancies. Br Med J *1*:552, 1975.

72. Matthews, T. G., and O'Herlihy, C.: Significance of raised immunoglobulin M levels in cord blood of small-for-gestational-age infants. Arch Dis Child *53*:895, 1978.

73. Meberg, A.: High hemoglobin levels and fetal risk during pregnancy. Acta Obstet Gynecol Scand *60*:224, 1981.

74. Mestyan, J., Soltèsz, G., Schultz, K., et al: Hyperaminoacidemia due to the accumulation of glycogenic amino acid precursors in hypoglycemic small-for-gestational-age infants. J Pediatr *87*:409, 1975.

75. Meyer, M., and Tonascia, J.: Maternal smoking: Pregnancy complications and perinatal mortality. Am J Obstet Gynecol *128*:494, 1977.

76. Moore, L. G., Rounds, S. S., Jahnigen, D., et al: Infant birth weight is related to maternal arterial oxygenation at high altitude. J Appl Physiol *52*:695, 1982.

77. Naeye, R.: Human intrauterine parabiotic syndrome and its complications. N Engl J Med *268*:804, 1963.

78. Naeye, R.: Abnormalities in infants of mothers with toxemia of pregnancy. Am J Obstet Gynecol *95*:276, 1966.

79. Naeye, R.: Fetal growth with congenital syphilis: a quantitative study. Am J Clin Pathol *55*:228, 1971.

80. Naeye, R., Benirschke, K., Hagstrom, J., et al: Intrauterine growth of twins as estimated from live-born birth-weight data. Pediatrics *37*:409, 1966.

81. Naeye, R., Diener, W., Dellinger, W., et al: Urban poverty: effects on prenatal nutrition. Science *166*:1026, 1969.

82. Olegard, R., Gustafson, A., Kjellmer, I., et al: Nutrition in low-birth-weight infants. III. Lipolysis and free fatty acid elimination after intravenous administration of fat emulsion. Acta Paediatr Scand *64*:745, 1975.

83. Ounsted, M., and Scott, A.: Social class and birthweight: a new look. Early Hum Dev *6*:83, 1982.

84. Ounsted, M., Moar, V., and Scott, W. A.: Perinatal morbidity and mortality in small-for-dates babies: the relative importance of some maternal factors. Early Hum Dev *5*:367, 1981.

85. Palmer, H., Ovellette, E., Warner, L., et al: Congenital malformations in offspring of a chronic alcoholic mother. Pediatrics *53*:490, 1974.

86. Papadatos, C., Papaevangelou, G. J., Alexiou, D., et al: Serum immunoglobulin G levels in small-for-dates newborn babies. Arch Dis Child *45*:570, 1970.

87. Papoz, L., Eschwege, E., Pequignot, G., et al: Maternal smoking and birth weight in relation to dietary habits. Am J Obstet Gynecol *142*:870, 1982.

88. Parkinson, C. E., Wallis, S., and Harvey, D.: School achievement and behavior of children who were small-for-dates at birth. Dev Med Child Neurol *23*:41, 1981.

89. Polani, P.: Chromosomal and other genetic influences on birth weight. *Size at Birth*. Ciba Foundation Symposium 27. Amsterdam, Associated Scientific Publishers, 1974.

90. Pratt, O. E.: Sex, alcohol and the developing fetus. Br Med Bull *38*:48, 1982.

91. Primhak, R. A., and Simpson, R. M.: Screening small for gestational age babies for congenital infection. Clin Pediatr *21*:417, 1982.

92. Public Health Service: *The Health Consequences of Smoking: A Report of the Surgeon General, 1973*. DHEW Publication No. (HSM) 73–8704. Dept. of Health, Education, and Welfare, 1973.

93. Qazi, Q., and Masakawa, A.: Altered sex ratio in fetal alcohol syndrome. Lancet *2*:42, 1976.

94. Reisman, L.: Chromosome abnormalities and intrauterine growth retardation. Pediatr Clin North Am *17*:101, 1970.

95. Remington, J., and Desmonts, G.: Toxoplasmosis. *In* Remington, J., and Klein, J. (eds.): *Infectious Diseases of the Fetus and Newborn*. Philadelphia, W. B. Saunders Co., 1976.

96. Report of the Committee on Environmental Hazards of the American Academy of Pediatrics: Effects of cigarette smoking on the fetus and child. Pediatrics *57*:411, 1976.

97. Rolschau, J.: Infarctions and intervillous thrombosis in placentas, and their association with intrauterine growth retardation. Acta Obstet Gynecol Scand Suppl *72*:22, 1978.

98. Saint-Anne Dargassies, S.: The full term newborn; neurological assessment. Biol Neonate *4*:174, 1962.

99. Shanklin, D.: The influence of placental lesions on the newborn infant. Pediatr Clin North Am *17*:25, 1970.

100. Shapiro, R., Beatty, D. W., Woods, D. L., et al: Serum complement and immunoglobulin values in small-for-gestational-age infants. J Pediatr *99*:139, 1981.

101. Shelley, H.: Carbohydrate reserves in the newborn infant. Br Med J *1*:273, 1964.

102. Sheppard, B. L., and Bonnar, J.: An ultrastructural study of utero-placental spiral arteries in hypertensive and normotensive pregnancy and fetal growth retardation. Br J Obstet Gynaecol *88*:695, 1981.

103. Sinclair, J.: Heat production and thermoregulation in the small-for-date infant. Pediatr Clin North Am *17*:147, 1970.

104. Sinclair, J., and Silverman, W.: Intrauterine growth in active tissue mass of the human fetus, with particular reference to the undergrown baby. Pediatrics *38*-48, 1966.

105. Smith, A., and McKeown, T.: Prenatal growth of mongoloid defectives. Arch Dis Child *30*:257, 1955.

106. Smith, C.: Effects of maternal undernutrition upon the newborn infants in Holland (1944–1945). J Pediatr *30*:229, 1947.

107. Stock, M., and Smythe, P.: Does undernutrition during infancy inhibit brain growth and subsequent intellectual development? Arch Dis Child *38*:546, 1963.

108. Sweet, A. Y.: Narcotic withdrawal syndrome in the newborn. Pediatr Rev *3*:285, 1982.

109. Thorburn, J., Drummond, M. M., Whigham, K. A., et al: Blood viscosity and haemostatic factors in late pregnancy, pre-eclampsia and fetal growth retardation. Br J Obstet Gynaecol *89*:117, 1982.

110. Tsang, R., Gigger, M., Oh, W., et al: Studies in calcium metabolism in infants with intrauterine growth retardation. J Pediatr *86*:936, 1975.

111. Ueda, H., Naganishi, A., and Ichijo, M.: Immunoglobulins in newborns, particularly in term SFD infants. Tohoku J Exp Med *132*:31, 1980.

112. Ulleland, C.: The offspring of alcoholic mothers. Ann NY Acad Sci *197*:167, 1972.

113. Usher, R.: Clinical and therapeutic aspects of fetal malnutrition. Pediatr Clin North Am 17:169, 1970.

114. Usher, R., and Ling, J.: Blood volume of the newborn premature infant. Acta Paediatr Scand 54:419, 1965.

115. Usher, R., and McLean, F.: Intrauterine growth of liveborn Caucasian infants at sea level: standards obtained in 7 dimensions of infants born between 25 and 44 weeks of gestation. J Pediatr 74:901, 1969.

116. Usher, R., McLean, F., and Scott, K.: Judgment of fetal age. II. Clinical significance of gestational age and an objective method for its assessment. Pediatr Clin North Am 13:835, 1966.

117. Van den Berg, B., and Yerushalmy, J.: The statistical approach to fetal growth. In Waisman, H., and Kerr, G. (eds.): Fetal Growth and Development. New York, McGraw-Hill, 1970.

118. Villar, J., Belizan, J. M., Spalding, J., et al: Postnatal growth of intrauterine growth retarded infants. Early Hum Dev 6:265, 1982.

119. Walther, F. J., and Ramaekers, L. H.: Neonatal morbidity of SGA infants in relation to their nutritional status at birth. Acta Paediatr Scand 71:437, 1982.

120. Warkany, J., Monroe, B., and Sutherland, B.: Intrauterine growth retardation. Am J Dis Child 102:249, 1961.

121. Williams, P., Fisher, R., Jr., Sperling, M., et al: Effects of oral alanine on blood glucose and insulin concentrations in small-for-gestational-age infants. N Engl J Med 292:612, 1975.

122. Wilson, M., Meyers, H., and Peters, A.: Postnatal bone growth of infants with fetal growth retardation. Pediatrics 40:213, 1967.

123. Winick, M.: Cellular growth of the human placenta. III. Intrauterine growth failure. J Pediatr 71:390, 1967.

124. Yeung, C. Y., and Hobbs, J. R.: Serum γ G-globulin levels in normal, premature, post-mature, and "small-for dates" newborn babies. Lancet 1:1167, 1968.

125. Yoshida, T., Metcoff, J., Morales M., et al. Human fetal growth retardation. II. Energy metabolism in leukocytes. Pediatrics 50:559, 1972.

126. Zackai, E., Mellman, W., Neiderer, B., et al.: The fetal trimethadione syndrome. J Pediatr 87:280, 1975.

5

The Physical Environment

MARSHALL H. KLAUS
AVROY A. FANAROFF
RICHARD J. MARTIN

The foetus was no larger than the palm of his hand, but the father ... put his son in an oven, suitably arranged ... making him take on the necessary increase of growth, by the uniformity of the external heat, measured accurately in the degrees of a thermometer.

LAURENCE STERNE
TRISTRAM SHANDY

Animal studies reveal that apparently minor changes in the environment may result in profound temporary or permanent developmental alterations in the organism. These studies suggest that the entire physical environment of the immature infant must be thoroughly explored.

The low-birth-weight infant is particularly dependent on the physician to provide the ideal "external milieu" in order to ensure optimal neurologic and physical development, not mere survival. Inasmuch as the ideal amounts of light, sound, cutaneous stimulation, humidity, and temperature at different ages are at present unknown, this is not a simple task.

In this chapter, the multiple aspects of the physical environment are considered.

THE THERMAL ENVIRONMENT

History

An understanding of the thermal requirements of the high-risk infant was slow to

develop. Pierre Budin,[10] historically the first neonatologist, had perhaps the earliest insight into the clinical importance of the thermal environment. In 1907, in his book *The Nursling*, he emphasized the need for temperature control, after noting a markedly increased survival rate when the infant's rectal temperature was maintained (Table 5–1). He recommended an air temperature of 30° C (86° F) for the small (1 kg), fully clothed infant. Sadly, his observations were neither fully understood nor appreciated in the first 50 years of this century.

Blackfan and Yaglou,[7] working between 1926 and 1933 with a group of infants fully clothed and weighing between 1360 and 2270 gm, observed that high relative humidity and an air temperature of about 25° C (77° F) were required to maintain equilibrium of body temperature. When comparable groups of infants were placed in a slightly higher thermal environment with a lower relative humidity, they noted wider fluctuations in temperature, an increase in weight gain, and an increased mortality.

Although their observations became the basis of care (and gospel), several significant but unstudied changes were made in the infants' environment during the next 29 years. Not only the humidity but also the particulate water was increased to such an extent that infants in incubators were often not visible. In the late 1940s, to improve observation, the infant was undressed and left nude without increasing the incubator temperature. In retrospect, the clinical value

96

TABLE 5–1 INFANT'S TEMPERATURE AND SURVIVAL RATE

32.5–33.5° C	10%
36.0–37.0° C	77%

of the two variables, temperature and humidity, was confused during these years.

The relative importance of incubator temperature and relative humidity was finally resolved by Silverman et al in three sequential analyses, the design of which has become a model for further studies of the neonate.[46, 47, 48] In the first study, they compared high and low humidity in two groups of infants. Infants in the high humidity group had a lower mortality but higher rectal temperatures. In the second study, to end the confusion caused by two variables, they controlled the humidity and examined the effect of varying environmental temperature. They noted a striking difference in survival rates. With only a 4° F increase in incubator temperature (from 85 to 89° F), they observed a 15 per cent increase in survival at the higher temperature (68.1 per cent vs. 83.5 per cent), with the biggest difference appearing in the smallest infants.

In a further study, controlling environmental temperatures but varying humidity caused no difference in survival.

About the same time, Cross et al,[13] working in England, observed a drop in oxygen consumption in normal full-term infants when they were placed in a low-oxygen environment (15 per cent) and suggested that this might explain the unusual ability of newborn mammals to survive prolonged periods of asphyxia. As a defense against asphyxia, oxygen consumption would be reduced. However, the infants breathing 15 per cent oxygen had lower body temperatures.

Hill,[30] working in Cross's laboratory with kittens and guinea pigs, in part clarified the exciting studies of Cross and explained the profound effects of environmental temperature on survival observed by Silverman. She found that, in 20 per cent oxygen, oxygen consumption and rectal temperatures varied with the environmental temperature (Figure 5–1). She noted *a set of thermal conditions at which heat production (measured as oxygen consumption) is minimal yet core temperature is within the normal range (neutral thermal environment).* When the animals were cooled while breathing room air, their oxygen consumption

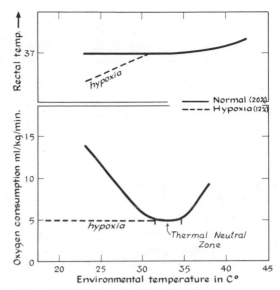

Figure 5–1. Effect of environmental temperature on oxygen consumption, breathing air or a hypoxic mixture.

markedly increased and body temperature was maintained. However, when they were given 12 per cent oxygen and cooled, oxygen consumption did not increase, and the animals' body temperatures dropped. This, as well as the work of Bruck[8] and others, has emphasized that the human infant is a homeotherm and not a poikilotherm, as is a turtle. When the infant is cooled and not hypoxic, he attempts to maintain body temperature by increasing the consumption of calories and oxygen to produce additional heat. Homeotherms possess mechanisms that enable them to maintain body temperature at a constant level more or less accurately despite changes in the environmental temperature. In contrast, the turtle drops its body temperature if placed in a cool environment.

The increased survival rate in the warmer environment observed by Budin and Silverman presumably resulted from the decreased oxygen consumption and carbon dioxide production as environmental conditions approximated the neutral thermal environment. *An immature infant with a minimal ability to transfer oxygen and excrete carbon dioxide across his lungs has the least chance of becoming hypoxic or developing a respiratory acidosis—increased $PaCO_2$—if maintained in an environment that minimizes oxygen consumption or metabolic rate.*

These observations became the stimulus for intense study of temperature control. The physiologic and clinical highlights of these investigations are summarized in the next section.

As pointed out by Dr. William Silverman in 1964, the presumption that neutral thermal conditions contribute to infant survival remains unproved.

Silverman, W.: Diagnosis and treatment: use and misuse of temperature and humidity in care of the newborn infant. Pediatrics 33:276, 1964.

P. Perlstein

Physiologic Considerations

Heat Production

The heat production within the body is a by-product of metabolic processes and must equal the heat that flows from the surface of the infant's body and the warm air from the lungs over a given period of time if the mean body temperature is to remain constant. A characteristic of the homeothermic infant is the ability to produce extra heat in a cool environment. In the adult, additional heat production can come from (1) voluntary muscle activity, (2) involuntary tonic or rhythmic muscle activity (at high intensities, characterized by a visible tremor known as "shivering"), and (3) nonshivering thermogenesis. The latter is a cold-induced increase in oxygen consumption and heat production, which is not blocked by curare, a drug that prevents muscle movements and shivering. *In the adult, shivering is quantitatively the most significant involuntary mechanism of regulating heat production, while in the infant, nonshivering thermogenesis is probably most important.* From animal and human studies it can be inferred that, in the human infant, the thermogenic effector organ—brown fat—contributes the largest percentage of nonshivering thermogenesis.

More abundant in the newborn than in the adult, brown fat accounts for about 2 to 6 per cent of total body weight in the human infant. Sheets of brown fat may be found at the nape of the neck, between the scapulae, in the mediastinum, and surrounding the kidneys and adrenals. Brown fat differs both morphologically and metabolically from the more abundant white fat. The cells are rich in mitochondria and contain numerous fat vacuoles (as compared with the single vacuoles in white fat). There is also an abundant blood and sympathetic nerve supply. Its metabolism is stimulated by norepinephrine released through sympathetic innervation, resulting in triglyceride hydrolysis to free fatty acids and glycerol.[17] Infusion of norepinephrine in the infant results in a marked increase in O_2 consumption without any appreciable increase in physical activity. During cold exposure of the human infant, the nape of the neck, which contains brown fat, is warmer than the rest of the skin.[49] The contribution of brown fat to extra heat production in the infant animal varies with the species.

Despite considerable enquiry, the precise mechanisms whereby the brown adipose tissue mitochondria release the chemical energy in fatty acids as heat are still not known. Also, the mechanisms that control the growth and the thermogenic performance of the tissue in the newborn period are not understood. Evidence suggests that the thermogenic capacity begins to decline soon after birth and that in the preterm infant it does not reach the performance level it might have achieved if intrauterine development had not been interrupted.

D. Hull

Heat Loss

Heat transfer within the body or loss to the environment can be divided into two types: (1) from within the body to the surface of the body (internal gradient), and (2) from the body surface to the environment (external gradient).

A third pathway must be considered today—that is, (3) from within the body into the cold gas stream introduced by a thoughtlessly managed respirator.

P. Perlstein

The physiologic control mechanisms of the infant may alter the internal gradient (i.e., vasomotor) to change skin blood flow. The external gradient is of a purely physical nature. Both the large surface/volume ratio of the infant (especially those below 2 kg) in relation to the adult and the thin layer of subcutaneous fat increase the heat transfer in the internal gradient.

The heat transfer from the surface of the body to the environment involves four means of loss: (1) by radiation, (2) by conduction, (3) by convection, and (4) by the evaporation of water. This heat transfer is complex, and the contribution of each component depends on the temperature of the surroundings (air and walls), air speed, and water vapor pressure. Of special clinical importance to the pediatrician is the considerable increase in radiant heat loss from the infant's skin to the cold walls of incubators. This is of major significance when the infant is nude and the incubator has only a single plastic wall. In this situation, the room temperature may have a major effect on the temperature of the inside wall of the incubator.

Radiant heat loss is related to the temperature of the surrounding surfaces, not air temperature. It is good to remember that when incubators are in cool surroundings—for example, during transfer—the inner surface temperature of the incubator will fall well below that of the air temperature in the incubator. In caring for the infant, this problem is easily solved by wrapping him in a light covering (transparent if necessary). The surrounding radiant temperature would then be close to body temperature and more under the influence of the incubator air temperature. **D. Hull**

The relative contributions of the various modes of heat loss are illustrated in Figure 5–2, under neutral thermal conditions (incubator wall warmed, minimal radiant losses) according to birth weight in the first week of life. The relative increase in evaporative heat loss in the very low-birth-weight infants may be related to increased permeability of the skin.[38]

The effect of environmental temperature on heat production (oxygen consumption) is considered in Figure 5–3. As the environmental temperature is decreased below point A (critical temperature), oxygen consumption increases. Body temperature, however, is maintained if heat production is adequate.

If cooling is severe and body temperature drops below point B, with cold paralysis of the temperature regulation center, oxygen consumption also drops—two to three times for every 10° fall in body temperature.

Homeothermy can also be abolished by hypoxia, sedative drugs, brain injury, polycythemia, and who knows what else. So not all babies are homeotherms all the time. Since babies are variable in their ability to make heat, good thermal protection of such babies can only be defined using variable terms. The real world *is* frustrating! **P. Perlstein**

From Figure 5–3 it can be seen that oxygen consumption is minimal in two areas: the neutral thermal environment and severe hypothermia. The cardiac surgeon works in the

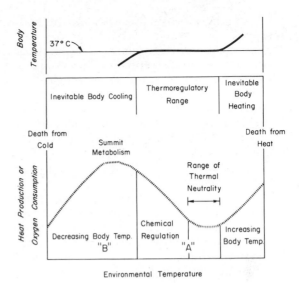

Figure 5–3. Effect of environmental temperature on oxygen consumption and body temperature. (Adapted from Merenstein and Blackmon.[37])

latter (temperatures below point B); the neonatologist attempts to maintain the infant in a warm environment (the neutral thermal environment, or the so-called zone of thermal comfort). *It is most important clinically to note that the infant may not be in a neutral thermal environment and yet the rectal temperature may be in the normal range.* As emphasized by Hey and Katz,[25] ". . . body temperature alone fails to indicate whether a baby is subjected to thermal stress: it can only alert us to situations in which the thermal stress has been so severe that the baby's normal thermoregulatory mechanisms have been at least partially overpowered." When the infant is in an environment above the neutral thermal zone, hyperthermia rapidly occurs.

It is important to realize that rectal temperature only drops when the baby's maximum effort to preserve and produce heat fails. The first mechanism to preserve heat is vasoconstriction, and this phenomenon can easily be detected by measuring skin temperature at a peripheral part of the body. A sensitive method to detect vasoconstriction is to measure both rectal and sole of the foot temperatures. (See p. 106.) **A. Okken**

Hyperthermia develops more rapidly in the neonate than in the adult. The infant has a lower capacity for heat storage because of the higher temperature of the body shell in relation to the environment and the larger surface/volume ratio. This is analogous to a warm pancake on a cold Sunday morning. Thus, the thermoregulatory system of the homeothermic infant adjusts and balances heat production, skin blood flow, sweating,

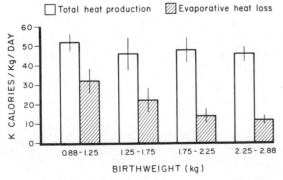

Figure 5–2. The relative role of evaporative heat loss at different birth weights.[38]

and respiration in such a way that the body temperature remains constant within a control range of environmental temperatures. The control range refers to the range of environmental temperatures at which body temperature can be kept constant by means of regulation. The control range of the infant is more limited than that of the adult because of less insulation. For the nude human adult, the lower limit of the control range is 0° C (32° F), while for the full-term infant it is 20–23° C (68–73.4° F).

It is necessary to note here that the insufficient stability of body temperature in the small premature infant does not indicate an immaturity of temperature regulation, for the system is intact. As pointed out by Bruck,[9] the insufficient stability "seems to be due to the discrepancy between efficiency of the effector systems and body size." The newborn infant has a well-developed temperature regulation but a narrower control range than the adult.

Reports and speculations on the ambient temperature range of thermoregulatory control by physiologic mechanisms cause me to reflect upon the newborn hamster. It, apparently, can neither increase its rate of heat production nor its rate of heat loss, but it does display the phenomenon of "thermotaxis." It drags itself to a comfortably warm spot!

Human infants certainly make postural adjustments to ambient temperature changes, and when I see a preterm infant apparently tugging at the restraining tubes and monitor lines and thrashing his way to a corner of his incubator, I often wonder if he is trying to say something to his attendants! Certainly we rely far more on behavioral than physiologic "thermoregulation"—we change our clothing, move out of draughts, switch heaters on and off—and we make sure we do not shiver or sweat unduly. Given the chance, these are the kinds of adjustments a mother would like to make for her baby.   **D. Hull**

In Utero

While in utero, the heat produced by the fetus is dissipated through the placenta to the mother. Normally, the core temperature of the fetus is higher than that of the mother. This system works well for the fetus except during periods when the mother has an increasing body temperature. During these febrile periods, the fetus's temperature will be raised even higher than the mother's temperature.[1]

After Birth

At birth, the infant's core temperature drops rapidly, owing mainly to evaporation from his moist body. The infant's small amount of subcutaneous tissue and large surface area/mass ratio compared with the adult, together with the cold air and walls of the delivery room, also result in large radiant and convective heat losses. Thus, under the usual delivery room conditions, deep body temperature of human newborns can fall 2–3° C unless special precautions are taken.

Small sick infants are at the highest risk of getting cold because of the heat loss mechanisms cited. But these infants also are more subject to central heat loss via a more direct route than the core to skin, skin to environment path. It must be recognized that the CO_2 that is removed by forcing cold oxygen in and out of the lungs is *warm* CO_2. In the act of resuscitation one can rapidly convert a warm, hypoxic, and therefore poikilothermic neonate with a profound respiratory acidosis into a cold, well-oxygenated homeotherm with just as profound metabolic acidosis.   **P. Perlstein**

Although moderate to severe cooling may result in metabolic acidosis, a lower arterial oxygen level, and hypoglycemia in the newborn infant, very slight cooling of the infant may be beneficial in his adaptation to extrauterine life. Cooling of the skin receptors may play a significant role in initiating respiration while probably stimulating thyroid function. The vasoconstriction and peripheral resistance observed with mild cooling also alter systemic vascular resistance, thereby reducing the right-to-left shunting of blood through the ductus arteriosus. With severe cooling a vicious circle can result in severe hypoxia and even death (Figure 5–4).

Despite the possible advantages of cooling, the neonatologist has chosen to keep the infant warm following delivery to prevent metabolic acidosis and possibly dangerous reflex responses to cooling. Many devices are now available that allow the newborn infant to be in a warm environment while still in

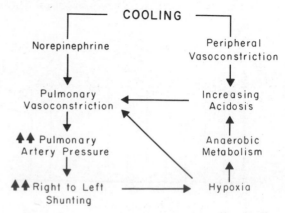

Figure 5–4. The vicious circle resulting from cooling in the neonate.

the delivery room, although the mother and obstetrician are cool.

Nutrition and Temperature

As a result of the relationship between metabolic rate and body temperature, both fluid and nutritional requirements for growth are intimately linked with temperature regulation. This is especially important to the small premature infant maintained in a slightly cool environment. His caloric intake is limited by the small capacity of his stomach. Fewer calories would be required for maintenance of body temperature if he were in a warmer environment; thus, in the neutral thermal environment, caloric intake can be more effectively utilized for growth.

The insensible loss of water parallels the metabolic rate, with 25 per cent of total heat produced being dissipated in this manner. Thus, an elevated metabolic rate results in elevated fluid losses and, hence, increased fluid requirements.

The neutral thermal temperature allows for smaller feedings and reduced caloric requirements for growth.

Glass et al[22] were able to quantitate the effect of temperature control on growth, comparing 12 matched, healthy, small infants aged 1 week and weighing between 1 and 2 kg. These infants were divided into a "warm" group (abdominal skin temperature maintained at 36.5° C [97.7°]) and a "standard" group (abdominal skin temperature maintained at 35° C [95° F]). Both groups received 120 kcal/kg/day. Those in the warm group showed a significantly more rapid increase in body weight and length; however, their cold resistance (ability to prevent a fall in deep body temperature in a cool environment) was diminished. Identical growth rates could be obtained by increasing caloric input in the standard group.

It is therefore difficult to decide if the premature infant, after the early neonatal period, should be maintained in the neutral thermal environment for optimal growth or be prepared for the rigors of a cold apartment.

Practical Applications

Delivery Room

Unfortunately, the temperature of the delivery room is frequently set for the comfort of the medical staff rather than for that of the newborn. Careful and immediate drying of the infant's entire body remains critical in minimizing evaporative heat loss. Many pieces of equipment are available to warm the infant—in particular, incubators and radiant warmers. However, the warm body of the mother is also suited to meet this need. It has been shown that if the dried infant, covered by a blanket, is cuddled by his mother, the temperature drop is similar to that when the infant is exposed to a standard heating unit.[41]

Heating in the Nursery

Although patting an infant dry helps diminish heat loss, it is not as effective as covering the infant with swaddling, which serves as a vapor barrier. Whether the material is cotton, wool, or aluminized Mylar makes little difference as long as the infant's undryable head of considerable surface area is included in the swaddle.

When the babe is born, immediate care
Includes the drying of body parts bare.
But the furry parts on the brand new heir
Also need swaddle, so cover the hair!

P. Perlstein

Maintenance of an infant in the neutral thermal environment minimizes heat production, oxygen consumption, and nutritional requirements for growth. Unfortunately, the equipment (usually incubators) presently available is not easily adjusted to maintain an infant in the neutral thermal environment.

INCUBATORS. In the United States, the most commonly used heating device for the nude infant is an incubator with a single plastic wall.[21] The infant is heated by convection. Because the temperature of the plastic walls cannot be controlled, the radiant heat loss of the infant to the wall of the incubator is variable. Figure 5–5 indicates how the

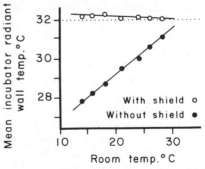

Figure 5–5. The effect of using a heat shield (see Figure 5–7) on the mean incubator wall radiant temperature at varying room temperatures.

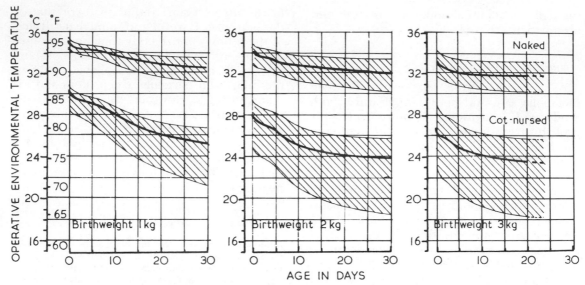

Figure 5–6. The range of temperature to provide neutral environmental conditions for a baby lying either dressed in a cot or naked on a warm mattress in draught-free surroundings of moderate humidity (50 per cent saturation) when mean radiant temperature is the same as air temperature. The hatched area shows the neutral temperature range for healthy babies weighing 1 kg, 2 kg, or 3 kg at birth. *Approximately 1° C should be added to these operative temperatures to derive the appropriate neutral air temperature for a single-walled incubator when room temperature is less than 27° C (80° F) and rather more if room temperature is very much less than this.*[25]

temperature of the inner wall of the incubator drops with cooler room temperatures—a major disadvantage when nursing a sick infant. If the nursery is cool (23.8 to 15.6° C, or 75 to 60° F) or if the incubator is placed near a cool window or wall, it will be difficult—usually impossible—to locate and maintain the neutral thermal environment. The infant will lose heat to the cold incubator wall and will needlessly increase oxygen and caloric consumption in his efforts to stay warm. The magnitude of this loss can be predicted if room temperature is known. Hey and Katz[25] found that operative temperature (true environmental temperature, taking into account radiation and convection) fell 1° below incubator temperature for every 7° that incubator air exceeded room temperature (Figure 5–6). Unless the incubator, room air, and radiant surfaces have similar temperatures, innumerable thermal conditions can exist.

Different types of adaptations will prevent radiant heat loss and allow a precise and controlled thermal environment.

One method is to warm the nude infant with warm air and heated incubator walls (using either a layer of warm water or electrically conductive plastic paneling).[28]

These expensive procedures have been obviated by Hey, who has developed a small clear plastic heat shield to be used within the traditional single-walled incubator (Figure 5–7). The warm incubator air heats the plastic wall of the shield to the same temperature as the air within the incubator. The infant radiates only to the warm inner plastic shield, since radiant waves from the infant (2–9 microns) will not penetrate the plastic wall.

When the thermal conditions can be described and controlled, the neutral thermal environment for any nude infant can easily be located by using the studies of Scopes and Ahmed.[44] Generally, the thinner, smaller, and younger the infant, the higher the environmental temperature required to achieve the neutral thermal environment.[24, 26]

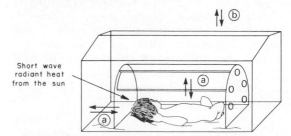

Figure 5–7. The inner heat shield provides warm inner walls to minimize radiant heat loss in a cool nursery. (a) Long wave radiant exchange between baby and heat shield and between inner wall of incubator and heat shield. (b) Long wave radiant exchange between incubator walls and surroundings.

Table 5–2 and Figure 5–6 are general guides for roughly locating the neutral temperature if the walls of the incubator are warm and within a degree of the incubator air temperature. When estimating neutral temperatures in single-walled incubators, add 1° C to all the temperatures in the table for every 7° that incubator air temperatures exceed room temperature.

If physics, common sense, and commitment to the task are combined, an even easier and more certain method for controlling incubator heating is possible. Since body temperature is only a measure of the balance between heat production and loss, then raising the incubator temperature to *just below* the degree that causes the body temperature to rise above the desired "normal" level will guarantee "neutral" thermal conditions.

P. Perlstein

If an incubator is placed in the sunlight, the short wavelength radiant emission goes through the plastic wall and can overheat the infant, since long wave reradiation through the plastic wall is prevented (the "greenhouse effect") (Figure 5–7).

RADIANT HEATERS. Radiant heat panels placed above the infant without a complete enclosure have been used.[4] Although there is a large increase in insensible water loss with radiant warmers, there is presently a debate on whether minimal rates of oxygen consumption can be achieved by servo controlling the heat panel according to the abdominal skin temperature and maintaining skin temperature between 36.2 and 36.8° C.[35, 55] Darnall et al, comparing radiant warmers with an incubator, found no difference in oxygen consumption, while LeBlanc and Wheldon et al found a significant increase in metabolic rate, of 9 and 20 per cent respectively. Under a radiant warmer, radiant losses are markedly reduced, or there is a net gain, while convective and evaporative losses are markedly increased. Cold infants can be warmed to a normal temperature, and net

TABLE 5–2 NEUTRAL THERMAL ENVIRONMENTAL TEMPERATURES*

Age and Weight	Range of Temperature (°C)	Age and Weight	Range of Temperature (°C)
0–6 hours		72–96 hours	
Under 1200 gm	34.0–35.4	Under 1200 gm	34.0–35.0
1200–1500 gm	33.9–34.4	1200–1500 gm	33.0–34.0
1501–2500 gm	32.8–33.8	1501–2500 gm	31.1–33.2
Over 2500 (and >36 weeks)	32.0–33.8	Over 2500 (and >36 weeks)	29.8–32.8
6–12 hours		4–12 days	
Under 1200 gm	34.0–35.4	Under 1500 gm	33.0–34.0
1200–1500 gm	33.5–34.4	1501–2500 gm	31.0–33.2
1501–2500 gm	32.2–33.8	Over 2500 (and >36 weeks)	
Over 2500 (and >36 weeks)	31.4–33.8	4–5 days	29.5–32.6
12–24 hours		5–6 days	29.4–32.3
Under 1200 gm	34.0–35.4	6–8 days	29.0–32.2
1200–1500 gm	33.3–34.3	8–10 days	29.0–31.8
1501–2500 gm	31.8–33.8	10–12 days	29.0–31.4
Over 2500 (and >36 weeks)	31.0–33.7	12–14 days	
24–36 hours		Under 1500 gm	32.6–34.0
Under 1200 gm	34.0–35.0	1501–2500 gm	31.0–33.2
1200–1500 gm	33.1–34.2	Over 2500 (and >36 weeks)	29.0–30.8
1501–2500 gm	31.6–33.6	2–3 weeks	
Over 2500 (and >36 weeks)	30.7–33.5	Under 1500 gm	32.2–34.0
36–48 hours		1501–2500 gm	30.5–33.0
Under 1200 gm	34.0–35.0	3–4 weeks	
1200–1500 gm	33.0–34.1	Under 1500 gm	31.6–33.6
1501–2500 gm	31.4–33.5	1501–2500 gm	30.0–32.7
Over 2500 (and >36 weeks)	30.5–33.3	4–5 weeks	
48–72 hours		Under 1500 gm	31.2–33.0
Under 1200 gm	34.0–35.0	1501–2500 gm	29.5–32.2
1200–1500 gm	33.0–34.0	5–6 weeks	
1501–2500 gm	31.2–33.4	Under 1500 gm	30.6–32.3
Over 2500 (and >36 weeks)	30.1–33.2	1501–2500 gm	29.0–31.8

*Adapted from Scopes and Ahmed.[44] For his table, Scopes had the walls of the incubator 1° to 2° warmer than the ambient air temperatures.

Generally speaking, the smaller infants in each weight group will require a temperature in the higher portion of the temperature range. Within each time range, the younger the infant, the higher the temperature required.

heat gain can occur. If the infant is covered with a small plastic chamber, insensible water loss will drop by 30 per cent.[57] When the infants are nursed under radiant warmers for more than short time periods, the increased insensible water loss must be considered in their overall management.

COT NURSING. An alternative approach that has been revived and studied in detail by Hey and O'Connell[29] is to care for the infant dressed (cot nursed) rather than naked. In a nude infant, the resistance to heat loss is 1.07 clo units, which is increased by 1.25 units when the infant is dressed in a shirt, diaper, and gown; an additional resistance of 0.61 unit only is added when a flannelette sheet and two layers of cotton blanket are added.

As emphasized by Hey, the major advantage of cot nursing is the larger latitude of safe environmental temperatures. If the incubator temperature drops 2° C, the naked infant must increase heat production by 35 per cent to prevent a fall in deep body temperature, while a 2° C increase would result in the infant's becoming febrile. Similar changes in room temperature would have a negligible effect on the cot-nursed infant. Hey calculated that for the same effects in the cot-nursed infant, the room temperature must fall to 19° C (66.2° F) or rise to 31° C (87.8° F). Lightly dressing the infant will minimize the effects of fluctuation in environmental temperature. Cot nursing is very inexpensive and is clinically useful when close, continuous observation is not required.

HATS. The relatively larger brain of the newborn is a major heat source. (The brain of the infant is 12 per cent of body weight compared with 2 per cent in the adult.) Fascinating studies by Stothers reveal that heat loss from the head is clinically important and can be significantly reduced with a three-layered hat made of wool and gauze.[14, 53] Figure 5–8 illustrates how the neutral thermal range is extended 1° and oxygen consumption reduced in a cool environment when a three-layered hat is worn by a nude 1200 gm infant. A tube gauze hat had no effect. We recommend the use of double-layered hats for all infants in home and hospital who would benefit by a controlled thermal environment.

SERVO CONTROL. A completely different approach to caring for an infant in the neutral thermal environment is to servo the heating device (whether it is a heat panel or

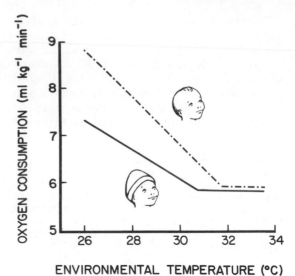

Figure 5–8. The extension of the neutral thermal range and reduction of oxygen consumption in a cool environment with the wearing of a three-layered hat by a nude 1200 gm infant.

incubator) to the infant's abdominal skin temperature. If the infant's skin temperature drops, the warming device increases its heat output. The temperature of the skin at which the incubator is servoed is critical. Silverman's studies showed that maintaining the abdominal skin temperature at 36.5° C (97.7° F) minimizes oxygen consumption; at an abdominal skin temperature of 35.9° C (96.6° F), oxygen consumption increases 10 per cent.[11, 45]

Two disadvantages of servo-controlled equipment are the increased expense and required reorientation of nurses and physicians when evaluating the infant's condition—both the infant and the incubator temperature must be compared together, lest the infant's true condition be masked. When an infant who is servo controlled starts to become febrile, the incubator temperature drops, but there is no change in body temperature. In the other direction, when an infant who is being servo controlled dies, his body temperature will be maintained because the incubator temperature will rise.

Servo control has been further refined by Perlstein et al[39] who developed a computerized system to control the heat input into the incubator. Their system was designed to maintain the infant in a thermoneutral zone, avoid wide temperature fluctuations that might induce apneic episodes, and recognize the point at which an infant can be weaned from the incubator. The use of this system led to a decreased mortality, although the impact of other portions of the computer information on the infant's survival could not be separated from the effect of incubator control.

When we use servo control, it means that we take over control of the infant's body temperature and, despite the infant's biologic and pathologic adjustments, hold the infant's temperature at a predetermined level. I don't think we know enough about thermoregulation in the newborn to know what surface or colonic temperature is desirable or whether or not it should be held constant. Certainly metabolic rates vary widely from one infant to another, even though the infants are of similar age, gestation, and weight and are nursed under similar ambient conditions. Metabolic rates will be influenced by the infants' responses to birth, their general well-being, and their plan of nutrition. Therefore, in all but the critically ill, I prefer to use systems that make the most of the infant's own thermoregulatory efforts by reducing heat losses to a minimum rather than adding extra heat.

D. Hull

Disorders of Temperature Regulation

Hypothermia

Hypothermia should be anticipated in low-birth-weight infants, and the routine use of low-reading thermometers (from 33.8° C, 85° F) is advocated in their care, since temperatures below 34.4° C (94° F) are frequently not immediately detected with the routine clinical thermometers. Hypothermia is seen particularly following resuscitation of asphyxiated premature infants. It may be an early sign of sepsis or evidence of intracranial pathology, such as meningitis, cerebral hemorrhage, or severe central nervous system anomalies.

Although infants may not respond to pyrogens as do older children, the popular myth notwithstanding, I know of no real evidence to conclude that septic babies who *are not in shock* become cold. Central nervous system disease can result in "hyper-" and/or hypothermia. When the controller of the balance between heat production and heat loss blows a fuse, the laws of physics are set free from the governance of physiology.

P. Perlstein

Neonatal Cold Injury

Neonatal cold injury following extreme hypothermia occurs under both warm and cool climatic conditions, particularly with domiciliary maternity services. Low-birth-weight infants are almost exclusively affected, except for full-term infants with problems such as intracerebral hemorrhage and major malformations of the central nervous system.

CLINICAL FEATURES. A slight drop in temperature may produce profound metabolic change;[3] however, a significant drop must occur before clinical features are evident.

The infants feed poorly, are lethargic, and feel cold to the touch. Mann and Elliott[36] describe an "aura" of coldness about the body and skin over the trunk; the periphery feels intensely cold and "corpse-like." Core temperatures will be depressed, often below 32.2° C (90° F).

The most striking feature is the bright red color of the infant. This red color (which may lead the physician astray, since the infant "looks so well") is due to the failure of dissociation of oxyhemoglobin at low temperatures. Central cyanosis or pallor may be present.

Respiration is slow, very shallow, irregular, and often associated with an expiratory grunt. Bradycardia occurs proportionate to the degree of temperature drop.

Activity is lessened. Shivering is rarely observed. The central nervous depression is constant, and reflexes and responses are diminished or absent. Painful stimuli (e.g., injections) produce minimal reaction, and the cry is feeble. Abdominal distension and vomiting are common.

Edema of the extremities and face is common, and sclerema is seen, especially on the cheeks and limbs. (Sclerema is hardening of the skin, associated with reddening and edema. It is observed particularly with cold injury and infection and near the time of death.)

Metabolic derangements include metabolic acidosis, hypoglycemia, hyperkalemia, elevated blood urea nitrogen, and oliguria.[36]

A problem encountered is massive intrapulmonary hemorrhage in association with a generalized bleeding diathesis (a common finding at autopsy).

TREATMENT. The infant should probably be warmed slowly, with the incubator temperature set approximately 1.5° C warmer than abdominal skin temperature, since oxygen consumption has been shown to be minimal when the temperature gradient between body surface and environment is <1.5° C, although the rectal temperature may be subnormal. (Skin temperature should be recorded every 15 minutes.) This part of the traditional mode of management has been challenged by Tafari and Gentz,[54] who saw no beneficial effect in slow versus rapid re-warming of 30 cold-stressed Ethiopian in-fants. The use of a saline push (20 ml/kg) early in the rewarming period, however, did significantly improve mortality.

In addition to the rewarming, oxygen is administered, blood sugar monitored closely, and the metabolic acidosis corrected with sodium bicarbonate as required.

The infant should be fed only by intrave-nous infusion or gavage of dextrose solution until the temperature is 35° C (95° F). Hy-pothermic infants should not be permitted to feed by nipple.

Antibiotics are only administered when in-fection is suspected or documented.

Hyperthermia

Elevation of the deep body temperature may be caused by an excessive environmental temperature, infection, dehydration, or alter-ations of the central mechanisms of heat control associated with cerebral birth trauma or malformations and drugs.

The question of systemic infection is in-variably raised in infants with elevated deep body temperatures. Due consideration should also be given to the environmental conditions that alter heat control. It is not uncommon to find an elevated core temper-ature following the increased heat input with the commencement of the use of bilirubin reduction lights. This can also occur if the incubator is placed in the sun (see Figure 5–7).

A febrile baby overheated by the environment will be vasodilated trying to lose heat, and the infant's extremi-ties and trunk will be at almost the same temperature. A septic baby will usually be vasoconstricted, and the ex-tremities will be colder than the rest of the body. Some-times called the "tummy-toe" gradient, when the feet are more than 2–3° colder than the belly, it's spinal tap time for a febrile neonate.[42]   **P. Perlstein**

Asphyxia

Research continues while arguments rage on the relationship between temperature and birth asphyxia. For many years it was believed that any asphyxiated infant should be main-tained at lower temperatures with a hope of diminishing permanent cerebral sequelae and increasing survival. Some experimental studies of animals cooled before asphyxia began support this view.

With newborn infants, prolonged resusci-tative attempts often are carried out on a damp towel, with precipitous drops in body temperature. Clinically relevant experimen-tal studies in which cooling was begun at the end of or during asphyxia show that a cool environment offers no advantage to the in-fant.

Temperature responses following delivery are sometimes a guide to the state of the infant during delivery.[12] If the infant was severely asphyxiated or hypoxic, temperature control is reflexively turned off, and body temperature is often not maintained imme-diately after delivery.

Resuscitative procedures should be per-formed with due attention to heat control.

1. Evaporative losses may effectively be reduced by immediately drying the infant.

2. Conductive losses can be eliminated by laying the infant on a dry, warm towel or cloth.

3. A radiant source of heat in the form of a radiant warmer will provide a heat-giving environment. This is ideal for resuscitation, since the infant can be maintained nude and is readily accessible. Abdominal skin temper-ature should be maintained.

4. Convection is to be controlled—no drafts in the room—and the oxygen is to be warmed.

And when placing the swaddled infant under the radiant warmer prior to initiating resuscitative measures, just keep saying over and over to yourself:

> When breathing for wee lads or lasses,
> Don't forget to warm the gases.
> And do not forget that fast flow will
> Decrease the heat by its wind chill.
> And don't dry out the son or daughter!
> Give them warm gas with some water.
> Resuscitation is not a trick
> Just make them well, don't make them sick.
> **P. Perlstein**

Apnea

Despite the beneficial effects of maintain-ing a warm environment, a possible disadvan-tage is its effect on respiratory control.

1. Immersing a normal infant in a bath equal to the maternal temperature sometimes stops respiration. Rapid warming is also as-sociated with apneic episodes.

2. Observations in a group of low-birth-weight infants[15] having apneic attacks re-vealed that lowering the servo-controlling temperature less than 1° C significantly re-duced the number of episodes.

We suggest, therefore, that a premature infant having apneic attacks should be maintained closer to the low range of neutral thermal environment, and most importantly, temperature fluctuations should be kept to a minimum.[40]

Has anyone else noticed that, thus far, no specific numbers defining the normal temperature of an infant have been offered in this chapter? Heck, I'll stick my neck out. I think babies should have core temperatures varying between 35.5 and 37.5° C (96–99.5° F). Whatever temperature range is accepted (no one knows what's acceptable) should be broad enough to allow for normal diurnal variations to occur. For example, heat production decreases with sleep and increases after feeding. The human body is not static and neither is its temperature! Of course, the true limits of "normal" are unknown and will likely remain so forever. And that's what makes the search for truth so endlessly interesting.

P. Perlstein

THE SENSORY ENVIRONMENT

Light, Sound, Touch, Movement

Historically, greater attention has been directed toward the thermal and bacteriologic aspects of the environment. A burst of studies of infant stimulation has appeared, suggesting that sensory stimuli may play a major role in neurologic and physical maturation and may be especially crucial in furthering the organization of many higher order processes.[19, 23, 32–34, 43]

These studies reveal that if a small, premature infant is touched, rocked, fondled, cuddled, or talked to daily during his stay in the nursery, he may have fewer apneic episodes and increased weight gain as well as progress more rapidly in some areas of higher central nervous system functioning, which persists for months after discharge from the hospital.

Simply fondling the premature infant for 5 minutes out of every hour for 2 weeks altered bowel motility, crying, activity, and possibly growth.[23, 52] Rocking one identical twin increased its growth rate above that of the unrocked twin.[20] When one experimental group of premature infants was provided with the increased sensory stimulation characteristic of thoughtful mothers during the early weeks of life, they were different from the controls in a learning situation 4 months later.[50] The stimulated infants at 4 months of age were more often able to control their own environmental visual inputs.

Anybody who takes care of sick, autonomically labile, and premature babies knows how often handling a baby can

lead to hypoxia. This has all been well documented using $tcPo_2$ as a measure.

> Before you start to touch and feel,
> See if the baby likes the deal.
> Touching is not the thing to do
> If touch makes falls in Po_2.
> It might be good to build a fence,
> To keep some infant bonders hence
> Until the infant makes it clear
> He means to live a life out here.
> Pray, oh Power, that you redeem us
> From messing with babies in extremis.
>
> **P. Perlstein**

With a shortage of personnel to provide stimulation, it seems logical to allow parents to help in this task. However, parents need encouragement, since they often do not appreciate that the small premature infant can see and hear. The prolonged periods of sleep with only short intervals of wakefulness further disconcert the parents. If the mother is able to stimulate the infant, she will take home a more responsive infant who will be closer in behavior to the full-term infant she had hoped to deliver.

Phototherapy for hyperbilirubinemia and increasing illumination in the nursery have focused attention on the light requirements of the newborn. It should be remembered that light has multiple effects, including a profound influence on biologic rhythm.

As we begin a major consideration of the effects of sensory stimuli, the most difficult criterion in every study will be: is the stimulus beneficial or harmful to the infant? The stimulation must be appropriate to his state of development and to his individual requirements, since there is danger in overstimulation of the immature organism. A recent suggestion is to permit the premature or newborn to decide on the amount of sensory stimulation. An example is allowing the rate of sucking to determine the intensity of light or the volume of a sound. Emphasizing our concerns in this area are the data on a group of full-term jaundiced infants treated with phototherapy.[51] The treated group, when compared with the jaundiced controls, showed decreased alertness and orientation to visual and auditory stimuli for many days after the treatment had been stopped. It was not determined whether this effect was secondary to the eye patches or to the phototherapy itself.

Noise levels are also of immediate concern, since present measurements of sound levels in the intensive care unit and incubator suggest that they approach potentially dangerous levels.[5] Of further concern are animal studies that reveal the immature of the species to be far more susceptible to damaging noise exposure than the adult. Additionally, these noise levels may potentiate the damaging effects of ototoxic drugs.

Thus, the bright lights and confusing noise of present-day intensive care nurseries will probably have to be changed in the future.

When attempting to determine the proper environment, we must evaluate the effects of sound, light, etc., not only on the immediate weight gain or activity but also on the later and long-term effects, such as age of sexual maturation, school performance, and length of survival.

The final environment, the ideal "external milieu," comprised of thermal and sensory considerations, must optimize both immediate and ultimate neurologic and physical development.

Editorial Comment: The significance of every aspect of the environment is emphasized by the observations of Glass et al who, in a sequentially designed trial, noted that the bright lights presently used in the intensive care nursery appear to affect the retina of the developing premature infant. They noted a significant reduction of retrolental fibroplasia in the experimental group of premature infants whose incubators were covered by a neutral density filter, compared with a control group exposed to the usual bright lights of the nursery. This effect was most noticeable in infants with birth weights under 1000 gm. It is important to note that they also observed behavioral differences between the two groups.

How do the many other elements of the complex environment of the nursery affect the developing premature infant?

Subramanian, K. N. S., Glass, P., Avery, G. B., Kolinjavadi, N., et al: Effect of bright light in the hospital nursery on the incidence of retinopathy of prematurity. N Engl J Med *313*:401, 1985.

Sisson, T. R. C.: Hazard to vision in the nursery [Editorial]. N Engl J Med *313*:444, 1985.

Questions

True or False

Provided that the rectal temperature is maintained between 36.5 and 37° C (97.7 and 98.6° F), the infant can be considered to be in the "neutral thermal environment."

A single measurement of temperature is of little value in defining the neutral thermal environment. The infant may have an elevated metabolic rate and be "working" to maintain normal body temperature. Therefore the statement is false.

When trying to produce a neutral thermal environment, take into account ambient air temperature, air flow, relative humidity, and temperature of surrounding objects.

The neutral thermal environment is that set of thermal conditions associated with minimal metabolic rate in a resting subject; thus, potential heat loss by conduction, convection, radiation, and evaporation must be considered. Therefore the statement is true.

Swaddling the infant should not influence the temperature of the incubator when it is set to achieve neutral thermal environment.

The use of the Scopes tables to achieve the neutral thermal environment refers to a set of specific conditions—namely, that the incubator wall temperatures are a degree higher than the air temperature and that the infants are nude. All the processes of heat exchange are altered and reduced by clothing the baby. The ambient air temperature inside the clothing is warmer than ambient incubator air, and humidity is higher, too. Therefore the statement is false.

Overheating the infant produces no noticeable clinical effects and can only be detected by monitoring deep body temperature.

Overheating will of course be documented by monitoring deep body temperature. However, the infant will be noted to be flushed and panting, and the extremities and trunk will be at the same temperature. He will hyperventilate and initially show irritability and may have apnea. Sweating may occur but is reduced in immature infants. With prolonged hyperthermia, stupor, coma, and convulsions may occur, and brain damage may be irreversible. The statement is false.

The stimulus for an increased metabolic rate begins immediately after onset of cold stimulus, even before the deep body temperature has fallen.

Bruck has shown that it is not necessary for body temperature to fall before there is an increase in metabolic rate. Therefore the statement is true. Even mild cold stress (e.g., blowing cold air on the face) may result in a significant increase in oxygen consumption. This occurs when unwarmed oxygen is blowing over the infant's face.

The lower end of the range of the neutral thermal environment is referred to as the "critical temperature." It varies with size, age, and clinical condition. Premature, appropriate-for-gestational-age infants have higher critical temperatures than term infants.

The above data are of value in using the charts of Scopes and Ahmed and Hey and Katz to place and maintain the infants in the neutral thermal environment. The statement is true.

Maintaining an infant with RDS in the neutral thermal environment plays an insignificant part in overall management.

Many infants with respiratory distress syndrome have a limited capacity to transfer oxygen, and the maintenance of the neutral thermal environment is most important in their care. Therefore the statement is false.

The rate of growth in body weight and length can be influenced by environmental temperature.

Infants kept at a warmer environment showed significantly greater increase in body weight and length over those maintained in a cooler environment when both groups had the same caloric intake. Infants in a cooler environment require more calories to regulate body temperature and thus have fewer available for growth. Therefore the statement is true.

When an infant who is being monitored in a servo incubator develops a fever, this is reflected by a rise in incubator temperature.

As the infant's temperature rises, the abdominal skin temperature that is controlling the infant will also rise, resulting in a fall in incubator temperature. Thus, a drop in incubator temperature reflects a rise in the temperature of the infant and vice versa. Therefore the statement is false.

Heat loss from the lungs may be diminished by maintaining the infants in supersaturated warm air.

Heat loss from the airways of the lung, due to evaporation of H_2O as inspired air is warmed and saturated with water vapor, can be diminished by increasing environmental humidity. Therefore the statement is true.

An elevated temperature during the first month of life is common and no cause for concern.

Too often an elevated temperature in a newborn has been attributed to environmental conditions, with disastrous consequences—for example, sepsis overlooked. A temperature elevation, particularly in infants at home, should be carefully evaluated (see Chapter 12). The answer is obviously false.

The newborn infant who has not been asphyxiated exhibits poikilothermic behavior when subjected to cold stress.

The newborn infant exhibits homeothermic behavior—that is, an elevation in metabolic rate (or oxygen consumption)—when subjected to cold stress. Therefore the statement is false. In the face of severe hypoxemia, metabolic rate is not increased with cooling.

In the usual incubator, the greatest source of heat loss in the immature infant is from the lungs.

Radiant heat loss is loss to immediately surrounding cooler solid objects (e.g., wall of incubator) and accounts for the majority of heat lost in the immature infant. Therefore the statement is false.

Radiant heat losses are similar in adults and immature infants, since they are both homeotherms.

Radiant heat loss is of less significance in adults because they are clothed and has no bearing on the question of homeothermy. A homeotherm is an animal that attempts to maintain a constant body temperature despite alterations in environment—for example, it increases metabolic rate in a cool environment. Therefore the statement is false.

The newborn infant loses equal amounts of heat per unit of body mass compared with the adult.

Although at birth the infant's body mass is about 5 per cent of that of the adult, the surface area is nearly 15 per cent. There is also less subcutaneous tissue, resulting in a higher thermal conductance and thus a higher skin temperature at lower ambient temperatures. Bruck has estimated that, because of these facts, the heat loss of the newborn infant per unit of body mass is about four times that of the adult. Therefore the statement is false.

Full-term infants who have been cold stressed at birth may have a normal pH and low HCO_3.

A compensated metabolic acidosis probably secondary to lactic acid production is sometimes observed. Therefore the statement is true.

Lowering the body temperature is beneficial in resuscitating asphyxiated newborns.

There is insufficient evidence to indicate that lowering the body temperature of depressed or asphyxiated newborns is of value in changing mortality or morbidity. Therefore the statement is false.

The duration of sleep is markedly reduced when small nude infants are exposed to an environmental temperature of only 1–2° C below the lower limit of the presumed range of thermal neutrality.

It has been suggested by some investigators that the temperature range in which the least amount of oxygen is consumed is also the temperature range of thermal comfort for the neonate. Therefore the statement is true.

Swaddled full-term babies may not cry or otherwise call attention to the fact that they are under severe cold stress.

This statement is true and is particularly important since the upper limit of heat production is reached for cot-nursed, full-term infants when the room temperature falls to about 10° C (50° F). In some situations at night, bedrooms get colder, and the infants become hypothermic.

The signs and symptoms of hypothermia shortly after delivery may imitate the clinical picture of the respiratory distress syndrome.

The signs of respiratory distress syndrome—notably grunting, acidosis, and an increased right-to-left shunt—can all be observed in a hypothermic infant. The statement is true.

CASE PROBLEMS

Case One

Baby D. O. was an 1160 gm male product of a 31 week gestation. No problems were encountered in the immediate neonatal period, and the pregnancy had been uncomplicated. Delivery was under caudal anesthesia by forceps. The Apgar score at 1 minute was 6. On the second day of life, the rectal temperature was noted to be 36.8° C (98.2° F). The incubator temperature at this time was 34.1° C (93.4° F).

What additional data would you require to define the neutral thermal environment?

To define the neutral thermal environment, you also require the temperature of the mattress with regard to conductive heat loss, the air flow in the incubator, the relative humidity, and the temperature of the inner walls of the incubator to determine the radiant heat losses that can occur to the surrounding walls of the incubator. A continuous recording of the abdominal skin temperature would permit a rough idea of whether or not the infant is in the neutral thermal zone. When a servo incubator is controlled to maintain an abdominal skin temperature of 36.5° C (97.7° F), oxygen consumption has been found to be minimal. In this case, the abdominal skin temperature

was 34.9° C (94.8° F), the side wall of the incubator was 32.5° C (90.5° F), and the relative humidity was 80 per cent. We can assume the temperature of the mattress to be the same as the incubator air temperature.

With these available data, would you say that the infant is in the neutral thermal environment?

No, the infant is not in the neutral thermal environment. Our indications of this are that the abdominal skin temperature is only 34.9° C (94.8° F), even with the incubator air at 34.1° C (93.4° F). If you refer back to the table of Scopes and Ahmed, the appropriate temperature for this infant to be in the neutral thermal environment is an environmental temperature of 34–35° C (93.2–95° F), provided that the walls are 1° C higher than the air. Note that the side wall temperature is only 32.5° C (86.5° F). He is losing heat by radiation.

How could you diminish radiant heat loss in this infant?

Radiant heat losses may be diminished by using a radiant warmer or by placing a plastic heat shield inside the single-walled incubator.

Case Two

Baby H. was a girl delivered after a 42 week pregnancy, weighing 1600 gm. No problems were noted in the immediate neonatal period. The neurologic examination was appropriate for an infant with a 42 week gestation, with the exception that there was diminished neck flexor tone. Head circumference was 33 cm. This infant was unable to increase her metabolic rate with cold stress.

How can the optimal thermal environment be found?

This is a difficult question to answer because no tables are available for this age and weight. The problem may best be managed by servo-controlling the incubator and maintaining the abdominal skin temperature at 36.5° C (97.7° F). Another approach is to use the "warmest" incubator possible to maintain a normal temperature in the infant.

REFERENCES

1. Adamsons, K., Jr.: The role of thermal factors in fetal and neonatal life. Pediatr Clin North Am *13*:599, 1966.
2. Adamsons, K., Jr., and Towell, M.: Thermal homeostasis in the fetus and newborn. Anesthesiology *26*:531, 1965.
3. Adamsons, K., Jr., Gandy, G., and James, L.: The

influence of thermal factors upon oxygen consumption of the newborn human infant. J Pediatr *66*:495, 1965.
4. Agate, F., and Silverman, W.: The control of body temperature in the small newborn infant by low-energy infra-red radiation. Pediatrics *31*:725, 1963.

5. American Academy of Pediatrics Commitee on Environmental Hazards. Noise pollution: neonatal aspects. Pediatrics *54*:476, 1974.

6. Benzinger, T.: Clinical temperature—the new physiologic basis. JAMA *209*:1200, 1969.

7. Blackfan, K., and Yaglou, C.: The premature infant: a study of the effects of atmospheric conditions on growth and development. Am J Dis Child *46*:1175, 1933.

8. Bruck, K.: Temperature regulation in the newborn infant. Biol Neonate *3*:65, 1961.

9. Bruck, K.: Heat production and temperature regulation. *In* Stave, U. (ed.): *Physiology of the Perinatal Period*. New York, Appleton-Century-Crofts, 1970.

10. Budin, P.: *The Nursling*. London, Caxton Publishing Co., 1907.

11. Buetow, K., and Klein, S.: Effect of maintenance of "normal" skin temperature on survival of infants of low birth weight. Pediatrics *34*:163, 1964.

12. Burnard, E., and Cross, K.: Rectal temperature in the newborn after birth asphyxia. Br Med J *2*:1197, 1958.

13. Cross, K., Tizard, J., and Trythall, D.: The gaseous metabolism of the newborn infant breathing 15 per cent oxygen. Acta Paediatr *47*:217, 1958.

14. Cross, K. W.: Review Lecture. La Chaleur Animale and the infant brain. J Physiol *294*:1, 1979.

15. Dailey, W., Klaus, M., and Meyer, H.: Apnea in premature infants: monitoring, incidence, heart rate changes, and effect of environmental temperature. Pediatrics *43*:510, 1969.

16. Darnall, R. A., Jr., and Ariagno, R. L.: Minimal oxygen consumption in infants cared for under overhead radiant warmers compared with conventional incubators. J Pediatr *93*:283, 1978.

17. Dawkins, M., and Hull, D.: Brown adipose tissue and the response of newborn rabbits to cold. J Physiol *172*:216, 1964.

18. Day, R.: Respiratory metabolism in infancy and childhood. Am J Dis Child *65*:376, 1943.

19. Freedman, D.: Personal communication, 1972.

20. Freedman, D., Boverman, H., and Freedman, N.: Effects of kinesthetic stimulation on weight gain and on smiling in premature infants. Paper presented at the Meeting of the American Orthopsychiatry Association, San Francisco, April 1966.

21. Gandy, G., Adamsons, K., Jr., and Cunningham, N.: Thermal environmental and acid-base homeostasis in human infants during the first few hours of life. J Clin Invest *43*:751, 1964.

22. Glass, L., Silverman, W., and Sinclair, J.: Effects of the thermal environment on cold resistance and growth of small infants after the first week of life. Pediatrics *41*:1033, 1968.

23. Hasselmeyer, E.: The premature neonate's response to handling. Am Nurs Assoc *11*:15, 1964.

24. Hey, E.: The relation between environmental temperature and oxygen consumption in the newborn baby. J Physiol *200*:589, 1969.

25. Hey, E., and Katz, G.: The optimum thermal environment for naked babies. Arch Dis Child *45*:328, 1970.

26. Hey, E., and Maurice, N.: Effect of humidity on production and loss of heat in the newborn baby. Arch Dis Child *43*:166, 1968.

27. Hey, E., and Mount, L.: Temperature control in incubators. Lancet *2*:202, 1966.

28. Hey, E., and Mount, L.: Heat losses from babies in incubators. Arch Dis Child *42*:75, 1967.

29. Hey, E., and O'Connell, B.: Oxygen consumption and heat balance in the cot-nursed baby. Arch Dis Child *45*:335, 1970.

30. Hill, J.: The oxygen consumption of newborn and adult mammals: its dependence on the oxygen tension in the inspired air and on environmental temperature. J Physiol *149*:346, 1959.

31. Hill, J., and Rahimtulla, K.: Heat balance and the metabolic rate of newborn babies in relation to environmental temperature; and the effect of age and of weight on basal metabolic rate. J Physiol *180*:239, 1965.

32. Katz, V.: Auditory stimulation and developmental behavior of the premature infant. Nurs Res *20*:196, 1971.

33. Korner, A., Kraemer, H., Haffner, M., et al.: Effects of waterbed flotation on premature infants. A pilot study. Pediatrics *56*:361, 1975.

34. Kramer, L., and Pierpont, M.: Rocking waterbed and auditory stimuli to enhance growth of preterm infants. J Pediatr *88*:297, 1976.

35. LeBlanc, M. H.: Relative efficiency of an incubator and an open warmer in producing thermoneutrality for the small premature infant. Pediatrics *69*:439, 1982.

36. Mann, T., and Elliott, R.: Neonatal cold injury due to accidental exposure to cold. Lancet, *1*:229, 1957.

37. Merenstein, G., and Blackmon, L.: *Care of the High-Risk Newborn*. San Francisco, Children's Hospital, 1971.

38. Okken, A.: Heat production and heat loss of low birth weight babies in an incubator with heated walls. Thesis. University of Groningen, Netherlands, 1976.

39. Perlstein, P., Edwards, N. Atherton, H., et al.: Computer-assisted newborn intensive care. Pediatrics *57*:494, 1976.

40. Perlstein, P., Edwards, N., and Sutherland, J.: Apnea in premature infants and incubator air temperature changes. N Engl J Med *282*:461, 1970.

41. Phillips, C.: Neonatal heat loss in heated cribs vs. mothers' arms. JOGN Nurs *3*:11, 1974.

42. Pomerance, J. J., Brand, R. J., and Meredith, J. L.: Differentiating environmental from related fevers in the term newborn. Pediatrics *67*:485, 1981.

43. Scarr-Salapatek, S., and Williams, M.: The effects of early stimulation on low birth-weight infants. Child Dev *44*:94, 1973.

44. Scopes, J., and Ahmed, I.: Range of critical temperatures in sick and premature newborn babies. Arch Dis Child *41*:417, 1966.

45. Silverman, W., and Agate, F.: Variation in cold resistance among small newborn animals. Biol Neonate *6*:113, 1964.

46. Silverman, W., and Blanc, W.: The effect of humidity on survival of newly born premature infants. Pediatrics *20*:477, 1957.

47. Silverman, W., Agate, F., and Fertig, J.: A sequential trial of the nonthermal effect of atmospheric humidity on survival of newborn infants of low birth weight. Pediatrics *31*:719, 1963.

48. Silverman, W., Fertig, J., and Berger, A.: The influence of the thermal environment upon the survival of newly born premature infants. Pediatrics *22*:876, 1958.

49. Silverman, W., Zamelis, A., Sinclair, J., et al.: Warm nape of the newborn. Pediatrics *33*:984, 1964.

50. Siqueland, E., and Lipsitt, L.: Learning ability and its enhancement. *In* Henkes, J., and Schain, R. (eds.): *Learning Disorders in Children.* Report of the 61st Ross Conference on Pediatric Research, Columbus, Ohio, Ross Laboratories, 1971, pp. 52–55.
51. Snyder, D., Telzrow, R., Tronick, E., et al.: Effects of phototherapy on neonatal behavior. Pediatr Res (Abstract) *10*:432, 1976.
52. Solkoff, N., Yaffe, S., Weintraub, D., et al.: Effects of handling on the subsequent development of premature infants. J Dev Psych *1*:765, 1969.
53. Stothers, J. K.: Head insulation and heat loss in the newborn. Arch Dis Child *56*:530, 1981.
54. Tafari, N., and Gentz, J.: Aspects of rewarming newborn infants with severe accidental hypothermia. Acta Paediatr Scand *63*:595, 1974.
55. Wheldon, A. E., and Ruller, N.: The heat balance of small babies nursed in incubators and under radiant warmers. Early Hum Devel *6*:131, 1982.
56. Wu, P. Y., and Hodgman, J. E.: Insensible water loss in preterm infants: changes with postnatal development and non-ionizing radiant energy. Pediatrics *54*:704, 1974.
57. Yeh, T. F., Anema, P., Lilien, L. D., et al.: Reduction of insensible water loss in premature infants under the radiant warmer. J Pediatr *94*:651, 1979.

6

Feeding and Selected Disorders of the Gastrointestinal Tract

AVROY A. FANAROFF
MARSHALL H. KLAUS

We have the baby weighed today
The nursing time is set,
At last we find we are so wise
We can begin to standardize
No baby now need fret;
In spite of this the baby grows
But why it does God only knows.

JOHN RUHRÄH
(1872–1935)

Since specific feeding practices alter mortality,[41] and probably morbidity, the feeding of a small infant presents a continuing challenge to those responsible for the care of low-birth-weight infants. Dietary mixtures for the low-birth-weight infant remain a highly controversial subject, and as noted by Barness:[19] "It is likely that no area in the care of the newborn infant is less critically or more controversially approached than his feeding. What, When, How, and How Often to Feed are questions surrounded by emotions, beliefs, fads, and even commercialism, all of which tend to obscure the basic goals of infant feeding."

Whereas the full-term healthy neonate will tolerate periods of prolonged starvation together with wide variation in both quantity and composition of formula, the low-birth-weight infant, as a result of limited nutritional reserves and gastrointestinal immaturity, is much more vulnerable.[13, 16, 37, 85, 92, 123, 152, 179] The food intake must satisfy the requirements for growth as well as replace mineral losses in the urine, feces, and sweat and nitrogen losses from tissue breakdown. There have been important advances in knowledge concerning development of the gastrointestinal tract, permitting more logical planning of feeding. Careful consideration must be given not only to the weight but also to the gestational age of the infant, because the gastrointestinal maturation, metabolic capabilities and rates, and requirements of fuel and water will differ with differing ages (see Chapter 4).

Improved perinatal care has resulted in the survival of large numbers of extremely precarious low-birth-weight infants requiring prolonged nutritional support. Guidelines for feeding the low-birth-weight infant and specific gastrointestinal problems are presented in this chapter; not included is a schema for feeding the healthy full-term neonate.

PHYSIOLOGIC CONSIDERATIONS

The objective of feeding is to meet the metabolic requirements of a number of de-

113

veloping organ systems. A major obstacle has been finding a yardstick with which to measure success. What represents optimum nutrition, and how should it be evaluated? At present, the adequacy of growth is judged according to increments of weight, length, total body fat, and head circumference as plotted on growth charts[15] (see Figure 6–1 and Appendices G–1, G–2, and G–3). Because the optimum positions on the charts are unknown, an attempt is made to maintain growth within or above the percentiles at birth.[16] The evaluation of nutrition should include not only short-term effects on growth

GROWTH CHART

Name_____ BD _____ Hosp #_____

Birthweight_____gms   Length_____cm   Head circ_____cm   Chest circ_____cm

Gestational Age_____

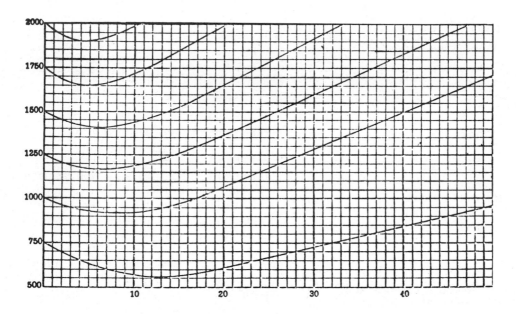

AGE IN DAYS

Date	Fluid Intake (ml)			Weight gms	ml/kgm	Calories			Calories per kgm	Head Circumference
	IV	P.O.	Total			IV	P.O.	Total		

Figure 6–1. Growth chart.

but also ultimate intelligence and length and quality of survival.[37, 49] Maintenance of a normal growth rate is associated with a minimal neurodevelopmental handicap rate.[78] This is difficult to achieve, and 71 of 150 surviving AGA infants were below the third percentile by their expected time of delivery. Nonetheless, provided that catch-up has occurred by 8 months corrected age, most of these infants will develop normally.[78, 79]

The exact quantity and combination of substances required by all the developing organ systems are unknown for the full-term infant.[45, 63, 92] For the immature or undernourished infant, the problem is even more complex. Nutritional problems of a preterm infant are compounded by a number of factors, including deficient or absent fat stores, minimal glycogen reserves, low serum albumin, and low levels of iron and calcium. The immaturity of the gastrointestinal tract and reduced gastric capacity, together with limited renal function, restrict the volume and composition of feedings that will be tolerated.

Nutritional Requirements

The caloric, water, electrolyte, mineral, and vitamin requirements of the low-birthweight infant are dependent upon body stores, absorption, rates of utilization and expenditure, and excretion of the substances. The metabolic rate and body composition of infants with similar weights but dissimilar gestational ages are different; hence their requirements will also differ.

Water[10, 23, 32, 57, 58, 101, 105, 143, 160]

The water content of the human infant decreases progressively from 85 per cent of body weight at 28 weeks' gestation to 70 per cent at full term. The usual weight loss of the newborn period appears to be mainly due to a loss of extracellular water. Low-birth-weight infants are particularly vulnerable to excess fluid losses in the early neonatal period because of a large surface/weight ratio, increased water content in the skin, a thinner epidermis, and increased skin permeability. This is compounded by renal immaturity (see Chapter 14) and impaired neuroendocrine control. The actual clinical requirements for water are highly variable and dependent on the state of the infant (Table 6–1). Very small and immature infants kept in a single-walled incubator who feed frequently have increased activity and may require large amounts of water.[58] The requirements are even greater if there are excessive losses via the gastrointestinal tract or insensibly by skin or lungs or if a large electrolyte load is given.

The fluid volume required to administer the necessary 100–140 cal/kg/day will depend on the caloric density (number of cal/ml) of the formula. Assuming a caloric density of 24 cal/30 ml, which may be achieved by the second week of life, the daily fluid requirement will be 120–180 ml/kg/day. Infants receiving 140–160 ml of water/kg/day are usually in positive water balance. Most infants can be adequately hydrated with 120 ml/kg/day. However, some tiny infants (<750 gm) may require from 180–200 ml/kg/day.

The ability of the low-birth-weight infant to take in this quantity of fluid is limited by the gastric capacity. Particularly in infants with birth weights below 1250 gm, it is easy to exceed this capacity inadvertently. Advancing the oral feeding too rapidly will result in abdominal distension and vomiting, frequently complicated by aspiration or even possibly necrotizing enterocolitis (NEC). This was probably a major factor in the increased mortality associated with early oral feeding of low-birth-weight infants.[173] A combined oral/IV regimen is invariably necessary during the first weeks of life.

Optimal management of fluid requirements in low-birth-weight infants can only be achieved with close monitoring of all intake and output, daily or twice daily determination of weight, and daily determination of serum electrolytes and glucose, urine specific gravity, and osmolarity. If the infant is not given adequate fluids, a number of physical and metabolic changes can be anticipated.

TABLE 6–1 FACTORS THAT INCREASE FLUID REQUIREMENTS

Increased insensible water loss in immature infants[30, 58, 83, 114]
Phototherapy[179]
Radiant warmers[111, 175]
Labile body temperature, labile ambient temperature
Increased urinary volume associated with glycosuria and acute tubular necrosis
Abnormal fluid losses—postsurgery, e.g., colostomy, chest tube drainage
Third space losses
Diarrhea or vomiting, etc.

These include evidence of excessive weight loss in association with hyperosmolarity, hypernatremia, and increased hematocrit and bilirubin as well as evidence of metabolic acidosis, dehydration, and frequently multiple apneic spells. Complications arising from excessive fluid administration to the low-birth-weight infant include hyponatremia, patent ductus arteriosus (PDA), congestive heart failure, bronchopulmonary dysplasia, and necrotizing enterocolitis.

Retrospective studies by Stevenson[160] and Brown et al[32] suggest an association between the volume of fluid intake and the development of symptoms of patent ductus arteriosus in premature newborn infants. Furthermore, in their randomized prospective study, Bell et al[23] found that the risk of patent ductus arteriosus and congestive heart failure was greater in infants receiving a high-volume regimen. Thirty-five of 85 infants in the high-volume group acquired murmurs consistent with patent ductus arteriosus and 11 had congestive heart failure. In contrast, only 9 of 85 infants in the low-volume group had murmurs consistent with patent ductus arteriosus. Surprisingly, there were significantly more infants with necrotizing enterocolitis in the high-volume group. The mean fluid intake in all infants in the high-volume group was 169 ± 20 ml/kg/day, and in all infants in the low-volume group it was 122 ± 14 ml/kg/day. Mean per cent weight loss in the high-volume group ($11.5 \pm 6.3\%$) was significantly less than in the low-volume group ($14 \pm 5.7\%$, $p < .005$). In studying the water balance in these same infants, a higher urine volume, higher water clearance, sodium retention, and less weight loss in the high-volume group compared with the low-volume group were noted by 8 days. Extracellular space as determined by inulin did not change in the high-volume group, whereas significant reduction occurred in the low-volume group. Bell and associates concluded that high fluid and sodium intake in low-birth-weight infants in the first week of life results in sodium retention and expanded extracellular volume despite appropriate renal attempts at compensation.

In a subsequent study, Lorenz et al[105] prospectively determined the effect of different degrees of negative water balance during the first 5 days of life in 88 very low-birth-weight infants. Fluid therapy was adjusted so that in Group 1 there was a 1–2 per cent loss of birth weight per day to a maximum loss of 8–10 per cent, whereas Group 2 lost 3–5 per cent of birth weight per day to a maximum loss of 13–15 per cent. Comparing Groups 1 and 2, there was no statistically significant difference in PDA, intracranial hemorrhage, bronchopulmonary dysplasia, dehydration, metabolic disturbances, or subsequent neonatal mortality. They concluded that the gradual loss of 5–15 per cent of birth weight during the first week of life did not adversely affect outcome.[105]

In considering water balance during the first weeks of life, it is desirable to achieve a consistent weight loss of up to 10 per cent to allow for the postnatal contraction of body fluid (primarily extracellular) that is part of the physiologic alteration of body composition. If the dose of fluid is greater than the infant's ability to excrete, positive balance will result in expansion of the extracellular fluid compartment, which in some instances adversely affects the infant's cardiopulmonary status. It has been shown that high fluid intake in the first few weeks of life in those infants with patent ductus arteriosus and left-to-right shunt may increase the magnitude of shunt and cardiac decompensation.[160] Another study has shown a direct correlation between high fluid intake and the development of bronchopulmonary dysplasia in artificially ventilated infants.[32] **W. Oh**

Calories[31, 33, 36, 39, 53, 129]

The caloric requirements are related to the cell mass and number. Thus, infants of the same weight may require different caloric intakes to achieve the same weight gain. In most instances, 100–120 cal/kg/day will provide maintenance for the normal infant and allow sufficient calories for growth.[72, 150] Some infants, particularly those who are small for gestational age and who have a higher metabolic rate, require more calories.[155]

The distribution of the caloric expenditure is outlined in Figure 6–2A. Table 6–2 shows daily weight gain in grams in infants of various gestational ages.

The partition of energy utilization in very low-birth-weight, formula-fed infants under thermoneutral conditions is shown in Figure 6–2.[128, 129] The energy requirements are partitioned between needs for maintenance (including resting metabolism, thermoregulation, and muscular activity) and needs for synthesis and storage of new tissue. In this study the energy cost of growth was determined as 4.9 cal/gm of weight gain. The caloric cost per gram of new tissue synthesis varies from 4–7 cal/gm/kg and depends on the fat composition of the tissue (fat synthesis requires 11.6 cal/gm of fat, whereas protein synthesis requires 7.5 cal/gm of protein). Recent data[128] suggest that prematurely born

Figure 6–2. *A,* Partition of energy utilization in very low-birth-weight, formula-fed infants (n = 22), under thermoneutral conditions. Results are expressed as mean kcal/kg/day and per cent of gross energy intake. (Reproduced with permission from Reichman, B. L., Chessex, P., Putet, G., et al: Partition of energy metabolism and energy cost of growth in the very low-birth-weight infant. Pediatrics *69:*446, 1982.) *B,* Fat deposition in preterm and term infants. The amount of accretion in the study subjects (5.4 ± 1.4 gm/kg/day, determined by 22 studies performed at a postconceptional age of 32.1 ± 1.6 weeks, mean ± SD) is contrasted with the range of accretion in fetuses (hatched area). *C,* Protein retention in preterm and term infants. The amount retained by the 13 study subjects (1.92 ± 0.37 gm/kg/day, determined by 22 metabolic studies performed at a postconceptional age of 32.1 ± 1.6 weeks, mean ± SD) is compared with the range of amounts retained by fetuses of the same age (hatched area). (*B* and *C* reproduced with permission from Reichman, B. L., Chessex, P., Putet, G., et al: Diet, fat accretion and growth in premature infants. N Engl J Med *305:*1495, 1981.)

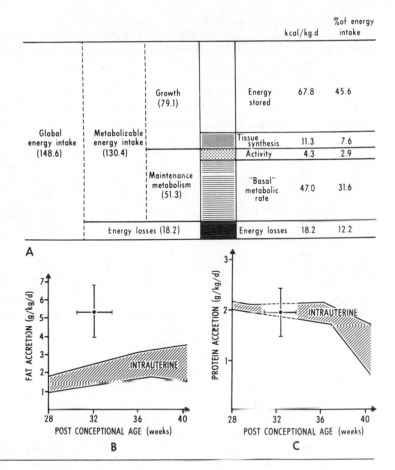

infants accumulate more fat than if they were still growing in utero. At usual rates of growth, 25–35 per cent of metabolizable energy is required for growth.

Considerable awe appears to be inspired by the determination for the infant to maintain the rate of intrauterine growth, even though he is no longer in the intrauterine state. The evidence that this is beneficial, mandatory, or necessary is not apparent; indeed, efforts to maintain this rate have often resulted in serious disturbances from excessive and overzealous nutritional attempts.

L. Stern

Most immature infants sleep approximately 60 per cent of the time and are in a state of quiet wakefulness for a further 25 per cent, during which metabolic rate will be low. Fifteen per cent of the time they are feeding and crying. If the metabolic rate is increased, so too are the caloric requirements necessary for growth. This is observed when the environmental temperature is outside the neutral thermal range[68] and with increased muscular activity, persistent respiratory problems, increased cardiac output, or infection.

Thus, environmental factors have a great influence in determining the total caloric requirements. Cold stress may increase oxygen utilization two and one half times compared with the resting state, and after the first week of life, the increased metabolic rate of nude infants maintained at subthermoneutral temperatures combined with relatively low caloric intake results in significantly retarded head growth.[67] Therefore, low-birth-weight infants should be maintained in a neutral thermal environment even after the first week of life because exposure to slightly cool temperatures may divert calories needed for brain growth into fuel for heat production (see Chapter 5). Handling or stroking the infant and nonnutritive sucking (see Sucking and Swallowing, below) may decrease caloric requirements or increase absorption. Addi-

TABLE 6–2 DAILY WEIGHT GAIN[185]

Gestational Age (weeks)	Gain (gm/day)
28	16.8
28–32	23.9
32–36	30.7
36–48	27.1

tionally, provision of as little as 60 cal/kg/day with added amino acids resulted in weight gain and positive nitrogen balance in some sick preterm infants.[6]

In practice, to achieve the recommended intake of calories takes at least a week to 10 days, and sometimes longer. Therefore we supplement with intravenous calories.

Protein

Precise requirements of preterm infants for most nutrients are not available, and the amount of protein required cannot be determined without consideration of the quality (i.e., the amino acid constituents) of the protein. Requirements for growth may be calculated from body composition analyses of reference fetuses of varying gestational ages.[185] The gain in specific substances (e.g., protein) is calculated between designated ages to estimate daily increments in body content of those substances. The nongrowth factors—utilization and per cent absorption—are considered in the calculation. (In term infants, the nongrowth level is between 0 and 1 gm of protein/kg/day.) For the reference fetus between 28 and 32 weeks' gestation with an estimated weight of 1200 gm, protein accounts for 12.2 per cent of the weight gained, and the rate of weight gain is 20 gm/day. Human fetal accumulation of nitrogen between 24 and 36 weeks is 320–350 mg/kg/day. Because of this net transplacental flux of amino acids, it has been estimated that the growing preterm infant (extrauterine) also requires the net retention of this quantity of amino nitrogen or 2.2 gm/kg/day of high quality protein (Figure 6–2C). Assuming 83 per cent absorption of protein[159] and allowing 0.5 gm/day for nongrowth, the daily protein requirement between 28 and 32 weeks is approximately 3–4 gm/day.

The optimal protein intake has not clearly been established. We presently aim for a protein intake of 2.5–4 gm/kg/day, where protein accounts for 10–15 per cent of caloric intake. A normal newborn will gain weight if provided with 2 gm of protein/kg/day. However, edema and low plasma protein levels are sometimes noted at this level of intake. Of special interest is the evidence that sick preterm infants can be maintained in positive nitrogen balance when provided with 60 cal/kg/day, 10 of these calories in the form of protein.

The distribution and kind of protein and amino acids given to the infant are critical.[94, 96] Low-birth-weight infants require some amino acids that are not essential for the term infant. Snyderman et al[159] demonstrated that the removal of cystine or tyrosine from the diet resulted in an impairment of growth and nitrogen retention and a depression of the level of that particular amino acid in the plasma. Because of a lack of cystathionase in the liver of preterm infants,[66] dietary methionine cannot be converted into cystine, and these infants are dependent on an exogenous supply.

Raiha et al[125] studied growth and biochemical changes in low-birth-weight infants fed five different formulae, including one of pooled breast milk (1.7 gm of protein/kg/day), two supplying 2.25 gm of protein/kg/day, and two supplying 4.5 gm of protein/kg/day and an equal number of calories. The whey/casein ratio was 60:40 and 18:82 at each protein level, with breast milk equal to 60:40. Although no differences were found in the growth parameters studied, striking differences in metabolism were found. The blood urea nitrogen (BUN) was markedly elevated in the groups receiving 3 per cent protein as compared with those receiving 1.5 per cent protein or breast milk. The lowest ammonia, tyrosine, and phenylalanine levels were noted in infants fed formula with whey/casein of 60:40 and the highest levels in those fed the high-protein formula with casein predominant. Elevated values of tyrosine and phenylalanine paralleling those found in phenylketonuria were observed in some of those infants fed the high-protein, casein-predominant formula. Late metabolic acidosis was also observed in some of the babies in this group. Serum protein levels were lowest in infants fed breast milk. The content of cystine in the breast milk and in the high whey protein formula was significantly higher than in the other preparations. In addition, the infants fed breast milk had higher taurine levels than those on other formulae. To prevent deficiencies, taurine has been added to low-birth-weight formulae.

Raiha's study demonstrated that low-birth-weight infants fed a diet high in casein-predominant protein had high concentrations of essential amino acids and tyrosine in the blood for long periods of time. In addition, they had high urea nitrogen and ammonia concentrations and tended to excrete a hyperosmolar urine and also to develop taurine deficiencies.[163] These metabolic imbalances may be harmful for the developing organism and are not found in infants fed breast milk or whey-predominant, low-protein formulae, which are now almost exclusively utilized for low-birth-weight infants (see Table 6–5, p. 127, and Table 6–7, p. 130). Furthermore, lactobezoars have been associated with casein-predominant formulae.[41, 51] Prior studies have demonstrated that infants fed high-protein diets had protein casts in the urine, became febrile more frequently, were often lethargic, fed poorly, and possibly had more apnea. The effects of the high protein intake in combination with abnormal amino acid profiles in the serum on brain maturation necessitate close follow-up of intellectual performance in these infants. Goldman et al[71] reported that the incidence of strabismus and children with low IQ scores was greater at 4–6 years of age among those infants who had received protein intakes in excess of 6 gm/kg/day.

We currently recommend the use of breast milk or humanized commercial formulae with whey-predominant protein for the feeding of preterm infants. Whether breast milk alone is adequate to meet the total protein requirements of these infants has yet to be proved. A number of hypothetic models, together with a limited number of clinical reports, suggest that breast milk is deficient in protein, calcium, sodium, etc. However, the high bioavailability of different substances (e.g., iron, zinc, and vitamin D), the presence of special carrier proteins, and the altered composition (i.e., higher nitrogen content) in the breast milk of mothers of preterm infants have led us to encourage the use of breast milk for sick preterm infants.

Carbohydrate

Carbohydrate provides 40–50 per cent of the calories in most formulae. Lactose is found in human and cow milk and supplies most or all of the carbohydrate in milk-based formulae. Intestinal disaccharidase is developed early in fetal life. Maltase and sucrase reach mature values by the sixth to eighth month of gestation; lactase is at mature levels only at term.[137] The delay in maturation of intestinal lactase may result in diarrhea and metabolic acidosis in some infants when challenged with lactose. However, in most preterm infants, lactase activity increases rapidly to the values in normal term infants soon after birth. Lactose enhances calcium absorption and reduces constipation. It also promotes development of fermentative, less putrefactive bacterial flora, which may provide some protection against infections. (*Lactobacillus bifidus* is enhanced by a factor present in breast milk.) Low-birth-weight infants develop satisfactorily when fed formulae in which the lactose of milk has been replaced with sucrose as well as when fed lactose-free formulae containing sucrose, dextrose-maltose, or dextrin as the carbohydrate.

Recently polycose, a glucose polymer, has been introduced as a carbohydrate source for low-birth-weight infants. Since alpha-glucosidase develops early in fetal life, it has been assumed that polycose is easily digested and absorbed. It provides the advantage of adding calories without increasing the formula's osmolar load.

Fat

The high fuel value of fat represents stored energy, and fat is responsible for transporting fat-soluble vitamins. It forms an integral part of cellular membranes and acts as an insulator. The fat content of the full-term infant is about 12 per cent of total body weight, most of which accumulates during the last 2 months of gestation.

Normal full-term infants fail to absorb 10–15 per cent of ingested fat, and fat malabsorption in excess of 30 per cent of intake has been observed during the first week of life in low-birth-weight infants.[18, 63, 96, 148]

Apart from gastrointestinal motor function, important factors relating to fat absorption are (1) the nature of the fat ingested, (2) the absorptive surface, (3) pancreatic function, and (4) hepatic function. The form of ingested fat alters absorption in the newborn. Human milk fat and certain mixtures of vegetable fat are better tolerated than butter fat. Medium-chain triglycerides are generally well tolerated by both normal and premature infants, whereas long-chain saturated fatty acids are poorly tolerated and are excreted as calcium soaps.[138] Medium-chain triglycerides included as part of the formula improve fat absorption in low-birth-weight infants, increase weight gain, and enhance calcium absorption and nitrogen retention.[149]

Deficiencies of the absorptive surface following surgery are often associated with fat malabsorption. Additionally, immaturity of mucosal function relative to the absorption of macromolecules and vitamin B_{12} has been demonstrated in some infants. Thus, ineffective fat absorption and transport cannot be ruled out as the cause of the steatorrhea in the newborn period.

Several recent studies suggest that exocrine pancreatic function is inadequate at birth and insufficient pancreatic lipolysis contributes to neonatal steatorrhea. Extrapancreatic lipase (lingual and gastric lipase) probably plays an important part in neonatal fat hydrolysis. Hepatic synthesis and secretion of bile acid are developed late in gestation and are still maturing at term.

Normal newborn infants have decreased rates of synthesis, decreased pool size, and decreased intraluminal concentrations of bile acid during the first weeks of life. Even more marked reductions of pool size and synthesis rate are demonstrable in premature infants. The ileal mechanism for active intestinal bile acid reabsorption is defective in the near-term fetus and newborn and may not develop for days or weeks after birth. Watkins et al,[171, 172] studying premature infants, found that there was a group with extremely low bile acid levels and a second group with levels matching those of full-term infants. The mothers of four fifths of the infants with levels matching the full-term infants had received adrenal corticosteroids during the 2 weeks before parturition.

To summarize, digestive function in the newborn is incompletely developed. Fat malabsorption, imposed primarily by a combination of relative pancreatic insufficiency and a small bile acid pool, may limit growth rates in premature infants as well as result in inadequate absorption of fat-soluble vitamins A, D, E, and K.

For low-birth-weight infants, formulae with fat contributing 40–50 per cent of the total calories are recommended. Three per cent of the total calories should be in the form of linoleic acid. This is equivalent to 300 mg of linoleic acid per 100 kcal and is usually easily achieved with proprietary formulae. Fatty acid deficiency is characterized by growth failure, dermatitis, diminished pigmentation, and hypotonia. Excessive linoleic acid produces excessive peroxidation and increases vitamin E requirements (see Chapter 15). In human milk, fat provides about 50 per cent of the calories, including 5 per cent

as essential fatty acids, principally linoleic acid. This fat is esterified differently, rendering it more readily absorbable.

Reichman et al[128] compared the growth and accumulation of protein, fat, and carbohydrate in the formula-fed premature infant and the fetus of a similar postconceptional age. Measurements combining nutritional balance and indirect calorimetry demonstrated the deposition rates of protein and fat. They found that the formula-fed, very low-birth-weight infant who gained weight comparably to the fetus retained the same amount of protein (1.92 ± 0.1 gm/kg of body weight per day) but accumulated fat at a rate of 5.4 ± 0.3 gm/kg/day—about three times that in the fetus, as confirmed by increased skin-fold thickness. (See Figure 6–2B.) The long-term significance of this finding is currently unknown.

Vitamins and Minerals

The low-birth-weight infant, in addition to taking in daily requirements, needs to replenish stores, since perinatal storage of many substances normally occurs during the last trimester of pregnancy. Body composition data[185] indicate that more than two thirds of the minerals acquired by the fetus are deposited in the last trimester of pregnancy. To allow for incomplete absorption, minerals must be supplied in excess of desired accretion rates. The daily nutritional and vitamin requirements are outlined in Table 6–3.

SODIUM.[8–10, 16, 18, 48, 56, 62, 105, 112, 140] Infants with birth weights less than 1.5 kg are prone to hyponatremia (sodium less than 130 mEq/l) during the first 6 weeks of life. Sodium balance studies reveal negative sodium balance below 32 weeks' gestation. This is due to the combined influence of (1) renal immaturity, which permits relatively high urinary sodium loss in the presence of low plasma sodium, (2) low sodium intake from formulae or breast milk, and (3) coprecipitation of sodium in bone during the active phase of bone growth. Sodium losses are accentuated in critically ill babies with respiratory distress syndrome, following diuretic therapy, and in the presence of glycosuria. Usually the hyponatremia is asymptomatic because of the chronicity in the development of this electrolyte abnormality. However, if these infants develop complications—such as sepsis or apnea—initiation of intravenous fluid therapy with acute expansion of body fluid may precipitate symptomatic hypona-

TABLE 6–3 DAILY NUTRITIONAL AND VITAMIN REQUIREMENTS FOR LOW-BIRTH-WEIGHT INFANTS*

Total Nutrients	Per 100 Cal	Per kg	Vitamins	Total (Vitamins) Per Day†
Calories	100	100–140	A	1400–2500 IU
Water	—	130–200 ml‡	Thiamine	0.4 mg
Protein	1.8	3–4 gm (10–15%)	Riboflavin	0.5 mg
Carbohydrate	—	10–15 gm (45–55%)	Pyridoxine	0.25 mg
Fat	3.3	5–7 gm (30–45%)	B_{12}	1.0 µg
Sodium	0.9	2–4 mEq	C	30–50 mg
Chloride	1.6	0.5–2 mEq	D	400 IU
Potassium	2.1	0.5–2 mEq	E	5–100 IU
Calcium	50 mg	4–6 mEq	Niacin	6.0 mg
Phosphorus	25 mg	2–4 mEq	Panthenol	—
Magnesium	6 mg	0.5–1.1 mEq	Folic acid	0.35 mg
Iron	—	6 mg/day	K	1.5 mg

*See Appendix J–1.
†Start vitamin supplementation between fifth and tenth days of life.
‡Adequate to maintain normal urine output of 1–3 ml/kg/hr.

tremia with water intoxication. Term babies require 1–1.5 mEq of sodium/kg/day, whereas preterm infants, especially those below 32 weeks' gestation, need 3–4 mEq/kg/day to prevent hyponatremia. Serum sodium and other electrolytes should be monitored at least weekly.

Calcium and magnesium are considered in Chapter 10.

VITAMINS. Because of rapid growth, the vitamin requirements of low-birth-weight infants may exceed intake, and supplementation is necessary. Most commercial formulae have vitamin supplements. However, to ingest the minimal daily requirements, the infant must be fed large quantities of formula each day. This is obviously impossible in the smaller infant, whose vitamin intake should be supplemented commencing on the fifth to tenth day of life.

Apart from vitamins D and E, most vitamin deficiencies are relatively rare in the absence of malabsorption syndromes. Nonetheless, folate and vitamin B_{12} deficiencies have been noted in low-birth-weight infants. Rickets may be seen in rapidly growing low-birth-weight infants not receiving vitamin supplements[103] (see Chapter 10). Vitamin E absorption, requirements, and deficiency are considered in detail in Chapter 15, as is vitamin K.

Functional Capacity—Gastrointestinal Tract

Sucking and Swallowing[59, 76, 77, 108, 152]

Sucking and swallowing are established prenatally but are not fully developed until after birth. The patterns of suck and esoph-

ageal and gastric motor function differ in the immediate neonatal period and the period thereafter. Gastric emptying is delayed in the first few hours. In the full-term infant, the esophageal response to deglutition is uncoordinated during the first day.

Normally, sucking precedes swallowing, which in turn inhibits respiration. At the time of swallowing, the nasal passages are open and the epiglottis closed, so that air enters the stomach. Thereafter, the epiglottis opens, and air goes into the trachea. The inhibition of respiration during swallowing safeguards against aspiration. Coordination of this mechanism develops at approximately 32–34 weeks' gestation. Before this time, the premature infant displays discoordinate activity, and aspiration is possible.

When presented with a stimulus, infants first "mouth" the nipple before making sucking attempts. Sucking varies with nipple flow and the type of food. Slower sucking is seen with glucose water than with formula. The "mature suck/swallow pattern" consists of prolonged sucking bursts with multiple swallows occurring simultaneously with sucking. *In immature infants, the suck pattern* is characterized by short sucking bursts that are preceded or followed by swallows. Simultaneous contractions are seen throughout the esophagus, but peristalsis is only evident with prolonged sucking bursts. This "immature suck pattern" persists for some time in the small premature infant and may represent a developmental protective mechanism that prevents overloading of an esophagus not yet ready to transmit a large bolus.

It had been postulated that in premature infants the use of a pacifier during gavage

TABLE 6–4 SOME TRACE ELEMENTS AND THEIR DEFICIENCIES

Element	Minimum Level Recommended	Human Milk	Neonatal Values in Human Plasma	Some Effects of Deficiency
[53]Chromium	—	11.6 ng/ml	5–17.5 ng/ml (serum)	Impaired glucose tolerance, poor growth
Copper	(60–90 μg/100 kcal)	(60–90 μg/100 kcal)	Newborn: <0.70 μg/ml	Neutropenia—anemia, osteoporosis
[71]Iodine	(5 μg/100 kcal)	(4–9 μg/100 kcal)	0.053–0.200 μg/ml	Endemic goiter, hypothyroidism
Iron	(1.0 mg/100 kcal)	(0.1 mg/100 kcal)	Newborn: 1.10–2.70 μg/ml	Anemia, impaired learning ability?
Manganese	(5 μg/100 kcal)	(1.5 μg/100 kcal)	—	In animals only—growth retardation, ataxia of newborn, bone changes
[49]Selenium	—	13–50 μg/ml	Newborn: 1 wk 80 ng/ml 2 wk 60 ng/ml 3 wk 40 ng/ml 4 wk 40 ng/ml 5 wk 35 ng/ml	Increased fragility of red cells
Zinc	(0.5 mg/100 kcal)	(0.5 mg/100 kcal)	Newborn: 1.10 μg/ml	Impaired appetite, impaired taste, growth retardation, acrodermatitis enteropathica

Modified from Hambidge.[81] (See also references 2, 82, and 110.)

feedings may accelerate the maturation of the sucking reflex and the transition to total oral feedings. Bernbaum et al[26] documented the addition of nonnutritive sucking as in fact accelerating the maturation of the sucking reflex, facilitating a more rapid transition from gavage to oral feedings. Furthermore, nonnutritive sucking decreased intestinal transit time and caused a more rapid weight gain as a result either of decreased energy expenditure or of more efficient nutrient absorption. They noted that sucking facilitates oxygenation measured transcutaneously and concluded that nonnutritive sucking appears to decrease energy expenditure by decreasing restless activity.

In the majority of term and premature infants, the inferior esophageal sphincter mechanism, which is located at or above the effective diaphragmatic hiatus, has poor tone. Barrie[20] demonstrated that all infants, even those fed through a nasogastric tube, regurgitated milk into the lower half of the esophagus and also showed altered or abnormal patterns of breathing associated with feeding. He noted an increase in respiratory rate and attributed this to mechanical interference with diaphragmatic movement. In contrast, Russell and Feather,[142] studying the effects of feeding on respiratory mechanics in healthy newborn infants, demonstrated no adverse effects of small feeds on the work of breathing, compliance, respiratory rate, and minute volume.

Shivpuri et al[151] studied the effect of oral feeding on ventilation in preterm infants 34–35.9 weeks of age and 36–38 weeks of age. The feeding pattern comprised an initial period of continuous sucking of at least 30 seconds followed by intermittent sucking bursts for the remainder of the feed. Minute ventilation fell during continuous sucking as the result of the decrease in both respiratory frequency and tidal volume, and this was associated with a fall in the transcutaneous oxygen level. Recovery occurred during intermittent sucking only in the more mature group. Oral feeding therefore results in an impairment of ventilation during continuous sucking, and the subsequent recovery during intermittent sucking is dependent on postconceptional age.

In immature infants, periodic breathing with apnea often occurs within 15 minutes following feeding.[44] Radiologically, large amounts of air are found in both the stomach and the esophagus. (For a further discussion of apnea, see Chapter 8.)

Gastric Activity in Emptying

At term, the human infant's stomach is round and holds about 10–20 ml. In the first 2 weeks of life, the infant's stomach grows more rapidly than the body as a whole, and as it enlarges, its rate of emptying slows. At birth, the stomach contains swallowed liquor amnii in addition to respiratory mucus, blood, and occasionally, meconium. Delayed gastric emptying in the first hours of life may also be due to elevated gastrin and glucagon levels, which delay emptying in adults. The thin gastric muscle coats and diminished motility often result in prolonged emptying time in the newborn.

Using a radioisotopic method in term infants (mean age 25 days) in the supine position, Signer and Fridrich[153] found that gastric emptying followed an exponential pattern with a half life of 87 ± 29 minutes in 24 of 28 normal infants. Gastric activity and emptying are dependent on the state and condition of the infant, the type of meal ingested, and the position when fed, as well as the volume of the feed. Yu[181] observed that the rate of gastric emptying is the same for the healthy term, the preterm, and the small-fordates infant.

In the supine position, infants with respiratory distress syndrome have delayed gastric emptying with a high incidence of abdominal distension and pooling of feeds in the stomach.[182] Furthermore, the risk of regurgitation and aspiration is greater than that in other positions. The prone or the right lateral position is thus preferred for feeding neonates, especially those in whom intolerance to the volume of feeds is anticipated. The stomach empties more rapidly in the prone than in the supine or left lateral positions, and higher arterial oxygen values are noted in the prone position. Moreover, gastric emptying is faster after tube feedings than after bottle feedings. (Incidentally, it is as necessary to burp infants after tube feeds as after bottle feeds.)

The higher the concentration of glucose solution, the slower the gastric emptying. However, despite the slow emptying of 10 per cent glucose, this solution may be preferable to 5 per cent glucose when oral glucose is used for intermittent feeding, because more glucose is being delivered to the small intestine per unit time.

Obviously, more calories can be delivered by the use of an equivalent volume of milk, and this form of oral nutrition is usually preferable to glucose and water solutions.   **L. Stern**

In summary, gastrointestinal function in the newborn, particularly those born preterm, may be characterized by (1) diminished smooth muscle mass and reflux from poor sphincteric development, (2) reduced gastric

propulsive activity, (3) less mature autonomic nervous system innervation, and (4) blunted hormonal and enzyme responses. The net result is inefficient intake, delayed digestion, and significant malabsorption.

Emptying is also retarded when more fat and larger protein particles are present in the formula. Isotonic food passes through the body more rapidly than extremely hypotonic or hypertonic foods.

PRINCIPLES

1. Energy reserves in the low-birth-weight infant are extremely small; therefore even brief periods of starvation should be avoided.

2. A new formula should not be used until it has been proved by adequate studies.[92] Experimental feeding practices should be limited to centers where critical analysis is available. When evaluating the results of any feeding study, one must distinguish the truly premature infants from those who are small for gestational age and also match birth weights, gestational ages, and sex. In comparing the results, one should study weight gain, increase in length, changes in head circumference, morbidity and mortality, and such difficult parameters to evaluate as school performance and length of life.

3. The institution of early feeding will shorten the period required to regain birth weight.

4. (a) Changes in metabolic rate with advancing postnatal age are modulated by energy intake and weight gain. (b) Metabolic rate is influenced by age, weight, sex, diet, hormones, and caloric intake. (c) There is a linear relationship between metabolic rate and weight gain.

5. Fifty-three per cent of energy intake is used for growth. The composition of weight gain can be manipulated by changes in energy and macronutrient intake.

6. In SGA infants there is increased basal energy utilization as a result of greater oxidation of fat. SGA infants absorb less protein and fat, but carbohydrate absorption is normal.

7. The optimal rate of growth is unknown.[40] Whereas efforts are directed to "prompt postnatal resumption of growth to a rate approximating intrauterine growth,"[39] this is usually impossible. Recent data suggest that, provided catch-up growth occurs prior to 8 months corrected age, neurodevelopment is unaffected.[78, 79]

8. While the protein, carbohydrate, fat, fluid, and electrolyte requirements necessary for increase in size are known, *bigger is not necessarily better*. The relationship between diet and longevity was established when it was demonstrated experimentally that a regimen of calorie restriction imposed throughout early postnatal life increased the length of life of rats. Actuarial analysis demonstrated that rats who had consumed large amounts of food were more likely to be short-lived.[135]

9. Low-birth-weight infants may require some amino acids that are not essential for term infants.

- Methionine cannot be converted to cystine, owing to absence of cystathionase. Cystine must therefore be supplied exogenously.[66]
- Taurine may be semiessential in the human infant. Taurine synthesized from cystine is involved in the synthesis of bile acids and in neurotransmission in various tissues.[163] Taurine deficiency produces degeneration of the developing retina in kittens. Human milk provides free taurine, thereby maintaining plasma and urine levels. Casein-predominant formulae, which contain no exogenous taurine, result in progressively low plasma and urine taurine levels in infants.
- Enzymatic capacity for degradation of some amino acids (e.g., phenylalanine and tyrosine) is impaired in low-birth-weight infants.[127, 159] Plasma levels of phenylalanine and tyrosine in infants receiving casein-predominant formulae are elevated to values similar to those associated with inborn errors of metabolism. Tyrosine, on the other hand, is essential for growth.
- Enzymatic detoxification of excess ammonia via production of urea is lower in these infants.

10. The term fetus receives large quantities of minerals during the last 2 months of gestation. Deficiency disease must be prevented by adequate supplementation of minerals and vitamins. Preterm infants are delivered before receiving these stores, which need to be repleted in addition to providing daily maintenance requirements.

11. Extrauterine adaptation should be normal *before the first feed*. The infant should be warm and breathing normally and should have good color, tone, and cry.[14] The technique of feeding will be determined by both birth weight and gestational age. The gag reflex is *not* complete until 8 months' gesta-

tion. Before this time, infants should be gavage fed, supplemented by IV feedings (see Practical Considerations). Note that the presence of normal sucking does not guarantee a completely adequate gag reflex. If the infant has a moderate to severe pulmonary problem, do not feed him orally.

12. The gastric capacity of the small infant is limited; thus, he may require small amounts of formula at frequent intervals. *Spitting should not be tolerated* in small infants (<1500 gm), in whom danger of pulmonary aspiration is great. If spitting is noted, reduce the volume of feed.

13. Because of the increased fluid content, the stomach of infants born by cesarean section and infants of diabetic mothers may be aspirated before the first feed.

14. Early feeding of low-birth-weight infants is associated with a higher blood sugar, lower bilirubin, less dehydration, and a more rapid return to birth weight.[22, 85, 93, 123, 156, 180]

In infants less than 2000 gm, maintain IV administration from approximately 3 hours of age until oral intake is around 110 ml/kg. In smaller infants, this may take a long period of time.

15. Although breast milk theoretically may not meet all the growth requirements of the preterm infant, we encourage mothers to breast feed their high-risk, low-birth-weight infants. Breast milk has unique physical and immunologic properties for the human infant.[69] It is better absorbed and causes fewer intestinal problems than other formulae. In developed countries, breast milk feeding is associated with reduced infant morbidity, and in developing countries, both morbidity and mortality are reduced.

16. While it has been clearly demonstrated that total parenteral nutrition can produce satisfactory growth and positive nitrogen balance without undue risk in low-birth-weight infants, the sequelae of total parenteral nutrition have not as yet been defined.

In infants receiving total parenteral nutrition, the line should be considered inviolate. Do not administer other medication, give blood, or take blood samples from the line, since this significantly increases the risk of infection.

17. Small-for-gestational-age infants are prone to hypoglycemia and cannot tolerate prolonged fasting.

18. Excessive fluid intake has been associated with patent ductus arteriosus, pulmonary edema, congestive heart failure, necro-

tizing enterocolitis, and bronchopulmonary dysplasia.

19. Nonnutritive sucking results in more rapid weight gain and facilitates the transition from gavage to oral feedings.

20. In the prone position, infants have less gastroesophageal reflux and maintain better oxygenation (see Chapter 8).

21. In premature neonates, deficiencies of calcium and phosphorus intake are a common problem that frequently results in osteopenia, rickets, and fractures (see Chapter 10).

22. Some basic problems in feeding the preterm infant include (a) lack of coordination between suck and swallow until 34 weeks' gestation; (b) limited gastric capacity; (c) gastroesophageal reflux (poor sphincter development); (d) diminished gastrointestinal motility; and (e) deficient enzymes and hormones and hence less efficient absorption.

23. Breast milk, obtained from mothers of infants delivered before term, if given in adequate volumes, may support macronutrient balance and growth in the early postnatal weeks. After this period, growth may be hindered in small infants if the expressed milk is neither fortified nor supplemented.

24. Low-birth-weight infants during the period of rapid catch-up growth may require increased vitamin intake to prevent deficiency diseases such as rickets.[103]

PRACTICAL CONSIDERATIONS

1. The commencement of feedings should be determined by the tone, color, and respiratory patterns of the immature infant and should be individualized. There should be no fixed feeding orders written for low-birth-weight infants. If the infant has respiratory distress or is hypothermic, oral feedings should be withheld and fluids and calories given by the intravenous route.

2. *The first feed*—Early feeding (IV and/or oral) of newborn infants, premature and full term, results in a reduction in the degree of hyperbilirubinemia, less hypoglycemia and dehydration, and a significantly higher survival rate (only in infants <1500 gm). Infants less than 1500 gm should probably receive all their fluids and calories intravenously for the first 24–48 hours. A most important controlled study revealed a steep reduction in mortality for infants weighing less than 1500 gm who received parenteral fluids early (at 6 hours of age) when compared with those given nasogastric fluids early or with those who were starved.[41]

Surprising to most pediatricians, Olson[116] found that 5 per cent glucose water instilled into the respiratory tree in rabbits caused changes similar to milk. Sterile water, which causes no pulmonary reaction, thus theoretically would be the choice for the first feed. However, when an infant aspirates, the lung is invaded not only by the feed but also by the other gastric contents, including HCl, which will cause a severe chemical pneumonia. We still use the traditional 5 per cent glucose water for the first feed (at 4–6 hours of age), exercising caution in selecting infants who have had normal extrauterine adaptation, using careful technique, and avoiding large volumes.

The finding by Olson that 5 per cent glucose and water appears to be as harmful to the lung in the newborn rabbit as milk casts serious doubt on the rationale that has made 5 per cent or 10 per cent glucose and water the first drink of the newborn infant. Since there appears to be no evidence to support it, there would seem to be little value in maintaining this so-called traditional initial feeding, and our own view therefore is to go immediately to a milk formula as the baby's first drink. **L. Stern**

3. A significant study evaluating the effect of a feeding gastrostomy on the survival of infants with birth weights between 750 and 1250 gm showed that the mortality with gastrostomy was higher than with routine feedings.[118] Gastrostomy should be reserved only for infants requiring surgical correction of anatomic malformations, such as tracheoesophageal fistula.

4. Infants over 34 weeks' gestation or those between 32 and 34 weeks who show an ability both to suck and swallow may be fed by nipple. Those who do not have an adequate gag reflex (<32 weeks) should be gavage fed.

Procedure for Gavage Feeding. Gavage feeding is indicated for all infants under 32 weeks' gestation, those with neurologic impairment, and those recovering from or with residual symptoms of respiratory distress. Use a No. 5 or 8 French polyethylene feeding tube.

- With the baby's head turned to the side, measure the length from xiphoid to tip of ear lobe plus ear to nose and mark tube.
- Pass the catheter through the nose or mouth to this mark.
- Check that the catheter is in the stomach by first placing the proximal end of the catheter under water to determine that air is not returned with each respiration and then injecting a small amount of air and

listening over the stomach for bubbling. Aspirate the contents of the stomach and test the reaction (pH 5 or less).

- If the gastric content is thick and/or contains blood and mucus, a small stomach washout with sterile water (5–10 ml) may be given.
- Feedings are to be introduced by gravity; they are not to be injected with a syringe under pressure.
- When removing the tube, pinch it closed as it is withdrawn to avoid dripping fluid into the pharynx.

5. To accommodate the relatively large fluid load and because of the diminished gastric capacity, we use frequent small feeds, feeding infants <1250 gm as often as hourly. The feeds are increased progressively per feeding schedule, making sure that a given amount is tolerated before increasing the amount. Oral feeding is supplemented initially by IV fluid.

An important practical consideration in daily management of feeding programs for the low-birth-weight infant receiving both oral and parenteral feedings is to reduce the amount of parenteral feeds proportional to the increment of the oral feeds. Failure to do this will often result in excessive fluid intake. **W. Oh**

Nasojejunal Feedings.[29, 50, 132] The use of nasojejunal feedings has been advocated for sick newborns and preterm infants.[34, 104, 130] A long silicone or polyvinyl nasojejunal tube is used with or without a weight to facilitate positioning of the tube. The tube is introduced through the nostril, allowing a generous length in the stomach so that it may pass through the pylorus to the duodenum. The infant is placed on the right side, and fluid is aspirated intermittently. When the pH of the aspirate rises to between 5 and 7, x-rays are obtained to confirm catheter position in the jejunum. Transpyloric passage usually takes between 1 and 4 hours. Once the catheter is in place, infusions may be commenced. Techniques including either continuous infusion or intermittent feedings have been successful. It is also advisable to place a gastric tube and monitor gastric residue. Complications resulting from the tube have included infection, perforation (the catheters tend to get stiff and should not be advanced once they have been correctly positioned), necrotizing enterocolitis, jejunal intussusception, and regurgitation with aspiration.[28, 35] Rhea et al[131] fed almost 500 patients by the nasojejunal route and did not encounter any serious complications. They stress the need

for isoosmolar feedings and use soft silicone tubing, which they lubricate with baby powder, wiping off the excess. However, they concluded from their studies that there was a slight but significant absorptive disadvantage to feeding via the nasojejunal route. We have rarely found it necessary to resort to this type of feeding and prefer the gastric route.[131]

Composition of Formula. The composition of some of the formulae used in our nursery is outlined in Tables 6–5 and 6–7. We use formula closely resembling breast milk (humanized milk) for feeding low-birth-weight infants.

A special formula, of which there are many available, may be required for infants with special dietary problems—galactosemia, milk intolerance, etc.

BREAST MILK[3, 4, 11, 12, 38, 70, 74, 75, 146, 164]

Human breast milk has probably been modified over many centuries so that it is geared to the full-term infant's particular needs, including protection from infection. While it has been shown that newborns may be adequately nurtured with artificial formulae, studies throughout the world reveal that breast milk markedly reduces morbidity and mortality, particularly as a result of reduced upper respiratory and gastrointestinal infections.[84] In addition to its nutrient and electrolyte components (Table 6–5), breast milk has a rich cellular and immunologic endowment (Table 6–6).

The cellular content of human milk has become the focus of intensive investigation. The majority of these cells are macrophages and immunocompetent B and T lymphocytes. Neutrophils have also been found in significant numbers early in lactation, and epithelial cells, possibly originating from the skin of the nipple, are occasionally present. The leukocytes, especially the macrophages, are active phagocytic cells and have been implicated as a factor in the protection that breast milk provides in laboratory animal models against necrotizing enterocolitis.[17] This cell is also responsible for the synthesis of several host resistance factors in milk, including lysozyme, C3 and C4 complement components, and lactoferrin. The B lymphocytes, in contradistinction to those in peripheral blood, synthesize only immunoglobulin A (IgA) and minimal IgM or IgG. The function of the breast milk neutrophil has not been well defined.[111, 119–121, 157]

W. Pittard

Renewed interest in the immunocompetent cellular components of breast milk has followed reports of colostrum halting otherwise uncontrollable epidemics of *E. coli* diarrhea in newborns and reports suggesting that

TABLE 6–5 COMPARISON OF INFANT FORMULAE

	Human Milk	SMA	Similac w/Whey	Similac w/Iron	Enfamil w/Iron
Protein (w/v)	1.2%	1.5%	1.5%	1.5%	1.5%
Casein	40%	40%	40%	82%	40%
Whey protein	60%	60%	60%	18%	60%
Fat (w/v)	3.6%	3.6%	3.6%	3.6%	3.8%
% Polyunsaturated	11	14	38	38	29
% Monounsaturated	40	41	15	15	16
% Saturated	49	45	47	47	55
Polyunsaturated: Saturated	0.2	0.3	0.8	0.8	0.5
Vitamin E (IU/qt)	5	9	18.9	18.9	20
E: Linoleate (IU/gm linoleate)	1.8	2.1	1.7	1.7	2.3
Minerals mg/dl (mEq/l)	210	250	340	330	300
Total (ash)					
Sodium	15 (6.5)	15 (6.5)	23 (10.0)	23 (10.0)	21 (9.1)
Potassium	55 (14.1)	56 (14.3)	75 (19.2)	80 (20.5)	69 (17.6)
Calcium	34 (17.0)	44 (22.1)	40 (20.0)	51 (25.4)	47 (23.2)
Phosphorus	14 (9.0)	33 (21.3)	30 (19.4)	39 (25.2)	32 (20.6)
Chloride	37 (10.4)	37 (10.6)	43 (12.1)	50 (14.1)	42 (11.8)
Iron (per qt)	0.8 mg	12 mg*	11.4 mg	11.4 mg*	12 mg*
Carbohydrate (w/v)	7.2% (lactose)	7.2% (lactose)	7.2% (lactose)	7.2% (lactose)	6.9% (lactose)

Courtesy of Wyeth Laboratories, Philadelphia, PA.

NOTE: All data for competitive products derived from product labels, *Physicians' Desk Reference* (Oradell, NJ, Medical Economics Company, 1985), or analyses.

*SMA lo-iron, Enfamil, and Similac contain 1.4 mg iron per quart. Infants fed these formulae should receive supplemental dietary iron from an outside source to meet daily requirements.

breast milk contains specific substances that neutralize both cholera and *E. coli* enterotoxin.[161] The specific antitoxin appears to be secretory IgA, which is the only immunoglobulin synthesized in vitro by human milk B lymphocytes. Secretory IgA is not destroyed by the gastrointestinal enzymes and carries most of the immunologic memory from the mother, containing her antibodies to viral and bacterial infection. During active swallowing, it is literally painted over the large mucosal surfaces of the pharynx and intestine and may act as a direct barrier against infection.

It is pertinent that the secretory IgA produced by milk B lymphocytes is largely directed against the microbial antigens of the mother's gastrointestinal tract (i.e., enterotoxin of pathogenic *E. coli*). This phenomenon is explained by a theory referred to as "homing." This theory proposes the B lymphocytes sensitized by gut antigens migrate from the intestinal Peyer's patches to the breast and then synthesize secretory IgA with specificity for antigens previously encountered in the gut.

W. Pittard

Additionally, interest in breast milk has been generated by the observation that colostral feeds stimulate growth and maturation

TABLE 6–6 HOST RESISTANCE FACTORS IN HUMAN MILK[69]

Components	Proposed Mode of Action
Growth factor of *L. bifidus*	*L. bifidus* interferes with intestinal colonization of enteric pathogens
Antistaphylococcal factor	Inhibits staphylococci
Secretory IgA and other immunoglobulins	Protective antibodies for the gut and respiratory tract
C4 and C3	C3 fragments have opsonic, chemotactic, and anaphylatoxic activities
Lysozyme	Lysis of bacterial cell wall
Lactoperoxidase-H_2O_2-thiocyanate	Killing of streptococci
Lactoferrin	Kills microorganisms by chelating iron
Leukocytes	Phagocytosis Cell-mediated immunity Production of IgA, C4, C3, lysozyme, and lactoferrin

of intestinal mucosa in beagle puppies[87] and that breast-fed infants develop higher concentrations of secretory IgA in their salivary and nasal secretions than do bottle-fed infants in the first 4 days of life.[133] The complex interactions of breast milk constituents resulting in immunoprotection, development, and maturation of the gastrointestinal tract of the newborn recipient represent an important area for further investigation.

For the immature infant, a revival of use of breast milk as a main source of nutrition follows a number of observations. Breast milk has an optimal distribution of calories, with 7 per cent provided as protein, 55 per cent as fat, and 38 per cent as carbohydrate.[63] In addition to the caloric distribution and easy digestibility, there is the favorable composition. The protein constituents are very different from humanized milk or cow's milk and provide essential amino acids, including cystine and taurine. The whey/casein ratio is 60:40, and whey proteins include alpha-lactalbumin, beta-lactoglobulin, serum albumin, lysozyme, and immunoglobulin A. The lipid-lipase system in fresh human milk is an important contributor to the fat and energy metabolism in the very low-birth-weight infant. The unsaturated fatty acids appear not only to be tolerated but even to enhance fat and energy balance in these small immature infants. Lactose in breast milk, which facilitates the growth of *Lactobacillus bifidus* upon hydrolysis, releases galactose, which may play a unique role in the synthesis of cerebrosides of myelin and the glycoproteins. Additionally, there is a special carrier protein for zinc. The small quantities of iron are bioavailable and well absorbed. There are also quantities of thyroid hormones in breast milk sufficient to delay the onset of hypothyroidism.

Previous calculations have suggested that the sodium, calcium, and protein contents of pooled maternal human milk are inadequate to achieve the growth potential of the small premature infant.[185] However, data on milk from mothers of premature infants reveal a significantly higher nitrogen concentration than is present in full-term infants' mother's milk during the first month of lactation.[3, 11, 12, 75, 146] Nonetheless, the conclusions from a number of studies suggest that, whereas large volumes of milk expressed from mothers who deliver prematurely will sustain growth during the early postnatal period, supplementation is required beyond then.

Schanler et al[146] recently fortified mother's fresh, preterm milk, augmenting both the energy and the nutrient content. Administering 120–160 ml/kg of this fortified milk per day resulted in growth, metabolizable energy, and nitrogen balance similar to intrauterine references and references for infants fed commercial formula. It should be emphasized that despite fortification the mineral content remained deficient.

Advances in human milk technology and lactoengineering will no doubt result in the development of a fortified human milk product that will meet the micro- and macronutrient needs of preterm growth.

Fresh but not frozen breast milk protects against a laboratory model of necrotizing enterocolitis. As yet, no human studies of breast milk demonstrate protection from necrotizing enterocolitis. Furthermore, there are many as yet unanswered questions concerning possible deleterious effects of human milk.

- With regard to the contamination of human milk, although it has been shown that the presence of DDT in human milk is in greater concentration than that in cow's milk, to date no harmful effects of such DDT have been demonstrated. It is likely that contamination of milk from the polluted environment is comparable in cow's milk and human milk.
- Knowledge of excretion of drugs and other substances in human milk is still inconclusive.
- Viral transmission in human milk remains a concern. To what extent are viruses such as cytomegalovirus, herpesvirus, and hepatitis transmitted via human milk?
- How should human milk be collected, processed, and stored? The cells in breast milk will stick to glass, so it is advisable that plastic containers be used for collection of human milk. Our own practice has been to use fresh milk, refrigerated for up to 48 hours. The initial sample is cultured, and only when the results of the cultures are available is this milk used for the mother's own infant.

Editorial Comment: Although breast milk is thought to offer the best nutrition, there remains a great deal of controversy about feeding very low-birth-weight (VLBW) infants banked human milk. Assessment of any new formulation of human milk and its components is a complex and possibly dangerous business.

Williams, A. F., and Baum, J. D.: *Human Milk Banking.* New York, Raven Press, 1984.

Heat treatment of milk may adversely influence fat absorption, functional carrier proteins, free amino acid availability, cellular immune function, and the content of lactoferrin, IgM, and IgA. The ability to inhibit bacterial overgrowth is lost if milk is heated excessively. We therefore avoid this practice.

Although the body of knowledge has expanded significantly, the question of the use of donor milk for preterm infants remains unanswered.

A SUGGESTED FEEDING SCHEDULE

The first feeding is 5–10 per cent glucose in water or sterile water. If the glucose is tolerated, formula is commenced. Formula feeding should be 20 or 24 calories/30 ml utilizing the preparations specially adapted for preterm infants (Table 6–7). For infants with a poor gag reflex (gestational age 32–34 weeks), it is most important that the chosen volume not result in any vomiting or spitting.

In the nursery where necrotizing enterocolitis (NEC) is observed (some centers have reported zero incidence of NEC), a routine monitoring protocol for early signs of NEC should be done in the high-risk infant. The factors making an infant at high risk for NEC include low birth weight and gestation, presence of patent ductus arteriosus with left-to-right shunt, evidence of thrombotic complication with indwelling umbilical arterial catheter, hyperviscosity, and previous episodes of hypoxia, acidosis, and shock. The monitoring protocol should include assessment of gastric residual before each feed, blood in stool, abdominal distension and tenderness, and emesis or regurgitation. When one or more of these signs are present, a plain abdominal roentgenogram should be obtained for radiologic evidence of NEC.   **W. Oh**

Supplement daily oral intake with IV infusion so that total fluid intake is between 120 and 150 ml/kg/day. To achieve minimum weight loss in some small infants, greater volumes may be required. The danger, however, of fluid overload and the association of large fluid intakes with PDA, bronchopulmonary dysplasia (BPD), or NEC have resulted in our efforts to reduce fluid losses and not to be forced to use mammoth intakes.

Maintain IV infusion of 10 per cent glucose, commencing at age 3–6 hours at a rate of 80–100 ml/kg/day. After 24 hours, add maintenance sodium chloride and potassium. Check urine every 8 hours, and if glycosuria develops, reduce concentration of IV fluids to 7.5 per cent or 5 per cent glucose, always calculating the rate of glucose derived in mg/kg/min. When oral feedings have reached 100–120 cal/kg/day, discontinue IV feedings.

The use of intravenous fluids, particularly in small infants, is clearly beneficial under these situations. Little attention, however, is usually paid to the question of calcium in these solutions; this, coupled with a tendency to hypocalcemia, may result in an augmented iatrogenic hypocalcemia from the use of calcium-free fluids. In our experience, this is frequently associated with apneic spells that can be abolished when the cause is recognized and calcium is administered, either orally or added to the intravenous fluids. It is our policy to monitor calcium along with the other electrolytes and to provide for its addition to either the intravenous or the oral portions of the feeding as indicated.   **L. Stern**

For Infants Weighing ≤1250 gm at Birth (after 24–48 hours of IV feeding)

The first feeding is 1 ml of 5 per cent glucose in water. If this is tolerated, give a second such feeding after 1 hour.

If the first two feedings are tolerated, the infant is scheduled to be fed every hour. Five per cent glucose in water is increased 1 ml every hour until 3 ml volumes have been given twice and tolerated.

Start the formula at 3 ml every hour, which may be slowly increased in volume by 1 ml until a maximum of 6 ml is given every hour. Then the quantity remains the same at least until 144 hours (6 days) of age. If the infant weighs less than 1100 gm, stop at 5–6 ml (120–144 ml/kg/day; 100–120 cal/kg/day), and continue this amount for 6–10 days. This is usually only achieved at between 7 and 14 days of age. Aspiration is a major problem in this group. Small infants may require hourly feedings for a long period of time.

Editorial Comment: The advantage of continuous over intermittent nasogastric infusion is still an open question. We have used both techniques, mostly the latter. The key, however, is to supplement oral intake with intravenous fluid and calories until adequate calories are tolerated orally.

An important factor in considering continuous nasogastric infusion of feeds versus intermittent nasogastric (or orogastric) feeding is the preference and experience of the nursing personnel in the nursery. For instance, in a nursery where the nursing team has been trained and accustomed to do orogastric intermittent feeding (and with good success), this method of feeding should become a routine practice. Allow the other mode of feeding only in those unusual instances when clinical indications dictate that the alternative method is more advantageous.

W. Oh

Aspirate the stomach before each feeding and measure the residue. Replace the aspirate plus the amount needed to achieve the desired volume. If residue is equal to the desired volume, no formula is added.

When an infant is gaining and tolerating hourly feeding well, increase up to 8 ml/hour,

TABLE 6–7 PREMATURE FORMULAE COMPARISON CHART

	Minimum Recommendations (per dl)	"Preemie" SMA (per dl)	Similac Special Care (per dl)	Enfamil Premature (per dl)
Protein (gm)	1.5	2.0	2.2	2.4
Whey protein: casein ratio		60:40	60:40	60:40
Fat (gm)	2.7	4.4	4.4	4.1
MCT (medium-chain triglycerides)		10%	50%	40%
Oleo oil		20%	0%	0%
Corn oil		0%	30%	40%
Oleic oil		25%	0%	0%
Coconut oil		27%	20%	20%
Soy oil		18%	0%	0%
Carbohydrate (gm)		8.6	8.6	8.9
Lactose		50%	50%	40%
Glucose polymers		50%	50%	60%
Minerals (ash) (total mg)		400	650	500
Calcium (mg)	41	75	144	95
Phosphorus (mg)	20	40	72	48
Sodium (mg)	16	32	35	32
Potassium (mg)	65	75	100	90
Chloride (mg)	45	53	65	69
Magnesium (mg)	5	7	10	9
Zinc (mg)	0.4	0.5	1.2	0.5
Iron (mg)	0.1	0.3	0.3	0.1
Copper (μg)	49	70	200	73
Manganese (μg)	4	20	20	21
Iodine (μg)	4	8.3	15	7
Vitamins	(per l)	(per l)	(per l)	(per l)
A (IU)	2030	3200	5500	2537
D (IU)	325	510	1200	507
E (IU)	5.7	15	30	16
K_1 (μg)	32	70	100	76
C (Ascorbic acid) (mg)	65	70	300	69
B_1 (Thiamine) (μg)	325	800	2000	624
B_2 (Riboflavin) (μg)	487	1300	5000	728
B_6 (μg)	284	500	2000	500
B_{12} (μg)	1.22	2.0	4.5	2.5
Niacin (mg)	2.0	6.3	24.0	10.1
Folic acid (μg)	32	100	300	63
Pantothenic acid (μg)	2436	3600	15,000	3800
Biotin (μg)	12.2	18	300	19
Choline (mg)	57	127	80	57
Calories (per l)		810	810	810
Calories (per fl oz)		24	24	24
Osmolality (mOsm/kg H_2O)	400 (maximum)	268	300	300
Potential Renal Solute Load (PRSL) (mOsm/l)		175.2	208.0	220.0
Ca:P ratio	1.1:1	1.9:1	2:1	2:1
$\frac{Na + K}{Cl}$ ratio	1.5	2.2	2.2	1.9

Courtesy of Wyeth Laboratories, Philadelphia, PA.

then move to a two-hourly schedule as follows: first hour—9 ml, second hour—7 ml, third hour—10 ml, fourth hour—6 ml, and so on, thus gradually changing to a larger volume. This should be done only when the calories or fluids are insufficient and the infant is taking the feedings easily.

If feeding is not tolerated, return to the next lower volume given, offer it times six, and start increasing volume again.

For Infants Weighing 1250–1500 gm at Birth

The first feeding is 3 ml of 5–10 per cent glucose in water. If this is tolerated, give 5 ml of 5–10 per cent glucose in water after 2–3 hours.

Thereafter formula is fed every 2–3 hours, starting with a volume of 5 ml and increasing it 1 ml every other feeding until the infant is getting 10 to 14 ml volumes. Then the amount stays the same for 72 hours.

If a feeding is not tolerated, go back one step.

For Infants Weighing 1501–2000 gm at Birth

The first feeding is 5 ml of 5–10 per cent glucose in water. If this is tolerated, give 8 ml of 5 per cent glucose in water after 2–3 hours.

Formula feedings may then be given every 2–3 hours, starting with 8 ml and increasing 1 ml every other feeding until 14 ml volumes are taken. Thereafter, increments of 2–4 ml may be made daily until calculated requirements are met.

If a feeding is not tolerated, go back one step.

For Infants Weighing ≥2001 gm at Birth

The first feeding is 15 ml of 5 per cent glucose in water. If tolerated, repeat 15 ml of 5 per cent glucose in water.

The third feeding is given 3 hours after the second and is formula. If the third feeding is tolerated, regular 3 hour feedings are given, starting with 15 ml and increasing 5 ml every other feeding until 30 ml feedings are given.

If a feeding is not tolerated, go back one step. Note: In small-for-gestational-age infants, 10–15 per cent glucose given orally may be utilized from soon after birth. (These infants usually feed well and will tolerate larger volumes than the immature infants.) Blood sugar must be carefully monitored (every 2 hours for 12 hours) and an IV instituted if

TABLE 6–8 POTENTIAL PROBLEMS OF ENTERALLY FED PRETERM INFANTS

General
Abdominal distension, gastric retention
Gastroesophageal reflux, regurgitation
Aspiration pneumonia, laryngospasm
Apnea, bradycardia
↓ PaO_2, ↓ FRC*
Necrotizing enterocolitis (NEC)

Specific
- Feeding tube–related
  Gastrointestinal perforation
  Nasopharyngeal irritation
  Otitis?
  Occult blood in stool
  Plasticizer toxicity?
  Reflux
- Formula-related
  Lactobezoars (MCT oil)
  Malabsorption/diarrhea
  Systemic metabolic intolerances
  Deficiency states (rickets: soy formula)
  NEC (hyperosmotic formula)
- Transpyloric feeds
  Abnormal upper GI tract colonization
  Jejunal-jejunal intussusception
  Fat malabsorption
  Pyloric stenosis

Modified from Kliegman, R. M., and Fanaroff, A. A.: Developmental metabolism and nutrition. *In* Gregory, G. A. (ed.): *Pediatric Anesthesia.* New York, Churchill Livingstone, Inc., 1983.
*FRC = functional residual capacity.

hypoglycemia develops and is not immediately controlled by oral feeding.

The oral intake is supplemented by intravenous fluid for at least a week in the smaller infants. With this technique, larger volumes can be fed, resulting in a more rapid weight gain.

Problems related to feeding preterm infants are tabulated in Table 6–8.

PARENTERAL NUTRITION[178]

The last decade has seen a marked increase in the use of parenteral protein, carbohydrate, and lipids. While their use in major neonatal surgical conditions (including necrotizing enterocolitis, gastric perforation and resections, giant omphalocele, gastroschisis, and tracheoesophageal fistula) has clearly been established, the role of parenteral nutrition in extremely low-birth-weight infants and those with chronic respiratory failure has yet to be clearly defined.[58, 88] The goals of total parenteral nutrition are to provide adequate calories for growth as well as to meet the protein, carbohydrate, fat, mineral, micromineral, and vitamin requirements of the infant. At all times, the benefits of the use of this technique must be clearly balanced against the many complications.[21, 42, 43, 115, 117, 118, 134, 144, 166, 170, 183] Total parenteral nutrition should not be utilized indiscriminately in all low-birth-weight infants.

In many centers, including ours, similar sentiments are expressed. In the very low-birth-weight infant, it is technically difficult to place a central venous catheter; the catheter size is proportionately too large for the vessel, the ability to metabolize the large dose of glucose is often impaired, resulting in hyperglycemia and glucosuria, and the rate of catheter-related infection is high. Therefore total parenteral alimentation with central venous catheter placement should be confined only to the term large-sized infant with indications for prolonged total parenteral nutritional support.　　**W. Oh**

Fluid used for total parenteral nutrition comprises a source of nitrogen containing both essential and nonessential amino acids, supplemented with nonprotein calories, usually in the form of glucose or fructose. Initially, solutions containing hydrolyzed casein or fibrin as well as synthetic amino acid solutions were utilized. Recently, however, only the amino acid solutions have been readily available commercially. Other required substances such as electrolytes, minerals, and vitamins must be provided by various additives to the infusate. Alcohol is occasionally used as an additional caloric source, but in view of its hepatotoxicity and the unpredictable blood alcohol level in infants, it is not recommended.

The usual composition of the nutritive fluid is listed in Table 6–9. Some complications associated with total parenteral nutrition are listed in Table 6–10. It should be

TABLE 6–10 COMPLICATIONS ASSOCIATED WITH PARENTERAL ALIMENTATION

Metabolic
 Hypo- and hyperglycemia
 Electrolyte imbalance
 Hypo- and hypercalcemia
 Hypophosphatemia
 Lower RBC, ATP, and 2,3-DPG
 Acquired phagocyte dysfunction
 Metabolic acidosis
 Hyperammonemia
 Isoosmolar coma
 Cholestasis
 Abnormal liver function
 Fatty acid deficiency
 Trace element deficiency

Infection
Candida sepsis is potentially the most dangerous
 Bacterial sepsis
 Fungal sepsis
 (If sepsis develops, the line must be removed)

Catheter Complications
Improper placement of catheter may lead to extravasation, hemorrhage, pneumothorax, and hydrothorax
 Superior vena caval thrombosis
 Pulmonary embolism
 Local irritation or slough

noted that full-strength fluid has nearly six times the isotonic value of plasma. Continuous infusion in a large vein is therefore mandatory if damage to the vein is to be avoided. The fluids are also excellent culture media for certain microorganisms, and for this reason meticulous aseptic technique is essential when mixing the fluid and placing the catheter to minimize the risk of sepsis. At many institutions, including our own, the fluid is modified for administration into peripheral veins. *Some practical hints related to total parenteral nutrition are as follows.*

- Fresh fluid should be prepared daily in the pharmacy, under rigidly sterile conditions using a laminar-flow hood.
- The filter, dressings, and connecting tubing should be changed daily, and cultures should be taken from filter fluid periodically.
- All connections should be taped, since disconnection may lead to serious hemorrhage.
- When connections are open, the distal lines should be clamped to prevent air embolism. Use a clamp with teeth that will not damage the tubing.
- If the line needs to be discontinued suddenly because of obstruction and/or infection, start peripheral IV glucose immedi-

TABLE 6–9 COMPOSITION OF SUITABLE INFUSATE FOR TOTAL PARENTERAL NUTRITION

Constituent	Amount
Nitrogen source*	2.5 gm/kg/day
Glucose	25–30 gm/kg/day
Sodium (NaCl)	3–4 mEq/kg/day
Potassium†	2–3 mEq/kg/day
Calcium (Ca gluconate)	1.0 mEq/kg/day
Magnesium (MgSO₄)	0.25 mEq/kg/day
Phosphorus	2.0 mM/kg/day
Total volume	130 ml/kg/day

Adapted from Heird, W., MacMillan, R., and Winters, R.: Total parenteral nutrition in the pediatric patient. *In* Fischer, J. E. (ed.): *Total Parenteral Nutrition.* Boston, Little, Brown and Co., 1976.

*Either protein hydrolysate or a mixture of crystalline amino acids.

†Two mEq/kg/day are provided as KH_2PO_4; remainder is provided as KCl.

ately, since the infant may be in danger of developing hypoglycemia. See Table 6–10 for complications associated with parenteral alimentation.

INTRALIPID[117, 147, 178]

Intralipid formula with 10 per cent soy bean oil emulsified with egg yolk, together with phospholipids in 2.5 per cent glycerol to attain isotonicity with serum, has been used for added calories. Intralipid provides 1.1 kcal/ml; it may be administered continuously along with dextrose–amino acid solutions through separate lines united by a terminal Y connector and may be fed into peripheral veins. Because the lipid emulsion is delicate, the two solutions are kept separate until just before they enter the needle. Nothing should be added to the emulsion that can interfere with stability.

Special features of triglycerides that make them desirable in parenteral nutrition include the following.

• They are a concentrated source of calories, providing 9 kcal/gm.
• They supply essential fatty acids in the form of linoleic acid.
• Fat emulsions for intravenous use are isotonic.
• Preliminary evidence suggests that because they do not excite secretions of massive amounts of insulin, they promote better nitrogen retention in catabolic patients.

Following the infusion of Intralipid, the fat particles are rapidly cleared from the blood stream through the action of a "post-heparin lipoprotein lipase activity." This activity is lower in premature infants, especially in small-for-dates infants, hence causing slower clearance.[7] It is important to check turbidity of the patient's serum daily to verify that the previous day's Intralipid has been cleared. If the serum is cloudy or milky, it has not been cleared, and further Intralipid should be withheld. Ideally, free fatty acids (FFA) and triglycerides as well as turbidity should be measured. Heparin may be added to the Intralipid to facilitate clearing.

Indications for Intralipid include those mentioned earlier for total parenteral nutrition.[33, 86, 88] It should be given to those infants with major bowel disorders and to selected preterm infants, particularly those who manifest features of essential fatty acid deficiency such as scaliness of the skin, poor wound

TABLE 6–11 COMPLICATIONS ASSOCIATED WITH INTRALIPID

Allergic reaction
Hepatomegaly
Adverse reaction: hyperthermia and shock
Eosinophilia
Blood hypercoagulability
Reduction of platelet adhesiveness
Interference with bilirubin measurement

healing, hair changes, and retardation of growth.

Intralipid should be used with extreme caution in preterm, SGA, and AGA infants in whom defective utilization of the liberated free fatty acids may cause displacement of unconjugated bilirubin from albumin, potentially increasing the risk of kernicterus. Additionally, the turbidity in the serum may cause a falsely elevated unconjugated bilirubin reading if a standard bilirubinometer is used.[150] A bilirubinometer equipped with a special yellow filter will eliminate this error.

Intralipid should not be used in patients with severely deranged liver function and should be used with extreme caution in those with respiratory diseases, including hyaline membrane disease, since the lipid may interfere with pulmonary diffusion of gases, particularly if it is infused rapidly (Table 6–11).

The Intralipid should be administered by continuous slow infusion over 24 hours and cannot be administered through an inline filter. A spun hematocrit tube should always be checked between administration, and liver function tests and lipid profile should be monitored during and prior to therapy.

The dose of Intralipid is increased starting at 0.5 gm/kg body weight/day. The infusion rate should not exceed 0.3 gm (3 ml/kg body weight/hour) or 3 gm/kg/day, with a minimum infusion time of 24 hours.

PRACTICAL HINTS

1. *Do not* starve infants for too long.
2. *Do not* nipple feed too early. All infants <32 weeks will require gavage feeding.
3. *Do not* increase the quantity too rapidly.
4. *Do not* nipple feed infants with respiratory rates above 60 per minute or those who are hypothermic. Do not feed those infants receiving assisted ventilation with mask and bag.
5. *Do not* feed infants delivered with maternal hydramnios or those who have excess

mucus until a tube has been passed into the stomach.

6. Weigh small infants (less than 1500 gm) twice daily during the first 2 weeks. Loss of weight is variable in rate and degree but can be measured accurately and is a useful clinical index of fluid requirements.

7. Keep accurate records of fluid and caloric intake. The basis for the infant's not gaining weight can then be readily established.

8. Test stool for reducing sugars at least daily in infants at risk for necrotizing enterocolitis.

9. Poor sucking after a period of normal feeding should be regarded as a danger signal and may be the first indication of serious infection. Infants who vomit, have aspirates, or become distended should have their intake reduced or discontinued and their stomach aspirated before the next feeding.

10. Attempt to maintain infants in the prone or right lateral position during feeding, since this accelerates gastric emptying and reduces risk of regurgitation and aspiration.

11. Most low-birth-weight infants achieve a satisfactory rate of growth when consuming 110–130 kcal/kg/day. Milk containing 67 kcal/dl supplies a suitable proportion of calories so that the water requirements are met.

12. Consult nurses before increasing volume or changing method of feeding.

13. Encourage the mother to come and feed her infant after he has taken easily from the nipple. Never ask the mother to do anything at which she will not succeed.

14. Offer nonnutritive nipple stimulus to infants receiving gavage feeding.

15. Beware of any new preparation—the use of new formulae has resulted in vitamin B, folic acid, and protein deficiency as well as hypernatremia.

16. Large-for-gestational-age preterm infants often are lethargic and feed poorly. They may be erroneously diagnosed as being infected or cerebrally damaged.

UNKNOWNS

1. Ideal timing and composition of the first and subsequent feeds are unknown. What are the effects associated with a higher protein intake (and its attendant elevated blood amino acids such as phenylalanine, tyrosine, etc.) on the subsequent neurologic development of low-birth-weight infants? Is the myelin composition different in artificially fed infants as compared with breast-fed infants?[46] (Galactose is necessary for the synthesis of sphingolipids, a principal lipid in myelin—there is less galactose in artificial formulae than in breast milk.)

2. Although intrauterine references have been used as the standard for postnatal growth, the "gold standard" for postnatal growth, particularly for low-birth-weight infants, has not been established. Should the growth of the premature infant fed human milk be considered the standard?

3. Do the differences in tissue composition stemming from the use of artificial formula as opposed to breast milk result in disease in adult life? For example, do present feeding practices and particularly overfeeding in early life relate to "those burdens of adult life—obesity, atherosclerosis, and hypertension . . . ?"[47]

4. What is the ideal thermal environment in which to raise and nourish the newborn infant? What are the proper criteria for assessing adequacy of nutrition? Should we only use increasing length, weight, and head circumference?

5. The sensory needs of the infant at feeding time are unknown. Feeding should represent a pleasurable experience and is the infant's major contact with the environment. Factors related to handling and technique of feeding may subsequently influence development. It is of interest that nonnutritive aspects of feeding—including the use of a pacifier during gavage feeds and rocking the baby between feeds—favorably influence the amount of weight gain, depress metabolic rate, and enhance absorption.[26, 59, 108]

6. Undernutrition due to uteroplacental dysfunction cannot be remedied by special oral feedings administered to the mother. It is not unreasonable that in the near future we will be able to influence the growth of undergrown fetuses in utero, and since 30–40 per cent of infants weighing less than 2.5 kg at birth are small for gestational age, this will involve a large number of infants. How can we give additional nutrition to the fetus in utero?

7. What is the significance of the high cholesterol content of human milk?

8. Is fat malabsorption a limiting factor in the growth of preterm infants?

9. Does the gastrointestinal mucosa of the immature infant allow the passage of immunologically intact foreign proteins and cells into the total circulation?

Congenital Anomalies Presenting with Obstructive Gastrointestinal Symptoms

HOWARD FILSTON
ROBERT J. IZANT

Anomalies of the gastrointestinal tract may involve any part of the primitive tube from the hypopharynx to the anal dimple. The common lesions are *atresias, stenoses, duplications,* and *functional obstructions.* Vascular occlusions, sometimes resulting from rotational anomalies and intussusceptions, may be in utero factors in atresias and stenoses.

Presenting findings include:
- History of hydramnios
- Increased salivation, cyanosis, and choking with feeds
- Large gastric aspirate in delivery room
- Vomiting, especially bile stained
- Abdominal distension
- Failure to stool.

Definitions

ATRESIA. Complete luminal discontinuity of the gastrointestinal tract ranging from the shortest segment web to complete loss of a major segment of bowel and mesentery. Multiple atresias may occur throughout the intestinal tract, especially in the jejunoileal segments.

STENOSIS. A narrowing that may involve the entire thickness of the bowel wall or be merely a partial web.

DUPLICATIONS. May vary from simple cystlike projections into the mesentery to complete replication of any length of the gastrointestinal tube, with or without luminal continuity with the inline segment. They may occur anywhere along the gastrointestinal tract and present as obstructions, as perforations, or simply as a palpable mass.

FUNCTIONAL OBSTRUCTIONS. Those not associated with anatomic malformation. They include achalasia, pyloric stenosis, and aganglionic megacolon, all of which have some component of myoneural dyscoordination in their etiologies. Other functional obstructions, such as meconium ileus and meconium plug syndrome, are caused by abnormalities of intraluminal contents.

We will not attempt to discuss each entity individually and at each level of the gastrointestinal tract; understanding of the basic entities and familiarity with some obvious yet essential principles will help to differentiate the lesions. Those lesions that are life-threatening in the newborn period will be discussed in greater detail.

These basic principles are helpful in evaluating neonatal and infant bowel problems.
- Green vomitus should be considered as indicating bowel obstruction until proved otherwise.
- Gastrointestinal obstruction between the pylorus and the ligament of Treitz is malrotation until proved otherwise.
- Once the continuity of the gastrointestinal tract is clearly demonstrated postnatally by the passage of "transitional stools" or air or contrast medium administered from above, congenital atresia has been excluded as the cause of the obstruction. Note that meconium may be passed from bowel distal to a complete obstruction.
- Before the age of 2 years, it is hazardous to attempt to differentiate large from small bowel on the basis of plain abdominal roentgenograms, particularly since the frequent errors in this evaluation may lead to delay in diagnosis and therapy for an obstructive bowel lesion.
- Multiple anomalies occur frequently.
- Any entity that can obstruct the bowel may also lead to perforation and the resulting signs and symptoms of peritonitis. Thus, when peritonitis is the presenting symptom, an obstructing lesion must be searched out and corrected.

Keeping these principles in mind, let us now approach some serious and frequently seen gastrointestinal anomalies, with illustrative cases.

CASE PROBLEMS

Case One

Pregnancy complicated by hydramnios—A full-term male infant presents with increased salivation and chokes with feedings. Vomitus is never bile stained. Subsequently he develops respiratory distress. On physical examination the infant is noted to be blue when crying and salivating excessively. The abdomen is distended. No obvious external malformation is noted. The x-ray from the referring hospital is reported to demonstrate aspiration pneumonia.

Author's Comment: With a history of hydramnios and increased salivation, the most likely diagnosis is esophageal atresia. The presence of abdominal distension suggests that the atresia is associated with a fistula. The absence of bile staining of the vomitus indicates obstruction proximal to the entry of the common duct into the duodenum.

Diagnostic Maneuver

Pass a radiopaque nasogastric tube until it stops, and take an x-ray, including neck, chest, and upper abdomen. When passing a nasogastric tube for diagnostic maneuver in suspected esophageal atresia, use as large a tube as will pass the nares. A small tube may enter the larynx and pass down the trachea, through the fistula to the esophagus, and into the stomach, giving the false impression of esophageal continuity. A large tube will not be tolerated in the larynx. If the tube passes through the esophagus to the stomach, esophageal atresia is ruled out.

Contrast medium should not be used in this evaluation until continuity of the esophagus has been demonstrated, because the inhalation of contrast medium from a blind esophageal pouch may produce pneumonia.

X-ray Findings in Esophageal Atresia

- There is a wide, air-filled pouch in the neck or upper mediastinum.
- The nasogastric tube is seen to stop in the upper mediastinum at about T3.
- Aspiration pneumonia may be noted, usually in the right upper lobe.
- Visible parts of the abdomen show air in the intestines (often an excess amount).
- Often skeletal anomalies are present (vertebral/ribs).

Management Considerations in Esophageal Atresia[1, 54, 91, 99, 167, 168]

Over 90 per cent of all patients with esophageal atresia will have the common variety of blind upper esophagus with the lower segment entering into the membranous posterior portion of the trachea above the carina as a fistula. This connects the acid-filled stomach to the tracheobronchial tree. A small percentage will have esophageal atresia without tracheoesophageal fistula, in which case the abdomen is airless. From the first suspicion that a fistula exists until complete separation of the esophagus from the trachea is achieved, proper management is essential to prevent the fatal complication of aspiration pneumonia. Aspiration from the proximal pouch into the larynx is prevented by withholding all feedings and continuously aspirating the pouch with a sump tube. Reflux of gastric juice into the fistula is more damaging and more difficult to prevent but can be offset by attention to optimal positioning and by early surgical intervention. The child should be maintained in the prone, head-elevated position, which allows the stomach to fall anteriorly away from the esophagus and provides an inclined esophagus as a retardant to reflux of gastric juice.

Once the diagnosis is confirmed, rapid evaluation of the child for tolerance of surgical correction should be undertaken. Our criteria for primary repair (transthoracic extrapleural fistula ligation and end-to-end esophageal anastomosis) include:

- Chest clear to auscultation and on roentgenogram.
- No major unevaluated cardiac anomalies.
- PaO_2 of 60 mm Hg or better in room air (usually from an established arterial cannula, such as umbilical).

If these criteria cannot be immediately satisfied, immediate gastrointestinal decompression by tube gastrostomy performed under local anesthesia should be achieved, and intensive respiratory care should be instituted. Established aspiration pneumonitis may require 2–3 weeks of intensive therapy to clear. If improvement is not rapid, tracheostomy may be an essential therapeutic component, since the fistula may interfere with effective coughing.

If prolonged preoperative care is required, nutritional support by total parenteral nutrition will be essential. Feedings by gastrostomy will rarely be tolerated as long as the tracheoesophageal fistula remains.

Cervical esophagostomy in esophageal atresia when initial repair cannot be made makes sham feeding necessary. This teaches the child the mechanics of swallowing as well as supporting the oral gratification so essential in this period for later motor development. An interposition procedure utilizing colon or stomach will be required but is usually delayed until after 6 months of age.

Case Two

An infant takes initial feedings and then vomits bile-stained material—he is otherwise asymptomatic. Examination may or may not reveal abdominal distension. The anus is patent, and meconium is usually present.

Any gastrointestinal obstruction distal to the entry of the common duct into the duodenum can lead to bile-stained vomiting. As a general rule, the earlier the onset of bile staining, the higher the level of obstruction. This is not infallible. Lower level obstructions usually present initially with failure to pass meconium and distension, with bile-stained vomiting occurring hours to days later.

X-ray findings will vary with the level and type of obstruction. They may be clearly diagnostic, as is the case with complete obstruction of the duodenum (double bubble) (duodenal atresia, annular pancreas, occasionally malrotation), or they may be equivocal, as in meconium ileus or Hirschsprung's disease.

Eventual diagnosis will be forthcoming in every case, given enough time and persistence. In the interim, effective nasogastric decompression and parenteral fluid, electrolyte, and nutritional support by vein will sustain most of these infants, even if significant time lapses prior to diagnosis and definitive therapy. Only those lesions that may lead to catastrophe require urgent diagnosis and treatment, so attention should be directed to recognizing these entities rapidly. These include malrotation, neonatal perforations, and aganglionic megacolon.

Case Three

Bilious vomiting, usually with some abdominal distension, occurs in a baby who passed normal meconium and has an open anus. X-rays may show duodenal obstruction and usually show some gas throughout the abdomen.

Diagnosis: Malrotation[24, 106, 154]

Malrotation is the most malevolent lesion of infancy because of its propensity toward volvulus with resultant strangulation of the superior mesenteric artery. This catastrophe can lead to total destruction of the digestive-absorptive segment of the intestinal tract—the jejunoileum. Furthermore, compared with any other single anomaly, this lesion is quite common. It must therefore always be in the differential diagnostic forefront to be rapidly ruled in or out. The most direct method for doing so is the upper gastrointestinal contrast study, which will demonstrate obstruction of the duodenum. If obstruction is incomplete, it will reveal that the duodenal C-loop fails to complete its normal course to a position in the left upper quadrant behind the stomach—the ligament of Treitz.

Contrast enemas, frequently recommended for diagnosis of malrotation in the past, may be confusing. The high-riding cecum with malpositioned appendix is diagnostic if clearly present, but often the cecal position is equivocal and difficult to locate clearly. Reflux of dye into the ileum may mask the position of the cecum. Therapeutic delay is intolerable here. Basically, one should quickly intervene operatively in any duodenal obstruction not *clearly* due to an entity other than malrotation.

Necrotizing Enterocolitis[97, 98]

AVROY A. FANAROFF
ROBERT M. KLIEGMAN

Necrotizing enterocolitis (NEC)[136] continues to be a major cause of morbidity in intensive care nurseries. The incidence varies from 2 to 15 per cent of admissions. Using data from a nationwide survey, Sweet[165] estimated an occurrence rate of 22 cases per 1000 admissions. Most infants with necrotizing enterocolitis are low birth weight, appropriately grown, and immature.

Although patent ductus arteriosus, sepsis,[145] low Apgar scores, and umbilical catheters were implicated in the etiology, matched studies do not support this.[63] Infection plays a prominent role, and the disease occurs in clusters with various outbreaks reported due to *E. coli*, *Klebsiella*, *Salmonella*, and the clostridial species. Viruses have also been implicated. A clinical classification and the pathogenesis of the disease are outlined in Table 6–12 and Figure 6–3. The initial precipitating event may be hypoxemia, sepsis, low cardiac output, or factors within the bowel, such as hypertonic feeding.[102] Feeding precedes the onset of symptomatology in the majority of cases. It remains unclear whether the major factor is the formula itself, the volume of the formula, or the effect of bacteria on the formula.

TABLE 6–12 CLINICAL CLASSIFICATION OF NEONATAL ENTEROCOLITIS

I. Classic NEC
- Endemic
- Epidemic
  Identifiable organism
  No organism identified
II. Benign NEC (pneumatosis coli)
III. NEC following exchange transfusion
IV. NEC following mucosal injury
- Hypertonic feeding
- Allergic enteritis
- Nonspecific diarrhea
- Polycythemia
- Polyvinylchloride?
V. Primary bowel pathology
- Spontaneous bowel perforation
- Congenital intestinal obstruction
VI. Neonatal appendicitis
VII. Neonatal pseudomembranous colitis

Adapted from Kliegman and Fanaroff.[97]
Each category is a distinct clinical and pathologic entity. The inclusive heading of neonatal enterocolitis includes classic idiopathic NEC (I, II), NEC associated with other factors (III, IV), and those newborn diseases that clinically resemble NEC (V, VI, VII). These disease processes may be distinguished from each other by history, clinical course, laboratory tests, and pathologic examination.

Clinical Features

The clinical features are variable, and the signs and symptoms may not be specific. Most often, the infants develop temperature instability, lethargy, abdominal distension, and retention of feedings. Occult blood is present in the stools, which may sometimes be frankly bloody. Reducing substances are often detected prior to the onset of necrotizing enterocolitis.[27] Apnea may be a prominent feature as well as bilious vomiting, increased abdominal distension, acidosis, and disseminated intravascular coagulopathy. The characteristic x-ray features are pneumatosis intestinalis with bubbles or layers of gas in the wall of the bowel as well as portal venous gas. Free air within the peritoneum is associated with perforation of a viscus.[127] Engel et al[55] demonstrated that about 30 per cent of the gas in the wall of the bowel is hydrogen, the product of bacterial fermentation of formula.

Medical management includes nasogastric suction, intravenous fluids, and broad-spectrum systemic antibiotics (Table 6–13). Frequent abdominal examinations as well as determination of abdominal girth and cross-table lateral x-rays are important to detect free air. We maintain the infants on a regimen of nothing per os for 2 weeks while they

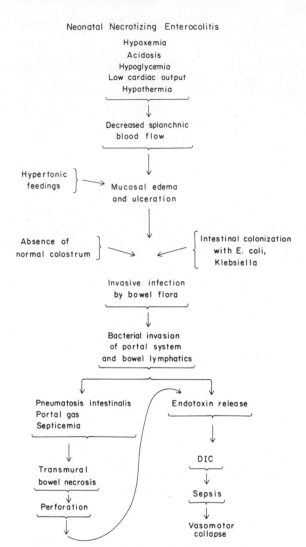

Figure 6–3. Possible factors in etiology and outcome of neonatal necrotizing enterocolitis. From Burrington, J. D.: Necrotizing enterocolitis in the newborn infant. Clin Perinatol 5:30, 1978.

receive all nutritional support intravenously. The main indication for surgery is perforation as demonstrated by free air in the peritoneum. The discovery of an abdominal mass and gas in the portal venous system are not necessarily indications for surgery. Some infants may require surgery at a later stage because of the development of strictures. With present vigorous medical and surgical management as outlined above, 75 per cent of infants should survive. Developmentally, at follow-up these infants usually do extremely well. Many complications relate to short bowel syndrome or infections and metabolic complications related to total parenteral nutrition. (See Tables 6–10 and 6–11.)

TABLE 6–13 APPROACH TO THE PATIENT WITH NEC

Cultures: blood, CSF, urine, stool, and paracentesis if indicated
Antibiotics: based on nursery's organisms and sensitivities; begin anaerobic coverage if peritonitis is present
NPO: with gastrointestinal decompression
Shock: maintain blood pressure and urine output
- Fluids; fresh/frozen plasma, whole blood
- Catecholamines—dopamine, dobutamine
- Steroids
DIC: exchange transfusion or specific factor replacement
X-rays: frequent abdominal x-rays to detect ascites or perforation
Supportive care:
- Maintain adequate HCT, pH, Po_2, Pco_2, electrolyte balance
- Mechanical ventilation for apnea, shock
Epidemics: institute infectious disease control measures (see Chapter 12)
Surgery: as indicated
Nutrition: once stabilized begin intravenous alimentation

Necrotizing enterocolitis is an entity that has emerged as a prominent factor in neonatal morbidity with the advent of neonatal intensive care. It is also known that the entity is seen in many neonatal intensive care centers and not observed at all in others. The phenomenon strongly suggests the multifactorial and perhaps iatrogenic nature of the disease. The incidence and/or occurrence is dependent on the presence or absence of the factors and nursery routines enumerated by the authors in the previous paragraph.   **W. Oh**

CASE PROBLEMS

Case One

C. K. weighed 1300 gm at 32 weeks' gestation; his Apgar scores were 4 at 1 minute and 6 at 5 minutes. He developed respiratory distress syndrome on the first day of life, had an arterial catheter placed at the level of T10, and required 60 per cent oxygen but no assisted ventilation. The RDS resolved by 48 hours of life, and the catheter was removed. Standard formula was first fed on the third day of life. On the eighth day, abdominal tenderness and distension were observed, and the nurses reported guaiac-positive stools, 5 ml residual from the last feeding, and that a higher incubator temperature was required to maintain body temperature.

What is the most likely preliminary diagnosis?
A. *Meconium plug syndrome*
B. *Necrotizing enterocolitis*
C. *Septicemia*
D. *Malrotation*
E. *Hirschsprung's disease*

Any neonate presenting with a triad of abdominal distension, Hematest- or guaiac-positive stools, and retention of gastric formula should be suspected of having and immediately evaluated for necrotizing enterocolitis. The initial manifestation of NEC may be indistinguishable from septicemia, and indeed a positive blood culture is obtained from 30 per cent of infants with NEC. The answer is B, necrotizing enterocolitis.

Initially, how would you evaluate this patient?
A. *Culture blood, urine, cerebral spinal fluid, and stool*
B. *CBC and clotting profile*
C. *Barium swallow*
D. *Gastrografin enema*
E. *AP and lateral film of abdomen*
F. *Blood gases and serum electrolytes*

A. Because sepsis is present in many if not all of these patients and many investigators feel that infection is directly related to the pathogenesis of the disease, blood, urine, stool, and cerebral spinal fluid cultures should be obtained.

B. A CBC blood smear and clotting profile should be ordered and the type and cross-match sent to the blood bank. Take specific note of fragmented red cells (disseminated intravascular coagulation, or DIC), neutropenia (margination of white cells), and thrombocytopenia.

C. Barium swallow is not indicated immediately. If there is evidence of obstruction without pneumatosis on the flat film, then a barium swallow may be necessary to exclude malrotation.

D. Gastrografin enema may be curative if there is a meconium plug but is contraindicated at this moment because the hyperosmolar contrast medium may produce further damage to already compromised bowel and result in perforation.

E. Abdominal x-rays, both KUB and cross-table lateral, should be ordered to detect the presence of pneumatosis intestinalis, hepatic portal gas, or free intraabdominal gas indicating a perforated viscus. If no free air is seen initially, but there is pneumatosis present, the cross-table lateral x-ray should be repeated every 4–6 hours, or sooner if there is clinical deterioration.

F. It is important to evaluate acid-base status and serum electrolytes in infants with suspected gastrointestinal disturbances. Correction of these metabolic derangements is crucial before submitting these precarious infants to major surgery.

The x-rays revealed pneumatosis intestinalis with no air in the liver or free intraperitoneal air. The blood pressure is 55/35, blood gases pH 7.32, Pao_2 65, Pco_2 40, bicarbonate 20, serum sodium 132, potassium 4.8, chloride 105, BUN 10, hematocrit 38, white blood cell count 14,900 with 70 per cent segmented cells, platelets adequate, clotting profile normal. Pediatric surgery was consulted and managed the baby with the nursery staff from here on.

True or False

The following treatment(s) should be instituted (true or false).
A. Nasogastric suction, intravenous fluids, and place patient on nothing per os (NPO)
B. Systemic and orogastric antibiotics
C. Laparotomy
D. Exchange transfusion
E. Place central hyperalimentation line

A. True. It is imperative to decompress the abdomen with a large oral or nasogastric tube. Carefully record all intake and output, weigh the baby twice daily, and measure abdominal girth frequently. Intravenous fluid therapy must take into consideration significant third space losses. We keep patients with documented necrotizing enterocolitis NPO for at least 14 days.

B. True. The patient was started on appropriate doses of intravenous carbenicillin and aminoglycosides. We no longer administer antibiotics per nasogastric tube since this has not proved to be efficacious.

C. False. There is no clear-cut indication for a laparotomy at this stage. While surgery is clearly indicated for intestinal perforation, some units operate when medical management fails to correct the shock-acidosis; if there is persistent cellulitis of the anterior abdominal wall or radiologically, a single dilated loop of bowel persists.

D. False. With normal clotting studies and no evidence of bleeding or significant hyperbilirubinemia, exchange transfusion is not indicated.

E. False. Total parenteral nutrition is going to be necessary for this infant. However, with septicemia likely, it is advisable to wait until the sepsis has been controlled and the general condition stabilized before placing a central line for feeding. Some centers will provide all nutritive support with peripheral lines, using glucose–amino acid mixtures supplemented with intravenous fat.

One hour later, the blood pressure has dropped from 55/35 to 40/0. The urine output has decreased to less than 1 ml/hour, and the abdomen is more distended, edematous, and tender. On physical examination, the infant is pink with a wide pulse pressure, tachycardia, and warm extremities. Repeat CBC reveals WBC 3.1, 10 per cent segs, 10 per cent bands.

These data should be interpreted as (true or false):
A. Septic shock
B. Perforated abdominal viscus
C. Patent ductus arteriosus with congestive heart failure
D. Pneumothorax
E. Third space loss

A and E. True. The patient as described—pink with wide pulse pressure, tachycardia, and warm extremities—has the classic features of warm shock. When such patients are untreated, the blood pressure will drop further and vasoconstriction will predominate, transforming the "warm" shock to "cold" shock. A major factor contributing to shock in patients with necrotizing enterocolitis is the massive third space that develops in the abdomen, secondary to the inflammatory response and bowel necrosis. These large fluid and protein losses result in hypovolemia and require urgent therapy. The mainstay of treatment is to raise the blood pressure by supporting the intravascular space with sufficient blood, plasma, or crystalloid to maintain the blood pressure and urine output. Whole blood is preferred because it will remain in the intravascular space, whereas other fluids will leak through the damaged capillaries and contribute to intestinal edema. Large volumes may be required.

Neutropenia may be documented in NEC without bacteremia. Margination of neutrophils had been assumed, since marrow reserves are not depleted. The role of white cells transfusion is undergoing evaluation (see Chapter 12).

B. False. While the sudden deterioration is suggestive of perforation and evaluation by transillumination and x-ray is certainly indicated, no perforation was present at this time. The wide pulse pressure is not usually detected at the time of perforation.

C. False. Tachycardia, edema, and wide pulse pressure are present with PDA and congestive heart failure. However, the striking abdominal findings, together with the diminished blood pressure, suggest that this is not the primary problem. Patent ductus arteriosus, however, is found frequently in infants with necrotizing enterocolitis.

D. False. This is unlikely, given the complete picture, particularly with a pink baby and wide pulse pressure.

Two hours later x-rays show increased distension and no evidence of free air but the appearance of bowel "floating" in the abdomen.

What is the significance of this? How would you react?

Bowel floating in the abdomen in a patient with sepsis and a distended tender abdomen indicates ascites due to peritonitis.[100] Because many cases of "intraabdominal sepsis" are caused by anaerobic bacteria, anaerobic antimicrobial coverage should be started following paracentesis. (That is why carbenicillin or clindamycin is instituted for infants with suspected NEC.)

On introducing a 22-gauge Medicut into the left lower quadrant, 10 ml of purulent fluid was removed. The cell count showed 90,000 WBC with 75 per cent polymorphonuclear neutrophil leukocytes (PMN). Gram stain showed gram-positive and gram-negative rods.

The patient was now noted to have blood oozing

from venipuncture sites, with petechiae and a falling hematocrit despite multiple blood transfusions.

Laboratory data

CBC HCT = 28; platelets 5000; smear shows fragmented RBCs and burr cells

Prothrombin time = patient 50 sec/control 10 sec

Partial thromboplastin time = patient 180 sec/control 30 sec

Fibrinogen = 50 mg/dl (normal 200 mg/dl)

Fibrin split products = 4+ (normal not present)

Disseminated intravascular coagulation has complicated the picture, and therefore an exchange transfusion with fresh blood was performed (see Chapter 15).

Blood pressure, urine output, and activity have been normal now for 3 days. The abdomen is softer, but there is still some edema of the abdominal wall. Repeated x-rays failed to reveal free intraabdominal air. After 5 days of relative stability, the patient becomes acutely distended with signs of respiratory embarrassment.

Which of the following management options would be appropriate?

A. Repeat clotting profile and exchange transfusion

B. Percuss abdomen and then transilluminate while awaiting x-ray

C. Repeat blood cultures and change antibiotics

D. Do blood gas and increase environmental oxygen

A. This acute episode following a period of stability cannot entirely be attributed to disseminated intravascular coagulation.

B. This acute change is probably due to intestinal perforation. Abdominal percussion used to demonstrate the absence of hepatic dullness and positive transillumination may confirm your suspicions before the cross-table lateral x-ray has been developed. The film in this instance demonstrated free air.

C. Blood culture should be repeated, but there is no reason to change antibiotics at this time.

D. This is only symptomatic management. The basic cause for the abdominal distension and respiratory embarrassment must be determined. The blood gas will indicate the need for ventilatory support.

The child was brought to the operating room where the perforated area of ileum was resected and an ileostomy and colostomy performed. Two days postoperatively a central intravenous catheter was placed in the operating room and total parenteral nutrition administered via this route for 21 days. After this period of being NPO, he was started on breast milk and has done well.

The danger of infection under conditions of intravenous hyperalimentation should not be underestimated. There is an extremely high incidence of infection, particularly with *Candida* and especially in situations in which high glucose-containing formulae are used. This infection appears to be only minimally affected by the use of small Millipore filters, and increasing reports have appeared of serious systemic candidiasis with meningitis, osteomyelitis, septic arthritis, and ensuing death. For the moment, it is our view that, unless specifically indicated because of surgical procedures that may limit the absorptive surface of the GI tract, intravenous hyperalimentation is not currently to be routinely recommended.

L. Stern

Case Two

L. M. is a 1200 gm, normal male born at 30 weeks' gestation who appeared in no distress during the first hours of life. By history and physical and neurologic examination, he appears appropriately sized for gestational age.

How and what should this infant be fed for the first 4 days of life? Please write your orders.

Intravenous maintenance should be begun by 3–4 hours of age, using a peripheral vein ideally, unless an umbilical catheter is otherwise justified. The solution should contain 10 per cent glucose.

At 24 hours of age, a solution of 10 per cent glucose with 20 mEq/l sodium chloride plus 20 mEq/l potassium chloride is substituted. The rate should be 4 ml/hour (100 ml/kg/day).

Oral feeding by nasogastric tube should begin at 36–48 hours of age with 2 ml of water and be repeated in 1 hour. Formula (20 cal/30 ml) may then be fed, 3 ml/hour, aspirating for gastric residue before each feeding. (Be sure to replace aspirate.)

Increase by 1 ml per feeding after 24 hours, then cautiously in 1 ml steps every other feeding. At 4 days of age, intake will *probably* be 4–5 ml/hour (80–100 ml/kg/24 hours) by nasogastric tube if all goes well. Intravenous fluids are tapered as oral intake increases.

Water needs vary and may be higher than these allowances in very small infants. If proper amounts of water are being provided:

- Weight loss should not exceed 8–10 per cent of birth weight at 4 days;
- Urine osmolarity should not exceed that of plasma;
- Plasma osmolarity and serum sodium values should remain normal.

Failure to achieve these goals calls for an increase in the intravenous water allowance.

Case Three

A 1740 gm female was born at 40 weeks' gestation to a primigravida who had no problems during pregnancy, labor, or delivery. A physical examination, including a neurologic examination for gestational age, agreed with the mother's dates. There were no physical abnormalities nor any suggestion of intrauterine infection.

What are this infant's nutritional requirements? How and what should she be fed during the first week of life?

Assuming this infant's low birth weight stems from intrauterine malnutrition, her caloric requirements will be high (120–150 cal/kg/day) for growth. She is at risk of hypoglycemia. Fortunately, she may feed well from a very early age.

Feedings should be started at 2–6 hours of age and offered on a 3 hour schedule. If she takes them well, there may be no further problem. If she does not, intravenous caloric supplements with 10 per cent glucose (see Chapter 10) and maintenance electrolytes should be given. Dextrostix monitoring at 2 hour intervals is sufficient guard against hypoglycemia as long as the baby remains well.

REFERENCES

1. Abrahamson, J., and Shandling, B.: Esophageal atresia in the underweight baby: a challenge. J Pediatr Surg 7:608, 1972.
2. AMA Department of Food and Nutrition: Guidelines for essential trace element preparations for parenteral use. J Am Med Assoc 241:2051, 1979.
3. Anderson, D., Williams, F., Kerr, D., et al: Length of gestation and nutritional composition of human milk. Am J Clin Nutr 37:810, 1983.
4. Anderson, G. H., Atkinson, S. A., and Bryan, M. H.: Energy and macronutrient content of human milk during early lactation from mothers giving birth prematurely and at term. Am J Clin Nutr 34:258, 1981.
5. Anderson, P.: Drugs and breast feeding—a review. Drug Intell Clin Pharm 11:208, 1977.
6. Anderson, T. L., Muttant, C. R., Bieber, M. A., et al: A controlled trial of glucose vs. glucose and amino acids in preterm infants. J Pediatr 94:947, 1979.
7. Andrew, G., Chan G., and Schiff, D.: Lipid metabolism in the neonate. J Pediatr 88:273, 1976.
8. Aperia, A., Broberger, O., Hern, P., et al: Sodium excretion in relation to sodium intake and aldosterone excretion in newborn preterm and full term infants. Acta Paediatr Scand 68:813, 1979.
9. Arant, B. S.: Nonrenal factors influencing renal function during the perinatal period. Clin Perinatol 8:225, 1981.
10. Arant, B. S.: Fluid therapy in the neonate—concepts in transition. J Pediatr 101:387, 1982.
11. Atkinson, S. A., Bryan, M. H., and Anderson, G. H.: Human milk from mothers of term and premature infants. J Pediatr 93:67, 1978.
12. Atkinson, S. A., Byran, M. H., and Anderson, G. H.: Human milk feeding in premature infants: protein, fat, and carbohydrate balances in the first two weeks of life. J Pediatr 99:617, 1981.
13. Auld, P., Bhangananda, P., and Mehta, S.: The influence of early caloric feeding with IV glucose on catabolism of premature infants. Pediatrics 37:592, 1966.
14. Avery, M., and Hodson, W.: The first drink reconsidered. J Pediatr 68:1008, 1966.
15. Babson, S.: Feeding the low birth weight infant. J Pediatr 79:694, 1971.
16. Babson, S., and Bromhall, J.: Diet and growth in the premature infant. The effect of different dietary intakes of ash-electrolyte and protein on weight gain and linear growth. J Pediatr 74:890, 1969.
17. Barlow, B., Santulli, T., Heird, W., et al: An experimental study of acute necrotizing enterocolitis—the importance of breast milk. J Pediatr Surg 9:587, 1974.
18. Barltrop, D., and Oppe, T.: Absorption of fat and calcium by low birth weight infants from milks containing butterfat and olive oil. Arch Dis Child 48:496, 1973.
19. Barness, L.: Infant feeding. Pediatr Clin North Am 8:639, 1961.
20. Barrie, H.: Effect of feeding on gastric and esophageal pressures in the newborn. Lancet 2:1158, 1968.
21. Beale, E. F., Nelson, R. M., Bucciarelli, R. L., et al: Intrahepatic cholestasis associated with parenteral nutrition in premature infants. Pediatrics 64:342, 1979.
22. Beard, A., Panos, T., Marasigan, B., et al: Perinatal stress and the premature neonate. 2. Effect of fluid and calorie deprivation on blood glucose. Pediatrics 68:329, 1969.
23. Bell, E. F., Warburton, D., Stonestreet, B. S., et al.: Effect of fluid administration of the development of symptomatic patent ductus arteriosus and congestive heart failure in premature infants. N Engl J Med 302:598, 1980.
24. Berdon, W., Baker, D., Bull, S., et al: Midgut malrotation and volvulus: which films are most helpful? Radiology 96:375, 1970.
25. Bergman, K., and Fomon, J.: Trace minerals. *In* Fomon, S. (ed.): *Infant Nutrition*. 2nd Ed. Philadelphia, W. B. Saunders Co., 1974.
26. Bernbaum, J. C., Pereira, G. R., Watkins, J. B., et al: Nonnutritive sucking during gavage feeding enhances growth and maturation in premature infants. Pediatrics 71:41, 1983.
27. Book, L., Herbst, J., and Jung, A.: Carbohydrate malabsorption in necrotizing enterocolitis. Pediatrics 57:201, 1976.
28. Boros, S., and Reynolds, J.: Duodenal perforation: a complication of neonatal transpyloric tube feeding. J Pediatr 85:107, 1974.
29. Brans, Y., Summers, J., Dweck, H., et al: Feeding the low birth weight infant: orally or parenterally? Preliminary results of a comparative study. Pediatrics 54:15, 1974.
30. Brice, J. E. H., Rutter, N., and Hull, D.: Reduction of skin water loss in the newborn. II. Clinical trial of two methods in very low birthweight babies. Arch Dis Child 56:673, 1981.
31. Brooke, O. G., Alveolar, J., and Arnold, M.: Energy retention, energy expenditures and growth in healthy immature infants. Pediatr Res 13:215, 1979.
32. Brown, E. R., Stark, A., Sosenko, I., et al: Bron-

chopulmonary dysplasia: possible relationship to pulmonary edema. J Pediatr 92:982, 1978.

33. Cashore, W., Sedaghatran, M., and Usher, R. P.: Nutritional supplements in small premature infants. Pediatrics 56:8, 1975.

34. Cheek, J., Jr., and Staub, G.: Nasojejunal alimentation in premature and full-term newborn infants. J Pediatr 82:955, 1973.

35. Chen, J., and Wong, P.: Intestinal complication in nasojejunal feeding in low-birth-weight infants. J Pediatr 85:109, 1974.

36. Chessex, P., Reichman, B. L., Verellen, G. J. E., et al: Influences of postnatal age, energy intake and weight gain on energy metabolism in the very low birth weight infant. J Pediatr 99:761, 1981.

37. Churchill, J.: Weight loss in premature infants developing spastic diplegia. Obstet Gynecol 22:601, 1963.

38. Committee on Nutrition: Commentary on breast-feeding and infant formulas, including proposed standards for formulas. Pediatrics 57:278, 1976.

39. Committee on Nutrition, American Academy of Pediatrics: Nutritional needs of low-birth-weight infants. Pediatrics 60:519, 1977.

40. Committee on Nutrition, Lewis A. Barnes, Chairman, American Academy of Pediatrics: Pediatric Nutrition Handbook. Evanston, Ill., 1979.

41. Cornblath, M., Forbes, A., Pides, R., et al: A controlled study of early fluid administration on survival of low birth weight infants. Pediatrics 38:547, 1966.

42. Craddock, P. R., Yawata, Y., VanSanten, L., et al: Acquired phagocyte dysfunction. A complication of the hypophosphatemia of parenteral hyperalimentation. N Engl J Med 290:1403, 1974.

43. Dahms, B. B., and Halpin, T. C.: Serial liver biopsies in parenteral nutrition–associated cholestasis of early infancy. Gastroenterology 81:136, 1981.

44. Daily, W., Klaus, M., and Meyer, B.: Apnea in premature infants—monitoring, incidence, heart rate changes and the effects of environmental temperatures. Pediatrics 43:510, 1969.

45. Davidson, M.: Formula feeding of normal term and low birth weight infants. Pediatr Clin North Am 17:913, 1970.

46. Davies, P.: Feeding the newborn baby. Proc Nutr Soc 28:66, 1968.

47. Davies, P.: Feeding. Br Med J 4:351, 1971.

48. Day, G., Radde, I., Balfe, J., et al: Electrolyte abnormalities in very low birth weight infants. Pediatr Res 10:522, 1976.

49. Drillien, C.: The Growth and Development of the Prematurely Born Infant. Edinburgh and London, E. and S. Livingstone Ltd., 1964.

50. Driscoll, J., Jr., Heird, W., Schullinger, J., et al: Total intravenous alimentation in low-birth-weight infants: a preliminary report. J Pediatr 81:145, 1972.

51. Duritz, G., and Oltorf, C.: Lactobezoar formation associated with high-density caloric formula. Pediatrics 63:647, 1979.

52. Dweck, H.: Feeding the prematurely born infant: fluids, calories, and methods of feeding during the period of extrauterine growth retardation. Clin Perinatol 2:183, 1975.

53. Editorial: Clostridia as intestinal pathogens. Lancet 2:1113, 1977.

54. Ein, S., and Therman, T.: A comparison of the results of primary repair of esophageal atresia with tracheoesophageal fistulas using end-to-side and end-to-end anastomosis. J Pediatr Surg 8:641, 1973.

55. Engel, R., Virnig, N., Hunt, C., et al: Origin of mural gas in necrotizing enterocolitis. Pediatr Res 7:292, 1973.

56. Engelke, S. C., Shah, B. L., Vasan, U., et al: Sodium balance in very low-birth-weight infants. J Pediatr 93:837. 1978.

57. Fanaroff, A. A., and Hack, M.: Fluid requirements of the low birthweight infant. In Sunshine, P. (ed.): Feeding the Neonate Weighing Less than 1500 Grams: Nutrition and Beyond. Report of the 79th Ross Conference on Pediatric Research. Columbus, Ohio, Ross Laboratories, 1980.

58. Fanaroff, A. A., Wald, M., Gruber, H., et al: Insensible water loss in low birth weight infants. Pediatrics 50:236, 1972.

59. Field, T., Ignatoff, E., Stringer, S., et al: Non-nutritive sucking during trial feedings: effects on preterm neonates in an intensive care unit. Pediatrics 70:381, 1982.

60. Filler, R. M., Eraklis, A. J., Rubin, V. G., et al: Long-term total parenteral nutrition in infants. N Engl J Med 281:589, 1969.

61. Filston, H., and Izant, R.: The Surgical Neonate, Evaluation and Care. New York, Appleton-Century-Crofts, 1978.

62. Finberg, L.: The relationship of intravenous infusions and intracranial hemorrhage: a commentary. J Pediatr 91:777, 1977.

63. Fomon, S.: Infant Nutrition. Philadelphia, W. B. Saunders Co., 1967.

64. Fomon, S., Ziegler, F., Vazques, H.: Human milk and the small premature infant. Am J Dis Child 131:463, 1977.

65. Gaull, G., Rassin, D., Raiha, N., et al: Milk protein quantity and quality in low-birth-weight infants: III. Effects on sulfur amino acids in plasma and urine. J Pediatr 90:348, 1977.

66. Gaull, G., Sturman, J., and Raiha, N.: Development of mammalian sulfur metabolism: absence of cystathionase in human fetal tissues. Pediatr Res 6:538, 1972.

67. Glass, L., Lala, R., Jaiswal, V., et al: Effect of thermal environment and calorie intake on head growth and low birth weight infants during the late neonatal period. Arch Dis Child 50:571, 1975.

68. Glass, L., Silverman, W., and Sinclair, J.: Relationship of thermal environment and caloric intake to growth and resting metabolism in the late neonatal period. Biol Neonate 14:324, 1969.

69. Goldman, A., and Smith, C.: Host resistance factors in human milk. J Pediatr 82:1082, 1974.

70. Goldman, A. S., Garza, C., Nichols, B., et al: Effects of prematurity on the immunologic system in human milk. J Pediatr 101:901, 1982.

71. Goldman, H., Goldman, J., Kaufman, I., et al: Late effects of early dietary protein intake on low-birth-weight infants. J Pediatr 85:764, 1974.

72. Gordon, H., Levine, S., Deamer, W., et al: Respiratory metabolism in infancy and in childhood. XXIII. Daily energy requirements of premature infants. Am J Dis Child 59:1185, 1940.

73. Gross, S.: Hemolytic anemia in premature infants: relationship to vitamin E, selenium, glutathione peroxidase, and erythrocyte lipids. Sem Hematol 13:187, 1976.

74. Gross, S. J.: Growth and biochemical responses of preterm infants fed human milk or modified infant formula. N Engl J Med 308:237, 1983.

75. Gross, S. J., David, R. J., Bauman, L., et al: Nutritional composition of milk produced by mothers delivering preterm. J Pediatr 91:641, 1980.

76. Gryboski, J.: The swallowing mechanism of the neonate. I. Esophageal and gastric motility. Pediatrics 35:445, 1965.

77. Gryboski, J.: Suck and swallow in the premature infant. Pediatrics 43:96, 1969.

78. Hack, M., Caron, B., Rivers, A., et al: The very low birth weight infant: the broader spectrum of morbidity during infancy and early childhood. JDBP 4:243, 1983.

79. Hack, M., Merkatz, I. R., McGrath, S. K., et al: Catch up growth in very low birth weight infants. Am J Dis Child 138:370, 1984.

80. Hambidge, M.: Chromium nutrition in the mother and the growing child. In Mertz, W., and Carnatzer, W. (eds.): Newer Trace Elements in Nutrition. New York, Marcel Dekker, Inc., 1971.

81. Hambidge, M.: The importance of trace elements in infant nutrition. Curr Med Res Opin 4:44, 1976.

82. Hambidge, M.: Trace elements deficiencies in childhood. In Suskind, R. M. (ed.): Textbook of Pediatric Nutrition. New York, Raven Press, 1981, p. 167.

83. Hammarlund, K., and Sedin, G.: Transepidermal water loss in newborn infants. III. Relation to gestational age. Acta Paediatr Scand 68:795, 1979.

84. Hansen, L., and Winberg, J.: Breast milk and defense against infection in the newborn. Arch Dis Child 47:845, 1972.

85. Haworth, J., and Ford, J.: Effect of early and late feeding and glucagon upon blood sugar and serum bilirubin levels of premature babies. Arch Dis Child 38:328, 1963.

86. Heird, W., and Driscoll, J., Jr.: Use of intravenously administered lipid in neonates: commentary. Pediatrics 56:5, 1975.

87. Heird, W., and Hansen, I.: Effects of colostrum on growth of intestinal mucosa. Pediatr Res 11:406, 1977.

88. Heird, W., and Winters, R.: Total parenteral nutrition: state of the art. J Pediatr 86:2, 1975.

89. Heird, W., Dell, R. B., Driscoll, J. M., Jr., et al: Metabolic acidosis resulting from intravenous alimentation mixtures containing synthetic amino acids. N Engl J Med 287:943, 1972.

90. Hodes, H.: Endotoxic shock in the critically ill child. In Smith, C. (ed.): The Critically Ill Child: Diagnostics and Management. Philadelphia, W. B. Saunders, Co., 1977.

91. Holder, T., Cloud, D., Lewis, J., Jr., et al: Esophageal atresia and tracheoesophageal fistula: a survey of its members by the Surgical Section of the American Academy of Pediatrics 34:542, 1964.

92. Holt, L., and Snyderman, S.: The feeding of premature and newborn infants. Pediatr Clin North Am 13:1103, 1966.

93. Hubbell, J., Drorbaugh, J., Rudolph, A., et al: Early versus late feeding of infants of diabetic mothers with respiratory distress syndrome. N Engl J Med 265:835, 1961.

94. Jarvenpaa, A. L., Raiha, N. C., Rassin, D. K., et al: Milk protein quantity and quality in the term infant. I. Metabolic responses and effects on growth. Pediatrics 70:214, 1982.

95. Jarvenpaa, A. L., Rassin, D. K., Raiha, N. C., et al: Milk protein quantity and quality in the term infant. II. Effects on acidic and neutral amino acids. Pediatrics 70:221, 1982.

96. Katz, L., and Hamilton, J. R.: Fat absorption in infants of birth weight less than 1300 gm. J Pediatr 85:608, 1974.

97. Kliegman, R. M., and Fanaroff, A. A.: Necrotizing enterocolitis. N Engl J Med 310:1093, 1984.

98. Kliegman, R. M., Horn, M., Jones, P., et al: Epidemiologic study of necrotizing enterocolitis among low birth weight infants. J Pediatr 100:440, 1982.

99. Koop, C., and Hamilton, J.: Atresia of the esophagus: factors affecting survival in 249 cases. Z Kinderchir 5:319, 1968.

100. Kosloske, A., and Lilly, J.: Paracentesis and lavage for diagnosis of intestinal gangrene in neonatal necrotizing enterocolitis. J Pediatr Surg 13:315, 1978.

101. Kurjak, A., Kirkinen, P., Latin, V., et al: Ultrasonic assessment of fetal kidney function in normal and complicated pregnancies. Am J Obstet Gynecol 141:266, 1981.

102 Lake, A., and Walker, W.: Neonatal necrotizing enterocolitis: a disease of altered host defense. Clin Gastroenterol 6:463, 1977.

103. Lewin, P., Reid, M., Reilly, B., et al: Iatrogenic rickets in low birth weight infants. J Pediatr 78:207, 1971.

104. Loo, S., Gross, J., and Warshaw, J.: Improved method of nasojejunal feeding in low birth weight infants. J Pediatr 85:104, 1974.

105. Lorenz, J. M., Kleinman, L. I., Kotagal, U. R., et al: Water balance in very low-birth-weight infants: relationship to water and sodium intake and effect on outcome. J Pediatr 101:423, 1982.

106. Louw, J., and Barnard, C.: Congenital intestinal atresia: observations on its origin. Lancet 2:1065, 1955.

107. Malvaux, P., Beckers, C., and DeVisscher, M.: Iodine balance studies in non-goiterous children and in adolescents on low iodine intake. J Clin Endocrinol Metab 29:79, 1977.

108. Measel, C. P., and Anderson, G. C.: Nonnutritive sucking during tube feeding: effect on clinical course in premature infants. JOGN Nurs Sept/Oct, 265, 1979.

109. Meites, S.: Pediatric Clinical Chemistry. Washington, American Association for Clinical Chemistry, Inc., 1977.

110. Michie, D. D., and Wirth, F. H.: Plasma zinc levels in premature infants receiving parenteral nutrition. J Pediatr 92:798, 1978.

111. Murillo, G., and Goldman, A.: The cells of the human colostrum. II. Synthesis of IgA and Bic. Pediatr Res 4:71, 1970.

112. Oh, W.: Renal functions and clinical disorders in the neonate. Clin Perinatol 8:215, 1981.

113. Oh, W., and Karecki, H.: Phototherapy and insensible water loss in the newborn infant. Am J Dis Child 124:230, 1972.

114. Okken, A., Jonxis, J. H. P., Rispens, P., et al: Insensible water loss and metabolic rate in low birthweight newborn infants. Pediatr Res 13:1072, 1979.

115. Olney, J. W., Ho, O. L., Rhee, V.: Brain-damaging potential off protein hydrolysates. N Engl J Med 289:391, 1973.

116. Olson, M.: Effects of water, 5 percent glucose, or milk on rabbits' lungs. Pediatrics 46:538, 1970.

117. Pereira, G. R., Fox, W. W., Stanley, C. A., et al: Decreased oxygenation and hyperlipemia during fat infusions in premature infants. Pediatrics, 66:26, 1980.

118. Pereira, G. R., Sherman, M. S., DiGiacomo, J., et al: Hyperalimentation-induced cholestasis. Increased incidence and severity in premature infants. Am J Dis Child 135:842, 1981.

119. Pitt, J., Barlow, B., and Heird, W.: Protection against experimental necrotizing enterocolitis by maternal milk. I. Role of milk leukocytes. Pediatr Res 11:906, 1977.

120. Pittard, W., Polmar, S., and Fanaroff, A.: The breast milk macrophage: a potential vehicle for immunoglobulin transport. J Reticuloendothel Soc 22:597, 1977.

121. Pittard, W., Polmar, S., Fanger, M., et al: Identification of immunoglobulin bearing lymphocytes in fresh human breast milk. Pediatr Res 10:359, 1976.

122. Rabinowitz, J., and Siegle, R.: Changing clinical and roentgenographic patterns of necrotizing enterocolitis. Am J Roentgenol 126:560, 1976.

123. Rabor, I., Oh, W., Wu, P., et al: Effects of early and late feeding of intrauterine fetally malnourished (IUM) infants. Pediatrics 42:261, 1968.

124. Raiha, N.: Biochemical basis for nutritional management of preterm infants. Pediatrics 53:147, 1974.

125. Raiha, N., Heinonen, K., Rassin, D. S., et al: Milk protein quantity and quality in low birth weight infants. I. Metabolic responses and effects on growth. Pediatrics 57:659, 1976.

126. Rassin, D., Gaull, G., Heinonen, K., et al: Milk protein quantity and quality in low birth weight infants. II. Effects on selected aliphatic amino acids in plasma and urine. Pediatrics 59:407, 1977.

127. Rassin, D., Gaull, G., Raiha, N., et al: Milk protein quantity and quality in low birth weight infants. IV. Effects on tyrosine and phenylalanine in plasma and urine. J Pediatr 90:356, 1977.

128. Reichman, B. L., Chessex, P., Putet, G., et al: Diet, fat accretion and growth in premature infants. N Engl J Med 305:1495, 1981.

129. Reichman, B. L., Chessex, P., Putet, G., et al: Partition of energy metabolism and energy cost of growth in the very low-birth-weight infant. Pediatrics 69:446, 1982.

130. Rhea, J., and Kilby, J.: A nasojejunal tube for infant feeding. Pediatrics 46:36, 1970.

131. Rhea, J., Ahmad, M., and Mange, M.: Nasojejunal (transpyloric) feeding: a commentary. J Pediatr 86:451, 1975.

132. Rhea, J., Ghazzawi, O., and Weidman, W.: Nasojejunal feeding: an improved device and intubation technique. Pediatrics 82:951, 1973.

133. Roberts, S., and Freed, D.: Neonatal IgA secretion enhanced by breastfeeding. Lancet 2:1131, 1977.

134. Roger, R., and Finegold, M.: Cholestasis in immature newborn infants: Is parenteral alimentation responsible? J Pediatr 86:264, 1975.

135. Ross, M., and Bras, G.: Food preference and length of life. Science 190:165, 1975.

136. Ross Symposium on Pediatric Research: Necrotizing enterocolitis in the newborn infant. Columbus, Ohio, Ross Laboratories, 1975.

137. Ross Symposium on Pediatric Research: Gastrointestinal development and neonatal nutrition. Columbus, Ohio, Ross Laboratories, 1977.

138. Roy, C., Ste-Marie, M., Chartrand, L., et al: Correction of the malabsorption of the preterm infant with a medium chain triglyceride formula. J Pediatr 86:446, 1975.

139. Roy, R., and Sinclair, J.: Hydration of the low birth weight infant. Clin Perinatol 2:393, 1975.

140. Roy, R., Chance, G., Radde, I., et al: Late hyponatremia in very low birth weight infants (1.3 kilograms). Pediatr Res 10:526, 1976.

141. Roy, R., Pollnitz, R., Hamilton, J., et al: Impaired assimilation of nasojejunal feeds in healthy low birth weight infants. J Pediatr 90:431, 1977.

142. Russell, G., and Feather, E.: Effects of feeding on respiratory mechanics of healthy newborn infants. Arch Dis Child 45:325, 1970.

143. Rutter, N., and Hull, D.: Reduction of skin water loss in the newborn. I. Effects of applying topical agents. Arch Dis Child 56:669, 1981.

144. Ryan, J. A., Jr., Abel, R. M., Abbott, W. M., et al: Catheter complications in total parenteral nutrition. A prospective study of 200 consecutive patients. N Engl J Med 290:757, 1974.

145. Santulli, T., Schullinger, J., Heird, W., et al: Acute necrotizing enterocolitis in infancy: a review of 64 cases. Pediatrics 55:376, 1975.

146. Schanler, R. J., Garza, C., Nichols, B. L.: Fortified human milk (FHM) feeding in very low birthweight (VLBW) infants. Evaluation of growth and metabolic balance. (Abstr) Pediatr Res 17:200A, 1983.

147. Schubert, W.: Fat nutrition and diet in childhood. Am J Cardiol 32:581, 1973.

148. Shaw, J.: Evidence for defective skeletal mineralization in low birth weight infants: the absorption of calcium and fat. Pediatrics 57:16, 1976.

149. Shenai, J. P., Reynolds, J. W., and Babson, S. G.: Nutritional balance studies in very-low-birth-weight infants: enhanced retention rates by an experimental formula. Pediatrics 66:233, 1980.

150. Shennan, A., Cherian, A., Angel, A., et al: Effect of intralipid on estimation of serum bilirubin. J Pediatr 88:285, 1976.

151. Shivpuri, C. R., Martin, R. J., Carlo, W. A., et al: Decreased ventilation in preterm infants during oral feeding. Pediatrics 103:285, 1983.

152. Siegel, M., and Lebenthal, E.: Development of gastrointestinal motility and gastric emptying during the fetal and newborn periods. In Lebenthal, E. (ed.): Textbook of Gastroenterology and Nutrition in Infancy. New York, Raven Press, 1981.

153. Signer, E., and Fridrich, R.: Gastric emptying in newborns and young infants. Acta Paediatr Scand 64:525, 1975.

154. Simpson, A., Leonidas, J., Krasna, I., et al: Roentgen diagnosis of midgut malrotation: value of upper gastrointestinal radiographic study. J Pediatr Surg 7:243, 1972.

155. Sinclair, J., Driscoll, J., Jr., Heird, W., et al: Supportive management of the sick neonate: parenteral calories, water, electrolytes. Pediatr Clin North Am 17:863, 1970.

156. Smallpiece, V., and Davies, P.: Immediate feeding of premature infants with undiluted breast milk. Lancet 2:1349, 1964.

157. Smith, C., and Goldman, A.: The cells of the human colostrum. I. In vitro studies of morphology and function. Pediatr Res 2:103, 1968.

158. Snyderman, S.: The protein and amino acid requirements of the premature infant. In Jonxis, J. H. P.: Processes in the Foetus and Newborn Infant. Nutricia Symposium. Baltimore, Williams and Wilkins, 1971.

159. Snyderman, S., Boyer, A., Kogut, M. D., et al: The

protein requirement of the newborn infant. I. Effect of protein intake on the retention of nitrogen. J Pediatr 74:872, 1969.

160. Stevenson, J. G.: Fluid administration in the association of patent ductus arteriosus complicating respiratory distress syndrome. J Pediatr 90:275, 1977.

161. Stoliar, O., Pelley, R., Kaniecki-Green, E., et al: Secretory IgA against enterotoxins in breast milk. Lancet 1:1258, 1976.

162. Sturman, J. Gaull, G., and Raiha, N.: Absence of cystathionase in human fetal liver: is cystine essential? Science 169:74, 1970.

163. Sturman, J., Rassin, D., and Gaull, G.: Taurine in development: is it essential in the neonate? Pediatr Res 10:415, 1976.

164. Sunshine, P. (ed.): Feeding the Neonate Weighing Less than 1500 Grams: Nutrition and Beyond. Report of the 79th Conference on Pediatrics. Columbus, Ohio, Ross Laboratories, 1980.

165. Sweet, A. Y.: Personal communication, 1982.

166. Touloukian, R.: Isoosmolar coma during parenteral alimentation with protein hydrolysate in excess of 4 gm/kg/day. J Pediatr 86:270, 1975.

167. Touloukian, R., Pickett, L., Spackman, T., et al: Repair of esophageal atresia by end-to-side anastomosis and ligation of the tracheoesophageal fistula: a critical review of 18 cases. J Pediatr Surg 9:305, 1974.

168. Ty, T., Brunet, C., and Beardmore, H.: A variation in the operative technique for the treatment of esophageal atresia with tracheoesophageal fistula. J Pediatr Surg 2:118, 1967.

169. Vengusamy, S., Pildes, R., Raffensperger, J., et al: A controlled study of feeding gastrostomy in low birth weight infants. Pediatrics 43:815, 1969.

170. Vileisis, R. A., Inwood, R. J., and Hunt, C. E.: Prospective controlled study of parenteral nutrition associated with cholestatic jaundice: effect of protein intake. J Pediatr 96:893, 1980.

171. Watkins, J., Ingall, D., Szcepanik, P., et al: Bile-salt metabolism in the newborn: measurement of pool size and synthesis by stable isotope technique. N Engl J Med 288:431, 1973.

172. Watkins, J., Szcepanik, P., Gould, J., et al: Bile salt metabolism in the human premature infant: preliminary observations of pool size and synthesis

rate following prenatal administration of dexamethasone and phenobarbital. Gastroenterology 69:706, 1975.

173. Wharton, B., and Bower, B.: Immediate or later feeding for premature babies: a controlled trial. Lancet 2:969, 1965.

174. Widdowson, E.: Chemical analysis of the body. In Brozek, J. (ed.): Human Body Composition: Approaches and Applications. Oxford, Pergamon Press, 1965.

175. Williams, P., and Oh, W.: Effects of radiant warmer on insensible water loss in newborn infants. Am J Dis Child 128:511, 1974.

176. Wilmore, D., and Dudrick, S.: Growth and development of an infant receiving all nutrients exclusively by vein. JAMA 203:860, 1968.

177. Winters, R. (ed.): The Body Fluids in Pediatrics. Boston, Little, Brown and Company, 1973.

178. Winters, R.: Total parenteral nutrition in pediatrics: the Borden Award address. Pediatrics 56:17, 1975.

179. Wu, P., and Hodgman, J.: Insensible water loss in preterm infants: changes with postnatal development and non-ionizing radiant energy. Pediatrics 54:704, 1974.

180. Wu, P., Teilmann, P., Cabler, M., et al: "Early" versus "late" feeding of low birth weight neonates. Pediatrics 39:733, 1967.

181. Yu, V.: Effect of body position on gastric emptying in the neonate. Arch Dis Child 50:500, 1975.

182. Yu, V., and Rolfe, P.: Effect of feeding on ventilation and respiratory mechanics in newborn infants. Arch Dis Child 51:310, 1976.

183. Yu, V. Y., James, B. E., Hendry, P. G., et al: Total parenteral nutrition in very low birth weight infants: a controlled trial. Arch Dis Child 54:653, 1979.

184. Ziegler, E., and Fomon, S.: Fluid intake, renal solute load, and water balance in infancy. J Pediatr 78:561, 1971.

185. Ziegler, E., O'Donnell, A., Nelson, S., et al: Body composition of the reference fetus. Growth 40:329, 1976.

186. Zlotkin, S. H., Bryan, H. M., and Anderson, G. H.: Cysteine supplementation to cysteine free intravenous feeding regimens in newborn infants. Am J Clin Nutr 34:914, 1981.

7

Care of the Parents

MARSHALL H. KLAUS
JOHN H. KENNELL

Unfortunately...a certain number of mothers abandon the babies whose needs they have not had to meet, and in whom they have lost all interest. The life of the little one has been saved, it is true, but at the cost of the mother.

PIERRE BUDIN
THE NURSLING

Study of the tie between parent and infant began as recently as 15–20 years ago, when the staffs of intensive care nurseries observed that sometimes, after extraordinary efforts had been made to save small premature infants, they would return to emergency rooms battered by their parents although they had been sent home intact and thriving. Careful examination of these phenomena has shown that prematurity or an infant's early hospitalization appears disproportionately frequently in the history of infants who are battered or who fail to thrive without an organic cause.

Lynch[49] noted six factors overrepresented in the history of abused children in England. These factors included abnormal pregnancy, abnormal labor and delivery, and neonatal separation. Reanalysis of a number of studies has shown an association between early separation and these disastrous conditions. The occurrence of these and other mothering disorders has provided a continuing stimulus to unravel the process by which a parent develops a close bond with his or her infant.

This chapter provides a historical background to explain why mothers have been isolated from their infants in the United States, describes recent studies of the process by which a parent becomes attached to the infant, and suggests applications of these findings to the care of the parents of a normal infant, a premature infant, a malformed infant, and a stillbirth or neonatal death.

HISTORY

The role of the mother in the hospital nursery for full-term and low-birth-weight infants has changed greatly during the last century.

The mother was welcomed into the premature nurseries of the Frenchman Pierre Budin (the first modern perinatologist) and was allowed to assist in her infant's care, for as Budin recognized in his book, *The Nursling,* published in 1907[12]: "Mothers separated from their young soon lost all interest in those whom they were unable to nurse or cherish."

Ironically, Budin's desire to publicize his methods resulted in the exclusion of the mother from the nursery. Martin Couney, a young pupil of Budin's, went to the Berlin Exposition of 1896, at which his "Kinderbrutanstalt" (child hatchery), where premature infants were brought and raised, became both commercially and clinically successful.[71] After exhibiting at fairs in England and the United States, Couney settled on Coney Island, successfully raising more than 5000 premature babies during the next 4 decades. Mothers were not permitted to participate in their infants' care at Couney's exhibits, and

147

it is of significance that on some occasions Couney experienced difficulty in persuading parents to take their infants back. Early hospital nurseries in the United States adopted many of his methods of newborn care.

The high rate of morbidity and mortality of hospitalized newborns in the early 1900s led to the development of strict isolation for patients with or without disease. Visitors were strongly discouraged. Unfortunately, Couney's example and the measures introduced to prevent the spread of infection were thus combined to exclude the mother totally from hospital nurseries.

The Sarah Morris Hospital in Chicago developed the first hospital center for premature care in 1923. Following the precepts of Budin, the director, Hess, encouraged the production of breast milk at home and invited mothers' assistance in caring for the infants.

However, in premature units created after the Sarah Morris Center, a standard set of stringent regulations was followed, including only essential handling of the infants, a policy of strict isolation, and the total exclusion of visitors.

During the period after World War II, several innovative approaches to newborn care appeared. In a study of the home nursing of prematures in Newcastle-on-Tyne, Miller[53] noted that the mortality rate was only slightly greater than that of a control group nursed in the hospital. A shortage of skilled personnel was the impetus for an arrangement created by Kahn et al[34] at Baragwanath Hospital, Johannesburg, South Africa. Here mothers were able to participate in supervised care and feeding of their infants while themselves remaining in the hospital. This innovation was accompanied by a sharp decline in infant mortality.

The creative work on rooming-in of Edith Jackson and her colleagues in the 1940s changed practices for a small percentage of mothers of full-term infants. However, it has only been in the last 10–15 years that large numbers of parents are able to care for their healthy infants a major part of each day.

PREGNANCY

It has been difficult to assess which factors determine the parenting behavior of an adult human who has lived for 20–30 years. A mother's and father's actions and responses toward their infant are derived from a complex combination of their own genetic endowment, the way the infant responds to them, a long history of interpersonal relations with their own families and with each other, past experiences with this or previous pregnancies, the absorption of the practices and values of their cultures, and probably most importantly, how each was raised by his or her own mother and father. The mothering or fathering behavior of each woman and man, his or her ability to tolerate stresses, and his or her need for special attention differ greatly and depend upon a mixture of these factors. Figure 7–1 is a schematic diagram of the major influences on paternal and maternal behavior and the resulting disturbances that we hypothesize may arise from them.

Included under *parental background* are the parent's care by his or her own mother, endowment or genetics of parents, practices of the culture, relationships within the family, experiences with previous pregnancies, and planning, course, and events during pregnancy.

Included under *care practices* are the behavior of physicians, nurses, and hospital personnel, care and support during labor, first days of life, separation of mother and infant, and rules of the hospital.

Included under *parenting disorders* are the vulnerable child syndrome,[20, 21, 27, 31, 41] child abuse,[49, 72] failure to thrive,[1, 24, 69] and some developmental and emotional problems in high-risk infants.[36] Other determinants—such as the attitudes, statements, and practices of the nurses and physicians in the hospital, whether the mother is alone for short periods during her labor, whether there is separation from the infant in the first days of life, the nature of the infant

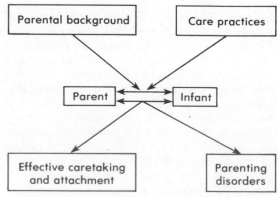

Figure 7–1. Diagram of the major influences on parent-infant attachment and the resulting outcomes.

himself, his temperament, and whether he is healthy, sick, or malformed—will obviously affect parenting behavior and the parent-child relationship.

The most easily manipulated variables in this scheme are the separation of the infant from his mother and the practices in the hospital during the first hours and days of life. It is here, during this period, that studies have in part clarified some of the steps in parent-infant attachment.

A wide diversity of observations are beginning to piece together some of the various phases and time periods that are helpful for this process (Table 7–1).

Pregnancy for a woman has been considered a process of maturation,[5, 8, 13] with a series of adaptive tasks, each dependent upon the successful completion of the preceding one. There are two general time periods in the pregnancy and another in the neonatal period during which a wide range of stressful factors may influence a woman's subsequent mothering behavior and possibly the developmental outcome of her child.

Many mothers are initially disturbed by feelings of grief and anger when they become pregnant, because of factors ranging from economic and housing hardships to interpersonal difficulties. However, by the end of the first trimester, the majority of women who initially rejected pregnancy have accepted it. This initial stage, as outlined by Bibring,[8] is the mother's *identification of the growing fetus as an "integral part of herself."*

The second stage is *a growing perception of the fetus as a separate individual,* usually occurring with the awareness of fetal movement. After quickening, a woman will generally begin to have some fantasies about what the baby may be like, will attribute to him some human personality characteristics, and will develop a sense of attachment and value toward him. At this time, further acceptance of the pregnancy and marked changes in attitude toward the fetus may be observed; unplanned, unwanted infants may now seem more acceptable. Objectively, the health worker will usually find some outward evidence of the mother's preparation in such actions as the purchase of clothes or a crib, selecting a name, and arranging space for the baby.

The increased use of amniocentesis and ultrasound has appeared to affect parents' perceptions of babies in a rather unexpected fashion. Many parents have discussed with us the disappointment they experienced when they discovered the sex of the baby. Half of the mystery was over. Everything was possible, but once the amniocentesis was done and the sex known, the range of the unknown was considerably narrowed. However, the tests have the beneficial result of removing some of the anxiety about the possibility of any abnormality. We have noted following the procedure that the baby is sometimes named, and parents often carry around a picture of the very small fetus. This phenomenon will require further investigation to understand the significance of these reactions to the bonding process.

Cohen[14] suggests the following questions to learn the special needs of each mother.

- How long have you lived in this immediate area, and where does most of your family live?
- How often do you see your mother or other close relatives?
- Has anything happened to you in the past (or do you currently have any condition) that causes you to worry about the pregnancy or the baby?
- What was your husband's reaction to your becoming pregnant?
- What other responsibilities do you have outside the family?

It is important to inquire about how the pregnant woman was mothered—did she have a neglected and deprived infancy and childhood or grow up with a warm and intact family life?

TABLE 7–1. STEPS IN ATTACHMENT

Prior to pregnancy
  Planning the pregnancy

During pregnancy
  Confirming the pregnancy
  Accepting the pregnancy
  Experiencing fetal movement
  Beginning to accept the fetus as an individual

Labor
Birth
After birth
  Seeing the baby
  Touching the baby
  Giving care to the baby
  Accepting the infant as a separate individual

DELIVERY

Newton and Newton noted that those mothers who remain relaxed in labor, who are supported, and who have good rapport with their attendants are more apt to be pleased with their infants at first sight.[57]

In two separate randomized controlled studies of a total of 560 mothers, women who had continuous social support during labor and birth had labors that were significantly shortened (8 hours vs. 14 hours) (p < 0.0001) compared with the control group. Likewise, in the experimental group, perinatal problems including cesarean sections and the number of infants admitted to intensive care were significantly reduced compared with the controls. Maternal attachment behaviors were more likely to be noted in the experimental mothers compared with the controls during a 20 minute observation period during the first hour of life.[39, 74] This low-cost intervention may be a simple way to reduce the length of labor and perinatal problems for women and their infants during childbirth, and it vividly illustrates the complicated interrelationships between social support, maternal behavior, and physiology, as well as medical complications.

The Day of Delivery

The environment in which the delivery takes place may be more important than has previously been realized. In sharp contrast to the woman who gives birth in the hospital, a woman delivering at home with a midwife will often be in control. She is an active participant during her labor and delivery rather than a passive participant. Although controlled studies have not yet been done to test the effects of this experience on the parent-infant relationship, it seems clear that the conditions surrounding delivery greatly affect the mother's initial mood and interaction with her infant.[43]

We do not favor home delivery but suggest that hospital deliveries be altered, as in alternative birth centers. Thus, the advantages of both home and hospital can be captured.[3]

Human mothers after delivery may have common patterns of behavior when they begin to care for their babies. Filmed observations[47] show that a mother presented with her nude, full-term infant begins with fingertip touching of the infant's extremities and within a few minutes proceeds to massaging, encompassing palm contact of the infant's trunk. Mothers of premature infants also follow this sequence but proceed at a much slower rate. Fathers go through some of the same routines.[67]

A strong interest in eye-to-eye contact has been expressed by mothers of both full-term and premature infants. Tape recordings of the words of mothers who had been presented with their infants in privacy revealed that 70 per cent of the statements referred to the eyes. The mothers said, "Let me see your eyes" and "Open your eyes and I'll know you love me." Robson[65] has suggested that eye-to-eye contact appears to elicit maternal caregiving responses. Mothers seem to try hard to look "en face" at their infants—that is, to keep their faces aligned with their babies' so that their eyes are in the same vertical plane of rotation as their babies', as shown by the mother in Figure 7–2. Complementing the mother's interest in the infant's eyes is the early functional development of his visual pathways. The infant is alert, active, and able to follow during the first hour of life[12] if maternal sedation has been limited and the administration of silver nitrate delayed.

Additional information about this early period was provided by Wolff,[80] who described six separate states of consciousness in the infant, ranging from deep sleep to screaming. (See Chapter 16 for further details of infant states.) The state in which we are most interested is state 4, the quiet, alert state. In this state, the infant's eyes are wide open, and he is able to respond to his environment. Unfortunately, he may be in this state for periods as brief as a few seconds. However, Emde et al[21] observed that the infant is in a wakeful state for a period of 38 minutes during the first hour after birth. It is now possible to demonstrate that an infant can

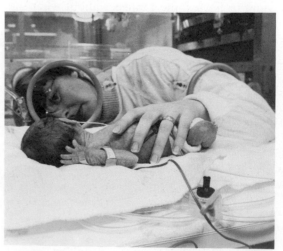

Figure 7–2. Mother in "en face" position with her premature infant.

see, that he has visual preferences, that he will turn his head to the spoken word, and that he moves in rhythm to his mother's voice in the first minutes and hours of life—a beautiful linking and synchronized dance between the mother and infant. After this, however, he goes into a deep sleep for 3–4 hours.

Therefore, during the first 60–90 minutes of his life, the infant is alert, responsive, and especially appealing. In short, he is ideally equipped to meet his parents for the first time. The infant's broad array of sensory and motor abilities evokes responses from the mother and begins the communication that may be especially helpful for attachment and the initiation of a series of reciprocal interactions.

Observations by Condon and Sander[15] reveal that newborns move in rhythm with the structure of adult speech. Interestingly, synchronous movements were found at 16 hours of age with both of the two natural languages tested, English and Chinese.

Nature has provided for the early union in a myriad of ways. MacFarlane[50] has shown that 6 days after birth, an infant reliably will be able to identify by scent his mother's breast pad from that of other women. The licking of the nipple induces a marked increase in the mother's prolactin and oxytocin, contracting the uterus and decreasing bleeding. Lind and associates[46] in Stockholm have noted a surprising increase in blood flow to the breast of a woman when she hears her baby cry. The alert infant follows his mother with his eyes, rewarding her and rekindling her fascination with him.

Figure 7–3 depicts a common situation—a mother feeding her infant in the first hour of life. The simplicity of the scene, however, is belied by the surrounding diagram, which presents the multiple simultaneous interactions between mother and child. Each is intimately involved with the other on a number of sensory levels. Their behaviors complement each other and serve to lock the pair together. The infant elicits behaviors from the mother that in turn are satisfying to him, and, vice versa, the mother elicits behaviors in the infant that in turn are rewarding to her. For example, the infant's hard crying is likely to bring the mother near and trigger her to pick him up. When she picks him up, he is likely to quiet, open his eyes, and follow. Looking at the process in the opposite direction, when the mother touches the infant's cheek, he is likely to turn his head, bringing him into contact with her nipple, on which he will suck. His sucking in turn is pleasurable to both of them. Actually, this is a necessarily oversimplified description of these interactions, for these behaviors do not occur in a chainlike sequence—rather each behavior triggers several others.

What we see is an immensely complex "fail-

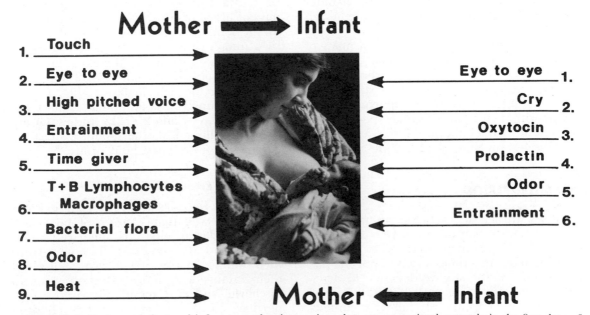

Figure 7–3. Mother-to-infant and infant-to-mother interactions that can occur simultaneously in the first days of life. (Klaus, M., Kennell, J., Plumb, N., et al: Human maternal behavior at the first contact with her young. Pediatrics 46:187, 1970.)

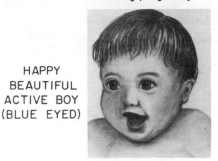
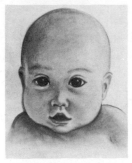

MOTHER'S
MENTAL IMAGE
(during pregnancy)

REAL BABY

HAPPY
BEAUTIFUL
ACTIVE BOY
(BLUE EYED)

QUIET GIRL
(BROWN EYED)

Figure 7–4. The mental image of the baby this mother planned to have is quite different from the baby she has.

safe" system designed to ensure the proximity of mother and child. Keeping the mother and baby together soon after birth is likely to initiate and enhance the operation of known sensory, hormonal, physiologic, immunologic, and behavioral mechanisms that possibly help lock the parent to the infant.[10, 11, 39]

Also, on the basis of our observations and the reports of parents, we believe that every parent has a task to perform during the postpartum period. The mother in particular must look and "take in" her real live baby and then reconcile the fantasy of the infant she imagined with the one she actually delivered (Figure 7–4). Many cultures recognize this need by providing the mother with a doula, or "aunt," who relieves her of other responsibilities so that she can devote herself completely to this task.[63]

There is suggestive evidence that many of these early interactions also take place between the father and his newborn child. Parkes[61] in particular has demonstrated that when fathers are given the opportunity to be alone with their newborns, they spend almost exactly the same amount of time as mothers in holding, touching, and looking at them.

SENSITIVE PERIOD

Many difficulties arise in attempting to determine whether or not there is a sensitive period in the human. Because so little was known about this time period in normal parents, most of the studies designed to determine the effects of early separation have focused on parents of full-term infants. These studies have addressed the question of whether there is a sensitive time period for parent-infant contact in the first minutes, hours, and days of life that may alter the parents' later behavior with that infant. In many biologic disciplines, these moments have been called sensitive periods, vulnerable points, or susceptible periods. However, in most of the examples of a sensitive period in biology, the observations are made on the young of the species rather than the adult.

The Hypothesis of a Sensitive Period

In the past 15 years, 17 separate studies have focused on whether additional time for close contact between the mother and full-term infant in the first minutes, hours, and days of life alters the quality of the maternal-infant bond over time. Figure 7–5 illustrates the timing of the contact in these studies. In three studies (Group A), the extra time was added not only during the first 2 hours but also during the next 3 days of life. In one study (Group B), the additional contact was added on days 1 and 2. In 13 studies (Group C), the additional mother-infant contact occurred only in the first hour of life.[39]

Early and Extended Contact

GROUP A STUDIES. In the first study, Klaus et al[40] observed that a group of poor, primarily single, primiparous, inner-city mothers who had 16 hours of extra contact with their infants in the first 3 days of life fed their infants with more affection prior to discharge and at 1 month were more supportive and affectionate with their children during a stressful office visit than control

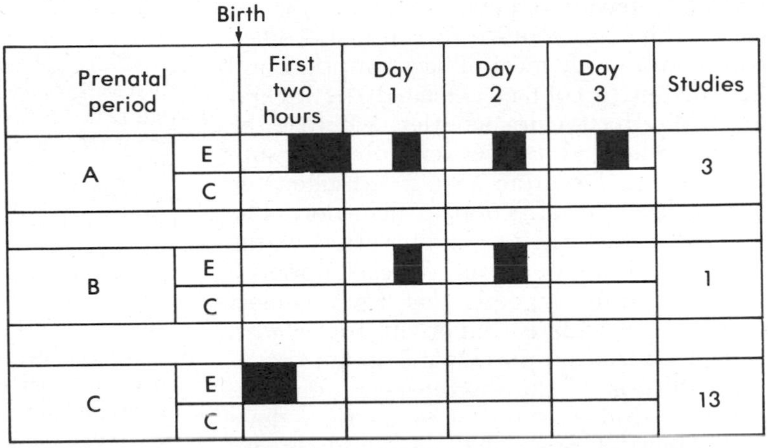

Figure 7–5. Three types of controlled studies in which one group of mothers have additional contact with their infants (E) compared with another group that have routine contact (C).

mothers. At 2 years, extra-contact mothers talked to their babies differently, using more complex sentences and fewer imperatives.

Extended Contact—No Early Contact

GROUP B STUDY. It is useful to compare the one study in this group by O'Connor and associates[58] with the large study by Siegel and associates[70] (Table 7–2). Siegel did not note any difference in parenting disorders, finding ten in the control group and seven in the extended contact groups. On the other hand, O'Connor noted significant differences in parenting disorders, child abuse, neglect, abandonment, and nonorganic failure to thrive, finding ten such cases in the control group and two of mothers who were given extended contact.

Because of the relatively small number of patients studied, the negative finding by Siegel does not answer the important question of whether extended contact for all mothers in the United States would prevent child abuse of some of the 100,000 infants presently abused each year. A study with about 1500 patients would be needed to detect a

TABLE 7–2. CHILD ABUSE OR NEGLECT IN THE FIRST YEAR OF LIFE

Study	Total	Abuse or Neglect
O'Connor et al, 1980		
Extended contact	134	2
Control	143	10*
Siegel et al, 1980		
Extended contact	97	7
Control	105	10

*p <0.05.

reduction in child abuse from 3 per cent to 1.5 per cent, 80 per cent of the time.

Early Contact

GROUP C STUDIES. Thirteen separate studies have looked at the effect of additional mother-infant contact in the first hour of life, with contact following this period being similar in both the experimental and the control groups. In nine of the studies, differences in either the mother or the infant were noted in the experimental group.

In six of nine studies it was striking that breast feeding continued for a significantly longer period for those mothers who had contact that involved suckling their babies in the first hour after birth.[39] It is difficult to distinguish whether it was simply the early contact or specifically the suckling that altered the length of time that these mothers continued to breast feed.

An important study in this group is that of Anisfeld and Lipper.[2] They found that the group of mothers given extra contact at delivery showed more affectionate behavior than the group who had had routine contact with their infants. They also found an interaction between early contact and the level of the mother's personal support system. All the mothers in the study were classified as having "higher" or "lower" levels of social support (based on marital status, receipt of public assistance, education, and presence of the father or other support person in the delivery room). The affectionate behavior scores for the extra-contact and routine-contact groups, subclassified by social support, were then compared. This analysis revealed that those women who had a higher level of social support showed the same amount of affectionate behavior, whether or not they received the extra contact. By contrast, women who had a lower level of social support and had the extra contact exhibited the highest level of affectionate behavior, whereas the women who had a lower level of social support and had routine contact exhibited the lowest level of affectionate behavior. The treatment thus had a significant effect on the women with a lower level of social support.

This finding suggests that early contact may be particularly important for women who lack social support. It also allows for the reconciliation of the discrepancies found in previous studies, some of which were done with middle-class populations and others with populations more likely to be lacking social support. For further details of these studies see Klaus and Kennell.[39]

Whereas the benefits of good apple pie are disputed by few, motherhood, bonding, and the importance of early contact with the newborn infant have generated a heated debate from which the ashes are still settling.

Anisfeld, E., Curry, M. A., Hales, D. J., et al: Maternal-infant bonding: a joint rebuttal. Pediatrics 72:569, 1983.

Klaus, M., and Kennell, J. H.: Parent to infant bonding: setting the record straight. J Pediatr 102:575, 1983.

Lamb, M.: The bonding phenomenon: Misinterpretations and their implications. J Pediatr 101:555, 1982.

A. Fanaroff

WHEN DOES LOVE BEGIN?

The first feelings of love for the infant are not necessarily instantaneous with the initial contact.

MacFarlane et al[51] helped to answer this question by asking 97 mothers, "When did you first feel love for your baby?" The replies were as follows: during pregnancy—41 per cent, at birth—24 per cent, first week—27 per cent, and after the first week—8 per cent.

In another study of two groups of primiparous mothers[66] (n = 112 and n = 41), 40 per cent recalled that their predominant emotional reaction when holding their babies for the first time was one of indifference. The same response was reported by 25 per cent of 40 multiparous mothers. Forty per cent of both groups felt immediate affection.

Donald Winnicott[78] made remarkably perceptive observations that suggest he was describing the sensitive period. From these observations Winnicott proposed that a healthy mother goes through a period of "Primary Maternal Preoccupation."

It is my thesis that in the earliest phase we are dealing with a very special state of the mother, a psychological condition which deserves a name, such as Primary Maternal Preoccupation. I suggest that sufficient tribute has not yet been paid in our literature, or perhaps anywhere, to a special psychiatric condition of the mother, of which I would say the following things: It gradually develops and becomes a state of heightened sensitivity during, and especially toward the end of, the pregnancy. It lasts for a few weeks after the birth of the child.

The mother who develops this state . . . provides a setting for the infant's constitution to begin to make itself evident, for the developmental tendencies to start to unfold, and for the infant to experience spontaneous movement and become the owner of the sensations that are appropriate to this early phase of life.

Only if a mother is sensitized in the way I am describing can she feel herself into her infant's place, and so meet the infant's needs.

Based on the available evidence, how strongly should physicians and nurses emphasize the importance of parent-infant contact in the first hour and extended visiting for the rest of the hospital stay? Obviously, in spite of a lack of early contact experienced by many parents in hospital births in the past 20 to 30 years, almost all these parents became bonded to their babies. The human is highly adaptable, and there are many fail-safe routes to attachment. Sadly, some parents who missed the bonding experience have felt that all was lost for their future relationship. This was (and is) completely incorrect, but it was so upsetting that we have tried to speak more moderately.

Obviously the infant should be with the mother and father only if the infant is known to be physically normal and if appropriate temperature control is utilized. We also strongly urge that the infant remain with the mother as long as she wishes throughout the hospital stay so that she and the baby can get to know each other. We believe that in the near future, placement in the large central nursery will be phased out for most babies. Leaving the infant with the mother will allow both mother and father longer periods in which to learn about their baby.

The Sick or Premature Infant

Although parental visiting has been permitted in the intensive care nursery, a number of studies[4, 6, 30, 54, 56] have revealed that most parents continue to suffer severe emotional stress. Harper et al[30] noted that even when parents have close contact with their infants in the intensive care nursery, they experience prolonged stress. Benfield and associates[6] also noted that most parents experienced grief reactions. The level of their response was unrelated to the severity of the baby's problems.

From interviews early in the course of pregnancy, Mason[52] found that if the mother expressed a moderately high level of anxiety, actively sought information about the condition of her baby, showed strong maternal feelings for the baby, and had strong support from the father, there was usually a favorable outcome. If the mother showed a low level of anxiety and activity, the chances were that her relationship with her child would be poor.

Newman[56] described "coping through commitment" as an intense yet variable involvement in the care of a low-birth-weight infant. In contrast, "coping through distance" was a slower acquaintance process in which the parents expressed fear, anxiety, and at times denial before they accepted the surviving infant. Minde et al,[55] in observations and interviews, noted that the most important variables were the mother's relationship to her own mother, her relationship to the father, and whether or not the mother had had a previous abortion. Highly interacting mothers visit and telephone the nursery more frequently while the infants are hospitalized and stimulate their infants more at home. Mothers who stimulate their infants very little in the nursery also visit and telephone less frequently and provide only minimal stimulation to them at home. Most perceptively, Minde et al noted that mothers who touched and fondled their infants more in the nursery had infants who opened their eyes more often.[55] He and his associates observed the contingency between the infant's eyes being open and the mother's touching and also between gross motor stretches and the mother's smiling. They could not determine to what extent the sequence of touching and eye opening was an indication of the mother's primary contribution or whether it was initiated by the infant. Thus Mason, Newman, and Minde et al predict that mothers who become involved with, interested in, and anxious about their infants in the intensive care nursery will have an easier time when the infant is taken home.

Field[24] has demonstrated the close connection between what a mother does and her infant's arousal level. While most mothers of full-term babies adopt a moderate level of activity that is associated with optimal arousal in their babies, some mothers of "premies" either over- or underreact. Field found that mothers of premature infants who were overreactive during early face-to-face interactions were more likely to be overprotective and overcontrolling during interactions with their infants 2 years later.[24]

Infant Stimulation or Imitation

As a result of studies by several perceptive researchers, our conceptual framework for stimulation of the infant after discharge home and possibly before discharge needs to be reconsidered and may have to be altered drastically.

From observation of normal full-term mothers and infants, Winnicott noted that what babies observe in their caretakers' faces in the early months of life helps them to develop a concept of themselves.[79] He suggested that ordinarily the baby sees himself or herself. The mother unconsciously imitates the infant's face—as Winnicott noted, the mother is a mirror for the baby. Pawlby[62] found that both mothers and infants imitate each other, and she observed this occurring during the entire first year of life.

Lastly, in the series of creative manipulations of infant-mother face-to-face interactions referred to above, Field[24] found that the mother and the normal *full-term* infant are each interacting about 70 per cent of the time in their spontaneous play (Figure 7–6). However, when the mother is asked to increase her attention-getting behavior (stimulation), her activity increases to 80 per cent of the time, and strikingly, the infant's gaze decreases to 50 per cent. When such mothers are told only to imitate the movements of their infant, which reduces their activity, the infant's gaze time greatly increases.

Field noted that in the spontaneous situation, mothers of *high-risk* infants are interacting up to 90 per cent of the time, whereas their infants are only looking 30 per cent of the time. If the mother is told to use attention-getting gestures, her activity increases even above 90 per cent of the time, but her infant's gaze decreases further. If the mother decreases her interactions when asked to imitate the baby's movements, there is then a striking increase in the infant's gaze. These experiments show that while much of parents' activity is aimed at encouraging more

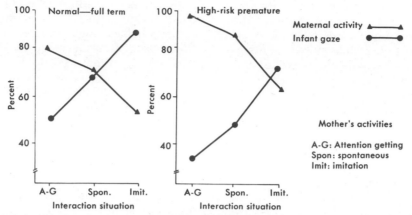

Figure 7–6. Relationship between maternal activity and infant gaze in three interaction situations: (1) mother attempting to get the infant's attention; (2) spontaneous interaction; and (3) mother imitating the baby. (Adapted from Field, T. M.[24] Copyright The Society for Research in Child Development, Inc.)

activity or responsivity from the premature infant, their approach may be counterproductive, leading to less instead of more infant responsiveness.

Once a person has a well-integrated self, imitation is an invasion of that individual's integrity. However, during the early months, when the infant's self is incompletely formed, imitation of the infant's gestures and facial expressions appears to be a help in the process of self-discovery. All these observations suggest that we should be careful about recommending increased stimulation for the premature infant. Instead, it would appear to be more appropriate to suggest that the mother attempt to find her infant's level and move at her infant's pace.

There is thus a great deal to be studied and defined about the mother's efforts to increase interaction with her premature infant. How should it be provided? By whom? When? Stimulation or imitation? In addition, there is the question of the long-term significance of the interaction.

In the next section we discuss specific interventions that have been used to help parents learn about their infants and prepare them for the early stressful weeks at home.

INTERVENTIONS FOR FAMILIES OF SICK INFANTS

Transporting the Mother to Be Near Her Small Infant

With the development of high-risk perinatal centers, there have been an increasing number of mothers who are transported to the maternity division of hospitals with a neonatal intensive care nursery just prior to delivery or shortly after. If there is not sufficient time to arrange for her transport prior to giving birth, we strongly recommend that the mother be moved during her early postpartum period. As yet we know little about how transportation of the mother may influence her relationship with her baby.

Rooming-in for the Parent of a Premature Infant

Baragwanath Hospital in South Africa provides another model of successful premature infant caretaking. Mothers of premature infants used to live in a room adjoining the premature nursery, and each feeding time they entered the nursery to feed and handle their babies. Kahn originally instituted this arrangement.[34] It allowed the mother to continue producing milk, permitted her to take on the care of the infant more easily, reduced nursing time, and allowed mothers time for mutual discussion and support.

When Tafari and Ross[75] in Ethiopia permitted mothers to live within their crowded premature unit 24 hours a day, they were able to care for three times as many infants in their premature nursery, and at the end of one year, the number of surviving infants increased 500 per cent. Mother-infant pairs were discharged when the infants weighed an average of 1.7 kg, and most infants were breast-fed. Previous to this most of the infants had gone home bottle-feeding and usually died of intercurrent respiratory and gastrointestinal infections. When the cost of prepared milk amounts to a high proportion of the parents' weekly income, policies in support of the mother rooming-in and breast feeding in premature nurseries have a direct relation to infant mortality. This procedure is probably appropriate for 50 per cent of the world.

Torres,[76] in a special care unit in the slums of Santiago, Chile, has achieved an excellent, low perinatal mortality and morbidity rate by placing special care units for low-birth-weight infants in the maternity unit and maintaining babies under professional observation for only as long as is necessary.

Garrow,[26] at a general hospital in High Wycombe, England, opened a 20 bed special infant care unit that can accommodate eight mothers at a time and 250 admissions each year. No matter how seriously ill they may be, some 70 per cent of the babies have their mothers with them from the first few days of life. Six of the mothers' rooms open directly into the infant special care unit so that the parents can easily see or care for their infants.

Whitby et al[77] have described a unit in Cambridge, England, in which a large proportion of infants over 1.80 kg can be cared for by the mothers on the postpartum wards.

Nesting

In the United States, James and Wheeler[32] first described the successful introduction of a care-by-parent unit to provide a homelike caretaking experience. Nursing support was available for parents of premature infants prior to discharge if they needed help. Earlier, Crosse[16] in England had provided a small room for mother and infant to live together before discharge.

For several years we have been studying "nesting"—namely, permitting mothers to live in with their infants before discharge. When babies reach 1.72–2.11 kg, each mother is given a private room with her baby where she provides all caregiving. Impressive changes in the behavior of these women are observed clinically. Even though the mothers had fed and cared for their infants in the intensive care nursery on many occasions prior to living-in, eight of the first nine mothers were unable to sleep during the first 24 hours. However, in the second 24 hour period, the mothers' confidence and caretaking skills improved greatly. At this time, mothers began to discuss the proposed early discharge of their infants and, often for the first time,

began to make preparations at home for their arrival. Several insisted on taking their babies home earlier than planned.

We suggest that early discharge, preceded by a period of isolation of the mother and infant, may help to normalize mothering behavior in the intensive care nursery. Encouraging the increasing possibilities for mother-infant interaction and total caretaking may reduce the incidence of mothering disorders among mothers of small or sick premature infants.

Early Discharge

Berg and Salisbury, Davies and associates, and Dillard and Korones discharged premature infants when they weighed about 2 kg.[7, 18, 19] Dillard and Korones found no deleterious effects associated with this early discharge.[19] Experienced personnel should visit the home to organize the families and, after discharge, to help supervise infant care. Recent studies of early discharge have not revealed any gross adverse effects on the physical health of the infants, but there have been no systematic observations of maternal behavior and anxiety or later infant development.

Parent Groups

In recent years, a number of neonatal intensive care units have formed groups of parents of premature infants who meet together once a week, or more often, for 1–2 hour discussions. Documented clinical reports from these centers suggest that parents find both support and considerable relief in being able to talk with each other and to express and compare their inner feelings.

Minde and colleagues, in a controlled study of a self-help group, reported that parents who participated in the group visited their infants in the hospital significantly more often then did parents in the control group.[54] The self-help parents also touched, talked, and looked at their infants more in the en face position and rated themselves as more competent on infant care measures. The mothers in the group continued to show more involvement with their babies during feedings and were more concerned about their general development 3 months after their discharge from the nursery.

Transporting the Healthy Premature Infant to the Mother—A New Intervention

Rather than bringing mothers into the neonatal intensive care unit, with its frightening sounds, strange equipment, and unfamiliar faces, we are studying the effects of bringing the baby to the mother in her own room in the maternity division of the hospital. In this way, the mothers have an opportunity to become acquainted with their premature newborns under circumstances similar to those experienced by mothers of full-term infants.

We include healthy infants whose birth weight is between 1.5 and 2.1 kg, whose gestational age is between 32 and 36 weeks, and whose medical status during the first day permits the infant to stay with the mother (for example, no continuing respiratory distress or hypoglycemia).

The early contact consists of 0.5–1 hour of mother-infant interaction on each of the first, second, and third days after birth. A nurse brings the baby to the mother's room in a transport incubator. The baby, clothed only in a diaper, is placed in the mother's bed with a radiant heat panel overhead. The nurse is present during the visit but seated out of the mother's view above the head of her bed. During the visit the nurse observes the infant's condition, particularly color and respirations. Resuscitation equipment is carried on the transport incubator for use in the event of apnea. As part of our research protocol, the nurse also made detailed observations of the mother's behavior during each of the three 1 hour visits. Verbal interaction between the mother and nurse was limited to a standard statement and answers to the mother's questions.

We monitor the babies' temperatures frequently and have found that on a single occasion one baby had a temperature less than 36° C, but that was the only episode of hypothermia. With the use of a heat panel and transport incubator, there have been no significant problems with temperature control. In addition, we have had no episodes of apnea, bradycardia, vomiting, or other unusual behavior. We appreciate that there may be times when difficulties with premature babies occur, so the nurses continue to monitor them closely. So far it appears to be a safe procedure; however, one infant died of late streptococcal septicemia. We have found that this procedure is increasingly acceptable to the nurses caring for the premature infants.

When the infants visited their mothers, the mothers spent a striking amount of time looking at them (84–90% of the time). These results are of special interest, since in our study of premature infants several years ago there was a strong correlation between the amount of time a mother looked at her infant during a feeding at discharge from hospital and the baby's development at 42 months.

In the current study, verbal communications have markedly increased to 40 per cent of the time at the first and second visits in the experimental group. The full impact of this intervention must await the results of long-term studies presently under way.

PRACTICAL SUGGESTIONS FOR PARENTS OF SICK OR PREMATURE INFANTS

1. The obstetrician of a high-risk mother should bring in the pediatrician early and continue to involve him in decisions and plans for the management of the mother and baby.

2. If the baby must be moved to a hospital with an intensive care unit, we have found it helpful to give the mother a chance to see and touch her infant, even if he has respiratory distress and is in an oxygen hood. The house officer or the attending physician stops in the mother's room with the transport incubator and encourages her to touch her baby and look at him at close hand. A comment about the baby's strength and healthy features may be long remembered and appreciated.

We encourage the father to follow the transport team to our hospital so he can see what is happening with his baby. He uses his own transportation so that he can stay in the premature unit for 3–4 hours. This extra time allows him to get to know the nurses and physicians in the unit, to find out how the infant is being treated, and to talk with the physicians about what we expect will happen with the baby in the succeeding days. We ask him to help act as a link between us and his family by carrying information back to his wife and request that he come to our unit before he visits his wife so that he can let her know how the baby is doing. We suggest that he take a Polaroid picture, even if the infant is on a respirator, so that he can show and describe to his wife in detail how the baby is being cared for. The mothers often tell us how valuable the picture is in allowing them to maintain some contact with the infant, even while physically separated.

3. Transporting the mother and baby together to the medical center that contains the intensive care nursery is now occurring more frequently and should be encouraged for its immediate and long-term benefits.

4. The intensive care nursery should be open for parental visiting 24 hours a day and be flexible about visits from others such as grandparents, supportive relatives, and on certain occasions siblings. Provided that proper precautions are taken, infection will not be a problem.

5. Communicate with the mother about her condition and about the baby's condition. This is important before, during, and after the birth of the baby. At times, this will be brief and incomplete, but communication is essential.

Clinically, we have been impressed and disturbed by the devastating and lasting untoward effects on the mothering capacity of women who have been frightened by a physician's pessimistic outlook about the chance of survival and normal development of an infant. For example, when the newborn infant is a 3 pound premature baby who is doing well but the mother is told by a physician that there is a reasonable chance the baby may not survive, the mother will often show evidence of mourning (as if the baby were already dead) and reluctance to "become attached" to her baby. We have repeatedly observed that such mothers may refuse to visit or will show great hesitation about any physical contact. When discussing such a situation with the physician who has spoken pessimistically with the mother, we have often been told that it is important to share all worries with her so that she will be prepared in case of a bad outcome. If there is a close and firm bond between the mother and infant (which occurs after an infant has been home for several months), there is no reason for the physician to withhold concern. However, while the ties of affection are still forming, they can be easily retarded, altered, or possibly permanently damaged. Physicians should not be untruthful because parents will quickly sense their true feelings, but they must base their statements on today's situation (infant mortality rates in low-birth-weight nurseries having decreased steadily year by year), not on yesterday's high mortality figures from the period during which

they were being trained. Today the vast majority of these infants will live.

We find it best to describe what the infant looks like to us and how the infant will appear physically to the mother. We do not talk about chances or survival rates or percentages but stress that most babies survive in spite of early and often worrisome problems. We do not emphasize problems that may occur in the future. We do try to anticipate common developments (e.g., the need for bilirubin reduction lights for jaundice in small premature infants).

6. If at all possible, mother and infant should be kept near each other in the same hospital, ideally on the same floor.

7. It is useful to talk with the mother and father together whenever possible. When this is not possible, it is often wise to talk with one parent on the phone in the presence of the other. At least once a day we discuss how the child is doing with the parents; we talk with them at least twice a day if the child is critically ill. It is necessary to find out what the mother believes is going to happen or what she has read about the problem. We move at her pace during any discussion.

The physician should not relieve his anxiety by adding his worries to those of the parents. If there is a possibility, for example, that the child has Turner's syndrome, it is not necessary to share this with the parents while the infant is still acutely ill with other problems and while affectional bonds are still weak. If the physician is worried about a slightly high bilirubin level, it is not necessary to dwell on kernicterus. Once mentioned, the possibility of death or brain damage can never be completely erased.

8. Before the mother comes to the neonatal unit, the nurse or physician should describe in detail what the baby and the equipment will look like. When she makes her first visit, it is important to anticipate that she may become distressed when she looks at her infant. We always have a stool nearby so that she can sit down, and a nurse stays at her side during most of the visit, describing in detail the procedures being carried out, such as the monitoring of respiration and heart rate.

9. The nurse should go into detail in describing all the equipment surrounding the infant. She should be nearby so that she may answer questions and give support during the difficult period when the mother first sees her infant.

10. It is important to remember that feel-

ings of love for the baby are often elicited through contact. Therefore, we turn off the lights and remove the eye patches from an infant under bilirubin lights, so that the mother and infant can see each other.

11. As soon as possible, we describe to both the father and the mother the value of touching the infant in helping them to get to know him, in reducing the number of apneic episodes (if this is a problem), in increasing weight gain, and in hastening his discharge from the unit. This encourages them to visit the baby frequently for extended periods.

12. We should continue to study interventions such as rooming-in, nesting, and early discharge as well as transporting a healthy premature infant to be with his mother. It is necessary to test these various interventions in different hospital settings and to evaluate their ability to reduce the severe anxiety that many parents experience during the prolonged hospitalization and the early days following discharge.

13. In all these interventions, it is critical that nurses take mothers under their wing, especially supporting and encouraging them during these early days and weeks. The nurse's guidance in helping a mother with simple caretaking tasks can be extremely valuable in helping her to overcome anxiety. In this sense, the nurse assumes the role of the mother's own mother and contributes much more than teaching her basic techniques of caretaking.

14. To begin an intervention with parents early, it is necessary to identify high-risk parents who are having special difficulties in adapting. Generally these parents will visit rarely and for short periods,[23] appear frightened, and do not usually engage the medical staff in any questioning about the infant's problems. Sometimes the mothers are hostile or irritable and show inappropriately low levels of anxiety.

15. As we develop a further understanding of the process by which normal mothers and infants interact with each other during the first months and year of life, it appears that some recommendations for stimulation may be detrimental to normal development. Rather than suggesting stimulation, it may be important for a mother naturally and unconsciously to use imitation to learn about and get to know her own infant.

It is possible that in the future several of these interventions will be combined so that a mother may have early contact with her premature infant if he is healthy and have the baby brought to her bedside in the maternity unit on several occasions early in the course of the infant's stay in the hospital. In addition, she will be a member of a parent group, and she will be living-in with the baby for 3 or 4 days before early discharge.

CONGENITAL MALFORMATIONS

The birth of an infant with a congenital malformation presents complex challenges to the physician who will care for the affected child and his family.[33] Despite the relatively large number of infants with congenital anomalies, our understanding of how parents develop an attachment to a malformed child remains incomplete. Although previous investigators agree that the child's birth often precipitates major family stress,[33, 68] relatively few have described the process of family adaptation during the infant's first year of life.[29, 33, 68] Solnit and Stark's conceptualization of parental reactions[73] emphasized that a significant aspect of adaptation is the mourning that parents must undergo, for the loss of the normal child they had expected. Other observers[81] have noted pathologic aspects of family reactions, including the chronic sorrow that envelops the family of a defective child.[59] Less attention has been given to the more adaptive aspects of parental attachment to children with malformation.

Parental reactions to the birth of a child with a congenital malformation appear to follow a predictable course. For most parents, initial shock, disbelief, and a period of intense emotional upset (including sadness, anger, and anxiety) are followed by a period of gradual adaptation, which is marked by a lessening of intense anxiety and emotional reaction (Figure 7–7). This adaptation is characterized by an increased satisfaction with and ability to care for the baby. These stages in parental reactions are similar to those reported in other crisis situations, such as occur with terminally ill children. The shock, disbelief, and denial reported by many parents seem to be an understandable attempt to escape the traumatic news of the baby's malformation, news so at variance with their expectations that it is impossible to register except gradually.

The intense emotional turmoil described by parents who have produced a child with a congenital malformation corresponds to a

Figure 7–7. Hypothetical model of a normal sequence of parental reactions to the birth of a malformed infant. (Adapted from Drotar, D., Baskiewicz, A., Irwin, et al: Adaptation of parents to birth of an infant with a congenital malformation. Pediatrics *51*:710, 1975.)

Intensity of Reaction

I. Shock

II. Denial

III. Sadness & Anger

IV. Equilibrium

V. Reorganization

Relative Time Duration

period of crisis (defined as "upset in a state of equilibrium caused by a hazardous event which creates a threat, a loss, or a challenge for the individual").[9, 64] A crisis includes a period of impact, a rise in tension associated with stress, and finally a return to equilibrium. During such crisis periods, a person is at least temporarily unable to respond with his usual problem-solving activities to solve the crisis. Roskies[68] noted a similar "birth crisis" in her observations of mothers of children with brain defects caused by thalidomide.

With the birth of a child with a malformation, the mother must mourn the loss of her expected normal infant.[73] In addition she must become attached to her actual living, damaged child (Figure 7–8). However, the sequence of parental reactions to the birth of a baby with a malformation differs from that following the death of a child in another respect. Because of the complex issues raised by the continuation of the child's life and hence the demands of his physical care, the parents' sadness, which is initially important in their relationship with the child, diminishes in most instances once they take over the physical care. Most parents reach a point at which they are able to care adequately for their children and to cope effectively with disrupting feelings of sadness and anger. The mother's initiation of the relationship with her child is a major step in the reduction of anxiety and emotional upset associated with the trauma of the birth. As with normal children, the parents' initial experience with their infant seems to release positive feelings that aid the mother-child relationship following the stresses associated with the news of the child's anomaly and, in many instances, the separation of mother and child in the hospital. Lampe et al noted a significantly

Figure 7–8. The change in mental image that a mother with a malformed baby must make following delivery. The normal mental portrait must be changed to the real baby.

MOTHER'S MENTAL IMAGE (during pregnancy)

REAL BABY

HAPPY BEAUTIFUL ACTIVE BOY (BLUE EYED)

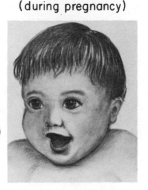

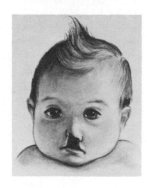

greater amount of visiting if an infant with an abnormality had been at home for a short while before surgery for a cleft lip repair.[42]

Practical Suggestions for Parents of Malformed Infants

1. We have come to believe that, if medically feasible, it is far better to leave the infant with the mother for the first 2–3 days or to discharge them. If the child is rushed to the hospital where special surgery will eventually be done, the mother will not have enough opportunity to become attached to him. Even if immediate surgery is necessary, as in the case of bowel obstruction, it is best to bring the baby to the mother first, allowing her to touch and handle him, and to point out to her how normal he is in all other respects.

2. The parents' mental picture of the anomaly may often be far more alarming than the actual problem. Any delay greatly heightens their anxiety and causes their imaginations to run wild. Therefore, we suggest that it is helpful to bring the baby to both parents when they are together as soon after delivery as possible.

3. We believe that parents should not be given tranquilizers, which tend to blunt their responses and slow their adaptation to the problem. However, a sedative at night is sometimes helpful.

4. Parents who are adapting reasonably well often ask many questions and indeed at times appear to be almost overinvolved in clinical care. We are pleased by this and are more concerned about the parents who ask few questions and who appear stunned or overwhelmed by the problem. Parents who become involved in trying to find out what the best procedures are and who ask many questions about care are sometimes annoying but often adapt best in the end.

5. Many anomalies are very frustrating to the physicians and nurses as well. There is a temptation for the physician to withdraw from the parents who ask many questions and then appear to forget and ask the same questions over and over.

6. We have found it best to move at the parents' pace. If we move too quickly, we run the risk of losing the parents along the way. It is beneficial to ask the parents how they view their infant.

7. Each parent may move through the process of shock, denial, anger, guilt, and adaptation at a different pace. If they are unable to talk with each other about the baby, their own relationship may be disrupted. Therefore, we use the process of early crisis intervention and meet several times with the parents. During these discussions, we ask the mother how she is doing, how she feels her husband is doing, and how he feels about the infant. We then reverse the questions and ask the father how he is doing and how he thinks his wife is progressing. The hope is that they will think not only about their own reactions but will begin to consider each other's as well.

STILLBIRTH OR DEATH OF A NEWBORN

In spite of the advances in obstetric and neonatal care, many mothers encounter a great disappointment with an early abortion or the perinatal loss of an infant. Until recently, it was not appreciated that a mourning reaction in both parents after the death of a newborn is universal.[38] Whether the baby lives 1 hour or 2 weeks, whether the baby is a nonviable 500 gm or weighs 4000 gm, whether or not the baby was planned, and whether or not the mother has had physical contact with her baby, clearly identifiable mourning will be present. Mothers and fathers who have lost a tiny newborn show the same mourning reactions as have been reported by Lindemann,[47] studying the survivors of the Coconut Grove fire, or by Parkes,[61] in his studies of individuals in England grieving the loss of a close adult friend or relative.

Lindemann has concluded that normal grief is a definite syndrome. It includes:
- Somatic distress with tightness of the throat, choking, shortness of breath, need for sighing, and an empty feeling in the abdomen, lack of muscular power, and an intense subjective distress described as tension or mental pain
- Preoccupation with the image of the deceased
- Feelings of guilt and preoccupation with one's negligence or minor omissions
- Feelings of hostility toward others
- Breakdown of normal patterns of conduct.

Although originally we believed that loss of an infant was similar to the loss of a close relative, we believe now, based on clinical studies and observations, that it fits far more closely with the concepts proposed by

Furman[25] and Lewis.[44, 45] Furman eloquently notes these reactions.

Internally, the mourning process consists of two roughly opposing mechanisms. One is the generally known process of detachment, by which each memory that ties the family to the person who is deceased has to become painfully revived and painfully loosened. This is the part of the process that involves anger, guilt, pain, and sadness. The second process is commonly called "identification." It is the means by which the deceased or parts of him are taken into the self and preserved as part of the self, thereby soothing the pain of loss. In many instances, a surviving marriage partner takes over hobbies and interests of the deceased spouse. These identifications soothe the way and make the pain of detachment balanced and bearable.

For the surviving parents, the death of a newborn is special in several ways. Because mourning is mourning of a separate person, the process can apply only to that small part of the relationship to the newborn that was characterized by the love of a separate person, but there has not been time to build up strong ties and memories of mutual living. It is also not possible for parents—adults functioning in the grown-up world—to take into themselves any part of a helpless newborn and make it adaptively a part of themselves; the mechanism of identification does not work. But what about the part of the newborn which was still part of the self and that cannot be mourned? To understand this part, one has to look at the different process by which individuals cope with a loss of a part of the self, for example amputation or loss of function. Insofar as the newborn remains a part of the parent's self, the death has to be dealt with as would the amputation of a limb or the loss of function of the parent's body. Detachment is the mechanism with which the victim deals with such tragedies, but it is detachment of a different kind. Acceptance that one will never ever again have that part of oneself is very different from the detachment that deals with the memories of living together with a loved one. The feelings that accompany this detachment are similar in kind and intensity: anger, guilt, fury, helplessness, and horror. In the case of the loss of a part of the self, however, they are quite unrelieved by identification.

Next, with such a tragedy there must be a readjustment in one's self image. It is, however, altogether different to have to readjust to thinking of oneself as an imperfect human being, a human being that cannot walk or cannot see. That is a pain of a different kind and the feelings that accompany it are emptiness, loss of self-esteem, and feeling low. Because the internal self never materialized in those arms and has not had a chance to be detached, it is very different from the process of mourning.

These feelings are made particularly difficult because people around the parents are not there to help. At a conscious level, people say they simply do not understand about losing part of the self, and indeed they do not. Unconsciously they understand it all too well. It fills them with fear the way an amputee fills many people with fear and anxiety and makes them shun him. This is the treatment that parents of dead newborns get. They are shunned, and they cannot rely upon the sympathy that is usually accorded the bereaved.

This syndrome may appear immediately after a death or may be delayed or apparently absent. Those who have studied mourning responses have indicated that a painful period of grieving is a normal and necessary response to the loss of a loved one and the absence of a period of grieving is not a healthy sign but rather a cause for alarm.

Without any therapeutic intervention, a tragic outcome for the mother has been shown in one third of the perinatal deaths. Cullberg[17] found that 19 of 56 mothers studied 1–2 years after the deaths of their neonates had developed severe psychiatric disease (psychosis, anxiety attacks, phobias, obsessive thoughts, and deep depressions). Because of the disastrous outcome in such a high proportion of mothers, it is necessary to examine in detail how to care for the family following a neonatal death.

In observations of parents who have lost newborns, the disturbance of communication between the parents has been a particularly troublesome problem. A husband and wife who have communicated well before the birth of a baby often have such strong feelings after an infant's death that they are unable to share their thoughts and therefore have an unsatisfactory resolution to their grieving. In America, it is expected that husbands will be strong and not show their feelings, so a physician should encourage a husband and wife to talk together about the loss and advise them not to hold back their responses—"Cry if you feel like crying." Unless told what to expect, their reactions may worry and perplex them, and this may tend further to disturb the preexisting husband and wife relationship.

At the time of the baby's death, it is important to tell the parents *together* about the usual reactions to the loss of a child and the length of time these last. It is desirable to meet a second time with both parents prior to discharge to go over the same suggestions, which may not have been heard or may have been misunderstood under the emotional shock of the baby's death. The pediatrician should plan to meet with the parents together again 3 or 4 months after the death to check on the parents' activities and on how the mourning process is proceeding. At the same time, he can discuss the autopsy findings and any further questions presented by the parents. At this visit the pediatrician should be alert for abnormal grief reactions, which, if present, may guide the physician to refer the parents for psychiatric assistance. Lindemann believes that pathologic mourning reactions represent distortion of normal grief. On the basis of his observations, he lists ten such reactions.

- Overactivity without a sense of loss
- Acquisition of symptoms belonging to the last illness of the deceased
- Psychosomatic reactions such as ulcerative colitis, asthma, or rheumatoid arthritis
- Alterations in relation to friends and relatives
- Furious hostility against specific persons
- Repression of hostility against specific persons
- Repression of hostility, leading to a wooden and formal manner resembling schizophrenic pictures
- Lasting loss of patterns of social interaction
- Activities detrimental to one's own social and economic existence
- Agitated depressions

CASE PROBLEMS

The clinical relevance of this subject can best be appreciated by the following case examples and the questions they raise. The words chosen in any discussion are dependent upon the needs and problems of individual patients at that moment. We have not given our answers as a specific formula but rather so that the reader may have an idea of how we approach parents.

Case One

Mrs. H. was happily married, had had a previous miscarriage, and had planned on having a baby for the past 3 years. She delivered a 3 lb, 2 oz male infant following a normal pregnancy. The infant cried immediately but then developed moderate respiratory distress, requiring arterial catheterization and a plastic hood placed over his head for administration of oxygen. At 36 hours of age, in an environment of 70 per cent oxygen, the pH was 7.31; $Paco_2$, 60 mm Hg; and Pao_2, 73 mm Hg.

The following questions must be answered when caring for this mother and infant.

Should the mother be permitted to go into the nursery?

The mother should be permitted to enter the nursery if she wants to. She will be relieved to see herself that the baby is well formed.

Should she be in a separate room on the maternity division?

The mother should be alone in a separate room on the maternity division if she so desires and as far away as possible from the sights and sounds of normal babies and more fortunate mothers whose healthy infants *come to them* every 4 hours.

What is the ideal method of communicating with both parents?

The best method of communicating with both parents is to have them sit down with you in a quiet, private room. You will be most effective if you can listen to the parents. Let them express their worries and feelings, then give simple, realistically optimistic explanations.

How should advice be given when discussing the situation with the parents? What should they be told about their infant and his chances for survival?

When first discussing the situation with the parents, advice should be given promptly, simply, and optimistically. As soon as possible after the birth, the mother can be told that the baby is small but well formed, that you will be doing routine tests and giving the usual treatment for a premature infant, and that you will report back to her when you have had time to complete more tests and observations.

When it is clear that the baby has respiratory distress and requires arterial catheterization, you can explain to the mother that the child has a common problem of premature infants ("breathing difficulty") owing to the complex adjustments he must make from life in utero to life outside. Furthermore, it should be stated that because it is common you know how best to treat it; that this treatment will involve putting a tube in the blood vessel through which she fed the baby while he was inside her; that you will use this tube to obtain tiny amounts of blood on frequent occasions to guide your therapy; that the baby will be transferred to a nursery for small babies; that, prior to his transfer, her husband can see the baby, and the baby will be brought to her in a special transport incubator for her to see; that babies sometimes get worse before they improve, but the outlook is good for complete recovery after several days; that you will keep her and her husband posted on the baby's progress and will tell them if problems arise; that you would like them to call at other times if they have questions; and that you would like her to come to the nursery to visit the baby.

At 36 hours, you have a firmer basis for an optimistic report, which should be kept simple but should include an explanation of the hood, apnea monitor, and other visible aspects of therapy. You might say something like "I'm pleased with your son's progress. He has responded well to our treatment, and his outlook is excellent. If you haven't been over to see him yet, I'd like to encourage you to do this today, because you will be pleased with his progress."

Can the nurses help the mother adapt to the premature infant?

The nurses can aid the mother in adapting to the premature infant by standing with her and explaining the equipment being used for him; by welcoming the mother by name and with personalized comments at each visit and encouraging her to come back soon; by carefully considering the mother's concerns and feelings; by explaining to her that the baby will benefit from her visits; and by showing her how she can gradually assume more of the baby's care and do the mothering better than the nurses. An example of the nurses' encouragement to mothers to continue visits later in the patient's course is the type of note our nurses put on the baby's crib. "My mother is coming to feed me at 1:30. Boy! Will I be happy to see her! —David."

Should the mother go home before the respiratory distress syndrome has subsided?

If the mother is confident that the infant will live, she can go home before the respiratory distress has subsided. Staying in a maternity unit and visiting her baby only one or two times a day is not tolerated very long by many mothers unless they can actively care for their babies or provide breast milk. It is particularly difficult for a woman if she has young children at home. Most mothers can return daily from home to visit the baby.

If she lives far away, is unlikely to return for many days, and is greatly concerned the baby will die, ideally the mother should not go home before the respiratory distress syndrome has subsided. It is helpful to reach a point at which both you and the mother are confident about the baby's survival.

If the infant lives, what problems will the mother face and how can she be helped?

When the infant survives, the mother may have withdrawn some of her attachment to the baby through anticipatory grief, in spite of all the steps having been taken that have been recommended. Under the best of circumstances, she will have had much less contact with her baby than a normal mother. The continuation of support to the mother—so that she will visit, touch, and provide increasing care for the baby (holding, feeding, bathing, and diapering)—is important during the hospital period. In the future the pediatrician should be alert to evidence that the baby is being handled differently from other children (delay in weaning, overprotection, excessive permissiveness, or excessively regimented management). A discussion at this time with the mother about her early experiences and her feelings and worries about the baby may be advisable. When specific questions have been answered, if appropriate, it may be best to reassure the mother that the baby's early problems are over and will not recur, that the baby was small in the beginning but is now normal in size and development, and that for his ultimate well-being he should be handled as normally as possible.

Case Two

Mrs. J., a 22 year old primiparous mother, delivered a full-term infant after a 12 hour uneventful labor. The infant was found to have a cleft lip and palate. The following questions should be answered concerning the care of this infant and mother.

Should the father be told about this before the mother has returned to her room?

Every effort should be made to tell the mother and father together about this problem; however, this is such an obvious defect that the father will notice it. If this is the case, the doctor should indicate that there is a problem, but that he wants to check the baby over thoroughly and he will then tell both parents about the problem and what will be done about it. It is popularly believed that the father is in much better condition to learn about difficulties right after delivery than his wife, but often a woman is better able to accept news about an illness or abnormality in her baby—in an emotional sense—than her husband. Any plan to give one bit of news or a different shading about the prognosis to one parent and not the other interferes with the communication between husband and wife, and it is extremely important to support and encourage this communication. The infant should be brought to the parents as soon as the mother and the infant are in satisfactory condition and after the caring physician (obstetrician or pediatrician) has the details of the baby's problem clearly in mind and is aware of the baby's health status. It is important for the baby to be brought to the mother's bed. It is worthwhile to repeat and emphasize the general good health and well-being of the baby.

Who should tell the mother: the obstetrician, the pediatrician, the nurse, or the father?

The obstetrician, whom the mother has known for many months, is usually the best person to tell the mother. He needs information from a pediatrician about the nature of the problem and the general health of the baby. Equally satisfactorily, the obstetrician and pediatrician may go together to tell the parents about the problem. If the obstetrician can speak briefly and calmly to the mother and place his mantle of acceptability upon the pediatrician's shoulders, then the pediatrician can continue with a brief explanation about the problem. Under most circumstances, neither the nurse nor the father will be in a position to provide enough reassurance to the mother to make this first encounter progress optimally.

How should the problem be presented to the parents?

It is desirable whenever possible to emphasize to the parents the normal healthy features of the baby. For example, "Mr. and Mrs. Jones, you have a strong 8 pound baby boy who is kicking, screaming, and carrying out all the normal functions of a healthy baby. There is one problem present that fortunately we will be able to correct, so it will not be a continuing problem for the baby. As far as I can tell, the baby is completely well otherwise. I would like to show the baby and this problem to you."

Should the baby be present?

Yes. As ugly as a cleft lip and palate may appear to a mother, exposure to the reality of the problem is important and is usually less disturbing than the mother's fantasies.

Case Three

The first infant of a 29 year old mother weighed 2 lbs, 8 oz at birth. The baby is now 4 days of age and is taking 6 ml of formula every 2 hours.

What are the normal processes that a mother goes through when she delivers an infant of this size, and how should the physician and nursing staff meet these requirements during the first 4 days?

The premature delivery often occurs before a mother is thoroughly ready to accept the idea that she is going to have an infant. Such a mother is faced, like the mother with a malformed infant, with a baby who is thin, scrawny, and very different from the ideal, full-sized baby she has been picturing in her mind. She may have to grieve the loss of this anticipated ideal baby as she adjusts to the reality of this premature baby with all of his problems.

In most hospitals, the mother has only a fleeting glimpse of the baby, who is then whisked away from her. If she has not seen the baby or has only viewed him briefly through a window, she may be picturing an infant who is fragile and much scrawnier than is actually the case. All of the equipment and activities of a premature nursery are new and may be frightening to a mother. The tubes, the flashing lights, the beepers, and other instruments used in a premature nursery are disturbing. If the functions of these items are explained to the mother, her concern will decrease. For example, "The two wires on the baby's chest and the beeping instrument tell us if the baby slows down in his respirations so we can rub his skin to remind him to keep breathing. This is frequently necessary during the first few days with a tiny infant."

There are some additional problems with a premature infant. Frequently, a mother is not able to see her infant the first day or two, and other members of her family may see and even touch and hold the infant. It is often quite upsetting to a new mother to think that others are getting an opportunity to become acquainted with and enjoy the baby while she, who produced the infant, has been kept away. It may be helpful for the mother and infant to be together as much as possible in the early days. The mother's guilt and anxiety, and the fear that touching the infant will harm him, sometimes lead her to turn down an offer to visit the infant. No mother should be forced to visit her infant against her wishes, but it is important for the hospital personnel to reassure her and encourage her visits. Move at the mother's pace.

What should the mother be told when she asks, "How is the baby doing?"

It is a common reflex in physicians and nurses to prepare patients for a possible poor outcome and to think in a problem-oriented manner. Because of the great importance of providing encouragement to the mother so that mother-infant affectional ties develop as easily as possible, it is desirable to approach this question in an optimistic but realistic manner. It is also wise to start out by asking the mother how *she* thinks the baby is doing, and then you know where to begin. For example, "We are using lights to help with the baby's yellowness, and we still have the infant on a respiratory monitor, which lets us keep track of the baby's breathing, but the baby is doing beautifully. We are confident that he will continue to improve and grow and gain. The baby is taking feedings nicely."

What arrangements should be made to keep the mother informed about the baby?

A physician should communicate with the mother about the baby's progress at least once a day. When the condition is more hazardous, more frequent contacts are indicated, such as morning and evening. The mother should have access to information about the baby by calling the nursery and talking to the nurses.

Should the nurses and nonprimary physicians talk with the parents?

Of course the nurses and nonprimary physicians should answer questions when asked by the parents. It is highly desirable for all who are concerned with the care of the baby to understand the general trend of the information that is being supplied to the parents. This can best be carried out if one individual takes this responsibility. The nonprimary physician and nurses can provide the parents with additional items without getting into questions of prognosis. These can usually be tactfully referred to the responsible physician.

What should the physician who is covering for the primary physician say?

Whenever possible, the covering physician should find out what the primary physician has been saying to the family and attempt to follow along in the same vein. There is no harm at all in his emphasizing the features that indicate improvement and a favorable outcome. Whenever possible, he should avoid statements that indicate differences in approach to the prognosis or management of the patient. All who are speaking to the parents should be certain to communicate before and after conversations with the parents so that a consistent picture is presented to them. Ideally, the Weed system of problem-oriented records and problem lists should be used to record on the chart what has been discussed with the parents, so that anyone covering for another physician can immediately know just where the family is in their understanding.

When should the mother take this baby home if the baby is eating well and gaining well at 4 lbs. 4 oz? Should there be a fixed weight at which the infant should be discharged? What factors determine the decision about the timing of discharge?

In the past, we have looked at the infant's weight, physical characteristics, and the presence of a clean bed at home. We must also look at the mother's ability to care for the infant in the hospital and her readiness and willingness to take the infant home. Her visiting pattern in the hospital and the preparations made at home have been helpful in making this decision. Preliminary observations of mothers living in with their 4 pound premature infants for 3 days suggest that this may be an ideal procedure to prepare mothers for routine caretaking.

If the infant has good heat control without an incubator, nipples easily, and is gaining weight, if the mother has experience in caretaking, and if the home is free of infection, early discharge may be beneficial.

Case Four

A 2½ lb infant of a 23 year old primiparous mother who has been married for 3 years died suddenly on the second day of life. The infant was planned. The mother did not handle the infant.

What are the processes this mother and father will go through?

The parents in this situation will go through the same intense mourning reactions that have been described in the text. If the parents can cry together, they themselves can best help each other. The use of drugs, except for a night's sleep, is therefore not indicated. Even though the mother did not handle the infant, she and her husband will be expected to show strong mourning responses, which will be intense for 2 or 3 weeks and under optimal circumstances will be markedly decreased by 6 months. In America, where the expression of emotion is not encouraged, the husband will often force himself to hold back his emotions to provide "strong support" for his wife. This is actually harmful, because a free and easy communication between the parents about their feelings is highly desirable for the resolution of mourning. On the basis of the studies that have been carried out, the stronger the mourning reaction in the early period, the more favorable the outcome.

How can the physician help them?

It is important for the physician to explain the details of the baby's death to both parents together within a few hours of the death of the baby. At that time, he should explain the type of mourning reaction they will go through. Then as a minimum, the physician should again meet with the parents 3–4 days later to find out how they are managing, to go over the details once more, and to indicate his availability for any questions or problems. At the postpartum checkup, the obstetrician should take time to ask how the parents are managing and should evaluate the normality of their mourning and their communications. If there are other children in the family, the pediatrician should inquire about their responses. Three or four months after the death of the baby, the physician should set aside a period of time to meet with both parents to review their present status, what has occurred since the death, their understanding of the death, and the normality of their reactions. If the mourning response is pathologic, he may then refer the parents for additional assistance.[39]

This short list of guidelines may incorrectly convey the impression of a mechanical quality to these discussions, which is not at all the authors' intent. Parents appreciate evidence of human concern and reactions in a physician at times such as these, so we would encourage physicians to show the sadness they feel and to allow the parents to express their pent-up feelings by making a statement such as "I know how sad and upset you both must feel."

UNKNOWNS

Observations of human mothers after periods of early separation from their infants force a thorough review and evaluation of our present perinatal care practices. The following unknowns remain to be answered.

- Is there a sensitive period in the human mother?
- What are the needs of most mothers with normal full-term infants in the first hours, days, and weeks after delivery?
- Are the diseases of failure to thrive, the battered child syndrome, and the vulnerable child syndrome in part related to hospital care practices?
- How should the minor problems, as well as the major ones, that the infant is born with or develops be handled with mothers of different backgrounds, cultures, and requirements?

Since in most instances the hospital now determines the events surrounding birth and death, these two most important events in the life of an individual have been stripped of the long-established traditions and support systems established over centuries to help families through these transitions.

Because the newborn baby is utterly dependent upon his parents for his survival and optimal development, it is essential to understand the process of attachment. Although we are only beginning to understand this complex phenomenon, those responsible for the care of mothers and infants would be wise to reevaluate the hospital procedures that interfere with early, sustained mother-infant contact and to consider measures that promote parents' experiences with their infant.

REFERENCES

1. Ambuel, J., and Harris, B.: Failure to thrive: a study of failure to grow in height or weight. Ohio Med J 59:997, 1963.
2. Anisfeld, E., and Lipper, E.: Early contact, social support, and mother-infant bonding. Pediatrics 72:79, 1983.
3. Ballard, R., Leonard, C. H., Irvin, N., et al: An alternative birth center in a hospital setting. In Klaus, M., and Kennell, J. (eds.): Parent-Infant Bonding. St. Louis, C. V. Mosby, 1982.
4. Barnett, C., Leiderman, P., Grobstein, R., et al: Neonatal separation: the maternal side of interactional deprivation. Pediatrics 45:197, 1970.
5. Benedek, T.: Studies in Psychosomatic Medicine: The Psycho-Sexual Function in Women. New York, Ronald Press Co., 1952.
6. Benfield, D. G., Leib, S. A., and Reutor, J.: Grief response of parents following referral of the critically ill newborn. N Engl J Med 294:975, 1976.
7. Berg, R. B., and Salisbury, A.: Discharging infants of low birth weight: reconsiderations of current practice. Am J Dis Child 122:414, 1971.
8. Bibring, G.: Some considerations of the psychological processes in pregnancy. Psychoanal Study Child 14:113, 1959.
9. Bloom, B.: Definitional concepts of the crisis concept. J Consult Psychol 27:42, 1963.
10. Bowlby, J.: Nature of a child's tie to his mother. Int J Psychoanal 39:350, 1958.
11. Brazelton, T., Koslowski, B., and Main, M.: The origins of reciprocity—the early infant interaction. In Lewis, M., and Rosenblum, L. (eds.): The Effect of the Infant on its Caregiver. Vol. I. New York, John Wiley and Sons, 1974.
12. Budin, P.: The Nursling. London, Caxton Publishing Co., 1907.
13. Caplan, G.: Emotional Implications of Pregnancy and Influences on Family Relationship in the Healthy Child. Cambridge, Harvard University Press, 1960.
14. Cohen, R.: Some maladaptive syndromes of pregnancy and the puerperium. Obstet Gynecol 27:562, 1966.
15. Condon, W., and Sander, L.: Neonate movement is synchronized with adult speech: Interactional participation and language acquisition. Science 183:99, 1974.
16. Crosse, V. M.: The Premature Baby. 4th ed. Boston, Little, Brown and Co., 1957.
17. Cullberg, J.: Mental reactions of women to perinatal death. In Morris, N. (ed.): Psychosomatic Medicine in Obstetrics and Gynecology. New York, S. Karger, 1972.
18. Davies, D. P., Herberts, S., Haxby, V., et al: When should pre-term babies be sent home from neonatal units? Lancet 1:914, 1979.
19. Dillard, R. G., and Korones, S. B.: Lower discharge weight and shortened nursery stay for low birth-weight infants. N Engl J Med 288:131, 1973.
20. Elmer, E., and Gregg, D.: Developmental characteristics of abused children. Pediatrics 40:596, 1967.
21. Emde, R., Swedberg, J., and Suzuki, B.: Human wakefulness and biological rhythms after birth. Arch Gen Psychiatry 32:780, 1975.
22. Evans, S., Reinhart, J., and Succop, R.: A study of 45 children and their families. J Am Acad Child Psychiatry 11:440, 1972.
23. Fanaroff, A., Kennell, J., and Klaus, M.: Follow-up of low-birth-weight infants—the predictive value of maternal visiting patterns. Pediatrics 49:287, 1972.
24. Field, T. M.: Effects of early separation, interactive deficits and experimental manipulations on infant-mother face-to-face interaction. Child Dev 48:763, 1977.

25. Furman, E. P.: The death of a newborn: care of the parents. Birth Fam J 5:214, 1978.
26. Garrow, D. H.: Personal communication, 197º
27. Green, M., and Solnit, A.: Reactions to the threatened loss of a child: a vulnerable child syndrome. Pediatrics 34:58, 1964.
28. Hales, D., Lozoff, B., Sosa, R., et al: Defining the limits of the maternal sensitive period. Dev Med Child Neurol 19:454, 1977.
29. Hare, E., Lawrence, K., Paynes, H., et al: Spina bifida cystica and family stress. Br Med J 2:757, 1966.
30. Harper, R. G., Sia, C., Sokal, M.: Observations on unrestricted parental contact with infants in the neonatal intensive care unit. J Pediatr 89:441, 1976.
31. Helfer, R., and Kempe, C. (eds.): The Battered Child. Chicago, University of Chicago Press, 1968.
32. James, V. L., Jr., and Wheeler, W. E.: The care-by-parent unit. Pediatrics 43:488, 1969.
33. Johns, N.: Family reactions to the birth of a child with a congenital abnormality. Med J Austral 7:277, 1971.
34. Kahn, E., Wayburne, S., and Fouche, M.: The Baragwanath premature baby unit—an analysis of the case records of 1,000 consecutive admissions. S Afr Med J 28:453, 1954.
35. Kaplan, D., and Mason, E.: Maternal reactions to premature birth viewed as an acute emotional disorder. Am J Orthopsychiatry 30:539, 1960.
36. Kennell, J., and Rolnik, A.: Discussing problems in newborn babies with their parents. Pediatrics 26:832, 1960.
37. Kennell, J. H., Chesler, D., Wolfe, H., et al: Nesting in the human mother after infant separation. Pediatr Res 7:269, 1973.
38. Kennell, J., Slyter, H., and Klaus, M.: The mourning response of parents to the death of a newborn. N Engl J Med 283:344, 1970.
39. Klaus, M., and Kennell, J.: Parent-Infant Bonding. St. Louis, C. V. Mosby Co., 1982.
40. Klaus, M., Jerauld, R., Kreger, N., et al: Maternal attachment: importance of the first post-partum days. N Engl J Med 286:460, 1972.
41. Klein, M., and Stern, L.: Low birth weight and the battered child syndrome. Am J Dis Child 122:15, 1971.
42. Lampe, J., Trause, M., and Kennell, J.: Parental visiting of sick infants: the effects of living at home prior to hospitalization. Pediatrics 59:294, 1977.
43. Lang, R.: Birth Book. Ben Lomond, Genesis Press, 1972.
44. Lewis, E.: Inhibition of mourning by pregnancy: psychopathology and management. Br Med J 2:27, 1979.
45. Lewis, E.: Mourning by the family after a stillbirth or neonatal death. Arch Dis Child 54:303, 1979.
46. Lind, J., Vuorenkoski, V., and Wasz-Hoeckert, O.: The effect of cry stimulus on the temperature of the lactating breast primipara: a thermographic study. In Morris, N. (ed.): Psychosomatic Medicine in Obstetrics and Gynecology. Basel, S. Karger, 1973.
47. Lindemann, E.: Symptomatology and management of acute grief. Am J Psychiatry 101:141, 1944.
48. Lozoff, B., Brittenham, G., Trause, M., et al: The mother-newborn relationship: limits of adaptability. J Pediatr 91:1, 1977.
49. Lynch, M. A.: Ill health and child abuse. Lancet 2:317, 1975.
50. MacFarlane, J.: Olfaction in the development of social preferences in the human neonate. In: The Parent-Infant Relationship. Ciba Foundation. Amsterdam, Elsevier, 1975.
51. MacFarlane, J. A., Smith, D. M., and Garrow, D. H.: The relationship between mother and neonate. In Kitzinger, S., and Davis, J. A. (eds.): The Place of Birth. New York, Oxford University Press, 1978.
52. Mason, E. A.: A method of predicting crisis outcome for mothers of premature babies. Public Health Rep 78:1031, 1963.
53. Miller, F.: Home nursing of premature babies in Newcastle-on-Tyne. Lancet 2:703, 1948.
54. Minde, K., Shosenberg, B., Marton, P., et al: Self-help groups in a premature nursery—a controlled evaluation. J Pediatr 96:933, 1980.
55. Minde, K., Trehub, S., Corter, C., et al: Mother-child relationships in the premature nursery: an observational study. Pediatrics 61:373, 1978.
56. Newman, L. F.: Parents' perceptions of their low birth weight infants. Paediatrician 9:182, 1980.
57. Newton, N., and Newton, M.: Mothers' reactions to their newborn babies. JAMA 181:206, 1962.
58. O'Connor, S., Vietze, P. M., Sherrod, K. B., et al: Reduced incidence of parenting inadequacy following rooming-in. Pediatrics 66:176, 1980.
59. Olshansky, S.: Chronic sorrow: a response to having a mentally defective child. Social Casework 43:190, 1962.
60. Parke, R.: Perspectives on father-infant interaction. In Osofsky, J. D. (ed.): The Handbook of Infant Development. New York, John Wiley and Sons, 1979.
61. Parkes, C.: Bereavement and mental illness. Part I. A clinical study of the grief of bereaved psychiatric patients. Br Med J Psychol 38:1, 1965.
62. Pawlby, S. J.: Imitative interaction. In Schaffer, H. R. (ed.): Studies in Mother-Infant Interaction. New York, Academic Press, 1977.
63. Raphael, D.: The Tender Gift: Breastfeeding. Englewood, NJ, Prentice-Hall, Inc., 1973.
64. Rappoport, L.: The state of crisis: some theoretical considerations. In Parad, H. (ed.): Crisis Intervention. New York, Family Service Association, 1965.
65. Robson, K.: The role of eye-to-eye contact in maternal-infant attachment. J Child Psychol Psychiatry 8:13, 1967.
66. Robson, K., and Kumar, R.: Delayed onset of maternal affection after childbirth. Br J Psychiatry 136:347, 1980.
67. Rodholm, M.: Father-infant interaction at the first contact after delivery. Early Hum Dev 3:21, 1979.
68. Roskies, E.: Abnormality and Normality: The Mothering of Thalidomide Children. New York, Cornell University Press, 1972.
69. Shaheen, E., Alexander, D., Truskowsky, M., et al: Failure to thrive—a retrospective profile. Clin Pediatr 7:225, 1968.
70. Siegel, E., Bauman, K. E., Schaefer, E. S., et al: Hospital and home support during infancy: Impact on maternal attachment, child abuse and neglect, and health care utilization. Pediatrics 66:183, 1980.
71. Silverman, W. A.: Incubator-baby sideshows. Pediatrics 64:127, 1979.
72. Skinner, A., and Castle, R.: Seventy-eight battered children: a retrospective study. Report by the National Society for the Prevention of Cruelty to Children, London, 1969.

73. Solnit, A., and Stark, M.: Mourning and the birth of a defective child. Psychoanal Study Child *16*:523, 1961.

74. Sosa, R., Kennell, J., Klaus, M., et al: The effect of a supportive companion on perinatal problems, length of labor, and mother-infant interaction. N Engl J Med *303*:597, 1980.

75. Tafari, N., and Ross, S. M.: On the need for organized perinatal care. Ethiop Med J *11*:93, 1973.

76. Torres, J.: Personal communication, 1978.

77. Whitby, C., DeCates, C. R., and Robertson, N. R. C.: Infants weighing 1.8–2.5 kg; should they be cared for in neonatal units or postnatal wards? Lancet *1*:322, 1982.

78. Winnicott, D. W.: Primary maternal preoccupation. *In: Collected Papers: Through Pediatrics to Psychoanalysis.* New York, Basic Books, Inc., 1958.

79. Winnicott, D. W.: The mirror role of mother and family in child development. *In: Playing and Reality.* London, Tavistock Publications, 1971.

80. Wolff, P.: Observations on newborn infants. Psychosom Med *21*:110, 1959.

81. Zuk, G.: Religious factors and the role of guilt in parental acceptance of the retarded child. Am J Ment Defic *64*:145, 1959.

8

Respiratory Problems

RICHARD J. MARTIN
MARSHALL H. KLAUS
AVROY A. FANAROFF

I observed that a few days after their admission infants frequently had attacks of cyanosis. They suddenly became blue.... If assistance was not immediately rendered, they died. If, however, en--ergetic measures were promptly taken, they usually revived, although many succumbed to subsequent attacks.

PIERRE BUDIN
THE NURSLING

Considering the complexity of the pulmonary and hemodynamic changes occurring after delivery, it is surprising that the vast majority of infants make the transition from intrauterine to extrauterine life so smoothly and uneventfully. Nonetheless, the staff working in the intensive care nursery will spend a lion's share of their time in caring for neonates with respiratory problems, diseases that are responsible for most of the morbidity and mortality in this period.

NORMAL PHYSIOLOGY

Before birth, the lung is a fluid-filled organ receiving 10–15 per cent of the total cardiac output. Within the first minutes of life, a large portion of the fluid is absorbed, the lung fills with air, and the blood flow through the lung increases 8- to 10-fold. This considerable increase is secondary to a decrease in pulmonary arterial tone and other physiologic changes that convert the circulation from a parallel arrangement to a series circuit.

The high vascular resistance in the fetal lung is due to pulmonary arterial vasoconstriction. The pulmonary arterial vasodilation observed following delivery results in part from the increased oxygen tension, from the decrease in CO_2 tension and change in pH, and only partially from the mechanical effect of the inflation.[32] Certain chemical mediators such as prostaglandin I_2 and bradykinin may be involved.

At the same time, an adequate functional residual capacity (FRC = volume of air in the lungs at end-expiration) is quickly attained. At 10 minutes, the FRC is the same as that found at 5 days. It is now clear that high opening pressures are not a prerequisite to lung expansion during the first breaths.[83] At 1 hour, the distribution of air with each breath in the newborn is already similar to that observed in the young adult. Specific lung compliance (lung distensibility/lung volume expressed in ml of air/cm of H_2O pressure change/ml of lung volume) and vital capacity increase briskly in the first hours of life, reaching values proportional to the adult at 8–12 hours.

Chemical control of respiration is in general similar in the newborn infant and the adult. As the inspired CO_2 is increased, the per cent increase in ventilation is similar in the infant and adult. The ventilation of the newborn is also transiently increased when breathing mixtures contain less than 21 per

171

cent oxygen; this response as well as other evidence[32] suggests that the aortic and carotid body chemoreceptors are active at birth. The infant, however, differs from the adult in that if hypoxia is severe or prolonged, respiration is depressed during the first 3 weeks of life. Marked hypoxia appears to depress the medullary respiratory center, negating the hypoxic stimulation of the aortic and carotid body chemoreceptors.

The effects of pulmonary stretch receptor activity on the timing of respiration are much more readily elicited in the newborn than in the adult via the Hering-Breuer reflex. A sustained increase in FRC causes a marked slowing of respiratory rate.[77] In the first day or two of life, the typical response to a brisk inflation of the lung with a pressure of 10–15 cm of water is a deep gasp (Head paradoxic gasp reflex—a pressure change from 20 to 40 cm H_2O) followed by a very prolonged apnea (Hering-Breuer inflation reflex). By the third and fourth days, greater pressure is required to produce the gasp and apnea, and a large number of infants no longer gasp. The deep gasp observed in the first day of life with low inflation pressures may explain the clinical observation that very low pressures (10–15 cm H_2O) are often effective in resuscitating the apneic newborn at birth by stimulating a gasp reflex.

The partial pressure of carbon dioxide (PCO_2) measures the ability of the lung to remove CO_2. The HCO_3^- concentration is controlled by the kidney. When the pH and HCO_3^- are determined, the arterial PCO_2 can be calculated by using the Henderson-Hasselbalch equation:

$$pH = 6.1 + \log \frac{HCO_3^-}{PCO_2 \times sol}$$

If only the pH is measured, the cause of the acidosis or alkalosis cannot be determined. With metabolic acidosis, HCO_3^- is decreased. To compensate for this, the infant hyperventilates, lowering arterial PCO_2. With pulmonary disease, apnea, or hypoventilation, the arterial PCO_2 increases. The kidney attempts compensation by retaining HCO_3^- and excreting hydrogen ions. Only by measuring the PCO_2 and HCO_3^- as well as the pH can the cause of an abnormality in acid-base balance be determined. The normal newborn quickly regulates his pH to near adult values. The low arterial PCO_2 of the healthy newborn infant during the first day of life is similar to the maternal values in the last months of pregnancy.

Physiologic Basis

Oxygen is carried in the blood in chemical combination with hemoglobin and also in physical solution. The oxygen taken up by both processes is dependent on the partial pressure of oxygen (PO_2).

At ambient pressures, the amount of dissolved oxygen is only a small fraction of the total quantity carried in whole blood (0.3 ml O_2/dl plasma/100 mm Hg at 37° C). Most of the oxygen in whole blood is bound to hemoglobin (1 gm of hemoglobin combines with 1.34 ml of oxygen at 37° C). The quantity of oxygen bound to hemoglobin is dependent upon the partial pressure and is described by the oxygen dissociation curve (Figure 8–1). The blood is almost completely saturated* at an arterial oxygen tension (PaO_2) of 90–100 mm Hg.

As an example, if the arterial PO_2 is 50 mm Hg, saturation is 90 per cent, and hemoglobin is 10 gm/dl, then 9.0 gm Hb is bound to oxygen. Thus the oxygen content of this 100 ml sample is 12.06 ml O_2 bound to Hb (1.34 × 9) + 0.15 ml O_2 (0.3 × 50/100) dissolved in plasma for a total of 12.21 ml O_2. Naturally, if the hemoglobin is doubled, then for the same saturation the O_2 transported by hemoglobin will also be doubled (1.34 × 18 = 24.12 ml O_2) without changing the amount dissolved. The dissociation curve of fetal blood is shifted to the left and, at any PaO_2 below 100 mm Hg, fetal hemoglobin binds to more oxygen. The shift is the result of the lower affinity of fetal Hb for diphosphoglycerate (DPG), although pH, PCO_2, and temperature also influence the position of the dissociation curve. There is a normal postnatal rise in DPG levels in healthy preterm infants that may be a compensatory response to the high oxygen affinity of fetal blood at birth; it contrasts with the marked fall in DPG that occurs in preterm infants with

---

*The arterial oxygen saturation is the actual oxygen bound to hemoglobin divided by the capacity of hemoglobin for binding oxygen.

$$\% \text{ sat.} = \frac{\text{ml } O_2 \text{ combined with Hb}}{\text{Hb (gm)} \times 1.34} \times 100$$

1.0 gm of hemoglobin can maximally bind to 1.34 ml of O_2.

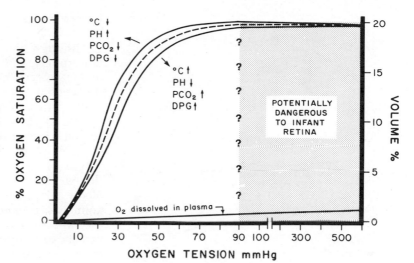

Figure 8–1. Factors that shift the oxygen dissociation curve of hemoglobin. (Fetal hemoglobin is shifted to the left as compared with that of the adult.)

respiratory distress, probably secondary to the accompanying acidosis.[117] Thus oxygen delivery to the tissues is determined by a combination of cardiac output, total hemoglobin concentration, arterial PO_2, and hemoglobin oxygen affinity.

Figure 8–2 illustrates that at an alveolar PO_2 of 100, the three different blood samples have very similar saturations and O_2 contents. However, if we assume a tissue PO_2 of 30, each sample will unload different amounts of oxygen/dl of plasma (A—3.0 ml, B—5.0 ml, C—7.0 ml) to the tissues. The clinical significance of this is that the sick neonates' blood (fetal) will take up more oxygen at an alveolar PO_2 of 40, but the tissue PO_2 will drop to a very low level to unload adequate amounts of oxygen.[36]

The shift makes clinical recognition of hypoxia (insufficient amount of oxygen molecules in the tissues to cover the normal aerobic metabolism) more difficult, since cyanosis will be observed at a lower oxygen tension. Cyanosis is first observed by physicians at saturations from 75–85 per cent, which are oxygen tensions of 32–42 mm Hg on the fetal dissociation curve. Cyanosis in the adult is observed at higher tensions. The flattening of the upper portion of the S-shaped dissociation curve makes it almost impossible to monitor oxygen tensions above 60–80 mm Hg by following arterial oxygen saturation.

The partial pressure of oxygen in arterial blood is not only dependent on the ability of the lung to transfer oxygen but also is modified by the shunting of venous blood into the systemic circulation through the heart or lungs. Breathing 100 per cent oxygen for a

prolonged time may partially correct desaturation secondary to alveolar hypoventilation, diffusion abnormalities, or ventilation/perfusion inequality. Measurements of PaO_2 while breathing 100 per cent oxygen are therefore useful diagnostically in determining whether arterial desaturation is caused by an anatomic right-to-left shunt, in which case oxygenation will fail to improve.

Immediately after birth, PaO_2 rises rapidly to between 60 and 90 mm Hg. During the first days of life, 20 per cent of the cardiac output is normally shunted from right to left. It is not known whether this shunt is in the heart or lungs. When the normal adult breathes 100 per cent oxygen, PaO_2 rises to 600 mm Hg as compared with around 300 mm Hg in healthy neonates owing to the substantial shunting in infants.

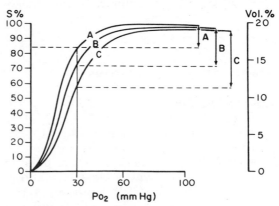

Figure 8–2. The effect of three different oxygen dissociation curves of hemoglobin on the oxygen delivered at a tissue PO_2 of 30 mm Hg.[36]

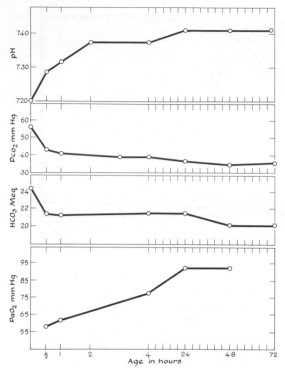

Figure 8–3. The arterial pCO_3, HCO_3, pH, and PO_2 during the first hours and days of life.[68]

At the end of the first hour of life, perfusion of the lung is distributed in proportion to the distribution of ventilation.[6] The effects of this rapid adaptation on the blood gases are illustrated in Figure 8–3, which shows the mean arterial pH, PaO_2, $PaCO_2$, and bicarbonate in normal infants during the early hours and days of life. The speed with which pulmonary ventilation and perfusion are uniformly distributed is an indication of the remarkable adaptive capacities of the newborn infant for the maintenance of homeostasis.

PRACTICAL CONSIDERATIONS

Oxygen Therapy

Oxygen supplementation is critical for the survival of many infants with respiratory problems. Previous restricted use resulted in an increase not only in mortality but also in neurologic handicaps.[30, 60] However, a recognition of the toxic effects of excessive or prolonged oxygen therapy is imperative when treating sick newborn infants.

OXYGEN TOXICITY

Although high concentration of oxygen at atmospheric pressures can affect the stability of the red cell membrane and possibly alter the neonatal brain, serious toxicity poses a major clinical problem in the lung and retina.

THE RETINA. The effect of oxygen on the retinal vessels is dependent upon (1) the stage of development of the retinal vessels, (2) the length of the exposure to oxygen, and (3) the partial pressure of oxygen in the arterial blood. (If just the eyes of susceptible young animals are exposed to oxygen by cupping the eye, no toxic effects are observed.) The vasoconstricting effects of very short periods of oxygen are reversible. If the vasoconstriction (first stage) lasts longer than several hours, it may not be reversible. Pronounced vasoconstriction is not observed when the retina is fully vascularized. In the full-term human neonate, the temporal portion of the retina is still sensitive at birth, but no lasting damage has been observed.

The second stage is the proliferative phase, in which new vessels grow from the capillaries and sprout through the retina into the vitreous. These vessels are usually permeable, and hemorrhages and edema sometimes follow. Organization of the hemorrhages that enter the vitreous can produce traction on the retina and may result in detachment and blindness.

In the human infant, retinal damage is observed when the gestational age is less than 36 weeks. A collaborative study[66] revealed changes in only a small number of infants if the ambient oxygen was below 40 per cent and administered for a short period of time. Significantly, prolonged exposure (10 days) to 30 per cent oxygen resulted in retrolental fibroplasia (RLF) in 10 per cent of small preterm infants. To prevent retinal damage, the arterial oxygen tension must be kept below the level that stimulates vasoconstriction. The exact concentration that is toxic is unknown. Other factors such as the volume of replacement blood transfusions have been associated with an increased risk of RLF.[120] Myopia frequently develops in infants with RLF. For the sick infant, the general practice is to maintain the PaO_2 between 50 and 80 mm Hg. For the healthy, small premature, 40–60 mm Hg may well be adequate.

We do not have any evidence that this recommendation is justified. In fact, it is possible that marginal hypoxemia may be a factor in the development of retinopathy of prematurity (ROP). The terms RLF and ROP are used interchangeably. While oxygen is certainly a critical factor for the disease, we have to admit that the cause of ROP (particularly the cicatricial stage) is not known. In over-emphasizing the role of oxygen in the past, neonatologists have created the false impression that ROP can be prevented, resulting in many unjustified malpractice claims.

Phelps, D. L., and Rosenbaum, A. L.: Effects of marginal hypoxemia on recovery from oxygen-induced retinopathy in the kitten model. Pediatrics 73:1, 1984.

G. Duc

Preliminary studies by Johnson suggested that the administration of the antioxidant vitamin E may reduce the incidence of RLF.[61] More recent studies have confirmed a modest benefit of vitamin E in decreasing the incidence of severe RLF, although current risk/benefit data are insufficient to justify routine prophylactic treatment of all infants at risk.[94]

The infant most at risk is not the premature with hyaline membrane disease in the first few days of life but rather the small premature infant who is repeatedly resuscitated for a period beyond that time for apneic spells, usually with a bag and mask into which a 100 per cent oxygen concentration is flowing. It is therefore recommended by the Fetus and Newborn Committees of both the Canadian Pediatric Society and the American Academy of Pediatrics that a self-inflatable (Ambu-type) bag be kept in the incubator of such a child and that when resuscitation is necessary it be carried out at the same oxygen concentration in which the infant is being kept at that time.

L. Stern

THE LUNG. (See also Bronchopulmonary Dysplasia, pp. 190–192.) Studies necessary for space flight have helped to clarify the pathogenesis of oxygen toxicity by exposing monkeys to one atmosphere of 100 per cent oxygen for varying periods of time.[62, 63] After 48 hours of breathing 100 per cent oxygen, only equivocal histologic changes were noted. When oxygen was continued for a longer period, a specific sequence of morphologic changes was observed: after 4 days, the alveolar epithelium was almost completely destroyed (exudative phase); after 7 days of high oxygen, Type I epithelial cells were replaced exclusively by Type II cells (proliferative phase). The vascular endothelium appears to constitute the target tissue in the early reaction, and the blood-air barrier becomes progressively thickened. After 12 days of 100 per cent oxygen, the animals required gradual weaning back to room air, similar in many ways to infants with supposed pulmonary oxygen toxicity. Eighty-four days after

the weaning, the lungs appeared surprisingly normal, but exact measurements revealed that a remodeling had occurred, with a large increase in the capillary bed but only a slight enlargement in the air-blood-tissue barrier.

The lung is the organ exposed directly to the highest partial pressure of inspired oxygen. The precise concentration of oxygen that is toxic to the lung probably depends on a large number of variables, including maturation, nutritional and endocrine status, and duration of exposure to oxygen and other oxidants. Although a safe level of inspired oxygen has not been established, concentrations in excess of 60 per cent carry a substantial risk of lung damage when administered over a period of many days. Continued exposure to high O_2 is accompanied by an influx of polymorphonuclear leukocytes containing proteolytic enzymes such as elastase. Bruce et al have observed that the antiproteinase defense system is significantly impaired in infants exposed to greater than 60 per cent inspired O_2 for 6 or more days.[16] Therefore proteolytic damage of structural elements in alveolar walls may be an important pathogenetic factor. Loss of mucociliary function may be an additional pathogenetic component, since exposure to 80 per cent oxygen has resulted in a cessation of ciliary movement after 48–96 hours in cultured human neonatal respiratory epithelium.[13]

Although the cellular basis for oxygen toxicity has not been completely elucidated, the principal mechanisms involve the univalent reduction of molecular oxygen and the formation of free radical intermediates. The latter can react with intracellular constituents and membrane lipids, thus initiating chain reactions that may result in tissue destruction.[34] To resist the detrimental effects of oxygen toxicity, the body has evolved various antioxidant enzymes such as superoxide dismutase, which eliminates the superoxide radical, whereas other components such as vitamin E and selenium also may offer endogenous antioxidant protection. Studies designed to enhance antioxidant protection by the administration of high doses of vitamin E, however, have failed to demonstrate any sustained beneficial effect in the neonate.

An observation especially disturbing to the physician using oxygen in the nursery is the altered developmental pattern observed in the infant rat lung when the rat was given as little as 46 per cent oxygen to breathe for 15 days.[9, 10] These data suggest that the growing lung is highly sensitive to oxygen exposure. With the rapid development that is observed in lung growth in early life and the known remodeling that occurs in the experimental animal following a prolonged period of high oxygen, the final anatomic resolution of the infant lung poisoned by oxygen is at present only speculation.

ARTERIAL OXYGEN ANALYSIS

Arterial oxygen tension measurements have, until recently, been based solely on *intermittent* sampling of blood (0.3–0.5 ml) from indwelling arterial catheters. Considerable interest has now focused on *continuous* PaO_2 monitoring via specially constructed catheters or the transcutaneous route (tcPO_2 measurements).[59] The latter consists of an electrode generally heated to 44° C that is easily attached to the skin and measures oxygen tension of the gas that has diffused from the arterialized capillary bed to the skin surface and through an O_2 permeable membrane. There is an excellent correlation between tcPO_2 and PaO_2 in normal and sick neonates with respiratory disease with PaO_2 values < 100 mm Hg (Figure 8–4).[79] By observing the effects on PaO_2 of procedures such as suctioning, bag ventilation, and altered respirator settings and the early recognition of complications such as pneumo-

thorax and endotracheal tube problems, it is possible to optimize the respiratory care quickly for each infant (Figure 8–5).[89] A major contribution of tcPO_2 monitoring has been the realization that excessive and vigorous handling of sick infants results in hypoxemia and that procedures such as lumbar punctures, when necessary, must be performed under optimal conditions (Figure 8–6).[48] It should be noted that tcPO_2 measurement remains an adjunct to and not a substitute for intermittent blood sampling in the very sick neonate.

Measurement of tcPO_2 may be a less accurate assessment of PaO_2 during severe hypotension with tissue hypoperfusion, which markedly alters skin blood flow. The temperature of the electrode must be carefully controlled to avoid burns to the skin, and the electrode is repositioned every 4 hours; transient areas of erythema, usually disappearing within hours, can be expected at the electrode site. Transcutaneous PCO_2 (tcPCO_2) offers a useful adjunct to tcPO_2 monitoring, via either separate or combined heated electrodes, although tcPCO_2 responds more slowly than tcPO_2 to changes in arterial blood gases. During profound hypoperfusion or shock, the normal elevation of tcPCO_2 levels[76] over the simultaneously measured $PaCO_2$ (as in Figure 8–4) will be further increased, presumably as a result of CO_2 accumulation in tissues.[18]

As newer techniques such as transcutane-

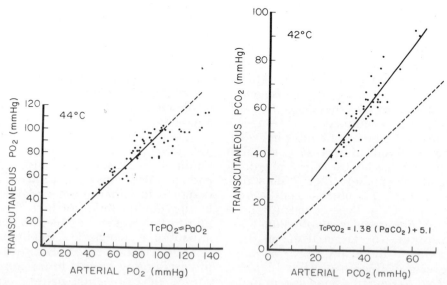

Figure 8–4. Correlation between transcutaneous and arterial values of oxygen tension *(left)* and carbon dioxide tension *(right)*. The regression line does not differ from the line of identity (dashed line) at values of PaO_2 less than 100 mm Hg.[79] For carbon dioxide the regression line clearly differs from the line of identity, and the appropriate correction must be made during either calibration or measurement of transcutaneous PCO_2.

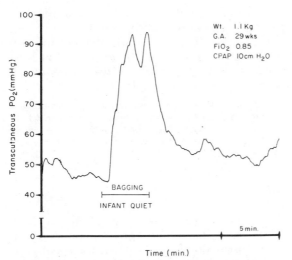

Wt.   1.1 Kg
G.A.   29 wks
FiO₂   0.85
CPAP   10 cm H₂O

BAGGING

INFANT QUIET

5 min.

Time (min.)

Figure 8–5. Transcutaneous oxygen measurements during 5 minutes of bag ventilation via nasal CPAP with the infant's mouth held closed.[89]

ous measurement of O_2 saturation evolve, their careful assessment is imperative so that they find their appropriate place in routine neonatal respiratory care.

As noted earlier, transcutaneous measurement of oxygen saturation is useful only to detect hypoxemia but not hyperoxemia.   **G. Duc**

We regard continuous monitoring of PaO_2 by an intravascular catheter-tip oxygen electrode (Conway et al) as mandatory in any infant with a serious respiratory illness. $TcPO_2$ electrodes are not really a satisfactory substitute for intravascular electrodes in the very ill, for a variety of reasons (le Souëf et al), particularly because they do not measure PaO_2 directly and one cannot always be quite sure that they are estimating PaO_2 accurately. Also, they need frequent resiting, which makes monitoring discontinuous and disturbs the infant. For infants with mild respiratory illnesses, $tcPO_2$ monitoring is extremely valuable, but even then it is important to be aware of the limitations in the performance of the different types of $tcPO_2$ electrodes. Some electrodes work better than oth-

ers, and the temperature setting is critical (le Souëf et al). Below 44° C, high PaO_2 values are often dangerously underestimated. Electrodes with a large cathode need resiting more frequently than those with microcathodes, because the skin is damaged more quickly (le Souëf et al).

Conway, M., Durbin, G., Ingram, D., et al: Continuous monitoring of arterial oxygen tension using a catheter-tip polarographic electrode in infants. Pediatrics 57:244, 1976.
le Souëf, P., Morgan, A., Soutter, L., et al: Continuous comparison of transcutaneous oxygen tension with arterial oxygen tension during prolonged monitoring of newborn infants with severe respiratory illnesses. Pediatrics 62:692, 1978.

E. Reynolds

OXYGEN ADMINISTRATION

Use a small hood or plastic cover to prevent fluctuation when opening the incubator (Figure 8–7). The temperature of the oxygen must be warmed to that of the incubator and monitored continuously. The flow into the hood must be at least 5 l/min to prevent CO_2 accumulation. Improper oxygen administration can be disastrous for the small infant and can result in death or brain, lung, or eye damage.[99]

1. Peripheral cyanosis may be present in a neonate with a normal or high arterial oxygen tension.

2. The environmental oxygen should be monitored at least hourly in all infants receiving supplementary oxygen or assisted ventilation. The oxygen analyzer should be calibrated at least once a day with high and low concentrations.

3. Management of oxygen therapy without arterial oxygen tension determinations is dangerous. We measure PaO_2 at least every

Figure 8–6. Transcutaneous oxygen and carbon dioxide measurements during the various stages of a spinal tap performed in the lateral flexed position in a preterm infant. Performing the procedure with the infant in the upright position can minimize the detrimental effect on blood gases.

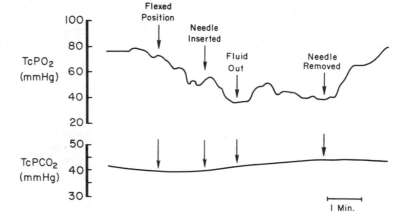

TcPO₂ (mmHg)

Flexed Position

Needle Inserted

Fluid Out

Needle Removed

TcPCO₂ (mmHg)

1 Min.

4 hours if the infant is receiving > 40 per cent oxygen.

4. Attempt to maintain arterial oxygen tension between 50 and 80 mm Hg during the acute phase of respiratory distress.

5. Some infants recovering from respiratory disease may require slightly increased oxygen concentrations (23–30 per cent) for many weeks. These infants should have an arterial or transcutaneous Po_2 determination or their O_2 saturation measured at least every day. When the environmental oxygen is to be lowered, observe these infants closely for pallor, tachycardia, tachypnea, abdominal distension, and a fall in body temperature; some of these symptoms are due in part to chemoreceptor stimulation secondary to hypoxia. If any of the symptoms appear, obtain blood gases and slightly raise the ambient oxygen concentration.

6. When infants receiving supplemental oxygen require intermittent mask and bag ventilation, both oxygen concentration and inflating pressures must be monitored closely.

7. Small infants with respiratory problems cannot usually maintain adequate tissue oxygenation for a prolonged period if Pao_2 falls to between 30 and 40 mm Hg, and they will require some change in treatment.

8. Long periods of time (3–10 days) at 25–40 per cent environmental oxygen can result in retrolental fibroplasia in the normal small premature infant.[58]

9. When the infant with respiratory distress syndrome (RDS) is improving (Pao_2 > 80 mm Hg), we lower environmental oxygen in 5 per cent increments and repeat Pao_2 before each further drop in concentration. This weaning process can be accelerated with continuous Pao_2 monitoring.

10. An environmental oxygen > 70 per cent can be damaging to pulmonary tissue if maintained longer than 4–5 days. It may be

harmful before this time. Oxygen at this level is continued only if absolutely necessary.

11. Every immature infant receiving additional oxygen should be examined at least once around the time of discharge by an experienced ophthalmologist.

Oxygenation should be monitored with continuous Po_2 recordings even if the infant is receiving less than 40 per cent inspired oxygen. This is particularly so in the weight group below 1500 gm in whom the risk of retinopathy of prematurity is high.   **G. Duc**

Alkali Therapy

Correction of severe metabolic acidosis with alkali has many physiologic benefits. With normalization of pH, myocardial contractility is increased, pulmonary vascular resistance is reduced, and the length of survival with asphyxia is prolonged. However, the rapid injection of hypertonic solutions of $NaHCO_3$ or tromethamine (THAM) is associated with a marked change in osmolality. (It is sometimes forgotten that although THAM does not contain Na, there is an equivalent cation—the amine—that has the same osmolal effect.) A brisk change in serum osmolality will alter many parameters. As water moves into the plasma, the vascular volume increases, and intracellular water is decreased. The rapid infusion of hypertonic solutions produces a sudden rise in cerebrospinal fluid (CSF) pressure and venous pressure followed by a steep fall in CSF pressure. As the plasma volume and venous pressures are increased, profound effects on the brain may result, including fatal hemorrhage. Since studies reveal that excessive and rapid $NaHCO_3$ administration may be associated with an increased incidence of intracranial hemorrhage, we closely control the use of alkali therapy.[42, 104] We use the following general rules for alkali therapy.

1. We exclusively use $NaHCO_3$ because of the possibility of hypoglycemia with THAM.

2. To reduce the corrosive effects of hypertonic solutions, we use $NaHCO_3$ solutions diluted with equal parts of distilled H_2O.

3. To prevent the toxic effects from large changes in osmolality, we attempt to limit alkali to 8 mEq/kg/day. In practice, we usually use a smaller dose.

4. Since other substances can also contribute to a significant increase in osmolality, we closely monitor glucose. (Each 18 mg/dl of glucose results in an osmolar rise of 1 mOsm/l.)

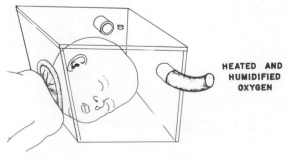

HEATED AND HUMIDIFIED OXYGEN

Figure 8–7. A plastic hood for oxygen administration.

5. We do not correct a respiratory acidosis with alkali, since the therapeutic value of $NaHCO_3$ depends on CO_2 removal by the lung.[91]

We would strongly support this recommendation. Respiratory acidosis is due to retention of CO_2, and its relief can be accomplished only by reduction of the CO_2 levels, usually with some form of controlled or assisted ventilation. **L. Stern**

6. The specific amount of bicarbonate cannot be determined from any of the widely used "recipes"; rather, treatment is empirical, with $NaHCO_3$ administration determined by serial blood gas studies.[33]

7. When an infant is severely asphyxiated, we administer alkali before the pH and HCO_3^- measurements have been completed (usually 2 mEq/kg $NaHCO_3$).

8. If the underlying cause of the metabolic acidosis is shock, etc., the primary treatment is to correct the basic problem, and alkali is only an adjunct.

NEONATAL PROBLEMS

Diagnosis

Even while administering emergency therapy, the initial objective is to establish an etiologic diagnosis for the respiratory symptoms. A major error in care can easily be made if other organ systems are not considered initially. *Not every cyanotic, rapidly breathing infant has the respiratory distress syndrome.* Hypovolemia, hyperviscosity, hypoglycemia, congenital heart disease, cerebral hemorrhage, hypothermia, or even the effects of drugs may all mimic primary respiratory disorders. Appropriate care depends on the diagnosis.

A working classification of some of these disorders is presented in Figure 8–8. Whenever faced with these respiratory symptoms, the next steps (following a history and physical examination) should be to obtain:

- X-ray of chest (plate under mattress).
- Intravascular hematocrit. (Peripheral hematocrits can be 25 per cent higher than intravascular hematocrits. All hematocrits should be central.)
- Blood sugar.

In many cases, blood gases will also be required, necessitating arterial catheterization (see Appendix I–2). The decision to catheterize the umbilical artery depends on the infant's condition. We catheterize the umbilical artery and/or vein during the first 15 minutes of life if metabolic resuscitation is required (as indicated in Chapter 1) or if the infant remains severely distressed (as defined by continued hypoxemia with or without hypotonia and severe respiratory efforts). On the other hand, if the infant has tachypnea and grunting with retractions but is active, pink, and weighs over 2000 gm, we catheterize only if there is deterioration or if the expiratory grunting continues for longer than 45–60 minutes of life. We base this on our experience and on the data of Rudolph et al,[102] who closely observed 549 immature infants immediately after delivery. They found a high incidence of continuing respiratory disease if grunting continued after 1

Figure 8–8. Differential diagnosis of neonatal respiratory disorders.

PULMONARY DISORDERS

Common	Less Common
Respiratory distress syndrome	Pulmonary hypoplasia
Transient tachypnea	Upper airway obstruction
Meconium aspiration	Rib cage abnormalities
Pneumonia	Space-occupying lesions
Pneumothorax	Pulmonary hemorrhage

EXTRAPULMONARY DISORDERS

Vascular	Metabolic	Neuromuscular
Persistent fetal circulation	Acidosis	Cerebral edema
Congenital heart disease	Hypoglycemia	Cerebral hemorrhage
Hypovolemia, anemia	Hypothermia	Drugs
Polycythemia		Muscle disorders
		Spinal cord problems
		Phrenic nerve damage

hour of life. Grunting sometimes stops when a cool infant is warmed.

At the time of arterial catheterization, a central blood pressure should be measured to check for acute blood loss. Although the newborn has a relatively larger cardiac output and a lower peripheral resistance and blood pressure than the older child and adult, measurements of blood pressure in this low-resistance circuit have been useful in diagnosing a large blood loss. (In the low-resistance circuit of the newborn kitten, the blood volume must be reduced by 40 per cent before blood pressure is observed to fall.) Nonetheless it has been shown that hypotension in sick preterm infants need not be associated with hypovolemia.[8] Hypothermia or acidemia results in severe peripheral vasoconstriction and will confound blood volume estimates from measurement of blood pressure. In a hypovolemic infant, blood pressure often drops only after acidemia and hypoxemia are corrected.

The mean blood pressure can be measured with a strain gauge[67] or alternatively with a cuff using the Doppler technique. A simple technique when these are not available is to use a saline column attached to the umbilical catheter. The zero point of the saline column must be the midclavicular line of the infant. Normal blood pressures and ranges are found in Figure 8–9.

If the initial hematocrit is below 35 without blood incompatibility or if blood pressure is reduced, we immediately start to correct the blood volume loss. We initially use saline or albumin and rush to obtain blood. We start with a push infusion of 10 ml/kg, observing blood pressure, heart rate, and the infant's general condition. In an emergency it is usually possible immediately after delivery to withdraw 20 ml of fresh heparinized blood from the fetal side of the placenta.

Perhaps one should be a little cautious about the very aggressive transfusion policy now adopted in some centers. No one doubts that urgent transfusion is indicated in the presence of definite evidence of serious hypovolemia, but there does not seem to be any good reason for transfusing infants merely because their arterial blood pressure is a little below the average. It may be that overtransfusion is one reason why patency of the ductus arteriosus is so common in some units in North America. We thus have rather a restrained transfusion policy. Another danger of acute overtransfusion is that it may be a cause of massive pulmonary hemorrhage and possibly also intraventricular hemorrhage.   **E. Reynolds**

Once the diagnosis has been made, it is necessary to determine if the neonatal unit has all of the facilities that might be needed during the course of the illness.

The ability to predict the course of the respiratory disease not only satisfies our instinct for gambling but permits the physician to determine which infant will require special respiratory therapy and must, therefore, be transferred.

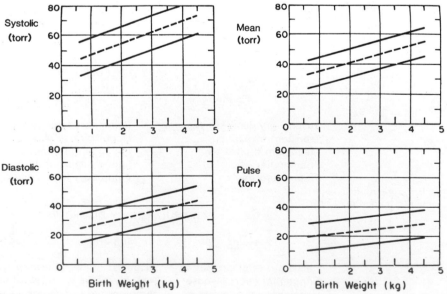

Figure 8–9. Linear regressions (dashed lines) and 95 per cent confidence limits shown for systolic, diastolic, and mean aortic blood pressure and pulse pressure during the first 12 hours of life. (From Versmold, H. T., Kitterman, J. A., Phibbs, R. H., et al.: Aortic blood pressure during the first 12 hours of life in infants with birth weight 610 to 4,220 grams. Pediatrics 67:607, 1981. Copyright American Academy of Pediatrics 1981.)

A low PaO$_2$ while breathing high O$_2$ concentrations usually means severe disease. As others have noted, mean arterial blood pressure is also a useful indicator of prognosis. We recommend transfer to a special center where all facilities are available while the infant is in reasonable physical condition before becoming damaged or moribund.

In the following section, respiratory distress syndrome will be discussed in great depth, because this is the major neonatal respiratory disorder and has been the primary focus of care and research in neonatal respiration.

Respiratory Distress Syndrome (Hyaline Membrane Disease)

Respiratory distress syndrome (RDS) is still the most common problem in the nursery and the major cause of mortality, occurring in 0.5–1.0 per cent of all deliveries and accounting for 15–20 per cent of all neonatal fatalities.[92] The disease is observed in roughly 10 per cent of all premature infants, with the greatest incidence in those weighing less than 1500 gm.

The following are lists of the common early symptoms, the physiologic abnormalities, and the pathologic findings at autopsy.

Early Signs and Symptoms

- Difficulty in initiating normal respiration—experienced by over half the infants. The disease should be anticipated if the mother is bleeding or has diabetes or if the infant is premature or has suffered perinatal asphyxia.[98]
- Expiratory grunting or whining—observed when the infant is not crying (due to partial closure of the glottis), a most important sign that sometimes may be the only early indication of disease; a decrease in grunting may be the first sign of improvement.[102]
- Sternal and intercostal retractions (secondary to decreased lung compliance).
- Nasal flaring.
- Cyanosis in room air (often).
- Respirations—rapid or often slow when seriously ill.
- Auscultation—diminished air entry.
- Extremities edematous—after several hours (altered vascular permeability).
- X-ray—reticulogranular, ground-glass appearance with air bronchograms.

- Pulsation of the umbilical cord—frequently observed after the age of 20 minutes.

Physiologic Abnormalities[6, 28]

- Lung compliance reduced to as much as one fifth to one tenth of normal (Figure 8–10).
- Large areas of lung not perfused (up to 50–60 per cent).[87, 95]
- Large right-to-left shunt of blood (30–60 per cent).[107]
- Pulmonary capillary blood flow decreased.[97]
- Alveolar ventilation decreased and the work of breathing increased.
- Lung volume reduced.

These changes result in hypoxemia, often hypercarbia, and, if hypoxemia is severe, a metabolic acidosis.

A fixed heart rate early in the disease is always associated with a severe course. (This is also noted by the obstetrician regarding fetal asphyxia.)   **S. Prod'hom**

Pathologic Findings (Anatomic, Biophysical, Biochemical)

- Gross—the lung is collapsed, firm, dark red, and liverlike.
- Microscopic—alveolar collapse, with overdistension of the dilated alveolar ducts, pink-staining membrane on alveolar ducts (composed of products of the infant's blood and destroyed alveolar cells). Muscular coat of pulmonary arteriolar walls thickened, lumen small. Distended lymphatic vessels.

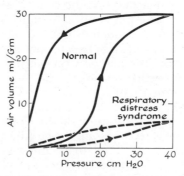

Figure 8–10. Air pressure volume curves of a normal and abnormal lung. Volume is expressed as milliliters of air per gram of lung. The lung of an infant with respiratory distress syndrome accepts a smaller volume of air at all pressures. Note also that the deflation pressure volume curve follows closely the inflation curve.[68]

- Electron microscopic
  (1) Damage and loss of alveolar epithelial cells.
  (2) Swelling of capillary endothelial cells.
  (3) Disappearance of lamellar inclusion bodies.
- Biophysical
  (1) Altered, deficient, or absent pulmonary surfactant.[5]
  (2) Abnormal pressure volume curve, as shown in Figure 8–10.[54]
  (3) Severely reduced arterial bed with blockage near the pulmonary arterioles revealed by perfusion studies of vascular tree.
- Biochemical—the lung contains decreased surface-active phospholipid (phosphatidylcholine) and lipoprotein fractions.[17]

ETIOLOGY

The distal respiratory epithelium responsible for gas exchange features two distinct cell types in the mature infant lung. Type I pneumocytes cover most of the alveolus, in close proximity to capillary endothelial cells. Type II cells have been identified in the human fetus as early as 22 weeks but become prominent at 34–36 weeks of gestation. These highly metabolically active cells contain the cytoplasmic lamellar bodies that are the source of pulmonary surfactant. The anatomic nervous system and its mediators appear to influence the rate of surfactant secretion or turnover. In particular β_2-adrenergic agents such as are used clinically to suppress premature labor appear to enhance the amount of phospholipid recovered from lung lavages. Surfactant synthesis is a complex process that requires an abundance of precursor substrates, such as glucose, fatty acid, and choline, and a series of key enzymatic steps that are regulated by various hormones, including corticosteroids.[41] The most widely held current theory to explain RDS is that the disease is the result of a primary absence, deficiency, or alteration of this highly surface-active alveolar lining layer (the pulmonary surfactant). The surfactant, a complex lipoprotein rich in saturated phosphatidylcholine molecules, binds to the internal surface of the lung and markedly lessens the forces of surface tension at the air-water interphase, thereby reducing the pressure tending to collapse the alveolus. By equalizing the forces of surface tension in alveolar

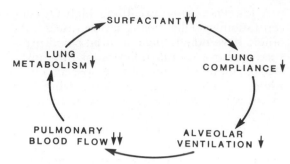

Figure 8–11. Alveolar function in the respiratory distress syndrome.

units of varying size, it is a potent antiatelectasis factor and is essential for normal respiration. Alteration or absence of the pulmonary surfactant would lead to the sequence of events shown in Figure 8–11; this results in decreased lung compliance (stiff lung) and thus an increase in the work of breathing. The additional work would soon tire the infant, leading to a sequence of reduced alveolar ventilation, atelectasis, and alveolar hypoperfusion.

There is no evidence that reduced pulmonary blood flow after birth reduces surfactant production. Pulmonary surfactant is always found in the lungs of infants who survive for 5 days or more and then die, even if they have had profound impairment of gas exchange, and presumably poor pulmonary perfusion, for the whole of their lives.

Adamson, T., Collins, L., Dehan, M., et al: Mechanical ventilation in newborn infants with respiratory failure. Lancet 2:227, 1968.

E. Reynolds

Asphyxia would induce pulmonary vasoconstriction; blood would bypass the lung through the fetal pathway (patent ductus, foramen ovale), lowering pulmonary blood flow; and a vicious circle would be promoted. The resulting ischemia would be an added insult and further reduce lung metabolism and surfactant production.[111]

The degree of pulmonary hypoperfusion and surfactant deficiency varies with each infant (Figure 8–12).

PREVENTION

A major effort in treating this disease should continue to focus on its prevention. Numerous studies have noted the inexcusably high incidence of this disorder following elective cesarean sections without adequate documentation of pulmonary maturity from

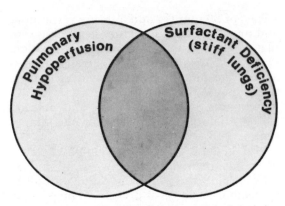

Figure 8–12. A schematic that may explain the varying manifestations of the respiratory distress syndrome.

amniotic fluid testing.[51, 55] The prolongation of pregnancy with bed rest and/or drugs that inhibit premature labor (e.g., tocolytic agents such as ritodrine), as well as the induction of pulmonary surfactant with maternally administered steroids, plays an important role in reducing the incidence of this disease[40] (see Chapter 1, page 17).

The collaborative trial on antenatal steroid therapy has convincingly shown that dexamethasone treatment can reduce the incidence of RDS. This effect was mainly attributed to its effectiveness in female infants, while the incidence of RDS in treated males was not decreased. Long-term follow-up of infants treated with steroids prenatally has shown no adverse effects. Prenatal steroid administration should thus be considered until other more effective ways to prevent or treat RDS are developed.

Collaborative Group on Antenatal Steroid Therapy: Effect of antenatal dexamethasone administration on the prevention of respiratory distress syndrome. Am J Obstet Gynecol 141:276, 1981.

W. Carlo

CLINICAL MANAGEMENT

Although much of the pathophysiology of the respiratory distress syndrome has been described and a multitude of treatments suggested and in some cases partially studied, the following approach appears most reasonable during this period of continuing research: for infants not moribund with the disease, the treatment should be of minimal risk to the infant and based on physiologic principles that are known to increase survival. Therapeutic regimens with increased risk (namely respiratory therapy) should only be used for infants whose chances of surviving

are diminished without their addition. The same basic care for RDS can be applied to infants with other neonatal pulmonary problems.

Since Avery and Mead postulated that infants with RDS were surfactant deficient, many investigators have attempted to treat RDS in premature infants with various exogenous surfactant preparations. Twenty years following the first trial to replace pulmonary surfactant in infants with hyaline membrane disease, several studies of animal models and clinical trials in human infants appear promising. Fujiwara et al documented that administration of a mixture of natural bovine surfactant enriched with synthetic phospholipids resulted in remarkable improvement in pulmonary status in a group of infants with RDS. Although controlled clinical trials of various surfactant preparations have revealed conflicting results, naturally derived surfactant appears to be superior to artificial mixtures. Whereas surfactant replacement offers great clinical promise, the ideal preparation and the amount, time, and method of administration remain under study. Nonetheless, surfactant therapy is anticipated to play a major role in the future management of RDS.

Egan, E. A., Notter, R. H., Kwong, M. S., et al: Natural and artificial lung surfactant replacement in premature lambs. J Appl Physiol 55:875, 1983.

Fujiwara, T., Chida, S., Watabe, Y., et al: Artificial surfactant therapy in hyaline membrane disease. Lancet 1:55, 1980.

Halliday, H., Reid, M. M., Meban, C., et al: Controlled trial of artificial surfactant to prevent respiratory distress syndrome. Lancet 1:476, 1984.

Hallman, M., Merritt, A., Jarvenpaa, A., et al: Exogenous human surfactant for treatment of severe respiratory distress syndrome: a randomized prospective clinical trial. J Pediatr 106:963, 1985.

Kwong, M. S., Egan, E. A., and Notter, R. H.: A double blind clinical trial of calf lung surfactant extract for prevention of hyaline membrane disease. Pediatrics 76:585, 1985.

Vidyasayar, D., Maeta, H., Raju, T. N. K., et al: Bovine surfactant (surfactant TA) therapy in immature baboons with hyaline membrane disease. Pediatrics 75:1132, 1985.

W. Carlo

In any regimen, the vicious circle noted in Figure 8–13 must be prevented or quickly blocked. The exquisite sensitivity of the pul-

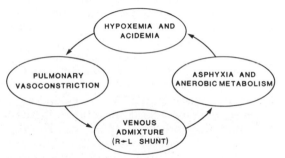

Figure 8–13. A vicious circle commonly observed in the neonatal period.

monary arterioles to hypoxia and the incompletely closed patent ductus and foramen ovale permit this vicious circle to perpetuate.

The clinical care can be divided into the acute and recovery phases. The acute phase lasts until it is reasonably certain the infant will survive. During the acute phase, every maneuver is directed to increasing the chance of recovery. The infant is placed in a neutral thermal environment (see Chapter 5) to reduce oxygen requirements and CO_2 production. For an infant with severe pulmonary involvement, this step alone may be lifesaving. To meet fluid and partial caloric requirements, dependent on environmental conditions, maturity, renal function, and hydration, the infant is given 65–150 ml/kg/day of 10 per cent glucose IV; because of poor gastric motility, he is not fed orally. To meet the immediate and changing oxygen, metabolic, and ventilatory requirements of the infant, we monitor color, activity, heart rate, and skin or rectal temperature at least hourly and pH, $PaCO_2$, PaO_2, and HCO_3 at a minimum of every 4 hours. Respiration and heart rate are monitored continuously to prevent a long apneic period.

Most important in the prescription are skilled nursing and physician management. Vital signs must be noted and observations made in such a fashion as not to disturb the infant continually, yet the patient must always be observed. Modern electronic monitoring of heart rate, respiration, and temperature now makes this easy. In many English units an essential part of the recipe is gentle, gentle care. Continuous PO_2 monitoring has confirmed the importance of minimizing simple maneuvers,[74, 106] such as (1) taking a rectal temperature, (2) vigorous oral and pharyngeal suctioning, (3) cleaning or positioning the face with a change in environmental oxygen lasting 2–3 minutes, and (4) vigorous auscultation of the chest. The real skills of a unit can be tested by closely noting the care given an infant with RDS. Is the environmental oxygen at the correct percentage, temperature, and flow rate? Is the arterial oxygen permitted to go too high or too low for a prolonged period? Is the unit anticipating the future needs of the infant or always treating complications? As an example, if, during the acute phase, an infant with RDS has an apneic episode, it usually signifies that the infant's condition is deteriorating and urgent intervention is indicated. Waiting for a PaO_2 of 30 mm Hg and a severe respiratory and metabolic acidosis before beginning ventilatory therapy is not adequate anticipation. Once the basic care has been arranged (metabolic rate minimized, fluid and electrolyte needs met), the essentials of care involve maintaining an adequate PaO_2 and pH and closely observing for a change in the infant's state.

Our general plan is to maintain the PaO_2 in the abdominal aorta between 50 and 80 mm Hg and the pH above 7.25, with alkali if metabolic acidosis is present. (The production of lecithin, the principal component of pulmonary surfactant, is maximal at a pH of 7.4.[80]) To prevent the toxic effects of hyperosmolar solutions, we are cautious about using $NaHCO_3$ and attempt to limit the total amount of alkali administered to 8 mEq/kg/day. In only rare instances do we administer this amount. Since clinical differentiation from group B streptococcal (or other bacterial) pneumonia is not possible, we take a blood culture and treat with antibiotics.

Around 10–30 per cent of infants with RDS will require further ventilatory support in the form of either continuous positive airway pressure (CPAP) or respirator treatment (see Chapter 9).

The most valuable prognostic laboratory measurement appears again to be the arterial oxygen tension. A PaO_2 below 40–50 mm Hg with the infant breathing 100 per cent oxygen is an indication for assisted ventilation; at this oxygen tension, the chance of survival without ventilatory assistance is probably less than 10 per cent.

For a complete discussion of mechanical ventilation and CPAP, see Chapter 9.

After 72 hours of age, most infants will start the recovery phase. Respiratory rate and retractions will decrease, and PaO_2 will rise without evidence of further CO_2 retention.

This recovery phase is preceded by a period of spontaneous diuresis during which there is an improvement in gas exchange, lung compliance, and functional residual capacity (Heaf et al).

Since the improved pulmonary function occurs after diuresis, it is important that the clinician anticipate the recovery phase and reduce ventilatory support in order to prevent barotrauma.

Heaf, D. P., Belik, J., Spitzer, A. R., et al: Changes in pulmonary function during the diuretic phase of respiratory distress syndrome. J Pediatr *101*:103, 1982.

W. Carlo

During this phase, expertise in oxygen management is required. PaO_2 should be kept below 90 mm Hg, but if environmental oxygen is dropped too rapidly and PaO_2 is not closely monitored, a condition termed "flip-flop" can occur. (Flip-flop is a larger than expected drop in PaO_2 when the ambient oxygen is lowered; the PaO_2 does not return to the original level when the ambient oxygen is again raised.) We rarely drop faster than 10 per cent every hour, checking PaO_2 before each drop in ambient oxygen, unless it is being continuously monitored.

We start oral feedings only during the recovery phase, when bowel sounds are present and the ambient oxygen has fallen to below 30 per cent. During the recovery phase, the umbilical arterial catheter is removed when PaO_2 has been adequate for several hours at an ambient concentration of about 30 per cent. It should be emphasized that an ambient concentration of 25–40 per cent oxygen can result in arterial oxygen tensions that are toxic to the retina if maintained for a prolonged period. We continue to lower ambient oxygen in 2–5 per cent increments, monitoring closely the infant's clinical state (i.e., respiratory rate, heart rate, and color, and observing for abdominal distension). Many very low-birth-weight infants require small amounts of additional oxygen for prolonged periods, and feeding may need to begin at a higher ambient oxygen concentration. As the infant recovers, apneic periods are now observed, but they do not have the ominous significance as when observed in the acute phase.[24]

The complications of RDS may occur spontaneously but more frequently result from well-intended therapeutic interventions. The major problems are consequent upon arterial catheter placement, oxygen administration, mechanical ventilation, and the use of endotracheal tubes, as discussed in Chapter 9. As the number of very low-birth-weight survivors has grown and the management of RDS become more complex, the time and effort devoted to preventing and treating the complications of RDS and its management have steadily increased.

During or following the recovery phase of RDS, cardiac failure secondary to a large left-to-right shunt through the patent ductus may occur as pulmonary vascular resistance falls. Bounding pulses and a systolic murmur are most useful in making the diagnosis. In most cases, conservative medical management with cautious fluid administration and diuretics will control the failure, and the patent ductus will close as the infant grows.[12] Although cardiomegaly is often noted on x-ray, an enlarged liver and edema are not always found with cardiac failure. Further evaluation of the magnitude of shunting by echocardiography (or in some instances contrast radiography via an umbilical arterial catheter) is indicated prior to initiating either surgical or pharmacologic closure of the ductus[114, 119] (see Chapter 13; for further details, see Table 8–1). The case problems and questions in this chapter further illustrate the care of these infants.

With reference to Table 8–1, we regard measurement of coagulation factors (they're often abnormal) and, if necessary, treatment of serious abnormalities—usually by a one-blood volume exchange transfusion with fresh adult blood—as another essential of care.   **E. Reynolds**

Persistent Fetal Circulation (PFC)

PFC describes the syndrome characterized by pulmonary hypertension resulting in severe hypoxemia secondary to right-to-left shunting through persisting fetal channels (foramen ovale and ductus arteriosus) in the absence of structural heart disease. Pulmonary hypertension in these infants is presumed to result from pulmonary vasospasm, possibly accompanied by an increase in muscle mass in the pulmonary vascular bed. The increase in pulmonary arterial smooth muscle tone may develop in response to intrauterine stress, whereas a decrease of a circulating pulmonary vasodilator such as bradykinin at the time of birth or an increase in the amount of circulating pulmonary vasoconstrictor during intrauterine or postnatal life may be responsible for vasospasm.

An initial report on this syndrome described term infants with respiratory distress and cyanosis without demonstrable cardiac, pulmonary, hematologic, or central nervous system disease.[47]

The same hemodynamic pattern occurs in both preterm and term infants with primary pulmonary disease (such as RDS, pneumonia, or meconium aspiration syndrome), polycythemia, hypocalcemia, hypotension, or congenital diaphragmatic hernia, or following neonatal asphyxia. The end result is cyanosis, tachypnea, and acidemia, which can superficially resemble cyanotic congenital heart dis-

TABLE 8–1 ESSENTIALS OF CARE FOR INFANTS WITH RESPIRATORY DISTRESS

Treatment	Logic
1. (A) Trained nurses (ratio of at least 1:1 or 2) and monitoring equipment. (B) Available trained physician.	1. Early management of complications and notification of change in course (e.g., apnea, bleeding from catheter).
2. Precise temperature control to maintain infant in neutral temperature (includes oxygen hood—see Chapter 5).	2. Maintains minimal oxygen consumption and carbon dioxide production.
3. (A) pH, Pao_2, $Paco_2$, and HCO_3^- measurements at least every 4 hours. Maintain Pao_2 50–80 mm Hg. *Continuous* Pao_2 is optimal. (B) Measure blood pressure. (C) Attempt to keep pH >7.25. If $Paco_2$ >55 or Pao_2 <50 mm Hg, consider changing treatment. (D) Lower environmental oxygen slowly when RDS infant is still ill. (E) Limit $NaHCO_3$ to 8 mEq/kg/day.	3. (A) To determine requirements for oxygen and additional HCO_3^-. Permits continual assessment of infant's condition and limits toxic effects of oxygen. (B) Rules out hypovolemia. (C) Same as (a). (D) Prevents "flip-flop" (greater than expected drop in Pao_2 when environmental oxygen is reduced) (Right-to-left shunt etiology?). (E) Prevents hypernatremia with brain damage.
4. No oral feeding (see Chapter 6).	4. Prevents aspiration in a sick infant; gastrointestinal motility reduced.
5. IV glucose 65 ml/kg 1st day, 80–100 ml/kg 2nd day with body weight determination for small infants to calculate if larger amounts of H_2O required. May require 150 ml/kg.	5. Meets a portion of the large caloric requirements, while reducing the risk of fluid overload problems (e.g., PDA).
6. Controlled oxygen administration: warmed and humidified, using a hood.	6. Prevents large swings in environmental oxygen concentration and temperature and decreases water requirements.
7. Continually monitor respiration, heart rate, and temperature.	7. Prevents hypoxemia and acidemia with apneic episodes.
8. Frequent determinations of blood sugar and Hct (Na, K, and Cl every 24–48 hr).	8. Necessary for calculating general metabolic requirements.
9. Transfuse if initial central Hct <40 or if Hct <40 during acute phase of illness.	9. For adequate oxygen-carrying capacity.
10. Record all observations (lab, nurse notes, etc.) on single form.	10. Permits immediate correlation of many variables.
11. Urinary output, blood urea nitrogen, and when indicated urinary pH, electrolytes, and osmolality.	11. Evaluation of renal function and blood flow to the kidney. An increase in output occurs as the infant starts to improve.
12. Obtain blood culture; treat with a penicillin and aminoglycoside until cultures available.	12. Cannot radiographically separate RDS from group B streptococcal pneumonia.[73]
13. Minimize routine procedures such as suctioning, handling, auscultation, etc.	13. Prevents iatrogenic drops in Pao_2[74, 101]

ease, primary pulmonary disease, or a cardiomyopathy. The initial roentgenographic descriptions of PFC stressed the absence of pulmonary parenchymal disease; however, meconium aspiration and streptococcal or *Listeria* pneumonia may be present as well as frank evidence of cardiomegaly and congestive heart failure. Pneumomediastinum or pneumothorax may also be present. Echocardiography has proved valuable as a guide to assessing elevated pulmonary artery pressure and pulmonary vascular resistance and more importantly as a means of excluding most anatomic cardiac malformations (see Chapter 13). Cardiac catheterization is very hazardous, but when necessary to exclude primary heart lesions, it will reveal normal cardiac structure, pulmonary hypertension, and evidence of right-to-left shunting at the level of the foramen ovale and ductus arteriosus.

The management of these infants is difficult. Polycythemia, hypoglycemia, hypocalcemia, and hypotension should be treated if present. These babies are exquisitely sensitive to changes in environmental oxygen. Most will require environmental oxygen of 100 per cent and show little improvement with continuous distending airway pressure. Assisted mechanical ventilation is usually needed to hyperventilate the infants to a $Paco_2$ of around 20–25 mm Hg and a pH of 7.5 so that the resultant respiratory alkalosis may relieve the intense pulmonary vasospasm and allow oxygenation to improve[35] (see Chapter 9).

Tolazoline (Priscoline) may be tried in infants in whom there is an elevation in pulmonary artery pressure in the presence of normal or elevated systemic pressure, no evidence of congenital heart disease, and failure of response to other management. Initially, 1–2 mg/kg of tolazoline is infused over 10 minutes via scalp vein, followed by continuous intravenous infusion of 1–2 mg/kg/hr and/or boluses administered when necessary. The aim is to infuse tolazoline into the superior vena cava (via a vein in the scalp or right upper extremity), hoping to avoid the right-to-left shunting of the inferior vena caval blood across the foramen ovale.

The relatively long half-life of tolazoline in neonates (3–10 hours) suggests that injection into veins that drain directly into the superior vena cava may not be necessary.

Monin, P., Vert, P., and Morselli, P.: A pharmacodynamic and pharmacokinetic study of Tolazoline in the neonate. Dev Pharmacol Ther 4:124, 1982.

W. Carlo

Unfortunately, responders cannot be distinguished from nonresponders by clinical or laboratory features prior to tolazoline therapy.[50] Complications possibly related to tolazoline include hypotension, abdominal distension, gastrointestinal hemorrhage, and renal insufficiency. Continuous transcutaneous or arterial P_{O_2} and systemic blood pressure must be closely monitored if tolazoline is used. In an infant whose oxygenation improves with tolazoline, systemic blood pressure may need to be maintained pharmacologically to prevent systemic hypotension and decrease right-to-left shunting.

Meconium Aspiration

Meconium is present in the amniotic fluid in 10 per cent of all births, and its presence suggests that the infant may have suffered some asphyxial episode in utero. It is doubtful that amniotic fluid alone can produce any airway obstruction. However, pulmonary disease is definitely observed in infants who have aspirated meconium (Figure 8–14), and there is significant mortality and morbidity without immediate aggressive management.

Editorial Comment: It has been proposed from autopsy data that the persistent pulmonary hypertension associated with fatal meconium aspiration may have originated antenatally. This is based upon the finding of severe structural abnormalities in the muscular walls of the pulmonary microcirculation in these patients.

Murphy, J., Vawter, G., and Reid, L. H.: Pulmonary vascular disease in fatal meconium aspiration. J Pediatr 104:758, 1984.

Multiple studies[25, 53, 110] strongly indicate that every infant with significant meconium aspiration requires the following:

1. Immediate suctioning of the nasopharynx should be done by the obstetrician as soon as the head appears on the perineum.

2. Immediately after delivery there should be visualization of the cords by laryngoscopy and direct suctioning of the trachea through an endotracheal tube if meconium is present. This is done prior to stimulation of the infant or positive-pressure ventilation.

Recent data in kittens indicate that meconium may remain in the trachea for periods exceeding 20 minutes despite spontaneous respirations, again underlining the importance of tracheal aspirations.[45] Figure 8–15 shows the remarkable impact of tracheal suctioning on morbidity and mortality. Studies of the efficiency of tracheal lavage and steroids do not support their use.

Because asphyxia is often the basis for the presence of meconium in the amniotic fluid, the infant who aspirates meconium at birth is often depressed and requires some resuscitation. Positive-pressure resuscitation should be avoided in these infants until an adequate laryngotracheal toilet has been performed, to prevent pushing meconium farther into the small airways. Interestingly, the

Figure 8–14. The pathophysiology of the cardiorespiratory problems accompanying meconium aspiration syndrome.[38]

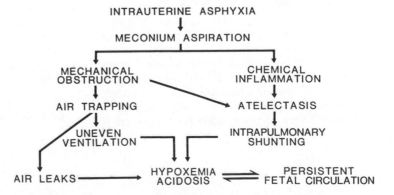

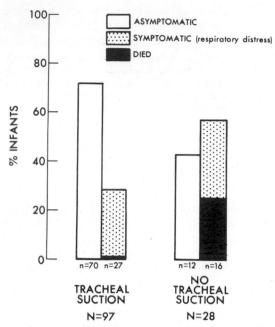

Figure 8–15. The effect of tracheal suctioning on morbidity and mortality in meconium aspiration.[110]

passage and aspiration of meconium in response to fetal stress are almost never seen prior to a gestational age of 34 weeks.

Gasping respirations are sometimes observed, the chest is enlarged, especially in the anteroposterior diameter, respirations are rapid, and rales may or may not be heard. A chest x-ray is helpful diagnostically and shows areas of increased density and areas of overexpansion irregularly distributed throughout the lung.

It is of interest that the lung can remove meconium rapidly. Studies with puppies in which meconium was instilled into the trachea revealed that it quickly moved to the periphery of the lung.[52] Marked recovery is usually noted after 48 hours of life, although a small number of infants with meconium aspiration recover over a prolonged period of time. In these sicker infants, persistent fetal circulation frequently becomes their major clinical problem, and management must be modified accordingly. One complication of the partially blocked, overexpanded areas of lung, occurring in 20–50 per cent of infants with meconium aspiration syndrome, is the development of air leaks, such as a pneumothorax. This should be suspected if the clinical status of the infant deteriorates suddenly.

Pneumothorax

Pulmonary air leaks comprise a spectrum of disorders that includes pneumomediastinum, pneumopericardium, and pulmonary interstitial emphysema. An asymptomatic pneumothorax is found in about 1 per cent of all routine newborn chest radiographic examinations. Considering the high intrathoracic pressures recorded during the first minutes of life, it is surprising that pneumothorax is not a more frequent occurrence. Macklin[75] described the path of the air after rupture: air from the ruptured alveolus dissects up the vascular sheath into the mediastinum and from there into the pleural cavity. In some series, as many as one half of the symptomatic patients aspirated meconium or blood. This suggests that obstruction with a ball-valve action may be the basis for the rupture. A pneumothorax frequently develops in infants with pulmonary interstitial emphysema, in whom there is a tracking of air from ruptured alveoli into the perivascular pulmonary tissues, usually during prolonged assisted ventilation.

Pneumothorax should be suspected in any newborn with respiratory distress or in a baby on a respirator whose condition suddenly worsens. In infants with RDS, a pneumothorax frequently develops when the severity of disease is decreasing and lung compliance is increasing. Bilateral pneumothoraces are often observed in infants with the hypoplastic lungs accompanying renal agenesis (Potter's syndrome), other forms of renal dysplasia, or congenital diaphragmatic hernia. In fact, the presence of otherwise unexplained extrapulmonary air in the early neonatal period should raise the question of an underlying renal malformation.

A high-intensity transilluminating light, using a fiberoptic probe, is especially helpful in quickly diagnosing a pneumothorax.[54] If the infant's clinical condition is relatively stable, it is wise to check the diagnosis radiographically prior to treatment. An anteroposterior film may underestimate the size of a large anterior pneumothorax, in which case a horizontal-beam lateral film of the supine infant will be very helpful.

Clinical Findings

Cyanosis, tachypnea, grunting, and flaring of the alae nasi are often observed. If the pneumothorax is unilateral, the cardiac impulse may be shifted away from the affected side and breath sounds decreased, although auscultation may be misleading because of wide referral of breath sounds. The sudden onset of a tense, distended abdomen with an easily palpable liver or spleen pushed down by the diaphragm is often a useful clinical feature signifying a pneumothorax.

Treatment

If the pneumothorax is asymptomatic, no specific therapy is necessary, but the infant's color, heart rate, and respiratory rate should be closely observed. If severe respiratory distress is noted or the infant has underlying pulmonary disease, a catheter should be placed in the pneumothorax and a continuous suction of 10–20 cm of water placed on the catheter. A high incidence of lung perforation has been described at autopsy following chest tube replacement, and thus a trocar should not be used to guide the catheter into the pleural space.[84] The catheter should be placed in the pleural space anterior to the lung—this is best achieved by insertion at the first to third intercostal space lateral to the midclavicular line.[3] Usually 24–72 hours of suction are necessary; it should be maintained until fluctuation of air in the tube with respiration and active bubbling have ceased.

Pneumopericardium will often present with profound hypotension and usually requires urgent intervention. Both pneumopericardium and pulmonary interstitial emphysema are almost invariably complications of assisted ventilation (see Chapter 9).

Transient Tachypnea of the Newborn

This syndrome (not always transient) usually follows an uneventful term pregnancy and is first detected in the transitional care nursery, because the infant is noted to have a persistently high respiratory rate.[7] Cyanosis is not prominent, although a few infants require 35–40 per cent oxygen to remain pink. Air exchange is good with no rales or rhonchi, an expiratory grunt is not heard, intercostal retractions are minimal, and arterial pH and $PaCO_2$ measurements should be within normal limits. The chest x-ray reveals central perihilar streaking, and often the cardiac silhouette is slightly enlarged.

The x-ray can usually be distinguished from that of meconium aspiration or the respiratory distress syndrome.

In most cases, respirations slow gradually during the first 5 days of life, and the infants are usually able to go home when their mothers are discharged from the hospital. The pathogenesis has not been clarified; however, it has been suggested that this syndrome may be secondary to slow absorption of lung fluid. The latter may be more prominent in infants born by elective cesarean section whose lungs contain less air and presumably more fluid over the first 6 hours than would be the case following vaginal delivery.[83] Fluid remaining in the periarterial tissue would explain the x-ray findings, and lung compliance would be decreased owing to the additional fluid. The infant's increased respiratory rate would then minimize respiratory work. The syndrome appears to be self-limited, and there have been no reported complications.

In our experience, grunting is extremely common in transient tachypnea. Probably it's useful in maintaining alveolar gas volume in liquid-loaded lungs. There is no rational explanation for transient tachypnea other than delayed removal of fetal alveolar liquid. The syndrome comes in two overlapping forms. In the first, streaky shadows can be seen on chest radiographs that are due to distended lymphatics and coalesce toward the hila. In the second, one or more lobes remain liquid-filled after birth and show up as dense shadows. The shadows disappear—often suddenly—within a few hours, when the infant has exerted sufficient transpulmonary pressure to transfer the liquid into the interstitium. CPAP or a brief period of mechanical ventilation solves the problem if it doesn't rapidly clear up spontaneously.   **E. Reynolds**

Hemorrhagic Pulmonary Edema and Massive Pulmonary Hemorrhage

E. O. R. Reynolds

Massive pulmonary hemorrhage has been found in about 10 per cent of neonatal autopsies,[43] but its incidence is probably now decreasing[26] because of improved perinatal care.

The illness occurs most commonly on the second to fourth days. It occasionally presents in low-birth-weight infants who have previously appeared well but more often affects infants who are already suffering from other life-threatening abnormalities or illnesses. A large number of predisposing factors have been implicated in the pathogenesis of the illness, including intrapartum asphyxia, infection, aspiration of gastric contents or maternal blood, hypothermia, severe rhesus isoimmunization, congenital heart disease, and defective hemostasis.[29, 37, 43, 59]

The usual mode of presentation is the development of bradycardia, apnea or slow gasping respirations, and peripheral vasoconstriction. Blood-stained liquid is then seen welling from the trachea. Once resuscitative measures have been undertaken, the flow of liquid usually ceases, although it sometimes continues or recurs.

Cole et al[29] analyzed the composition of the lung effluent in infants with massive pulmonary hemorrhage and found that, although it looked like blood, in most cases it was a filtrate of plasma with a small admixture of whole blood; in other words, it was hemorrhagic edema fluid, formed as a result of increased pulmonary capillary pressure. The likely reason for the increase in pressure is that a severe asphyxial episode (of whatever etiology) causes acute left heart failure or centralization of the circulation. An acute rise in filtration pressure in the pulmonary capillaries may be expected to have far more serious consequences in newborn infants than in adults for gravitational reasons. For example, an adult with a failing left heart filters excess fluid into the bases of the lungs, but ventilation can proceed normally at the apices. In a newborn infant, the height of the column of blood in the lung is by comparison much smaller, and a similar rise in filtration pressure will cause the formation of edema in the whole lung more or less simultaneously.

Factors identified by Cole et al[29] that might have predisposed infants in their series to develop hemorrhagic pulmonary edema, if they sustained an episode of increased capillary pressure in the lung, included those favoring filtration of fluid (hypoproteinemia, overtransfusion, increased surface tension at the air-liquid interface) and those causing damage to lung tissue (infection, hyaline membrane disease, mechanical ventilation, and oxygen breathing). Abnormalities of coagulation were present in some of the infants, but it was concluded that although these abnormalities probably did not initiate the hemorrhage, they could have exacerbated it by allowing continued bleeding through ruptured capillaries.

By comparison with hemorrhagic pulmonary edema, frank bleeding into the lung seems relatively unusual and probably occurs only in association with profound hemostatic failure, severe pneumonia, or direct trauma due, for example, to passing an endotracheal tube too far into the lung.

Treatment

Hemorrhagic pulmonary edema can be successfully treated by prompt mechanical ventilation[112] and transfusion of fresh blood. Prevention is more important, though, by avoidance of asphyxia at birth and subsequently, together with proper management of the underlying illnesses or abnormalities that predispose infants to develop the condition.

SPECIAL PULMONARY PROBLEMS IN THE IMMATURE NEONATE

Bronchopulmonary Dysplasia

For some infants with respiratory distress, the use of assisted ventilation in conjunction with high concentrations of oxygen has resulted in a clinical syndrome first described by Northway et al,[88] called bronchopulmonary dysplasia (BPD). Their patients had been on respirators using greater than 70 per cent oxygen for longer than 5 to 6 days. During the prolonged recovery, the infants exhibited persistent respiratory difficulty and a characteristic radiographic progression that resulted in cystic lung changes. Increased concentrations of oxygen were required for several weeks before slow improvement was noted. In those infants who expired, autopsy revealed that their lungs were diffusely involved, although it was not possible to implicate solely the toxic effects of high oxygen since these infants had also received respiratory therapy with endotracheal intubation (see also page 174, Oxygen Toxicity).

Since Northway et al's original description of BPD, the problem of chronic respiratory disease in infants has steadily increased, because of both more aggressive respiratory management and increased survival of very low-birth-weight infants. Bronchopulmonary dysplasia can be regarded as a clinicopathologic symptom complex associated with prolonged oxygen and respiratory therapy initiated for RDS, or less commonly for other acute neonatal respiratory problems. Controversy remains regarding the individual contributions of inhaled oxygen, respirator pressures, endotracheal tube injury, infection, and immaturity to the overall pathologic picture of BPD. The end result is a coarse pattern of scarring mixed with regions of overdistension. Parts of the vascular bed are condensed in the scars, and these arteries develop smaller than normal arterial diameters and thicker muscular walls.

The radiographic sequence initially described by Northway et al is no longer commonly seen, and stage I is essentially indistinguishable from uncomplicated RDS. Dense parenchymal opacification, as seen in stage II BPD, may commonly simulate another process, such as congestive heart failure from a patent ductus arteriosus (PDA), fluid overload, or pulmonary hemorrhage. The bubbly pattern of stage III BPD is not necessarily seen, and when it does appear, it may not follow a period of parenchymal opacity. Finally, the roentgenographic development of chronic lung disease (stage IV) may be more insidious than originally described. The characteristic picture of chronic lung disease ultimately appears at around 20 or 30 days of age. The major features of stage IV disease include hyperinflation and nonhomogeneity of pulmonary tissues, together with multiple fine, lacy densities extending to the periphery.

Of all the differential diagnostic possibilities, Wilson-Mikity syndrome (or pulmonary dysmaturity) has probably engendered the greatest confusion with BPD. Patients with Wilson-Mikity syndrome generally have an initially benign course, frequently with normal early chest x-rays, and an insidious onset of respiratory difficulty. Burnard et al have proposed that the unequal air distribution seen in these infants results from the increased collapsibility of their airways[19, 21] (Figure 8–16). In contrast, patients who develop BPD initially have severe respiratory disease (usually RDS) and a need for high inspired oxygen concentrations and assisted ventilation. Thus, even though the radiographic appearance of the two can be indistinguishable, the characteristic clinical histories usually will permit these conditions to be differentiated.

By analogy with animal studies it would be very surprising if breathing high concentrations of oxygen did not produce some pathologic changes in the lungs. Nevertheless, there is no convincing evidence in the literature that oxygen per se is an important factor in causing any form of chronic pulmonary insufficiency in infants. Rather than try to make a sharp distinction between the Wilson-Mikity syndrome or pulmonary dysmaturity and bronchopulmonary dysplasia—neither of which has a clear definition—it might be more profitable to think etiologically

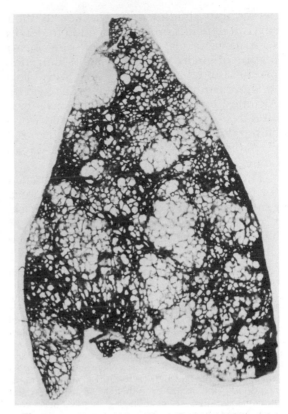

Figure 8–16. A section of lung from an infant dying with pulmonary dysmaturity. The lung was inflated at 15 cm of water and fixed in formalin for 48 hours. Note the uneven aeration.[58]

about known or presumed insults predisposing to chronic lung disease and devise a more rational classification. An abbreviated outline of such a classification could look as follows.

Chronic pulmonary insufficiency

A. Congenital
   Hypoplastic lungs (various sorts)
B. Acquired
   1. Airway lesions

   Aspiration of feed
   Inspissated secretions } = ? "Wilson-Mikity
   Floppy airways   syndrome"

   Infection
   Trauma from mechanical
      ventilation   } = ? "BPD"
   ? O_2
   2. Interstitial lesions
   Interstitial emphysema
   ? O_2
   Massive pulmonary hemorrhage

Treatment

With skillful and patient management, most of these infants will recover, although abnormalities in pulmonary function may persist into childhood.[105] The key to their survival depends on close attention to details such as vigorous treatment of right heart failure (digitalis, frequent use of diuretics, precise fluid balance, and very, very slow weaning from raised environmental oxygen). At times, lowering environmental oxygen as little as 2 per cent can lead to marked worsening. We have found transcutaneous Po_2 monitoring for 1–2 hours every other day to be helpful in this process.

These infants need to be closely watched for early signs of infection since pneumonia generally results in a profound setback. Bronchodilators have been reported to be of benefit when there are clinical signs of bronchospasm.[100]

Editorial Comment: Since infants with BPD have both clinical and radiographic evidence of airway obstruction, therapeutic efforts have been directed to decreasing airway resistance even in the absence of wheezing. Control trials of both diuretic therapy and isoproterenol inhalation have revealed encouraging short-term improvements in airway resistance.

Other modalities of treatment such as steroids and superoxide dismutase have also been utilized either to ameliorate or prevent BPD or to assist in weaning these infants from the ventilator. Although the reports in and of themselves are very encouraging, they will need confirmation in larger clinical trials to define the optimal role and timing of these interventions.

Avery, G. B., Fletcher, A. B., Kaplan, M., et al: Controlled trial of dexamethasone in respirator-dependent infants with bronchopulmonary dysplasia. Pediatrics 75:106, 1985.

Kao, L., Warburton, D., Platzker, A., et al.: Effect of isoproterenol inhalation on airway resistance in chronic bronchopulmonary dysplasia. Pediatrics 73:509, 1984.

Kao, L., Warburton, D., Sargent, C., et al.: Furosemide acutely decreases airway resistance in chronic bronchopulmonary dysplasia. J Pediatr 103:624, 1983.

Mammel, M. C., Green, T. P., Johnson, D. E., et al: Controlled trial of dexamethasone therapy in infants with bronchopulmonary dysplasia. Lancet 1:1356, 1983.

Rosenfeld, W., Evans, H., Concepcion, L., et al: Prevention of bronchopulmonary dysplasia by administration of bovine superoxide dismutase in preterm infants with respiratory distress syndrome. J Pediatr 105:781, 1984.

Many of these infants require prolonged hospitalization, and a well-organized program of infant stimulation may help the child achieve maximum potential. Parents must be encouraged to assume some of the responsibility for medical procedures, such as chest physiotherapy, and where possible a consistent medical team should oversee the infant's care and be available for continuing parental support. Finally, adequate nutritional management is the key, since malnutrition will delay somatic growth and the development of new alveoli in these infants who may already have an elevated level of oxygen consumption.[115]

Apnea in the Immature Infant

Periodic breathing (short, recurring pauses in respiration) of 5–10 seconds' duration is common in the immature infant and should be considered a normal respiratory pattern at this age. Apnea, on the other hand, has been defined as either (1) a given time period with complete cessation of respiration (> 10–15 seconds), or (2) the time without respiration after which functional changes are noted in the infant, such as cyanosis, bradycardia, hypotonia, or metabolic acidosis. Although the use of a standard, set time period appears to simplify routine nursery management, some small infants (usually < 1200 gm) appear to suffer if the apneic period extends beyond as little as 5–10 seconds. The problem increases substantially in both incidence and severity with decreasing gestational age.

Hypoglycemia, mild dehydration, hypocalcemia, temperature fluctuations, sepsis, anemia with a patent ductus, and severe brain lesions can be heralded by apneic spells and should be ruled out when apneic episodes first begin (Figure 8–17).[20, 38] In a very small number of infants, usually close to term, apneic spells may be the equivalent of a convulsion. However, the vast majority of apneic periods occur in infants who are immature and have no organic disease. An exception is an apneic episode in an infant with severe RDS, which usually indicates the presence of hypoxia and acidemia and is a clear indication for immediate intervention, such as assisted ventilation.[24]

When respirations and heart rate are closely monitored, it has been noted that about 30 per cent of all infants below 1750 gm birth weight will have an apneic period, commonly in the beginning of sleep immediately after eating.[31] These spells are usually limited to the first 2–4 weeks of life. In 90 per cent of these infants, heart rate starts dropping within 10–15 seconds after the onset of apnea and is usually below 100 beats per minute within 30 seconds. In some infants, heart rate falls within a few seconds of

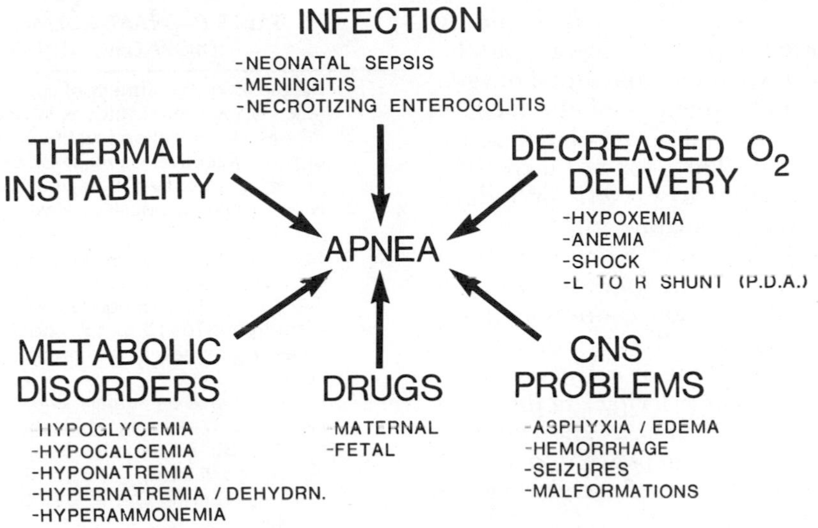

INFECTION

-NEONATAL SEPSIS
-MENINGITIS
-NECROTIZING ENTEROCOLITIS

THERMAL INSTABILITY

DECREASED O₂ DELIVERY

-HYPOXEMIA
-ANEMIA
-SHOCK
-L TO R SHUNT (P.D.A.)

APNEA

METABOLIC DISORDERS

HYPOGLYCEMIA
-HYPOCALCEMIA
-HYPONATREMIA
-HYPERNATREMIA / DEHYDRN.
-HYPERAMMONEMIA

DRUGS

-MATERNAL
-FETAL

CNS PROBLEMS

-ASPHYXIA / EDEMA
-HEMORRHAGE
-SEIZURES
-MALFORMATIONS

Figure 8–17. Specific causes of apnea.

onset of apnea, suggesting that bradycardia results primarily from vagal influences on central cardiorespiratory control.

In clinical observations, it has been noted that metabolic acidosis at times follows short repeated episodes of apnea. This may be the result of slightly reduced oxygen delivery secondary to altered perfusion or a short period of hypoxemia.

Although no good physiologic or chemical explanation completely describes these apneic spells,[64] Table 8–2 lists factors that singly or together make the immature infant more susceptible to apnea.

Treatment

If undetected, the first apneic episode can result in catastrophe. Therefore, because these spells occur so commonly, we suggest that all premature infants below 1750 gm or 34 weeks' gestation be routinely and continuously monitored during the first 10–14 days of life, until no apneic episode has occurred for 5–7 days.[5] Since heart rate does not regularly drop in all infants with apnea, respiration monitors should not depend solely upon a change in heart rate to signal an alarm. Conversely, since apnea with an obstructive component may not trigger a respiration alarm, simultaneous heart rate must always be monitored. We recommend diffuse cutaneous stimulation rather than painful stimuli to reinstitute breathing. Stimulation alone will stop 80–90 per cent of apneic spells if begun early. However, a mask and bag should be set up near every monitored infant,

to be used if breathing does not begin promptly after stimulation. (Room air or 30–40 per cent oxygen should be used in the bag.)

We should stress again that the use of a mask and bag in resuscitating a premature infant from apnea needs to be carried out within the oxygen concentration limits in which the infant has previously been kept.　**L. Stern**

TABLE 8–2 FACTORS RELATED TO APNEA IN THE IMMATURE INFANT

Observation	Explanation
1. Hypoxemia results in hypoventilation in the neonate instead of sustained hyperventilation as in the adult.[96]	1. Hypoxemic depression of respiration in the young infant is not overridden by stimulation from peripheral chemoreceptors.
2. Obstructed inspiratory efforts may occur during apnea and may be misdiagnosed as primary bradycardia when breathing movements persist.	2. Upper airway respiratory muscles (genioglossus, alae nasi) play a role in maintaining pharyngeal patency during inspiration.[15, 23]
3. Apnea most common during active sleep.[44]	3. During active sleep respiration is irregular, rib cage collapses, lung volume drops 30%, and Pao₂ falls.[56, 78]
4. Delayed auditory evoked responses.[57]	4. There may be fewer dendritic synaptic connections in the brain stem, leading to instability of respiratory control.

Miller et al[81] noted a decreased frequency of apneic episodes but an increase in the length of apnea when environmental oxygen was increased. (The memory of the medical disaster in using oxygen to regularize respirations is strong evidence for not increasing oxygen concentration to prevent or reduce apnea in a normal premature infant.)

A marked reduction in apnea has been noted with a variety of treatments, such as a pulsating water bed, a low continuous positive airway pressure, and respiratory stimulants such as theophylline or caffeine.[65, 70, 103]

Table 8–3 illustrates principles in the management of idiopathic apnea. The order in which these therapeutic steps are undertaken is based on the assessment of each individual patient.

A reasonable principle is to commence with a therapy that carries a low potential for short- or long-term side effects. Nasal CPAP at 3–5 cm of water is particularly effective in treatment of apneic episodes with an obstructive component[82] (Figure 8–18). The most probable mechanisms for the beneficial effect of CPAP include maintenance of upper airway patency, increase in FRC and PaO_2, and stabilization of the chest wall. The use of xanthines (theophylline, caffeine) has become increasingly widespread in the management of neonatal apnea. Theophylline is metabolized to caffeine in substantial amounts in neonates, although the precise mechanism whereby these xanthines increase respiratory drive remains unclear.[46, 86] While long-term sequelae of their use have not appeared, care must be taken to avoid short-term side effects such as tachycardia and diuresis.

TABLE 8–3 MANAGEMENT OF IDIOPATHIC APNEA

1. Diagnosis and treatment of specific causes (e.g., hypoglycemia, etc., as in Figure 8–17).
2. Increased stimulation (cutaneous, vestibular, or proprioceptive; via nurses, parents, pulsating water bed or its equivalent).[70]
3. Nasal continuous positive airway pressure (4 cm H_2O).[65, 82]
4. Theophylline (oral or intravenous); loading dose of 5 mg/kg followed by maintenance at 1–2 mg/kg/dose (8 hourly). Monitor serum theophylline (6–13 µg/ml) and serum caffeine (5–20 µg/ml) levels with theophylline administration.[4, 14, 103]
5. Increased environmental oxygen only as necessary to maintain a baseline PaO_2 between 50–60 mm Hg. (PaO_2 *must* be closely monitored.)
6. Artificial ventilation for as short a period as possible.

PRACTICAL HINTS

1. Prompt resuscitation possibly prevents respiratory disease.

2. Grunting is the most valuable clinical sign in diagnosing RDS. It is not normally heard beyond 60 minutes after delivery in a normothermic infant.

3. Although close observation of temperature control, respiration, and acid-base balance is necessary, frequent handling and manipulation of a sick infant may be harmful.

4. When using high concentrations of oxygen (> 40 per cent), arterial oxygen tension should be measured continuously or at least every 4 hours. Even concentrations of oxygen between 21 and 40 per cent, when adminis-

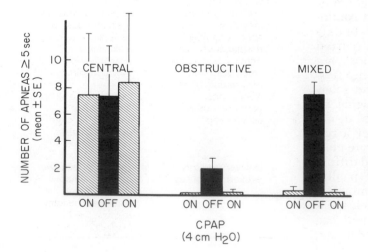

Figure 8–18. Apneas may be classified as central (airflow and chest wall movements cease simultaneously), obstructive (airflow ceases although chest wall movements continue throughout the apnea), or mixed (chest wall movements occur intermittently during the apnea). CPAP decreases the frequency of obstructive and mixed apnea but has no effect on central apnea.[82]

tered for prolonged periods (3–10 days), can damage the eyes of small immature infants.

5. Do not start early feeding in an infant with respiratory distress. Gastrointestinal motility is reduced, and there is a risk of aspiration and necrotizing enterocolitis. We start feeding when the respiratory rate is below 60 and bowel sounds are present.

Questions

True or False

As long as the arterial Pao$_2$ remains below 130 mm Hg, there will be no retinal damage when using high concentrations of oxygen (> 40 per cent) for the treatment of the respiratory distress syndrome.

When Pao$_2$ is measured every 4 hours and is less than 130 mm Hg, a small number of infants have been observed with retinal damage. Therefore the statement is false. There are several possible explanations: (1) a large right-to-left ductal shunt is directed to a sampling site in the lower aorta, while retinal vessels receive blood with a higher Pao$_2$; (2) Pao$_2$ actually varies between measurements; and (3) factors other than Pao$_2$ are involved in retinal injury. Continous monitoring should always detect (2) and should detect (1) if a skin Po$_2$ electrode is sited over the right upper thorax (preductal blood) and compared with postductal Pao$_2$. Nevertheless, even with very close monitoring of the oxygen level, retinopathy of prematurity still occurs.

Editorial Comment: A new international classification of retinopathy of prematurity has been adopted and rapidly introduced into the neonatal arena. This classification allows for a more dynamic yet consistent reporting of the evolution of the retinopathy. Furthermore, in contrast to previous classification systems, the new system permits reporting of location and extent in addition to the grade of the retinopathy.

An international classification of retinopathy of prematurity. Pediatrics *74*:127, 1984.
Lucey, J. F., and Dangman, B.: A reexamination of the role of oxygen in retrolental fibroplasia. Special article. Pediatrics *73*:82, 1984.
Phelps, D. L.: Neonatal oxygen toxicity—is it preventable? Symposium on the newborn. Pediatr Clin North Am *29*:1233, 1982.

Sensory stimulation in the form of multiple examinations and routine nursing measurements of pulse, rectal temperature, heart rate, and so forth may be harmful to an infant with severe RDS.

Striking changes have been recorded in heart rate and Pao$_2$ with standard nursing manipulations. This has been suspected for some time by several English physicians who strongly recommend minimal handling. Continuous Pao$_2$ moni-

toring has confirmed these suspicions. Therefore the statement is true.

While we would agree that minimal handling is desirable, it has in too many institutions become a euphemism for simply doing nothing for the infant. Gentleness and avoidance of unnecessary trauma are mandatory, but minimal handling should not and must not be allowed to become an excuse for failure to initiate and carefully apply adequate therapy when indicated. **L. Stern**

B. W. is a 2 day old, 1200 gm male infant with moderate respiratory distress syndrome. During the first 2 days of life he has not been apneic and has maintained a reasonable pH, Paco$_2$, and Pao$_2$ in 40 per cent oxygen. However, the most recent Pao$_2$ has dropped to 35 mm Hg (breathing 40 per cent oxygen). This environmental oxygen concentration should be left the same, since raising the concentration may be harmful to the retina.

A drop in Pao$_2$ 35 mm Hg suggests worsening of the infant's condition. He may deteriorate rapidly if he remains in 40 per cent oxygen. If the arterial oxygen is monitored closely (continuously or at least every 4 hours), raising the inspired oxygen concentration to maintain the Pao$_2$ between 50 and 80 mm Hg should not result in retinal disease. Therefore the statement is false. The oxygen concentration should be raised.

The occurrence of 20 apneic periods (no respiration >20–30 seconds) during the first 10 days of life in a premature infant without respiratory distress is commonly associated with brain damage.

In years past, when respiration was not closely monitored and apneic episodes were not promptly terminated with either stimulation or short-term mask and bag ventilation, frequent apneic periods were associated with brain damage. Today this should not occur. Although there may be a slightly increased incidence of damaged infants, most of them do quite nicely. Therefore the statement is false.

If apneic periods are noted after several feedings, it is recommended that oral feeding be stopped.

Apneic periods are more commonly noted after feedings and are not an indication to stop feedings. Therefore the statement is false, although manipulating the quantity and frequency of the feeds and the position of the infant may help. It is not clear whether such apneic episodes following feeds represent a vagal reflex or hypoxemia, in response to swallowing or gastric distension.

Maintaining the arterial Pao$_2$ between 50 and 90 mm Hg will prevent pulmonary oxygen toxicity.

Pulmonary oxygen toxicity is related to the inspired concentration of oxygen, not the arterial oxygen concentration. Therefore the statement is false.

BLOOD GAS RECORD SHEET (to be used in conjunction with Cases One through Five)

Start _____
Date _____ Time _____

Finish _____
Date _____ Time _____

ACTIVITY
++ = ACTIVE
+ = ACTIVE (STIMULATED)
− = LIMP
A = IRRITABLE
S = TWITCHY

COLOR
P = PINK
W = PALE
D = DUSKY
B = BLUE

S = SKIN
R = RECTAL
M = MEAN

	Time	Age (Hrs.)	O₂ conc.	TEMPERATURE (°C) Hood / Inc.	S / R	B.P. (M)	P.	R.	Hct. / Hgb.	Dext. / Sug.	Bil.	#	pH	pO₂	pCO₂	Act. HCO₃
Case One		8	70	34 / 34	36⁶ / 37¹							5	7.28	50	60	27.3
		12	70	34 / 34	36⁶ / 37²	160	50					6	7.29	40	62	29
Case Two		½	40	33⁶ / 33⁶	33 / 32	39			43	>90		1	7.14	30	35	11.4
		1		33⁶ / 33⁶	34 / 33	22			43				7.28	90	36	16.4
Case Three		8	40	32 / 34	36² / 36⁶	38			50	>90		6	7.40	60	32	19.5
		11	40	32 / 34	36¹ / 36	39						7	7.40	30	38	23.2
		13		32 / 34	36 / 36⁶	39						8	7.40	60	42	25.6
		18	50	32 / 34	36 / 35	48						10	7.20	25	50	18.8
Case Four		3	70	33⁶ / 33⁶	36⁵ / 36⁷	40			54	>90		2	7.36	280	40	22.2
		4½	60	33⁶ / 33⁶	36⁵ / 36⁷	39						4	7.35	250	42	22.8
		5	40	33⁶ / 33⁶	36⁶ / 37	39						5	7.36	30	43	23.9
		5½	60	33⁶ / 33⁶	36⁵ / 37¹	38						6	7.37	70	33	18.7

(Record sheet continued on opposite page.)

BLOOD GAS RECORD SHEET (to be used in conjunction with Cases One through Five) (*Continued*)

Start _____ ACTIVITY   COLOR

Date   Time   ++ = ACTIVE   P = PINK   S = SKIN

Finish _____ + = ACTIVE (STIMULATED)   W = PALE   R = RECTAL

Date   Time   − = LIMP   D = DUSKY   M = MEAN

    A = IRRITABLE   B = BLUE

    S = TWITCHY

	Time	Age (Hrs.)	O₂ conc.	TEMPERATURE (°C) Hood / Inc.	TEMPERATURE (°C) S / R	B.P. (M)	P.	R.	Hct. / Hgb.	Dext. / Sug.	Bil.	#	pH	pO₂	pCO₂	Act. HCO₃
Case 5	6		100	34 / 34	36 / 36.5	54	140	80	52 /	>90 /		4	7.4	32	29	19
	6½		100	34 / 34	36 / 36.5				/	/			7.35	30	32	18
				/	/				/	/						

CASE PROBLEMS

(When studying each case, refer to the blood gas sheet, on the opposite page and above.)

Case One

A. B. is a 1500 gm growth-retarded female with aspiration pneumonia. At 8 hours of age, she is in an oxygen concentration of 70 per cent. She has meconium-stained nails and a good urine output.

At 12 hours, the left leg turns white. What should be done?

If the blanching does not quickly disappear with warming of the contralateral extremity, remove the umbilical artery catheter. Sometimes no problems arise when another catheter is inserted into the same artery. Otherwise, attempt to catheterize the other umbilical artery.

If you decide to remove the catheter, how do you manage the infant's environmental oxygen concentration?

There is no substitute for continuous intraarterial Po_2 monitoring and/or intermittent arterial blood sampling in an acutely ill infant, although transcutaneous monitoring may suffice. Placement of an arterial line in an extremity is another solution for intermittent arterial sampling, since the infant has a respiratory acidosis and pH and Pco_2 should be measured in addition to Po_2.

Heel stick or venous blood sampling is useful for monitoring pH and $Paco_2$ but cannot be used to control ambient oxygen.

Case Two

C. D. is a 2100 gm male, who has been grunting since birth. X-ray shows no pneumothorax but is technically of poor quality.

What are this infant's obvious problems?

(a) Hypothermia, (b) hypoxemia, and (c) metabolic acidosis. He may have been resuscitated without good thermal control, which hastened his drop in body temperature. Infants with prenatal asphyxia have been noted to have a greater drop in body temperature during the first hours of life. His $Paco_2$ is not elevated, but he is not making a respiratory adjustment for the metabolic acidosis as one might expect in the "normal" infant.

How should these problems be handled?

Provide an increased oxygen concentration, treat with bicarbonate (2 mEq/kg), and repeat the blood gas.

What problem is noted at 1 hour?

The blood pressure has dropped (but the hematocrit has not).

How do you explain what happened?

Hypoxemia or acidemia alone or in combination may result in an elevation of blood pressure. Partial correction of the metabolic acidosis and raising the $Paco_2$ probably reduced the increased peripheral vascular resistance. The low blood pressure suggests a severely reduced blood volume. Blood volume should be expanded.

Case Three

E. F. is an 1100 gm female. Her Apgar score at 1 minute is 1. She was bagged at 10 minutes and has been grunting since that time. The chest x-ray was compatible with the diagnosis of respiratory distress syndrome.

Should NaHCO$_3$ be given 1 hour after Blood Gas #6?

No. Her pH, Paco$_2$, and HCO$_3^-$ are within the normal range.

Should anything else be changed?

Yes. The hood temperature is too low. At this level, metabolic rate (oxygen consumption) is increased. It should be raised to her neutral temperature (incubator temperature).

At 11 hours, should anything be changed?

Yes. The hood temperature is still ignored. Also, the environmental oxygen should be increased. At this low oxygen tension, metabolic acidosis and death often quickly ensue. The infant should be on antibiotics because pneumonia cannot be excluded.

At 18 hours, after Blood Gas #10, should anything be changed?

Yes—hood temperature, environmental oxygen, and in addition a short period of bagging to control the respiratory acidosis. Check x-ray for pneumothorax; repeat the hematocrit. In view of the marked hypoxemia and CO$_2$ retention, we would consider early administration of continuous positive airway pressure, although we usually wait until greater than 70 per cent O$_2$ is required to maintain a Pao$_2$ above 60 mm Hg. Unless she promptly improves, mechanical ventilation should be started.

Case Four

G. H. is a 2000 gm male, who has been grunting since birth. His x-ray reveals questionable respiratory distress syndrome. He has been placed in 70 per cent oxygen.

At 3 hours, what would you do, if anything?

Decrease environmental oxygen to 60 per cent immediately and if possible start transcutaneous Po$_2$ monitoring for rapid weaning. Inspired oxygen should then be lowered in steps of 2–5 per cent at least every 15 minutes during continuous Po$_2$ monitoring and a repeat blood gas obtained when tcPo$_2$ approaches 100 mm Hg. This is a dangerous level of oxygen.

What happened at 5 hours? What now?

This patient demonstrated the "flip-flop" phenomenon, which sometimes occurs when environmental oxygen is decreased and can generally be avoided with continuous Po$_2$ monitoring. First, return the baby to an oxygen concentration of 60–70 per cent. Second, transilluminate the chest to rule out the possibility of pneumothorax. Determine another blood oxygen tension in 15–20 minutes after the environmental oxygen has been increased.

What is the explanation for what happened between 4½ and 5½ hours of life?

There is not a complete physiologic explanation underlying the "flip-flop" phenomenon. It is assumed that in some infants the pulmonary vessels are particularly sensitive to changes in oxygen tension and lowering the environmental oxygen results in pulmonary vasoconstriction and an increased right-to-left shunt. Under these circumstances, the Pao$_2$ will drop out of proportion to what might ordinarily be expected when the environmental oxygen is reduced.

Case Five

M. L. weighed 3000 gm at 41 weeks and was covered with thick meconium. Apgar scores were 2 and 5 in the delivery room. Immediate suctioning via endotracheal tube produced thick meconium from the trachea. Chest x-ray at 2 hours showed bilateral patchy infiltrates.

What is the main problem at 6½ hours?

The infant has marked hypoxemia in 100 per cent O$_2$. It would be unusual for such a degree of hypoxemia without CO$_2$ retention to be attributable to meconium pneumonitis alone in a well-resuscitated infant. It appears that persistent fetal circulation secondary to neonatal asphyxia has complicated the course of this infant.

How should this be handled?

The response of the hypoxemia to ventilatory support in such an infant is variable; nonetheless, assisted ventilation should be administered and a respiratory alkalosis induced in an attempt to improve oxygenation. If this is not satisfactory, we would use a tolazoline (Priscoline) infusion while continously monitoring Po$_2$.

REFERENCES

1. Ablow, R., Driscoll, S., Effmann, E., et al: A comparison of early-onset group B streptococcal neonatal infection and the respiratory distress syndrome of the newborn. N Engl J Med 294:65, 1976.

2. Aherne, W., Cross, K., Hey, A., et al.: Lung function and pathology in a premature infant with chronic pulmonary insufficiency (Wilson-Mikity syndrome). Pediatrics 40:962, 1967.

3. Allen, R. W., Jung, A. L., and Lester, P. D.: Effectiveness of chest tube evacuation of pneumothorax in neonates. J Pediatr 99:629, 1981.

4. Aranda, J., Sitar, D., Parsona, W., et al.: Pharmacokinetic aspects of theophylline in premature newborns. N Engl J Med 295:413, 1976.

5. Avery, M., and Mead, J.: Surface properties in relation to atelectasis and hyaline membrane disease. Am J Dis Child 97:517, 1959.

6. Avery, M., Frank, N., and Gribetz, I.: The inflationary force produced by pulmonary vascular distention in excised lungs. The possible relation of this force to that needed to inflate the lungs at birth. J Clin Invest 38:456, 1959.

7. Avery, M., Gatwood, O., and Brumley, G.: Transient tachypnea of newborn. Possible delayed resorption of fluid at birth. Am J Dis Child 111:380, 1966.

8. Barr, P. A., Bailey, P. E., Sumners, J., et al: Relation between arterial blood pressure and blood volume and effect of infused albumin in sick preterm infants. Pediatrics 60:282, 1977.

9. Bartlett, D., Jr.: Postnatal growth of the mammalian lung. Influence of exercise and thyroid activity. Resp Physiol 9:50, 1970.

10. Barlett, D., Jr.: Postnatal growth of the mammalian lung. Influence of low and high oxygen tensions. Resp Physiol 9:58, 1970.

11. Behrman, R.: Persistence of fetal circulation. J Pediatr 89:636, 1976.

12. Bell, E. F., Warburton, D., Stonestreet, B. S., et al: Effect of fluid administration on the development of symptomatic patent ductus arteriosus and congestive heart failure in premature infants. N Engl J Med 302:598, 1980.

13. Boat, F. F., Kleinerman, J. I., Fanaroff, A. A., et al: Toxic effects of oxygen on cultured human neonatal respiratory epithelium. Pediatr Res 7:607, 1973.

14. Boutroy, M. J., Vert, P., Royer, R. J., et al: Caffeine, a metabolite of theophylline during the treatment of apnea in the premature infant. J Pediatr 94:996, 1979.

15. Brouillette, R. T., and Thach, B. T.: A neuromuscular mechanism maintaining extrathoracic airway patency. J Appl Physiol 46:772, 1979.

16. Bruce, M., Boat, T., Martin, R. J., et al: Proteinase inhibitors and inhibitor inactivation in neonatal airways secretions. Chest 81(Suppl):44, 1982.

17. Brumley, G., Hodson, W., and Avery, M.: Lung phospholipids and surface tension correlations in infants with and without hyaline membrane disease. Pediatrics 40:13, 1967.

18. Brunstler, I., Enders, A., and Versmold, H. T.: Skin surface Pco_2 monitoring in newborn infants in shock: effect of hypotension and electrode temperature. J Pediatr 100:454, 1982.

19. Burnard, E.: The pulmonary syndrome of Wilson and Mikity and respiratory function in very small premature infants. Pediatr Clin North Am 13:999, 1966.

20. Burnard, E., and Grauaug, A.: Dyspnoea and apnoea in the newborn: some results of investigation. Med J Aust 1:445, 1965.

21. Burnard, E., Grattan-Smith, P., Picton-Warlow, C., et al: Pulmonary insufficiency in prematurity. Aust Paedr J 1:12, 1965.

22. Campiche, M., Jaccottet, M., and Juillard, E.: La pneumonose à membranes hyalines. Observations au microscope électronique. Ann Pediatr 199:74, 1962.

23. Carlo, W. A., Martin, R. J., Abboud, E. F., et al.: Alae nasi activation (nasal flaring) decreases nasal resistance in preterm infants. Pediatrics 72:338, 1983.

24. Carlo, W. A., Martin R. J., Versteegh, F. G. A., et al: The effect of respiratory distress syndrome on chest wall movements and respiratory pauses in preterm infants. Am Rev Respir Dis 126:103, 1982.

25. Carson, B., Losey, R., Bowes, W., et al: Combined obstetric and pediatric approach to prevent meconium aspiration syndrome. Am J Obstet Gynecol 126:712, 1976.

26. Chamberlain, R., Chamberlain, G., Howlett, B., et al: British Births 1970; First Week of Life, Vol. I, London, Heinemann, 1975.

27. Chu, J., Clements, J., Cotton, E., et al: The pulmonary hypoperfusion syndrome. Pediatrics 35:733, 1965.

28. Chu, J., Clements, J., Cotton, F., et al: Neonatal pulmonary ischemia. Pediatrics 40:709, 1967.

29. Cole, V., Normand, I., Reynolds, E., et al: Pathogenesis of hemorrhagic pulmonary edema and massive pulmonary hemorrhage in the newborn. Pediatrics 51:175, 1973.

30. Cross, K.: Cost of preventing retrolental fibroplasia. Lancet 2:954, 1973.

31. Daily, W., Klaus, M., and Meyer, H.: Apnea in premature infants: monitoring, incidence, heart rate changes, and an effect of environmental temperature. Pediatrics 43:510, 1969.

32. Dawes, G.: Foetal and Neonatal Physiology. Chicago, Year Book Medical Publishers, 1968.

33. Dell, R., and Winters, R.: Acid-base effects of hypertonic sodium bicarbonate solutions: a commentary. J Pediatr 80:681, 1972.

34. Deneke, S. M., and Fanburg, B. L.: Normobaric oxygen toxicity of the lung. N Engl J Med 303:76, 1980.

35. Drummond, W. H., Gregory, G. A., Heymann, M. A., et al: The independent effects of hyperventilation, tolazoline, and dopamine on infants with persistent pulmonary hypertension. J Pediatr 98:603, 1981.

36. Duc, G.: Assessment of hypoxia in the newborn: suggestions for a practical approach. Pediatrics 48:469, 1971.

37. Esterley, J., and Oppenheimer, E.: Massive pulmonary hemorrhage in the newborn. I. Pathologic considerations. J Pediatr 69:3, 1966.

38. Fanaroff, A. A., and Martin, R. J.: The respiratory system. In: Behrman's Neonatal-Perinatal Medicine. 3rd ed. St. Louis, C. V. Mosby Co., 1983.

39. Fanaroff, A. A., Aladjem, S., France, F., et al: Identification of the high-risk infant from placental phase microscopy. Pediatr Res 5:411, 1971.

40. Farrell, P., and Avery, M.: Hyaline membrane disease. Am Rev Respir Dis 111:657, 1975.

41. Farrell, P. M., and Perelman, R. H.: The developmental biology of the lung. In Fanaroff, A. A., and Martin, R. J. (eds.): Behrman's Neonatal-Perinatal Medicine. 3rd ed. St. Louis, C. V. Mosby Co., 1983.

42. Finberg, L.: The relationship of intravenous infusions and intracranial hemorrhage. A commentary. J Pediatr 91:77, 1977.

43. Frederick, J., and Butler, N.: Certain causes of neonatal death. IV. Massive pulmonary hemorrhage. Biol Neonate 18:243, 1971.

44. Gabriel, M., Albani, M., and Schulte, F. J.: Apneic spells and sleep states in preterm infants. Pediatrics 57:142, 1976.

45. Gage, J. E., Taeusch, H. W., Treves, S., et al: Suctioning of upper airway meconium in newborn infants. JAMA 246:2590, 1981.

46. Gerhardt, T., McCarthy, J., and Bancalari, E.: Effect of aminophylline on respiratory center activity and metabolic rate in premature infants with idiopathic apnea. Pediatrics 63:537, 1979,

47. Gersony, W., Duc, G., and Sinclair, J.: "PFC" syndrome (persistence of fetal circulation). Circulation 39:111, 1969.

48. Gleason, C. A., Martin, R. J., Anderson, J. V., et al: Optimal position for a spinal tap in preterm infants. Pediatrics 71:31, 1983.

49. Gluck, L., Kulovich, M., and Borer, R., Jr.: Diagnosis of the respiratory distress syndrome by amniocentesis. Am J Obstet Gynecol 109:440, 1971.

50. Goetzman, B., Sunshine, P., Johnson, J., et al: Neonatal hypoxia and pulmonary vasospasm: response to tolazoline. J Pediatr 89:617, 1976.

51. Goldenberg, R., and Nelson, K.: Iatrogenic respiratory distress syndrome: an analysis of obstetric events preceding delivery of infants who develop respiratory distress syndrome. Am J Obstet Gynecol 123:617, 1975.

52. Gooding, G., Gregory, G., Taber, P., et al: An experimental model for the study of meconium aspiration of the newborn. Radiology 100:137, 1971.

53. Gregory, G., Gooding, C., Phibbs, R., et al: Meconium aspiration in infants—a prospective study. J Pediatr 85:848, 1974.

54. Gribetz, P., Cook, C., O'Brien, D., et al: Studies of respiratory physiology in the newborn infant. II. Observations during and after respiratory distress. Acta Paediatr 43:397, 1954.

55. Hack, M., Fanaroff, A., Klaus, M., et al: Neonatal respiratory distress following elective delivery: a preventable disease? Am J Obstet Gynecol 126:43, 1976.

56. Henderson-Smart, D., and Read, D.: Depression of intercostal and abdominal muscle activity and vulnerability to asphyxia during active sleep in the newborn. In Guilleminault, C., and Dement, W. C. (eds.): Sleep Apnea Syndromes. New York, Alan R. Liss, 1978.

57. Henderson-Smart, D. J., Pettigrew, A. G., and Campbell, D. J.: Clinical apnea and brain-stem neural function in preterm infants. N Engl J Med 308:353, 1983.

58. Hodgman, J., Mikity, V., Tatter, D., et al: Chronic respiratory distress in the premature infant: Wilson-Mikity syndrome. Pediatrics 44:179, 1969.

59. Huch, R., Huch, A., Albani, M., et al: Transcutaneous PO_2 monitoring in routine management of infants and children with cardiorespiratory problems. Pediatrics 57:681, 1976.

60. James, L., and Lanman, J. (eds.): History of oxygen therapy and retrolental firbroplasia (Supplement). Pediatrics 57:591, 1976.

61. Johnson, L., Schaffer, D., and Boggs, T.: The premature infant, vitamin deficiency and retrolental fibroplasia. Am J Clin Nutr 27:1158, 1974.

62. Kapanci, Y., Weibel, E., Kaplan, H., et al: Pathogenesis and reversibility of the pulmonary lesions of oxygen toxicity in monkeys. II. Ultrastructural and morphometric studies. Lab Invest 20:101, 1969.

63. Kaplan, H., Robinson, F., Kapanci, Y., et al: Pathogenesis and reversibility of the pulmonary lesions of oxygen toxicity in monkeys. I. Clinical and light microscopic studies. Lab Invest 20:94, 1969.

64. Kattwinkel, J.: Neonatal apnea: pathogenesis and therapy. J Pediatr 90:342, 1977.

65. Kattwinkel, J., Nearman, H., Fanaroff, A., et al: Apnea of prematurity: Comparative therapeutic effects of cutaneous stimulation and continuous positive airway pressure. J Pediatr 86:588, 1975.

66. Kinsey, V., Jacobus, J., and Hemphill, F.: Retrolental fibroplasia: cooperative study of retrolental fibroplasia and the use of oxygen. AMA Arch Ophthalmol 56:481, 1956.

67. Kitterman, J., Phibbs, R., and Tooley, W.: Aortic blood pressure in normal newborn infants during the first 12 hours of life. Pediatrics 44:959, 1969.

68. Klaus, M.: Respiratory function and pulmonary disease in the newborn. In Barnett, H. (ed.): Pediatrics. 15th ed. New York, Appleton-Century-Crofts, 1972, pp. 1255–61.

69. Klaus, M., and Meyer, B.: Oxygen therapy for the newborn. Pediatr Clin North Am 13:731, 1966.

70. Korner, A., Draemer, H., Haffner, M., et al: Effects of waterbed flotation on premature infants: a pilot study. Pediatrics 56:361, 1975.

71. Kuhns, L., Bednarek, F., Wyman, M., et al: Diagnosis of pneumothorax or pneumomediastinum in the neonate by transillumination. Pediatrics 56:355, 1975.

72. Lauweryns, J.: Pulmonary arterial vasculature in neonatal hyaline membrane disease. Science 153:1275, 1966.

73. Leonidas, J., Hall, R., Beatty, E., et al: Radiographic findings in early onset neonatal group B streptococcal septicemia. Pediatrics 59:1006, 1977.

74. Long, J. G., Philip, A. G. S., and Lucey, J. F.: Excessive handling as a cause of hypoxemia. Pediatrics 65:203, 1980.

75. Macklin, C.: Transport of air along sheaths of pulmonic blood vessels from alveoli to mediastinum. Arch Intern Med 64:913, 1939.

76. Martin, R. J., Herrell, N., Pultusker, M., et al: Transcutaneous measurement of carbon dioxide tension: effect of sleep state in term infants. Pediatrics 67:622, 1981.

77. Martin, R. J., Okken, A., Katona, P. G., et al: Effect of lung volume on respiratory time in the newborn infant. J Appl Physiol 45:18, 1978.

78. Martin, R. J., Okken, A., and Rubbin, D.: Arterial oxygen tension during active and quiet sleep in the normal neonate. J Pediatr 94:271, 1979.

79. Martin, R. J., Robertson, S. S., and Hopple, M. M.: Relationship between transcutaneous and arterial oxygen tension in sick neonates during mild hyperoxemia. Crit Care Med 10:670, 1982.

80. Merritt, T., and Farrell, P.: Diminished pulmonary lecithin synthesis in acidosis: experimental findings as related to the respiratory distress syndrome. Pediatrics 57:32, 1976.

81. Miller, H., Behrle, F., and Smull, N.: Severe apnea and irregular respiratory rhythms among premature infants. Pediatrics 23:676, 1959.

82. Miller, M. J., Carlo, W. A., and Martin, R. J.: Continuous positive airway pressure selectively reduces obstructive apnea in preterm infants. J Pediatr 106:91, 1985.

83. Milner, A. D., and Vyas, H.: Lung expansion at birth. J Pediatr 101:879, 1982.

84. Moessinger, A. C., Driscoll, J. M., and Wigger, H. T.: High incidence of lung perforation by chest tube in neonatal pneumothorax. J Pediatr 92:635, 1978.

85. Möller, E.-B.: Studies in Diabetic Pregnancy. Boras, Sweden,, Lund. Dept. of Obstetrics and Gynecology, Central Hospital, 1970.

86. Murat, E., Moriette, G., Blin, M. C., et al: The efficacy of caffeine in the treatment of recurrent idiopathic apnea in premature infants. J Pediatr 99:984, 1981.

87. Nelson, N., Prod'hom, L., Cherry, R., et al: Pulmonary function in the newborn infant. II. Perfusion—estimation by anaylsis of arterial alveolar carbon dioxide difference. Pediatrics 30:975, 1962.

88. Northway, W., Rosan, R., and Porter, D.: Pulmonary disease following respirator therapy. N Engl J Med 276:357, 1967.

89. Okken, A., Rubin, I., and Martin, R.: Intermittent bag ventilation of preterm infants on continuous positive airway pressure: the effect on transcutaneous Po₂. J Pediatr 93:279, 1978.

90. Oski, F., and Naiman, J.: Hematologic Problems in the Newborn. 3rd ed. Philadelphia, W. B. Saunders Co., 1982.

91. Ostrea, E., and Odell, G.: The influence of bicarbonate administration on blood pH in a "closed system": clinical implications. J Pediatr 80:671, 1972.

92. Perelman, R. H., and Farrell, P. M.: Analysis of causes of neonatal death in the United States with specific emphasis on fatal hyaline membrane disease. Pediatrics 70:570, 1982.

93. Perlstein, P., Edwards, H., and Sutherland, J.: Apnea in premature infants and incubator-air temperature changes. N Engl J Med 282:461, 1970.

94. Phelps, D. L.: Vitamin E and retrolental fibroplasia in 1982. Pediatrics 70:420, 1982.

95. Prod'hom, L., Levison, H., Cherry, R., et al: Adjustment of ventilation, intrapulmonary gas exchange and acid-base balance during the first day of life: infants with early respiratory distress. Pediatrics 35:662, 1965.

96. Rigatto, H., and Brady, J.: Periodic breathing and apnea in preterm infants. II. Hypoxia as a primary event. Pediatrics 50:219, 626, 1977.

97. Riggs, T., Hirschfeld, S., Fanaroff, A., et al: Persistence of fetal circulation syndrome: an echocardiographic study. J Pediatr 91:626, 1977.

98. Robert, M., Neff, R., Hubbell, J., et al: Association between maternal diabetes and the respiratory distress syndrome in the newborn. N Engl J Med 294:357, 1976.

99. Roberton, N., Gupta, J., Dahlenberg, G., et al: Oxygen therapy in the newborn. Lancet 1:7556, 1968.

100. Rooklin, A. R., Moomjian, A. S., Shutack, J. G., et al: Theophylline therapy in bronchopulmonary dysplasia. J Pediatr 95:882, 1979.

101. Rowe, S., and Avery, M.: Massive pulmonary hemorrhage in the newborn. II. Clinical considerations. J Pediatr 69:12, 1966.

102. Rudolph, J., Desmond, M., and Pineda, R.: Clinical diagnosis of respiratory difficulty in the newborn. Pediatr Clin North Am 13:669, 1966.

103. Shannon, D., Gotay, F., Stein, I., et al: Prevention of apnea and bradycardia in low birthweight infants. Pediatrics 55:589, 1975.

104. Simmons, M., Adcock, E., Bard, H., et al: Hypernatremia and intracranial hemorrhage in neonates. N Engl J Med 291:6, 1974.

105. Smyth, J. A., Tabachnik, E., Duncan, W. J., et al: Pulmonary function and bronchial hyperreactivity in long-term survivors of bronchopulmonary dysplasia. Pediatrics 68:336, 1981.

106. Speidel, B.: Adverse effects of routine procedures on preterm infants. Lancet 1:864, 1978.

107. Strang, L., and MacLeish, M.: Ventilatory failure and right-to-left shunt in newborn infants with respiratory distress. Pediatrics 28:17, 1961.

108. Swyer, P., Delivoria-Papadopolous, M., Levison, H., et al: The pulmonary syndrome of Wilson and Mikity. Pediatrics 36:374, 1965.

109. Thach, B. T., and Stark, A. R.: Spontaneous neck flexion and airway obstruction during apneic spells in preterm infants. J Pediatr 94:295, 1979.

110. Ting, P., and Brady, J.: Tracheal suction in meconium aspiration. Am J Obstet Gynecol 122:767, 1975.

111. Tooley, W.: Hyaline membrane disease: telling it like it was. Am Rev Respir Dis 115:19, 1977.

112. Trompeter, R., Yu, V., Aynsley-Green, A., et al: Massive pulmonary hemorrhage in the newborn infant. Arch Dis Child 50:123, 1975.

113. Versmold, H. T., Kitterman, J. A., Phibbs, R. H., et al: Aortic blood pressure during the first 12 hours of life in infants with birth weight 610 to 4,220 grams. Pediatrics 67:607, 1981.

114. Vick, G. W., Satterwhite, C., Cassady, G., et al: Radionuclide angiography in the evaluation of ductal shunts in preterm infants. J Pediatr 101:264, 1982.

115. Weinstein, M. R., and Oh, W.: Oxygen consumption in infants with bronchopulmonary dysplasia. J Pediatr 99:958, 1981.

116. Wilson, M., and Mikity, V.: A new form of respiratory disease in premature infants. Am J Dis Child 99:489, 1960.

117. Wimberly, P. D.: Fetal hemoglobin, 2,3-diphosphoglycerate and oxygen transport in the newborn premature infant. Scand J Clin Lab Invest 42(Suppl):160, 1982.

118. Workshop on bronchopulmonary dysplasia. J Pediatr 95(Suppl):815, 1979.

119. Yeh, T. F., Luken, J. A., Thalji, A., et al: Intravenous indomethacin therapy in premature infants with persistent ductus arteriosus—a double-blind controlled study. J Pediatr 98:137, 1981.

120. Yu, V. Y., Hookman, D. M., and Nave, J. R. Retrolental fibroplasia—controlled study of four years' experience in a neonatal intensive care unit. Arch Dis Child 57:247, 1982.

9

Assisted Ventilation

JUNE P. BRADY
GEORGE A. GREGORY

But that life may, in a manner of speaking, be restored to the animal, an opening must be attempted in the trunk of the trachea, into which a tube or reed or cane should be put; you will then blow into this so that the lung may rise again and the animal take in air. Indeed, with a single breath in the case of this living animal, the lung will swell to the full extent of the thoracic cavity and the heart become strong and exhibit a wondrous variety of motions ... when the lung long flaccid has collapsed, the beat of the heart and arteries appears wavy, creepy, twisting, but when the lung is inflated, it becomes strong again and swift and displays wondrous variations ... as I do this, and take care that the lung is inflated at intervals, the motion of the heart and arteries does not stop.

ANDREAS VESALIUS
DE HUMANI CORPORIS FABRICA (1543)

The primary objective of assisted ventilation is to support ventilation until the patient can adequately do so for himself. Ventilation may be required during immediate care of the asphyxiated or apneic infant, prior to evaluation and disposition, or for prolonged periods for treatment of respiratory failure. Ventilation during emergency care should be available in *every* delivery room and newborn nursery. Prolonged ventilation will only be available in special units in which continuous expert nursing, respiratory therapy, and medical care are available.[16, 28]

This chapter is intended as an introduction to assisted ventilation. Before undertaking assisted ventilation of any form, one must recognize that the techniques are demanding of time and resources and require experienced personnel.

RESPIRATORY FAILURE

The most common reason for assisting ventilation is respiratory failure, the inability to remove CO_2 by respiratory efforts. This results in a rising arterial PCO_2 and a falling pH. Hypoxemia is usually (but not invariably) present; in some instances arterial oxygenation is normal if the inspired oxygen is increased. Respiratory failure occurs because of disease in the lungs, the thorax, the airways, the respiratory muscles, or the central nervous system (Table 9–1).[28]

Clinical Manifestations of Respiratory Failure in the Newborn

1. Increase or decrease in respiratory rate
2. Decrease in respiratory efforts
3. Periodic breathing with increasing prolongation of respiratory pauses
4. Apnea
5. Cyanosis unrelieved by oxygen
6. Falling blood pressure with tachycardia associated with pallor, circulatory failure, and ultimately, bradycardia

Cardiac versus Pulmonary Disease

Differential diagnosis between cardiac and pulmonary disease may be very difficult to make in the sick newborn infant. Cyanotic heart disease may mimic severe respiratory distress. One way of differentiating between the two is to obtain an arterial PO_2 after 10

TABLE 9–1 INDICATIONS FOR ASSISTED VENTILATION

Infants with respiratory failure severe enough to elevate the $Paco_2$ above 60–65 mm Hg ($>$1500 gm) or 50 mm Hg ($<$1500 gm) with a pH below 7.25–7.20 or with a Pao_2 below 50 mm Hg when breathing 80% O_2 may need assisted ventilation. This often occurs in the following diseases.

Pulmonary
- Respiratory distress syndrome (RDS)
- Aspiration syndromes
- Pneumonia
- Pulmonary hemorrhage
- Pulmonary edema
- Wilson-Mikity syndrome
- Bronchopulmonary dysplasia
- Pulmonary insufficiency of prematurity

Loss of Lung Volume
- Pneumothorax
- Tumor
- Diaphragmatic hernia

Airway
- Choanal atresia
- Pierre Robin syndrome
- Micrognathia
- Nasopharyngeal tumor

Abnormalities of Muscles of Respiration
- Phrenic nerve palsy
- Spinal cord injury
- Myasthenia gravis

Central Problems
- Apnea of prematurity
- Drugs: morphine, magnesium, mepivacaine
- Seizures
- Birth asphyxia
- Hypoxic encephalopathy
- CNS hemorrhage
- Ondine's curse

Miscellaneous
- Patent ductus arteriosus with congestive heart failure
- Postoperative
- Asphyxia neonatorum
- Tetanus neonatorum
- Extreme immaturity
- Shock
- Sepsis

minutes' ventilation with bag and mask using 100 per cent oxygen and 5 cm H_2O end-tidal pressure. If this is done during the first hours of life, infants with severe respiratory distress will usually raise their arterial Po_2 over 100 mm Hg, while infants with cyanotic heart disease show little change in arterial Po_2 breathing room air or 100 per cent oxygen. However, infants with severe pulmonary hypertension may fail to raise their Po_2 with 100 per cent oxygen,[14] and infants with total anomalous venous return may raise their Po_2 over 100 mm Hg early in life.

The hyperoxia test, while useful diagnostically, can occasionally be misleading or even hazardous. Pulmonary hypertension frequently accompanies acute pulmonary disease, such as meconium aspiration, thus leading to a false-positive test for heart disease. Conversely, some forms of cyanotic heart disease associated with high pulmonary blood flow beyond the first few days of life (e.g., transposition of great vessels) can result in a relatively high Pao_2 and thus a false-negative test. Also, if the high concentration of oxygen used for the test is reduced too rapidly in a baby with reactive pulmonary vasculature, arterial oxygenation may be abruptly compromised. Use of a transcutaneous oxygen monitor during the test can be helpful in improving both the interpretation and the safety of the test. **J. Kattwinkel**

The optimal way of assisting respiration is ventilation via an endotracheal tube and anesthesia bag by an experienced person. However, most infants *can and should* be ventilated with a bag and mask plus 100 per cent oxygen prior to attempting tracheal intubation. This improves oxygenation and decreases arterial Pco_2, decreasing the likelihood of cardiac arrest during endotracheal intubation. Hand ventilation is impractical for prolonged periods of time but should always be used:

- For immediate resuscitation
- For stabilization following tracheal intubation
- In an infant whose condition is deteriorating without obvious cause
- During transport to intensive care facilities when mechanical ventilation is unavailable.

In certain instances assisted ventilation should not be used because intact survival will not occur. These are listed in Table 9–2.

CONTINUOUS DISTENSION OF LUNGS

Respiration can also be assisted by expansion of the lungs with continuous positive airway pressure (CPAP). This technique is of value when respiratory drive is normal and pulmonary disease is not overwhelming.

Studies by Gregory and colleagues[17] demonstrated that gas exchange can be significantly improved in respiratory distress syndrome by applying a constant positive pressure to the airway. CPAP is now the first method we use to assist the ventilation of infants severely ill with RDS who weigh more than 1750 gm at birth (Figure 9–1). Those who weigh less are mechanically ventilated.

Because of surfactant deficiency in RDS, alveoli tend to collapse easily. The resulting atelectatic areas of lung are the sites of shunt-

TABLE 9–2 CONTRAINDICATIONS FOR ASSISTED VENTILATION

Mechanical ventilation is not warranted when there is no reasonable chance of intact survival, as in the following diagnoses.
- Anencephaly
- Trisomy 13–15 or 16–18
- Werdnig-Hoffmann paralysis
- Potter's syndrome
- Intracranial hemorrhage with marked cerebral extension
- Hypoxic encephalopathy with absent reflexes or absent cerebral blood flow

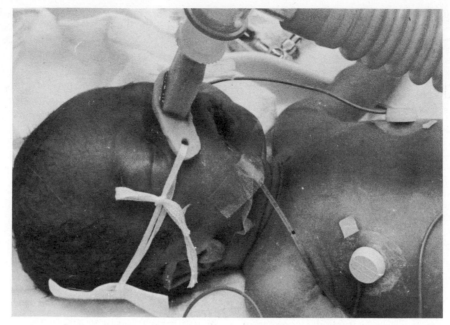

Figure 9–1. Nasal CPAP unit in place on infant.

ing from right to left. When alveoli are prevented from closing by maintaining a continuous positive transpulmonary pressure throughout the respiratory cycle, functional residual capacity increases. In addition, there is improved ventilation of perfused areas of lung, which decreases intrapulmonary shunt.

CPAP can be applied by a number of techniques. All of them have their advantages and disadvantages (Table 9–3).

General Guidelines for CPAP

1. In most centers the indications for application of CPAP are a PaO_2 below 50–60 mm Hg breathing more than 60–70 per cent oxygen and/or recurrent apnea.

2. Initially a CPAP of 6 cm H_2O is used. If this fails to produce improvement within 10 minutes, the pressure can be increased in 2 cm H_2O increments to 15 cm H_2O by endotracheal tube or 12 cm H_2O with a "noninvasive technique."

3. Arterial blood gases should be measured within 20 minutes of each change of pressure or oxygen. Continuous measurement of transcutaneous PO_2 ($tcPO_2$) or oxygen saturation with a Nellcor pulse oximeter is of great value.

4. These positive pressures are not completely transmitted to the pleural space because of reduced compliance. Hence, venous return and cardiac output are usually not compromised and may be improved. However, if $PaCO_2$ rises and PaO_2 falls, a reduction in CPAP pressure is indicated and may reverse these changes.

5. Inspired oxygen should be increased by 5–10 per cent increments if PaO_2 remains below 50 mm Hg at pressures of 12–15 cm H_2O.

Several studies have demonstrated that early use of CPAP will decrease the requirement for high oxygen concentrations. Since low levels of CPAP (e.g., < 6 cm H_2O) probably have little effect on cardiac output, we are tending to use CPAP earlier than previously recommended. If a baby clearly has decreased pulmonary compliance (he is grunting and/or retracting), we will begin nasal CPAP when only 40 per cent O_2 is required. If the baby is extremely preterm (e.g., 29 weeks' gestation or less), we may begin nasal CPAP even earlier. Thoracic wall elastic recoil is almost nonexistent in such babies, so that the resting volume of the lung is very close to the collapse volume. Also, the compliant chest wall tends to collapse as the diaphragm descends, resulting in an ineffective tidal volume. Early use of CPAP may improve the efficiency of ventilation in these very immature babies (Table 9–3). **J. Kattwinkel**

While low CPAP may be beneficial in infants with RDS, very high levels decrease lung compliance, which may result in an elevation of $PaCO_2$. **W. Carlo**

The technique for applying endotracheal CPAP has been developed primarily by Gregory et al (Figure 9–2).

A suitable air-oxygen mixture passes

TABLE 9–3 TECHNIQUES OF APPLYING CONTINUOUS DISTENDING PRESSURE

Method	Advantages	Effective for Infants <1500 gm?	Disadvantages
Endotracheal	Effective	Yes	Requires intubation, nursing, and medical skills as for ventilator[17]
Head box	Noninvasive	No	Neck seal a problem; suction difficult; nerve palsies[17, 40]
Face mask	Simple, inexpensive	Yes	Abdominal distension, pressure on face and eyes, CO_2 retention, cerebellar hemorrhage[2, 15, 33, 36]
Nasal prongs	Simple	No	Trauma to turbinates and septum, excessive crying, variation in Fio_2 increased work of breathing[15, 22, 23]
Nasopharyngeal prongs	Relatively simple, fixation easy	Yes	May become blocked or kinked[6, 25, 31]
Face chamber	Good seal, minimal trauma to face	Yes	Expensive, baby inaccessible[1]

We would take exception to several statements in Table 9–3. First, we have found CPAP by nasal prongs to be quite effective in the <1500 gm baby when the requirements for a small diameter, high resistance endotracheal tube often render endotracheal CPAP ineffective. It can be calculated that the resistance to air flow through a 10 cm long 2.5 mm diameter endotracheal tube is nearly seven times that encountered with a pair of 1.0 cm long 2.0 mm diameter nasal prongs. Nasal trauma can be completely avoided if care is taken to assure proper orientation of the nasal device. High cerebral venous pressures, perhaps leading to hydrocephalus, have been reported with head chambers that require tight-fitting neck seals. All of the various chambers and masks restrict accessibility of the patient for routine nursing care and/or airway cleansing. In our nursery, we use the nasal cannulae for delivering CPAP to all weight categories and reserve endotracheal intubation for those babies who require intermittent positive pressure ventilation.

J. Kattwinkel

Editorial Comment: In most tertiary centers today, infants appear to be managed preferentially with mechanical ventilators. The art of sustaining infants with continuous distending airway pressure supplemented by intermittent positive pressure has been lost. However, the vastly improved ventilators especially designed for babies have allayed the concerns of those who went to great lengths to avoid endotracheal intubation and mechanical ventilation. Whereas it is sad to observe the attrition of a skill, the quality of care with end-expiratory pressure applied via mechanical ventilators is superb and the outcome excellent.

through a humidifier. Gas passes the elbow, which is attached to an endotracheal tube. The screw clamp on the reservoir bag is used to control the flow of gas and maintain a constant positive pressure within the system, as indicated on the pressure manometer. The side-arm ends under a column of water (15 cm). This acts as an underwater safety valve.[17]

Nursing and medical management, tube care, etc., are as exacting as during mechanical ventilation. Similar systems can be used to apply noninvasive CPAP. Problems with CPAP are similar to those seen with the ventilator (see *Changes in Blood Gas Status*, page 213).

Weaning from CPAP

1. Inspired oxygen can be reduced by 2–3 per cent when the PaO_2 exceeds 70 mm Hg.

2. CPAP is reduced when the PaO_2 is above 70 mm Hg and the inspired oxygen is less than 40 per cent.

With small babies (< 1500 gm), if recurrent apneic spells are a problem, we may continue low-pressure CPAP (< 6 cm H_2O) until inspired oxygen concentrations have been reduced to 21–30 per cent. (See Chapter 8 for a discussion of the use of CPAP for apnea of prematurity.)

J. Kattwinkel

INTERMITTENT POSITIVE PRESSURE VENTILATION (IPPV)

Although ventilation with nasal mask, face mask, and nasopharyngeal prongs has been used for sick infants, mechanical ventilation with an endotracheal tube is preferable and is the only way of assuring effective ventilation.

Mechanical ventilation should be instituted when the criteria in Table 9–1 are met or

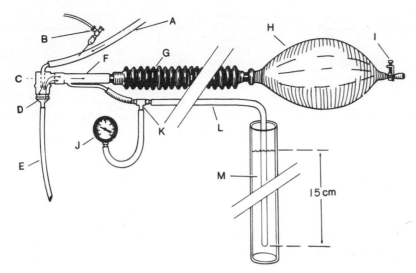

Figure 9–2. System for applying continuous positive airway pressure (CPAP) through an endotracheal tube. (Adapted from Gregory et al.[17]) A = gas flow. B = oxygen sampling port. C = Normal elbow (modified T piece). D = endotracheal tube connector. E = endotracheal tube. F = Sommers T piece, G = corrugated anesthesia hose. H = reservoir bag (500 ml) with open tail piece. I = screw clamp. J = aneroid pressure manometer. K = plastic T connector. L = plastic tubing (1 cm internal diameter). M = underwater "pop-off." Arrows indicate direction of gas flow.

when PaO_2 cannot be corrected by endotracheal CPAP of 15 cm H_2O and 60–80 per cent oxygen.

Ventilators

The principle of all mechanical ventilators is to achieve a pressure gradient between lungs and mouth producing a flow of gas into the lung. This is created by intermittently building up a positive pressure in the airway.

Several mechanical ventilators are commercially available. The clinician is advised to learn about and understand one or two ventilators and circuits available rather than use several types.

INTERMITTENT POSITIVE PRESSURE VENTILATORS

All ventilators in use should have the following features.

1. *Gas mixing,* to allow easy adjustment of the inspired oxygen concentration between 21 and 100 per cent. This reduces the likelihood of inadvertent high oxygen concentrations.

2. *Inspiratory-expiratory time adjustment* (I/E ratio), to allow altering of the inspiratory time, permitting its prolongation in cases of widespread atelectasis or its shortening if the lungs are normal. These two independent adjustments permit respiratory rates of 1–150 breaths/minute.

3. *Expiratory relief valve,* to limit the peak inspiratory pressure. When used in combination with the inspiratory time adjustment, it allows the peak pressure to be held, generating a pressure plateau (see Figure 9–3b). This valve also allows one to limit the peak pressure to reduce the likelihood of pulmonary air leak.

4. *Pressure gauge,* to measure the applied airway pressures accurately. It should have a small amount of inertia. At ventilator rates over 40, most pressure gauges have too much inertia and are very inaccurate. A Pneumogard (Novametrix Co.) or 18 gauge needle connected by stiff tubing to a differential pressure gauge and recorder must be placed in the inspiratory line of the ventilator, close to the endotracheal tube, to measure correct peak and end-expiratory pressures.

5. *Alarms,* to warn of inadvertent disconnections, pressure loss, and failure of the ventilator to cycle at the proper time. Alarms should also be provided to warn of inadvertent high gas temperatures and low or high oxygen concentrations.

6. *Humidification* or nebulization, to saturate the inspired gases with water at 32–37 degrees C. Ultrasonic nebulizers should *not* be used in infants because they frequently cause inadvertent fluid overload and pulmonary edema. The temperature of the inspired gas should be measured continuously and adjusted when necessary.

Precise regulation of the temperature of inspired air is extremely important. We have found it helpful to place a thermistor in the incoming gas flow; the humidifier heater can then be electronically servocontrolled to adjust the temperature of inspired gases to the baby's neutral thermal environment.

J. Kattwinkel

7. *End-expiratory pressure* should be obtainable when desired. It should be adjustable between 0 and 15 cm H_2O. Occasionally, infants with very stiff lungs will require high end-expiratory pressures to survive.

Editorial Comment: We rarely use an end-expiratory pressure above 6 cm H_2O in newborn infants.

8. *Exhalation assist,* to reduce the end-expiratory pressure to desired levels when rapid rates are used. Inadvertent positive end-expiratory pressure (PEEP) is a problem with most pediatric ventilators because they have a high expiratory resistance (40–60 cm H_2O/l/sec) with gas flows greater than 5 liters/minute. The greater the gas flow, the greater the resistance to exhalation.

FEATURES NOT NECESSARY FOR INFANT VENTILATORS

1. *Tidal volume adjustment* is not attainable unless a pneumotachograph is inserted between the endotracheal tube and ventilator. The larger compression volumes of the ventilator and its circuit make it impossible to deliver a constant tidal volume when lung compliance and resistance change. In addition, to prevent subglottic stenosis, there should always be a leak between the endotracheal tube and trachea. Even the most expensive ventilators cannot deliver a constant tidal volume.[38]

2. *Patient triggering* of the ventilator is not possible in most ventilators nor is it desirable since most infants requiring mechanical ventilation are too ill and weak to cycle the ventilator. Devices that are designed to allow patient cycling of the machine increase the cost significantly.

3. *Bacterial filter.*

TYPES OF VENTILATORS USED FOR INFANTS

Ventilators for infants are usually:

1. *Time cycled.* A constant flow of gas passes through the ventilator. Intermittently a valve closes, and the gas flows to the infant. When the valve has been closed for the preset period of time, the valve opens, and inspiration ceases. Examples of this type of ventilator include the Baby Bird II, Bourns BP 200, Bear-Cub, and Sechrist.

2. *Volume cycled.* A preset volume of gas is delivered to the system (patient and ventilator circuit). When this gas has been delivered by the piston, inspiration is terminated. Examples of this type of ventilator include the

Starling Pump, Siemens-Elema 900B and 900C, Vickers, and Engstrom.

SPECIAL CONSIDERATIONS

The ventilator chosen should deliver an adequate volume of gas to ventilate the lung and to oxygenate and remove CO_2 from the blood while compensating for compression volume, dead space, and leaks. In a large ventilator circuit, the volume of gas compressed (compression volume) may be excessively high, even with moderate inflation pressures. For example, a compression volume of 2 ml/cm H_2O will compress 2 ml of gas for each cm H_2O airway pressure generated. This volume of gas is lost from the circuit and never ventilates the patient. To reduce this problem, the circuit volume should be kept low with low-volume, noncompressible tubing. A constant volume of water in the humidifier is helpful.

GENERAL CONSIDERATIONS

The *respiratory pattern* can be described by the duration of the inspiratory gas flow, the tidal volume, and the pressure required to produce them. They are interrelated:

$$\text{volume/pressure} = \text{compliance}$$
$$\text{resistance} = \text{pressure/flow}$$
$$\text{volume} = \text{flow} \times \text{time.}$$

Positive pressure ventilators cause tidal ventilation by altering the pressure in the airway relative to atmospheric pressure. The respiratory cycle generated consists of four elements: (1) inspiration, (2) expiration, (3) inflation hold, and (4) the pressure at end-expiration (Figure 9–3). Tidal volume is the result of a pressure difference between the mouth and the alveoli and is dependent on peak inspiratory and end-expiratory pressure.[19] It is independent of inspiratory or expiratory time (Figure 9–3).

Depending on the time constant of the respiratory system (and the endotracheal tube and ventilator circuits), very short inspiratory and expiratory times may limit tidal volume delivery and completion of exhalation, respectively.

Chatburn, R. L., Primiano, F. P., and Lough, M. D.: Mechanical ventilation. *In* Lough, M. D., Chatburn, R. L., and Schrock, W. A. (eds.): *Handbook of Respiratory Care.* Chicago, Year Book Medical Publishers, 1984, pp. 73–75. **W. Carlo**

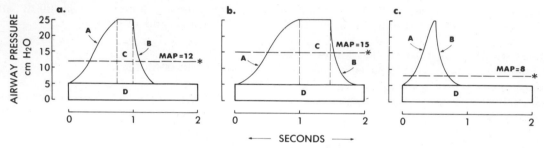

Figure 9–3. Respiratory wave forms obtained from ventilator pressure tracings, at pressures of 25/5 cm H_2O and rate of 30 breaths/minute. *a*, I/E is 1:1, inspiratory hold is 0.25 second, and mean airway pressure is moderately high, at 12 cm H_2O. *b*, I/E is reversed, 3:1, inspiratory hold is long, 0.50 second, and mean airway pressure is 15 cm H_2O. *c*, Inspiratory time is decreased; I/E is 1:3, inspiratory time is 0.5 second, and mean airway pressure is low, at 8 cm H_2O. MAP (*) = mean airway pressure. A = inspiratory phase; B = expiratory phase; C = inflation hold; D = end expiratory pressure.

Increasing end-expiratory pressure decreases tidal volume, and decreasing end-expiratory pressure increases tidal volume, when the peak inspiratory pressure is not altered. Changes in peak inspiratory pressure will have the opposite effect. Increasing tidal volume usually lowers $PaCO_2$ and improves PaO_2 and vice versa. All four elements of the respiratory cycle affect the lung volume by increasing or decreasing the mean airway (or alveolar) pressure. The area under the curve divided by the duration of the cycle is the mean airway pressure (Figure 9–3). Thus, a long inflation hold (Figure 9–3*b*) creates a high mean airway pressure and increased lung volume. A short inspiratory time and no inflation hold create a low mean airway pressure and smaller lung volume (Figure 9–3*c*). The duration of inspiration and expiration affects mean airway pressure by increasing or decreasing the area under the curve. Arterial PO_2 rises linearly with increasing mean airway pressure.[5] However, if pressure is excessive, PO_2 may fall because of overdistension of well-ventilated alveoli and because redistribution of blood flow to poorly ventilated areas of lung increases the right-to-left shunt. Figure 9–3*c* shows the effects of shortening the inspiratory time. Note that when this is done, the gas flow must be increased to reach the required inspiratory pressure and deliver the desired tidal volume. Very rapid flows may cause turbulence and further increase the mean airway pressure. If the expiratory time is shortened excessively (Figure 9–3*b*), there may be inadequate time for exhalation. This can cause gas trapping and inadvertent PEEP, which can also result in hypoxemia. This problem can be offset by increasing the expiratory

flow gradient. However, this does *not* usually change the end-expiratory pressure within the lung. The faster inspiration and expiration are achieved, the less these factors contribute to the mean alveolar pressure and to ventilation, and vice versa.

In high-frequency ventilation, inspiration and expiration become extremely short, and tidal gas exchange will be the result of a mean alveolar pressure. High-frequency ventilators are still experimental. They make use of gas exchange by diffusion, using rates of 1800–2000 breaths/minute with very low tidal volumes (often less than the dead space of the ventilator and airways) and reduced mean airway pressures.[13, 21, 30] After several hours of high-frequency ventilation, atelectasis and lung damage may occur.[30] The techniques still need to be perfected.[13] Positive pressure ventilators are usually able to achieve the mean and peak alveolar pressures necessary for tidal ventilation, but they may do so by producing high alveolar pressures, which increase the likelihood of barotrauma.[41] There may be a place for high-frequency ventilation in the management of severe pulmonary interstitial emphysema or bronchopleural fistula.[21, 30]

The improved survival rate accomplished with assisted ventilation has been accompanied by an increased incidence of pulmonary complications.

Newly developed techniques of high-frequency ventilation that deliver tidal volumes smaller than those of conventional ventilators at very fast rates may reduce barotrauma. These techniques include: (1) high-frequency positive pressure ventilation consisting of modified conventional ventilators that effectively deliver small volumes of gas at rates over 60/minute; (2) high-frequency jet ventilation that employs a solenoid valve and an injector to deliver small jets of gas at rates of approximately 100–600/minute; and (3) high-frequency oscillation and high-frequency flow interruption that consist of a piston pump or flow interruptor that generates sine or quasi-sine wave pressure changes at extremely elevated rates of up to 3000/minute or even higher. These high-frequency ventilators maintain adequate gas exchange in neonates with RDS or pulmonary interstitial emphysema at airway pressures lower than conventional ventilation and may thus be advantageous in reducing barotrauma. Clinical trials are under way to determine if high-frequency ventilation reduces acute or chronic ventilator-related lung injury.[3, 30] **W. Carlo**

Carlo, W. A., Chatburn, R. L., Martin, R. J., et al.: Decrease in airway pressure during high-frequency jet ventilation in infants with respiratory distress syndrome. J Pediatr *104*:101, 1984.

Frantz, I. D., Werthammer, J., and Stark, A. R.: High-frequency ventilation in premature infants with lung disease: adequate gas exchange at low tracheal pressure. Pediatrics *71*:483, 1983.

The technique of high-frequency ventilation (HFV) requires major changes in the concept of gas flow in the lung. Currently it is believed that by vibrating the gas column, gas exchange is promoted by a process of facilitated diffusion rather than by convection, which is the predominant mechanism of conventional IPPV. Early studies suggest that HFV may improve ventilation:perfusion matching throughout the respiratory cycle, thus permitting lower peak inflation pressures and lower inspired oxygen concentrations. Both high pressure and high oxygen have been implicated in the development of bronchopulmonary dysplasia. Although HFV is an exciting new concept, technical problems (e.g., provision of adequate humidification) and physiologic questions (e.g., what is the effect on pulmonary and cerebral blood flow) remain. Many investigative studies are required before this technique is ready for widespread use.

J. Kattwinkel

SETTING UP THE POSITIVE PRESSURE VENTILATOR

It is essential that the clinician understand the circuit, the capabilities, and the principles of the ventilator being used. Prior to starting mechanical ventilation:

1. Check that the circuit to be used is leakproof. This may be done by cycling the ventilator with a finger over the patient outlet. At this time set the pressure relief valve at the maximum pressure desired.

2. Ensure that the nebulization of inspired gas is adequate and that the heated nebulizer is functioning. Temperature gradients between the air outside the infant's incubator and inside the incubator will tend to result in condensation of water in respirator tubing. This should be caught in a water trap. Keep the volume of tubing outside the incubator minimal. Heat the tubing to avoid condensation.

3. Be aware that the assist/controlled mode is seldom used in infants.

4. Select ventilator settings suitable for the patient. There are no absolute rules. Although there has been very little assessment of the effect of altering ventilator settings on gas exchange, we recommend the following:

VOLUME-CYCLED. The tidal volume delivered by the ventilator must be adequate to normalize arterial oxygen and carbon dioxide and consist of:

- Infant's tidal volume (7 ml/kg).
- Compression loss in the ventilator tubings (if ventilator tubing volume is large, this may be appreciable). These volumes must be known either from manufacturer's instructions or preferably from direct measurement prior to using the ventilator.
- Volume losses by leaks from the tubing system around the endotracheal tube.

PRESSURE-CYCLED. The peak inflation pressure will depend on the compliance of the lungs.

- A pressure of 25/5 cm H_2O, a rate of 40/minute, and an I/E ratio of 1:1 are a reasonable starting point. This will give a mean airway pressure of approximately 12 cm H_2O.
- Lower pressures and rates should be used for apnea and for diseases in which lung compliance is normal.
- Current evidence suggests that increasing airway pressure improves oxygenation but increases the risk of pneumothorax and bronchopulmonary dysplasia.
- Frequency: Rapid (80 +) cycling frequencies may be associated with a lower PaO_2 than low cycling frequencies (30).[10,12] Frequency is closely associated with I/E ratio, which is also related to inspiratory flow rate. Optimal I/E ratios vary from patient to patient.[32] Herman and Reynolds[19] found that a progressive increase in inspiratory phase resulted in a progressive rise in PaO_2 in infants with RDS. However, very small infants (<1250 gm) often do better with rapid rates and low pressures.[3] Their mortality is improved and barotrauma reduced.[18]

We agree that Reynold's suggestions for prolonging inspiratory time constitute a valuable technique for ventilating babies with RDS. Prolonged inspiratory times allow more time for alveolar filling and thus less time for alveolar collapse. Therefore, intrapulmonary shunting decreases, and arterial oxygenation improves. However, it does not necessarily follow that because lower pressures are employed, the risk of pneumothorax is decreased. The volume of gas delivered is dependent upon not only inflation pressure but also inflation time. One is probably much more likely to encounter a pneumothorax at a pressure of 30 and an I/E of 4:1 than at the same pressure with an I/E of 1:2. Since we have begun to utilize more prolonged inspiratory times, it is our impression that although the survival from severe RDS has increased, so too has the incidence of pneumothorax and bronchopulmonary dysplasia. **J. Kattwinkel**

● Inspired oxygen should initially correspond to the oxygen necessary to maintain adequate PaO_2 (50–70 mm Hg). Effective mechanical ventilation may result in sudden reduction in oxygen requirements; hence, watch for a high PaO_2 after starting IPPV.

It is important to consider the disease process when considering initial ventilator settings. If alveolar collapse is anticipated (e.g., RDS or pneumonia), inspiratory time should be relatively long, expiratory time short, and PEEP should be added. If airway disease and air trapping are predominant (e.g., meconium aspiration syndrome), expiratory time should be long and PEEP kept relatively low. If pulmonary vascular resistance is high (e.g., persistent pulmonary hypertension of the newborn), high cycling frequencies may be required to achieve alkalosis and hence pulmonary vasodilatation. **J. Kattwinkel**

CARE OF THE VENTILATOR

After use, ensure:

1. Adequate sterilization (ideally by soaking detachable tubings in bactericidal solution or by gas sterilization of ventilator unit).

2. Maintenance by an experienced technician.

3. Routine cultures to check sterilization and mode of storage.

Endotracheal Intubation

The endotracheal tube should fit loosely enough to allow a leak of gas between tube and trachea when 10 cm H_2O inspired pressure is generated.

SIZE

If birth weight is <1250 gm, use 2.5 mm internal diameter; if 1250–2000 gm, use 3.0 mm internal diameter; if >2000 gm, use 3.5 mm internal diameter.

ORAL TUBES

The advantages of an oral endotracheal tube are the relative ease of insertion and the fact that a stylet can be used to aid insertion. Oral tubes should always be used in emer-

gency situations. The disadvantages are the increased tube mobility if the tube is inadequately taped to the upper lip, the greater difficulty in keeping the tube in position, and the tendency to distort the hard palate following prolonged oral intubation, which may cause dental problems later in life.[4]

NASOTRACHEAL TUBES

The advantage of a nasotracheal tube is the reduced likelihood of its slipping into the right main stem bronchus or esophagus. The disadvantages are trauma to the nares and nasal septum, greater difficulty in insertion of the tube, possibility of an increased number of gram-negative nasal superinfections, and potential trauma to the developing eustachian tubes and sinuses.

Nasotracheal intubation is always an elective procedure and should not be done for acute emergencies. A stylet is never used.

INTUBATION

Insertion of an endotracheal tube should be performed as a sterile procedure under a radiant heat lamp to keep the infant warm.

ORAL TUBES. Use a laryngoscope with a Miller 0 or 1 blade; visualize the glottis by leaving the head in a neutral position and inserting the blade above the epiglottis. Pull upward and outward at a 45° angle. Do not traumatize the gums and tooth buds. The heart rate should be monitored continuously, and preferably audibly and visibly on an oscilloscope, during attempts at intubation. Continuous $tcPO_2$ monitoring is invaluable.

NASOTRACHEAL TUBES. Insert the lubricated endotracheal tube through the nares until visualized in the oropharynx. Grasp the tip with a McGill forceps to guide it into the glottis. It is helpful if the endotracheal tube has been previously curved and lubricated with a nontoxic, water-soluble lubricant.

General Guidelines for Intubation

Do not make repeated attempts at intubation without allowing the infant to recover. Ventilate the infant with a bag and mask and high oxygen between attempts.

The tip of the tube should be midway between the carina and the glottis (Figure 9–4).[27] Check air entry bilaterally after inser-

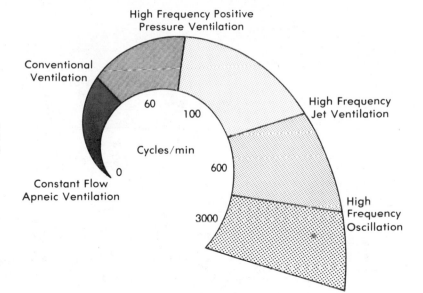

Figure 9–4. Frequency spectrum for assisted ventilation. (From Rainbow Babies and Childrens Hospital.)

tion. It is easy to allow the tube to pass into the right main stem bronchus. The position should always be checked radiologically at the completion of the procedure.

The tube should be secured so that movement of the head and neck will not dislodge it (Figures 9–5 and 9–6). Use lightweight plastic connectors to avoid kinking the tube. Do not use adapters with narrow tips, since the resistance is high.

Suctioning. This is potentially dangerous because it may result in an anoxic episode by discontinuing ventilation, extracting gas from small airways, and producing atelectasis. It may also produce lesions in the trachea at the site of the suction catheter tip. The use of a Novametrix endotracheal tube connector reduces hypoxemia during suctioning because assisted ventilation is not discontinued. However, this adapter has a very high resistance.

Suctioning should be done every hour if

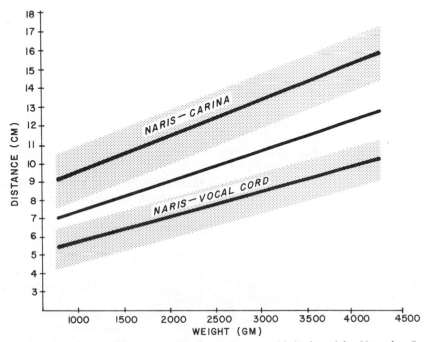

Figure 9–5. The relation of naris-carina and naris-glottis distance with body weight. Note that for oral tubes the lower line is used for mouth to mid-trachea position[11,27]

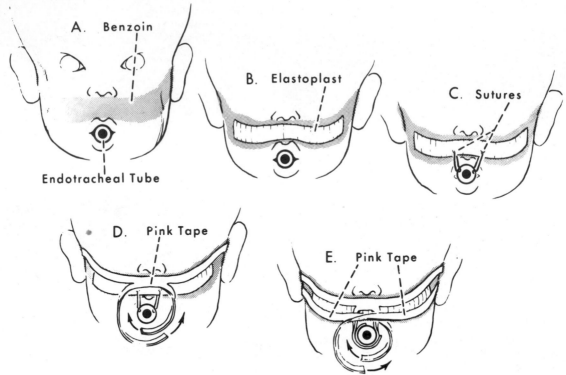

Figure 9–6. Technique for securing an oral tracheal tube. *A,* Benzoin is applied liberally from ear to ear and over the upper lip. *B,* A ¼-inch width of Elastoplast* is applied over the benzoin. *C,* A 4–0 silk suture is passed into the edge of the endotracheal tube without entering its lumen. The suture is then passed through the Elastoplast and tied so that the endotracheal tube is securely held against the upper lip. This process is repeated on the opposite side of the tube. If the suture enters the lumen of the endotracheal tube, it may obstruct passage of suction catheters. *D,* Pink tape cut in the form of an "H" is applied first to the upper edge of the Elastoplast to help secure it to the upper lip. The other "arms" of the "H" are then wrapped around the tube as shown. *E,* Single ⅜-inch strips of pink tape are then fastened to the lower edge of the Elastoplast and wound around the endotracheal tube. These help secure the lower edges of the Elastoplast to the face and lip. (From Gregory, G[16]).

*Duke Laboratories, South Norwalk, Connecticut

there are copious amounts of secretions or every 2–4 hours if the amount of secretions is sparse. Failure to suction often results in an occluded endotracheal tube and atelectasis. Use a strict sterile technique with disposable gloves and suction tubes. Allow the infant to recover between episodes of suctioning by reexpanding the lung with 20 per cent more pressure than used for routine ventilation.

Routine Instillation of Saline. This is done to facilitate removal of secretions when secretions are thick or meconium or blood has been aspirated.

Changing an Endotracheal Tube. This is only indicated if the tube becomes dislodged or occluded or if the infant outgrows it. Routine changing is *not* indicated.

Fox et al have shown that suctioning of the endotracheal tube will decrease oxygenation and pulmonary function.

We would advocate increasing inspired oxygen concentration by 10–15 per cent immediately prior to and following the period of suctioning and avoiding the practice of "routine" suctioning except as secretions warrant. **J. Kattwinkel**

MONITORING THE INFANT DURING MECHANICAL VENTILATION

When you initiate mechanical ventilation, you undertake the responsibility for the infant's gas exchange. Hence, monitoring the patient's condition is vital and requires ideally one nurse per patient for continuous observation.[16]

Frequent arterial blood gas estimations should be performed:
● Within 10 minutes of initiating mechanical ventilation.

- Within 10 minutes of altering any ventilator setting.
- Immediately, if the infant's condition changes markedly; otherwise, every 4 hours.
- The goal should be to maintain PaO_2 between 50 and 70 mm Hg, $PaCO_2$ between 35 and 45 mm Hg, and pH between 7.30 and 7.45.

Continuous monitoring with transcutaneous PCO_2 and PO_2 electrodes or a catheter electrode is invaluable during intubation, stabilization procedures, or weaning.

Changes in Blood Gas Status

1. *A sudden fall in PaO_2 accompanied by a rise in $PaCO_2$ associated with rapid clinical deterioration of the infant.* This may be due to a problem with the ventilator or with the infant. These may be differentiated by disconnecting the ventilator from the infant and by manually inflating the lungs.

If the infant's condition improves there is a ventilator problem. Check:
- Concentration of inspired oxygen going to ventilator
- Presence of leaks or disconnected tubing
- Mechanical or electric failure.

If no clinical improvement occurs with manual inflation, there is a problem with the infant. Check air entry bilaterally by auscultation, listen over the stomach, and determine the position of the heart and trachea.

If air entry is diminished bilaterally, look for the cause:
- Tube displaced into nasopharynx. There may be air entry heard over stomach, and air may be visibly escaping at the mouth or via a nasogastric tube; to check, place end under water. *Action*—Replace tube.
- Tube blocked. This occurs especially from the third day of ventilation onward owing to increased secretions. *Action*—Suction tube briefly. If this has no effect, replace the tube.
- Tension pneumothorax. Results in abdominal distension and an easily palpable liver and spleen; the condition is usually critical. Transillumination is invaluable in small infants.[24] *Action*—Emergency relief of tension pneumothorax by inserting a No. 25 scalp needle attached to a three-way stopcock and a 20 ml syringe into the third intercostal space at the midclavicular line or the fourth intercostal space at the an-

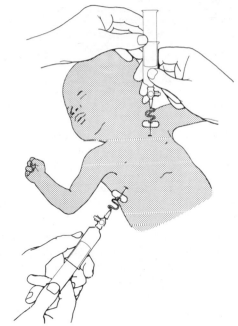

Figure 9–7. Positions for needling chest for tension pneumothorax and for chest tube positioning. (For small infants, lateral position is preferred.) (From Brady, J. P., and Lewis, K.[8])

terior axillary line. Remove air until the condition improves. Insert a chest tube and check its position with a chest radiograph (Figure 9–7).[6]

If air entry is diminished unilaterally, ascertain the cause:
- Tube in main stem bronchus. It is usually in the right main stem bronchus, producing diminution of air entry on the left. *Action*—Withdraw tube 0.5 cm–1 cm. Immediate improvement in air entry will result. Recheck position by x-ray.
- Unilateral pneumothorax.

Radiologic confirmation of clinical diagnosis is obtained if the condition of the infant warrants a delay in initiating therapy. If not, treat as for tension pneumothorax, above.

If air entry is not diminished and the infant does not improve with manual lung inflation, this suggests intraventricular or periventricular hemorrhage, pneumopericardium, convulsions, hypoglycemia, or overwhelming sepsis. It is important to note that the incidence of intraventricular and periventricular hemorrhage is greatly increased in infants who have had a pneumothorax.[26]

Airway sounds are easily transmitted across a small chest, and therefore evaluation of breath sounds can be terribly misleading in small infants. Even with "adequate" breath sounds, we would transilluminate the chest, check the placement of the endotracheal tube with a laryngoscope, and perhaps replace the endotracheal tube before attributing the problem to a nonrespiratory etiology.

J. Kattwinkel

Pneumothorax is frequently associated with pneumomediastinum, which gives a classic butterfly appearance to the thymus on the AP projection and can often be seen as a collection of air on the lateral x-ray film. The pneumomediastinum is rarely responsible for any of the debility, but does reflect the usual associated presence of the pneumothorax. Of interest also is the occasional occurrence of pneumoperitoneum as a result of forcing air through the diaphragm in the periaortic spaces. This can seriously mislead the clinician into the assumption that a ruptured viscus has occurred and abdominal surgery is indicated.

L. Stern

2. *Gradual fall in PaO$_2$ accompanied by a rise in PaCO$_2$ associated with gradual deterioration of the infant.* This suggests inappropriate ventilator settings, although the factors just outlined should be considered. A fall in PaO$_2$ suggests increasing intrapulmonary shunting due to progressive atelectasis.

To improve PaCO$_2$, increase minute ventilation by:

- Increasing peak inflation pressure by 5 cm H$_2$O (pressure-cycled ventilator)
- Increasing tidal volume by 3–5 ml (hence increasing peak inflation pressure) (volume-cycled ventilator)
- Increasing rate by 10 breaths/minute
  To improve PaO$_2$, consider:
- Increasing the end-expiratory pressure
- Decreasing the rate
- Altering I/E ratio to a longer inspiratory phase

The responses to these three maneuvers are variable, and blood gases must be obtained.

3. *Changes in PaCO$_2$ without gross changes in PaO$_2$.* A rise in PaCO$_2$ is due to increased ventilation of dead space, in either the ventilator tubings and the connectors, or "physiologic" dead space of the infant (i.e., nonperfused but ventilated alveoli).

This is an indication for an increase in overall minute volume by increasing peak inflation pressure or decreasing end tidal pressure if pressure-cycled, by increasing tidal volume if volume-cycled, or by increasing cycling frequency.

4. *A fall in PaCO$_2$ due to overventilation.* It is potentially dangerous, since it will produce a respiratory alkalosis and rise in pH. Alkalosis is associated with a fall in cardiac output, cerebral blood flow, and tissue oxygen delivery, especially if the infant is also hypotensive. Hence, it is an indication for a reduction in overall minute volume (provided oxygen-

ation is adequate). The insertion of artificial dead space to increase "dead space ventilation" is unnecessary and potentially harmful. It should always be possible to reduce total ventilation until PaCO$_2$ returns to normal.

5. *Rise in PaO$_2$ unaccompanied by changes in PaCO$_2$.* This suggests a fall in intrapulmonary shunting and reduction in degree of atelectasis. Because of the toxic effect of oxygen on lung tissue, it is generally believed that the concentration of inspired oxygen should be reduced to below 70 per cent before attempting to reduce any ventilator parameter.

Routine Care of the Infant

Remember that monitoring of blood gases is only one aspect of supportive treatment. Due attention must also be paid to temperature control, caloric and fluid intake, and metabolic balance (see Table 8–2).[16, 20, 37, 39]

Avoid excessive and unnecessary handling of the infant.

Special Instances

Pulmonary interstitial emphysema (PIE). Small infants with severe RDS and those who have PIE on x-ray may respond better to a rapid ventilating rate (60–180/min), low peak pressure (usually less than 20 cm H$_2$O), and low PEEP (less than 2 cm H$_2$O).[3]

Meconium aspiration syndrome. Infants with severe meconium aspiration syndrome and pulmonary hypertension may need very high distending pressures (50–60/4–6 cm H$_2$O), short inspiratory times, and rapid ventilating rates (60–100/min). Respiratory alkalosis appears to be of value in reducing the severe pulmonary vasoconstriction in these infants and may result in a rise in PaO$_2$. We therefore like to keep the pH at 7.45–7.55 and the PCO$_2$ at 22–30 mm Hg.[7, 8] It may be necessary to use dopamine to keep the arterial blood pressure in the normal range.

Neonatal surgery. We like to intubate the very low-birth-weight infant in the intensive care nursery and use a ventilator during surgery. In this way, inspired oxygen and inspired gas temperature can be carefully controlled. The anesthetic can be "bled" into the nebulizer in low concentrations. However, it may not be possible to ventilate patients adequately with a time-cycled flow generator during abdominal or thoracic surgery because they may not be able to compensate for the increased resistance to gas flow or the decreased lung and chest compliance caused by retractors and surgeons' hands. The only solution is to use a modified Ayres T-piece. Arterial blood gases are obtained frequently throughout surgery to maintain the infant in acid-base balance and PaO_2 within normal limits. Transcutaneous PO_2 should be monitored continuously. The infant is slowly weaned after surgery (see Weaning from Ventilator).

Drug Therapy

The use of muscle paralysis with curare, pancuronium bromide (Pavulon), or metocurine may be invaluable in infants who "fight" the ventilator when $PaCO_2$ is rising and PaO_2 is falling on "maximum" ventilation.[35] Curare may cause relaxation of the pulmonary vascular bed, resulting in increased oxygenation and improvement in gas exchange.

Muscle paralysis for babies on ventilators must be viewed with caution. The histamine-releasing effect of competitive neuromuscular blocking agents (particularly curare) can cause hypotension and, rarely, bronchospasm. Some patients may require *higher* ventilator settings after paralysis as their own respiratory efforts are eliminated. Also, a system failure (e.g., extubation, tubing disconnection, etc.) in a paralyzed patient will be rapidly fatal.

J. Kattwinkel

A recent well-controlled study suggests that elimination of a fluctuating cerebral blood flow velocity pattern induced by muscle paralysis with pancuronium reduces both the incidence and the severity of intraventricular hemorrhage.

Perlman, J. M., Goodman, S., Kreusser, K. L., et al: Reduction in intraventricular hemorrhage by elimination of fluctuating cerebral blood-flow velocity in preterm infants with respiratory distress syndrome. New Engl J Med *312*:1353, 1985.

W. Carlo

Antibiotics should be used whenever there is any question of a combination infection and RDS. A Wright stain for neutrophils may be useful in recognizing superinfection, and culture of the endotracheal tube secretions should be performed every 3 or 4 days. However, the appearance of neutrophils is also a sign of early bronchopulmonary dysplasia.[41]

Racepinephrine (Vaponefrin) has been used postextubation when there is laryngeal edema. However, if the tube is not too large, is well positioned, and is not mobile during ventilation, it is rare to have problems with the glottis following extubation.

Weaning from Ventilator

This should be attempted when the concentration of inspired oxygen is 40 per cent or less and the peak inflation pressure $\leq$20 cm H_2O. Slowly decrease the time on the venilator by reducing the ventilator rate and allowing the patient to breathe spontaneously. Initially, the infant is placed in a concentration of oxygen 5 per cent higher than that used during ventilation and allowed to breathe spontaneously through the endotracheal tube, at a CPAP level of 2–4 cm H_2O.[16]

Do not distress the infant just prior to weaning.

Extubate when CPAP has been reduced to 2 cm H_2O and the patient has been breathing spontaneously for 1–2 hours without significant changes in blood gases or clinical condition.

After extubation, a brief period of manual inflation with a face mask or mask ventilation may be helpful.

Infants less than 800 gm. These infants frequently will not tolerate endotracheal CPAP because the resistance of the 2.5 mm tube is too high. They should be weaned to 21–25 per cent oxygen, pressures of 12/2, and rates of <10 and extubated from these settings.[20]

In our experience, babies can be weaned from the ventilator much sooner if they are placed on nasal CPAP rather than directly in an oxygen hood. The resistance to gas flow and therefore inhibition of spontaneous ventilation through a small endotracheal tube may be too great for some babies. Any baby with an endotracheal tube should be given at least 2 cm H_2O CPAP, since glottic closure and grunting are prohibited by the tube. In selected babies who are particularly difficult to wean (e.g., with bronchopulmonary dysplasia), administration of theophylline may help, perhaps by lessening diaphragmatic fatigue. **J. Kattwinkel**

Editorial Comment: When weaning any infant from assisted ventilation—respirator, bagging, or CPAP—change one variable at a time and check blood gases. For example, do not reduce oxygen concentration and respirator pressure at the same time. Our practice is to reduce environmental oxygen until it is 40 per cent and then reduce pressure.

Technique for Extubation

1. The baby should receive postural drainage and suctioning of the tube followed by a few "puffs" of positive pressure to reexpand atelectatic areas of lung.

2. The tube should only be withdrawn during inspiration. This stimulates coughing, which reduces the likelihood of aspirating any material around the endotracheal tube.

3. The baby should be placed immediately in a warm humidified hood with an oxygen concentration 5–10 per cent higher than that used with endotracheal CPAP.

4. A postextubation x-ray should be obtained within 4 hours of extubation to be sure there is no collapse of the lobes. If there is, these areas should receive special attention during chest physical therapy and postural drainage.

Brief suctioning using a flexible infant bronchoscope (only with a skilled operator) can often quickly open collapsed airways.

5. Infants who have been intubated for more than a week may benefit from the use of nasal prongs or mask CPAP for 24–48 hours to reduce the incidence of right upper lobe atelectasis.

6. Postural drainage should be done every 2–4 hours as long as secretions are obtained.

SUMMARY

Survival of very low-birth-weight infants has dramatically improved with the introduction of techniques of assisted ventilation with continuous distension of the lungs. Meticulous care with placement of endotracheal tubes, frequent blood gas determinations, continuous monitoring of $tcPO_2$ and $tcPCO_2$, and careful attention to fluid, caloric, and thermal balance are essential. However, it should be understood that most of the difficulty with adequately ventilating small infants resides not in the ventilator but in the infant's lungs and airways. Remove secretions and correct atelectasis, and/or increased airway resistance. Do not look for a better ventilator. Look for a way to correct the patient's pulmonary problems. Mechanical ventilators are still not ideal, and long-term morbidity is still a major problem.

Questions

True or False

If you set a pressure-limited safety valve on a volume-cycled ventilator at 40 cm H_2O, a pneumothorax will not occur.

Although pneumothorax is particularly associated with high inflation pressures, it can occur at any time during either mechanical or spontaneous ventilation. Therefore the statement is false. The fine airways of the infant lung reduce the pressure applied to the lung tissue. Also, the noncompliant lung of the infant with RDS reduces the possibility of a pneumothorax at this pressure.

The larger the volume of ventilator tubings, the less the compression volume at any given pressure.

During positive pressure ventilation, a proportion of the gas delivered by the pump ("compression volume") does not reach the alveoli. The larger the volume of ventilator tubings, the greater the compression volume. Hence, ventilator tubings should be low volume and nondistensible. The statement is false.

Condensation of water in ventilator inspiratory tubings can be reduced by placing as much tubing as possible inside the incubator.

A temperature gradient exists between air outside and inside the incubator. Water tends to condense out at lower temperatures, and droplets will appear in tubing outside the incubator (not reaching the baby). Therefore the statement is true. In addition, care must be taken to avoid an excessive water load to the infant during humidification. Water intoxication has been described following the use of an ultrasonic nebulizer.

If a small leak develops in a ventilator, there will be adequate compensation, provided the ventilator is volume-cycled.

A volume-cycled ventilator delivers a preset volume regardless of the pressure developed in the system. Recycling will occur even if no pressure is developed and all the gas is lost through a leak. Therefore the statement is false. A pressure-cycled ventilator delivers gas until a preset pressure is attained. Hence, it is possible to compensate for a small leak (e.g., around the endotracheal tube); a large leak causes failure of cycling.

During IPPV in 80 per cent oxygen (for RDS), an increase in peak inflation pressure may increase the Pao_2 by 200 mm Hg without altering $Paco_2$ significantly.

When breathing a high concentration of oxygen, a low Pao_2 is indicative of venous admixture or shunting. This shunting is thought to occur primarily through areas of atelectatic lung. Effective positive pressure ventilation may open some of these atelectatic areas, reducing the degree of shunting, with an ensuing increase in Pao_2. However, a large right-to-left shunt will not alter $Paco_2$, since the A-V difference for CO_2 is only 4 mm Hg. Therefore $Paco_2$ will not rise, so that statement is true.

During mechanical ventilation, provided the $Paco_2$ does not change, pH will remain constant.

The pH depends on both the $Paco_2$ and the bicarbonate level. Metabolic and respiratory factors are often closely associated (e.g., a period of apnea is associated with both a rise in $Paco_2$ and a fall in Pao_2, the latter leading to tissue anoxia and anaerobic metabolism). However, they may operate quite independently. Therefore the statement is false.

(This paragraph pertains to the next three questions.) Prior to mechanical ventilation using a pressure-cycled ventilator, the Pao_2 is 30 mm Hg and the $Paco_2$ is 60 mm Hg in 100 per cent oxygen. Thirty minutes after initiating therapy, a blood gas estimation is performed.

1. The Pao_2 has risen to 140 mm Hg. This is a dangerous level, and the concentrations of inspired oxygen should be reduced at once.

In immature infants, arterial oxygen tensions in that range have been associated with retrolental fibroplasia. Since the infant is breathing 100 per cent oxygen, the lung may also be affected. Therefore the statement is true. Priority should be given to reducing the concentration of inspired oxygen in this situation rather than altering other ventilator settings. However, beware of reducing inspired oxygen concentrations too quickly. This can result in a sudden deterioration in the infant's condition possibly due to pulmonary vasoconstriction. We decrease environmental oxygen 5–10 per cent every 10–15 minutes and obtain a blood gas measurement after each change.

Five to 10 per cent every 10–15 minutes may be too fast or too slow. A transcutaneous oxygen monitor can be very useful for titrating the appropriate Fio_2 to Pao_2. A blood gas determination should then be made once the transcutaneous monitor shows that a steady state has been reached. **J. Kattwinkel**

2. Pao_2 has risen to only 35 mm Hg, and Pco_2 is still 60 mm Hg. It is advisable to switch to a volume-cycled ventilator, since the lungs are too stiff to be adequately ventilated by a pressure-cycled machine.

The statement is false. The initial ventilator settings were probably quite arbitrary and should now be adjusted to the infant's requirements. The high Pco_2 indicates hypoventilation, and an attempt should be made to increase minute ventilation by increasing peak ventilation pressure. Pao_2 can be increased by raising end-tidal pressure 2–3 cm H_2O or by increasing inspiratory time. Adjustments should be made every 10 minutes, checking blood gases until Pao_2 is > 60 mm Hg and $Paco_2$ is < 50 mm Hg.

3. Pao_2 is only 35 mm Hg and $Paco_2$ is 35 mm Hg. It might be helpful to try adding positive expiratory pressure before increasing peak inflation pressure further.

A positive expiratory pressure of 5–6 cm H_2O will help to prevent small airway closure. This may prevent atelectasis and hence reduce the degree of right-to-left shunt. Therefore the statement is true.

(This paragraph pertains to the next three questions.) A blood gas estimation is performed during mechanical ventilation in 80 per cent oxygen. There has been no change in the clinical condition of the infant since the previous estimation.

1. It is found that $Paco_2$ has changed from 36 to 24 mm Hg and pH has risen from 7.38 to 7.56. This is a sign that the infant is recovering and ventilator settings should remain unchanged.

A $Paco_2$ of 24 mm Hg suggests overventilation. The resulting alkalosis is dangerous, because it causes a reduction in cardiac output and cerebral blood flow. The $Paco_2$ should be brought back to a more physiologic range by reducing minute volume (i.e., by reducing peak inflation pressure, tidal volume, or cycling frequency). The statement is therefore false.

2. The arterial oxygen tension is 39 mm Hg, pH is 7.36, and $Paco_2$ is 35 mm Hg. The ventilator should not be changed.

$Paco_2$ and pH are satisfactory, oxygenation is unsatisfactory. Both peak inflation and end-expiratory pressure should be increased to keep tidal volume (and minute ventilation) constant and increase mean airway pressure. The statement is false.

3. The arterial oxygen tension is 46 mm Hg, pH is 7.30, and $Paco_2$ is 26 mm Hg. Although pH is within normal range, there is some degree of metabolic acidosis, which should be corrected with intravenous sodium bicarbonate.

Hyperventilation on the ventilator is compensation for a metabolic acidosis. Correction of metabolic acidosis is indicated with intravenous bicarbonate and the measures outlined above to handle the low Pco_2. Therefore the statement is true. A search should be made for the etiology of the acidosis, such as reduced cardiac output, patent ductus arteriosus, or pneumothorax. Fio_2 should also be increased.

(The following pertains to the next three questions.) During mechanical ventilation, an infant becomes cyanosed.

1. He is noted to be making very vigorous respiratory efforts with considerable intercostal and sternal retractions out of phase with the ventilator. This is a good indication for sedation and attempting to adjust the ventilator to accommodate the infant's respiratory pattern.

Although "out of phase" respiration could account for this clinical picture, an obstructed airway must first be excluded. Vigorous respiratory efforts with cyanosis suggest an obstructed endotracheal tube. Therefore the statement is false.

2. Air entry is diminished over the left lung field. The diagnosis is pneumothorax, which should be relieved immediately.

Diminution of air entry over the left lung field may be due to (1) the endotracheal tube slipping into the right main stem bronchus or (2) pneumothorax.

The procedure should be to withdraw the endotracheal tube slightly. If this fails to improve the infant's condition, a chest x-ray is indicated unless the infant is deteriorating rapidly and the left side of the chest is tympanic and the heart displaced. Emergency relief of a pneumothorax is then indicated.

3. A blood sample for gas estimation is taken immediately and resuscitative measures started.

When the blood sample is estimated 1 hour later, the results show Po_2 to be 127 mm Hg and Pco_2 to be 8 mm Hg. This suggests that the infant had been crying prior to this cyanotic spell.

The most likely explanation for these bizarre blood gas findings is that an air bubble was left in the syringe and equilibration has occurred between gas in the blood and gas in the air. In the ensuing 1 hour, the values tend to approximate the Po_2 and Pco_2 of room air. (Samples drawn for blood gases must be bubble-free, capped and iced, and analyzed immediately.) The statement is false.

After extubation following prolonged IPPV, an infant may have some stridor and copious secretions. The stridor usually decreases spontaneously.

Despite the use of nontoxic nasotracheal tubes, there is almost always some laryngeal edema. This, together with large quantities of secretions and lack of tracheal cilia, may lead to some degree of upper airway obstruction, which will decrease in 2–3 days. Therefore the statement is true.

REFERENCES

1. Ahlström, H., Jonson, B., and Svenningsen, N. W.: Continuous positive airways pressure treatment by a face chamber in idiopathic respiratory distress syndrome. Arch Dis Child *51*:13, 1976.
2. Allen, L. P., Reynolds, E. O. R., Rivers, R. P. A., et al: Controlled trial of continuous positive airway pressure given by face mask for hyaline membrane disease. Arch Dis Child *52*:373, 1977.
3. Bland, R. D., Kim, M. H., Light, M. J., et al: High frequency mechanical ventilation in severe hyaline membrane disease. An alternative treatment? Crit Care Med *8*:275, 1980.
4. Boice, J., Krous, H., and Foley, J.: Gingival and dental complications of orotracheal intubation. J Am Med Assoc *236*:957, 1976.
5. Boros, S. J., and Campbell, K.: A comparison of the effects of high-frequency low tidal volume and low-frequency high tidal volume mechanical ventilation. J Pediatr *97*:108, 1980.
6. Boros, S. J., and Reynolds, J. W.: Hyaline membrane disease treated with early nasal end-expiratory pressure: one year's experience. Pediatrics *56*:218, 1975.
7. Brady, J. P., and Goldman, S. L.: Management of meconium aspiration syndrome. *In* Thibeault, D., and Gregory, G. (eds.): *Neonatal Pulmonary Care.* 2nd ed. Menlo Park, Addison-Wesley, 1984.
8. Brady, J. P., and Lewis, K.: Newborn emergencies. *In* Pascoe, D. J., and Grossman, M. (eds.): *Quick Reference to Pediatric Emergencies.* 3rd ed. Philadelphia, J. B. Lippincott, 1984.
9. Cabatu, E. E., and Brown, E. G.: Thoracic transillumination: aid in the diagnosis and treatment of pneumopericardium. Pediatrics *64*:958, 1979.
10. Cave-Smith, P., Daily, W. J. R., Fletcher, G., et al: Mechanical ventilation of newborn infants. I. The effect of rate and pressure on arterial oxygenation of infants with respiratory distress syndrome. Pediatr Res *3*:244, 1969.
11. Coldiron, J. S.: Estimation of nasotracheal tube length in neonates. Pediatrics *41*:823, 1968.
12. Daily, W. J. R., and Cave-Smith, P.: Mechanical ventilation in the newborn infant. Part I. Curr Probl Pediatr *1*:16, 1971.
13. deLemos, R. A., Null, D. M., Jr., and Meredith, K. S.: High-frequency ventilation: panacea or problem? Pediatrics *69*:240, 1982.
14. Drummond, W. H., Gregory, G. A., Heymann, M. A., et al: The independent effects of hyperventilation, tolazoline, and dopamine on infants with persistent pulmonary hypertension. J Pediatr *98*:603, 1981.
15. Goldman, S. L., Brady, J. P., and Dumpit, F. M.: Increased work of breathing associated with nasal prongs. Pediatrics *64*:160, 1979.
16. Gregory, G. A.: Respiratory care of newborn infants. Pediatr Clin North Am *19*:311, 1972.
17. Gregory, G. A., Kitterman, J. A., Phibbs, R. H., et al: Treatment of the idiopathic respiratory-distress syndrome with continuous positive airway pressure. N Engl J Med *284*:1333, 1971.
18. Heicher, D. A., Kasting, D. S., and Harrod, J. R.: Prospective clinical comparison of two methods for mechanical ventilation of neonates: rapid rate and short inspiratory time versus slow rate and long inspiratory time. J Pediatr *98*:957, 1981.
19. Herman, S., and Reynolds, E. O. R.: Methods for improving oxygenation in infants mechanically ventilated for severe hyaline membrane disease. Arch Dis Child *48*:612, 1973.
20. Hirata, T., Epcar, J. T., Walsh, A., et al: Survival and outcome of infants 501 to 750 gm: a six-year experience. J Pediatr *102*:741, 1983.
21. James, L. S.: High frequency ventilation for immature infants. Report of a conference March 2–4, 1982. Pediatrics *71*:280, 1983.
22. Kattwinkel, J., Fleming, D., Cha, C., et al: A device

for administration of continuous positive airway pressure by the nasal route. Pediatrics 52:131, 1973.

23. Krouskop, R. W., Brown, E. G., and Sweet, A. Y.: The early use of continuous positive airway pressure in the treatment of idiopathic respiratory distress syndrome. J Pediatr 87:263, 1975.

24. Kuhns, L. R., Bednarek, F. J., Wyman, M. L., et al: Diagnosis of pneumothorax or pneumomediastinum in the neonate by transillumination. Pediatrics 56:355, 1975.

25. Levene, M. I.: Hazard of nasal continuous positive airway pressure. Lancet 1:1157, 1977.

26. Lipscomb, A. P., Thorburn, R. J., Reynolds, E. O. R., et al: Pneumothorax and cerebral haemorrhage in preterm infants. Lancet 1:114, 1981.

27. Loew, A., and Thibeault, D. W.: A new and safe method to control the depth of endotracheal intubation in neonates. Pediatrics 54:506, 1974.

28. Lucey, J. F. (ed.): Problems of Neonatal Intensive Care Units. Report of 59th Ross Conference on Pediatric Research. Columbus, Ohio, Ross Laboratories, 1969.

29. Mansfield, P. B., Graham, C. B., Beckwith, J. B., et al: Pneumopericardium and pneumomediastinum in infants and children. J Pediatr Surg 8:691, 1973.

30. Marchak, B. E., Thompson, W. K., Duffty, P., et al: Treatment of RDS by high-frequency oscillatory ventilation: a preliminary report. J Pediatr 99:287, 1981.

31. Novogroder, M., MacKuanying N., Eidelman, A. I., et al: Nasopharyngeal ventilation in respiratory distress syndrome. J Pediatr 82:1059, 1973.

32. Owen-Thomas, J. B., Ulan, O. A., and Swyer, P. R.: The effect of varying inspiratory gas flow rate on arterial oxygenation during IPPV in the respiratory distress syndrome. Br J Anaesth 40:493, 1968.

33. Pape, K. E., Armstrong, D. L., and Fitzhardinge, P. M.: Central nervous system pathology associated with mask ventilation in the very low birth weight infant: a new etiology for intracerebellar hemorrhages. Pediatrics 58:473, 1976.

34. Peabody, J. L., Gregory, G. A., Willis, M. M., et al: Transcutaneous oxygen tension in sick infants. Am Rev Respir Dis 118:83, 1978.

35. Pollitzer, M. J., Reynolds, E. O. R., Shaw, D. G., et al: Pancuronium during mechanical ventilation speeds recovery of lungs of infants with hyaline membrane disease. Lancet 1:346, 1981.

36. Rhodes, P. G., and Hall, R. T.: Continuous positive airway pressure delivered by face mask in infants with the idiopathic respiratory distress syndrome: a controlled study. Pediatrics 52:1, 1973.

37. Shaw, J. L. C.: Parenteral nutrition in the management of sick low birth weight infants. Pediatr Clin North Am 20:333, 1973.

38. Simbruner, G., and Gregory, G. A.: Performance of neonatal ventilators: the effects of changes in resistance and compliance. Crit Care Med 9:509, 1981.

39. Spitzer, A. R., Fox, W. W., and Delivoria-Papadopoulos, M.: Maximum diuresis—a factor in predicting recovery from respiratory distress syndrome and development of bronchopulmonary dysplasia. J Pediatr 98:476, 1981.

40. Turner, T., Evans, J., and Brown, J. K.: Monoparesis: complication of constant positive airways pressure. Arch Dis Child 50:128, 1975.

41. Workshop on bronchopulmonary dysplasia. J Pediatr 95(Suppl):815, 1979.

10

Problems in Metabolic Adaptation: Glucose, Calcium, and Magnesium

ROBERT M. KLIEGMAN
MICHAEL K. WALD

These infants are remarkable not only because like foetal versions of Shadrach, Meshach and Abednego, they emerge at least alive from within the fiery metabolic furnace of diabetes mellitus, but because they resemble one another so closely that they might well be related. They are plump, sleek, liberally coated with vernix caseosa, full-faced and plethoric. . . . They convey a distinct impression of having had such a surfeit of both food and fluid pressed upon them by an insistent hostess that they desire only peace so that they may recover from their excesses. And on the second day their resentment of the slightest noise improves the analogy while their trembling anxiety seems to speak of intrauterine indiscretions of which we know nothing.

JAMES W. FARQUHAR,
THE CHILD OF THE DIABETIC WOMAN*

The newborn emerges from a uterine environment where glucose, calcium, and magnesium have been continuously provided and fetal plasma levels closely regulated by maternal metabolic homeostasis and placental exchange. Abrupt termination of supply at birth requires profound changes in energy and mineral metabolism, depending upon regulatory mechanisms that are immature.

*Farquhar, J. W.: The child of the diabetic woman. Arch Dis Child *34*:76, 1959.

The result is rapid changes in plasma glucose and calcium during the first days of life. The infant who is premature, growth retarded, stressed, or born to a diabetic mother is at increased risk for problems with homeostasis and can develop hypoglycemia or hypocalcemia.

Historically, glucose and calcium problems have undergone similar evolutions in recognition and understanding of them. To summarize:

1. Initial identification of hypoglycemia and hypocalcemia as infrequent neonatal emergencies requiring dramatic intensive treatment.

2. Broad surveys with better analytic methods showing glucose and calcium problems to be very common, and frequently unrecognized, in high-risk infants.

3. Changing routines of care, with prevention, early identification, and metabolic support of the sick newborn, which has made severe hypoglycemia and hypocalcemia infrequent problems.

This chapter outlines the basis for, and types of, glucose and mineral disturbances commonly seen in neonates. Emphasis is on identification of infants at risk for these common problems and on anticipatory management. Differential diagnosis of more unusual and profound disorders is then discussed.

The reader will note an overlap in pathogenic factors (prematurity, maternal diabetes, asphyxia, etc.), which frequently cause glucose and calcium problems to coexist.

GLUCOSE

FETAL AND NEONATAL ENERGY METABOLISM[1, 2, 5, 9–11, 17, 22, 23, 27, 32, 40]

A composite picture of fetal and neonatal fuel metabolism has emerged from studies in animals[1] and humans. Fetal energy consumption is high, deriving from growth needs and energy storage as well as metabolic maintenance. The fetus receives energy continuously as glucose, lactate, free fatty acids, ketones, and surplus amino acids. Hepatic gluconeogenesis from lactate may occur in utero and is certainly active at birth. Gluconeogenesis from alanine has been reported shortly after birth.[17] Neither fatty acids nor ketones supply significant energy in utero in normal states of maternal nutrition.

Energy is stored rapidly near term. Fat storage exceeds 100 calories/day in the ninth month. Glycogen stores, a vital source of energy in the first hours of life, rise toward term to reach about 5 per cent by weight in liver and up to 4 per cent in heart muscle. These energy stores are compromised by prematurity and by intrauterine growth retardation. Perinatal anoxia can particularly diminish glycogen stores.

Insulin appears in the fetal pancreas and plasma by 12 weeks' gestation. There is a poor insulin response to glucose infusion early in gestation and a blunted response near term. Insulin does not cross the placenta.

In the normal fetus, insulin is permissive in the accumulation of hepatic glycogen stores. The presence of maternal hyperglycemia and fetal hyperinsulinemia as seen in the infant of a diabetic mother (IDM) is associated with macrosomia and elevated liver glycogen and total body fat stores. Macrosomia in the presence of fetal hyperinsulinemia without maternal hyperglycemia is seen with Beckwith's syndrome and in the rare infants with nesidioblastosis, suggesting that fetal insulin and *not maternal hyperglycemia* may be the important growth-promoting factor. Furthermore, infants born with pancreatic aplasia and those with transient neonatal diabetes mellitus have little or no insulin present and demonstrate severe intrauterine growth retardation, suggesting that insulin is an important hormone for fetal growth.

At birth, cold stress, work of respiration, and muscle activity all cause increased energy demands. The newborn must now call upon stored fuels to defend blood glucose.

The first response is rapid glycogenolysis; hepatic glycogen falls to low levels within 24 hours. Because the newborn has a two-fold greater basal fasting glucose utilization than the adult, gluconeogenesis must supplement glycogenolysis.[22] Lipolysis begins at birth, and plasma free fatty acids treble, subsequently remaining high. The respiratory quotient then drops to less than 0.8 during the first day as most tissues switch to burning fat. High growth hormone, glucagon, and catecholamine levels may help this fat mobilization.

Neonatal catecholamine secretion is such that there is very little epinephrine but a great preponderance of norepinephrine. Accordingly, catecholamine-induced glycogenolysis would be expected to be minimal.

L. Stern

The brain requires continued glucose supply. Hepatic glucose production in fasted healthy newborns is 4 mg/kg/min. The additional energy comes from fat metabolism.[22] Brain metabolism may be supported only in part by the oxidation of ketones and lactate.[23]

Blood glucose at birth, transported by facilitative diffusion, is 60–70 per cent of the simultaneous maternal level. Glucose then falls over 1–2 hours, stabilizes at a minimum of 35–40 mg/dl, and rises by 6 hours to 45–60 mg/dl in healthy unstressed newborns (see "normal" curve, Figure 10–1). In fasting premature infants, glucose averages 40–45 mg/dl in the first 24 hours. With intravenous glucose or early feeding, higher average values (60–70 mg/dl) are seen (Figure 10–2).

METHODOLOGY—A FEW PITFALLS[9]

Sampling Problems. Capillary samples from unwarmed heels may lead to underestimation of venous glucose due to stasis. Glucose level falls as much as 18 mg/dl/hour at room temperature while awaiting analysis. Thus all samples should be immediately placed on ice. Plasma glucose exceeds whole blood glucose by 15 per cent, more when hematocrit is very high.

Analysis Problems. True glucose or true hexose methods are essential in newborns;

FUEL METABOLISM IN INFANTS OF "CONTROLLED" DIABETIC MOTHERS

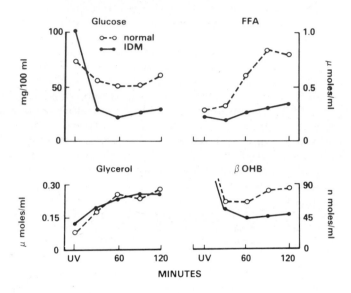

Figure 10–1. Glucose, free fatty acids (FFA), glycerol, and beta-hydroxybutyrate (BOHB) in normal infants (o---o) and infants of diabetic mothers (IDM) (●---●). Note that not only does blood glucose decline more abruptly in the IDM, but FFA and ketones rise less. With more time the blood glucose spontaneously rises over the next 4–6 hours.[34]

Figure 10–2. Plot of mean blood glucose as a function of age in both IV and fasted groups. Bars indicate range of 1 standard deviation.[27]

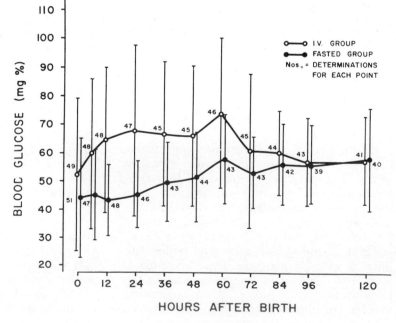

plasma non–glucose reducing substances are high. Fortunately, specific methods (glucose oxidase or AutoAnalyzer) are now standard in almost all laboratories.

Dextrostix. Used with the Eyetone Reflectance Meter,* Dextrostix have achieved a generally satisfactory precision for *screening* and following newborn glucose levels, *provided* they are fresh, the instrument properly functioning and calibrated, the blood spot generous, and the operator experienced and careful. Used otherwise, Dextrostix can give disastrous false reassurance. At least one or two laboratory glucose determinations should be done as a check with any established glucose problem.[4, 16]

Amen. It has been our experience as well that such reliance on Dextrostix alone has often led not only to difficulty but on occasion to dire consequences.

L. Stern

Hypoglycemia

Definition

Blood glucose in newborns should be maintained above 40 mg/dl.

The definition of hypoglycemia proposed by Cornblath et al[9, 10] is two whole blood glucose values less than 20 mg/dl in preterm infants and two whole blood glucose values less than 30 mg/dl in full-term infants less than 72 hours old. After this time 40 mg/dl is the accepted lower limit of normal. If plasma is measured, the lower limits are 25, 35, and 45 mg/dl, respectively. These recommendations are the result of statistical analyses of many blood glucose values, with approximately only 2 per cent of the populations having values below these levels. Compatible symptoms relieved by glucose administration at higher glucose levels should also be considered as hypoglycemia.

Symptoms[9, 23]

Hypoglycemia in newborns is often asymptomatic but can cause jitteriness or convulsions; apathy, hypotonia, refusal to suck, apnea, congestive heart failure, or cyanosis; high-pitched cry or abnormal eye movements; or temperature instability with hypothermia. In small sick infants, symptoms may easily be missed (Table 10–1.)

*Ames Co., Elkhart, Indiana.

TABLE 10–1 NEONATAL SYMPTOMATIC HYPOGLYCEMIA IN 56 INFANTS[10]

Clinical Manifestations	No.	Presenting Sign
Tremors ("jitteriness")	42	20
Cyanosis	43	19
Convulsions	29	9
Apnea, irregular respiration	23	6
Apathy	16	2
Cry—high pitched or weak	10	1
Limpness	13	4
Refusal to eat	5	1
Eye rolling	2	2

Age of Onset (hours)

<6	6–24	24–48	48–72	>72
8	6	18	18	6

Many newborns with one or more of these symptoms are normoglycemic and have another problem (Table 10–2). Hypoglycemia must therefore always be confirmed chemically and by response to treatment.

TABLE 10–2 DIFFERENTIAL DIAGNOSIS IN NEONATE WITH EPISODES OF TREMORS, CYANOSIS, CONVULSIONS, APNEA, IRREGULAR RESPIRATION, APATHY, HIGH-PITCHED OR WEAK CRY, LIMPNESS, REFUSAL TO FEED, EYE ROLLING[10]

Central nervous system
  Congenital defect
  Birth injury, anoxia
  Infection
  Kernicterus

Sepsis

Heart disease
  Congenital
  Acquired
  Arrhythmias

Iatrogenic
  Drugs to mother
  Overheating

Adrenal hemorrhage

Polycythemia

Metabolic
  Hypocalcemia
  Hyponatremia
  Hypernatremia
  Pyridoxine dependency
  Magnesium deficiency
  Uremia

Neonatal Symptomatic Hypoglycemia

Transient Neonatal Hypoglycemia[2, 11, 25, 27, 32, 40]

This syndrome is the most common type of hypoglycemia in an intensive care nursery. It occurs in low-birth-weight infants, particularly in those with intrauterine growth retardation. Males are more susceptible. The smaller of discordant twins is frequently affected. Maternal toxemia, perinatal asphyxia, hypothermia, and respiratory distress all increase the incidence. It may occur early, within 1–2 hours of birth, or classically later during the first week of life. Asymptomatic patients exceed those with symptoms.

The pathogenesis involves multiple factors affecting glucose supply and demand: low total body energy reserves; high energy requirement—particularly a large, glucose-requiring brain; and inordinate energy demands imposed by disease. There is an association with CNS injury or anomaly, which may reflect a subtle control problem (Table 10–1).

Hypoglycemia should be *anticipated* and preventable in this large group of infants, which will include most admissions to the intensive care nursery. Providing caloric support with early feeding or intravenous glucose by age 2–4 hours and maintaining continuous energy supply through the neonatal period dramatically reduce the incidence of hypoglycemia.[27] Such support should provide, at a minimum, glucose at rates normally generated by the liver of a healthy newborn: 4–9 mg/kg/min. Therapeutic measures that reduce energy needs also help.

With such support, hypoglycemia will be uncommon, but high-risk infants should still be screened for hypoglycemia at intervals of 1–2 hours initially and then 2–4 hours until their condition is definitely stabilized.

Hyperinsulinemic Hypoglycemia

INFANTS OF DIABETIC MOTHERS.[15, 22, 23, 28, 34, 35] Hypoglycemia occurs regularly in infants of diabetic mothers soon after birth, with the nadir at 1–2 hours of age frequently below 10 mg/dl (see Figure 10–1). Spontaneous rise in glucose usually follows, reaching acceptable levels by age 4–6 hours. Very few IDMs become symptomatic. Infants of gestational diabetic mothers have a less dramatic fall in glucose.

Fluctuating maternal hyperglycemia results in fetal hyperglycemia, pancreatic beta cell hyperplasia, and hyperinsulinism. After birth, hyperinsulinemia persists, as evidenced by accelerated utilization of exogenous glucose and diminished endogenous glucose production.[22] Furthermore free fatty acids and ketones are low (see Figure 10–1).[34]

Hyperinsulinism may not totally explain the hypoglycemia. Glucagon and catecholamine levels and responses may be low.

Careful metabolic control of pregnant diabetics, with prevention of hyperglycemia in labor, ameliorates excess fetal weight and helps prevent perinatal deaths but may not prevent neonatal hypoglycemia.[28] Early oral feeding is both prophylactic and therapeutic.

Beware of hypoglycemia following exchange transfusion with ACD-preserved blood because of the hyperglycemia induced by this procedure.

Additional problems of the IDM are listed in Table 10–3.

OTHER SYNDROMES.[12, 14, 21, 24, 36, 49]

Erythroblastosis. Infants with erythroblastosis show islet cell hyperplasia, increased cord blood insulin, and hypoglycemia both shortly after birth and reactive following exchange transfusion. The severity of the problem relates inversely to cord hemoglobin level.[36]

The etiology of the hyperinsulinemia in severe erythroblastosis is still not completely understood, although it is clearly related to the degree of anemia (i.e., the severity of the erythroblastosis itself). One proposal that bears consideration is that the glutathione released as a product of broken-down red cells occurring in intrauterine hemolysis acts as a stimulus toward insulin production and release in the fetus.

ACD-preserved blood contains 300 mg/dl of glucose. As a result insulin production rises throughout the exchange. At its termination, when the glucose load is suddenly withdrawn, there is continued production of insulin with a resultant hypoglycemic fall, usually at about 2 hours after exchange. Substitution of heparin as the anticoagulant may result in hypoglycemia as well. There is very little glucose in heparinized blood, since no glucose is added in preparation of the anticoagulant mixture. Characteristically, however, the hypoglycemia occurs during the exchange transfusion and not following it, as it does with ACD blood.   **L. Stern**

Islet Cell Dysplasias (nesidioblastosis and islet cell adenoma). These infants have a primary disorder of islet cell formation with hyperinsulinism. Their hypoglycemia tends to be profound, symptomatic, unremitting, resistant to virtually all medical management, and best handled by surgical removal of most or all abnormal islet tissue. Hyperinsulinemia may be difficult to document. Plasma ketones, free fatty acids, branch chain amino acids, and the insulin/glucose ratio may help establish the diagnosis.[12, 21, 24]

TABLE 10–3 PATHOPHYSIOLOGY OF MORBIDITY AND MORTALITY OF THE IDM

Problem	Pathophysiology
Fetal demise	Acute placental failure? Hyperglycemia–lactic acidosis–hypoxia?
Macrosomia	Hyperinsulinism
RDS	Insulin antagonism of cortisol Variant surfactant biochemical pathways
Wet lung syndrome	Cesarean section
Hypoglycemia	↓ Glucose and fat mobilization
Polycythemia	Erythropoietic "macrosomia"? Mild fetal hypoxia? ↓ O_2 delivery to fetus—HbA_{1c}?
Hypocalcemia	↓ Neonatal parathyroid hormone ↑ Calcitonin?
Hyperbilirubinemia	↑ Erythropoietic mass ↑ Bilirubin production Immature hepatic conjugation? Oxytocin induction
Congenital malformations	Hyperglycemia? Genetic linkage? Insulin as teratogen? Vascular accident?
Renal vein thrombosis	Polycythemia? Dehydration?
Neonatal small left colon syndrome	Immature GI motility?
Cardiomyopathy	Reversible septal hypertrophy ↑ Glycogen? ↑ Muscle?
Family psychologic stress	High-risk pregnancy Fear of diabetes in infant

Adapted from Kliegman, R. M., and Fanaroff, A. A.: Developmental metabolism and nutrition. *In* Gregory, G. A. (ed.): *Pediatric Anesthesiology.* New York, Churchill Livingstone, 1983.

Beckwith's Syndrome (or hyperplastic fetal visceromegaly). This is associated with macroglossia and umbilical hernia.[8]

Maternal Drugs (e.g., beta sympathomimetics, beta blockers, chlorpropamide). In chlorpropamide treatment, hypoglycemia may be prolonged for days; exchange transfusion may be helpful.[49]

Other Hypoglycemia Syndromes

Hyperviscosity. An increased rate of glucose disposal without hyperinsulinemia is part of the syndrome of hyperviscosity; it responds to exchange transfusion to reduce hematocrit.

Failure of glycogen storage or release, gluconeogenic blocks, galactose or fructose intolerance, carnitine deficiency, congenital heart disease, and endocrine deficiencies. These disorders are all very rare.[32]

Treatment of Hypoglycemia

Prophylactic care (to be instituted as soon as an infant is determined "at risk") consists of early oral or enteral tube feeding if appropriate or 10 per cent dextrose and water, IV 70–80 ml/kg in the first 24 hours increasing to 100–120 ml/kg/24 hours thereafter (4–5 mg, increasing to 7–8 mg glucose/kg/min). Glucose infusion should be continuous and steady, by pump, and continued until replaced calorically by enteral feeding.

Treatment is indicated for all hypoglycemic infants. Asymptomatic infants with transient hypoglycemia and *no* other medical illness may be given enteric D5W or milk.

Blood glucose should be monitored every 30 minutes to determine a response. If glucose does not rise or if enteric alimentation is contraindicated, intravenous glucose, 4–5 mg/kg/min, should begin. If symptoms are present, a "minibolus" of 2 ml/kg of D10W should be infused to prevent excessive hyperglycemia and rebound hypoglycemia (Figure 10–3). This should be followed by 8 mg/kg/min of glucose together with vigilant blood glucose monitoring. The minibolus and infusion should be adequate for almost all infants. However, on rare occasions refractory hypoglycemic may require as much as 20 mg/kg/min in addition to hydrocortisone, 10/mg/kg/day bid. More severely ill patients may require somatostatin plus glucagon replacement to alleviate hyperinsulinemic hypoglycemia. Diazoxide has also benefited some of these patients.

Additional or alternative treatment

- Reduce energy needs: correct acidosis, place infant in neutral thermal environment, etc.
- Monitor treatment at least half-hourly until the infant's condition is stable.
- Titrate glucose infusion. Consider sepsis. Avoid iatrogenic hyperinsulinism from arterial glucose infusion into the pancreatic artery.

The use of a constant infusion pump when glucose is being delivered for therapeutic purposes in the newborn is of critical importance. It has been our experience that most of the so-called "intractable" hypoglycemic episodes are in fact due to an inconstant rate of delivery and can be either corrected or ameliorated if the infusion rate is kept constant. In the absence of an absolutely constant infusion rate, glucose delivery and its reactive insulin response become out of phase with each other with resultant wide swings to both hypoglycemic and hyperglycemic levels. **L. Stern**

My bias is that it is relatively easy to maintain normoglycemia with early intervention. When an infant of a diabetic mother has serum glucose concentrations that fall below 40 mg/dl, early institution of constant glucose infusion of 4–8 mg/kg/min is very effective. If the serum glucose is not raised in half an hour on 4 mg/kg/min, the dose is raised to 6 mg/kg/min; if that does not increase the serum glucose in another half hour, it can be raised to 8 mg/kg/min. It is rare, with this management, to need any "bolus" glucose infusions or other therapeutic agents. Prevention and/or early intervention appears to be the key in this equation.

Tsang, R. C., Ballard, J., and Braun, C.: The infant of the diabetic mother: today and tomorrow. Clin Obstet Gynecol *24*:125, 1981.

R. Tsang

Prognosis

Symptomatic hypoglycemia can cause specific central nervous system damage. It commonly occurs in sick small infants with other factors affecting outcome, such as anoxia or severe intrauterine malnutrition. Infants with hypoglycemia with seizures have the poorest outcome.

Survivors of symptomatic neonatal hypoglycemia have shown a 30–50 per cent incidence of neurologic impairment and a 10 per cent incidence of recurrent hypoglycemia. Infants with asymptomatic hypoglycemia do well. Infants with Beckwith's syndrome or with inborn metabolic errors do poorly as a group.

Prompt diagnosis and treatment of hypoglycemia should prevent CNS injury from this cause.

Hyperglycemia[13, 23, 30, 33]

Hyperglycemia (glucose greater than 150 mg/dl) is a common, serious, iatrogenic problem of very immature infants on intravenous support. One cause appears to be the reduced insulin response to glucose characteristic of extreme immaturity. Hepatic glucose release also may fail to decrease when exogenous glucose is given. Most affected infants are also stressed by respiratory, infectious, or other metabolic problems. Thus, catecholamines may further raise glucose levels and inhibit glucose use and insulin release. In anticipating hyperglycemia, four factors are paramount.

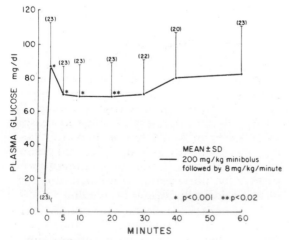

Figure 10–3. Minibolus therapy of neonatal hypoglycemia achieves euglycemia without excessively high glucose levels, which may further stimulate insulin release and later result in rebound hypoglycemia.[25]

- Immaturity: infant almost always below 30 weeks' gestation and 1.0 kg birth weight.
- Age: usually less than 3 days.
- Glucose infusion rates: exceed 8 mg/kg/min (equivalent to 10 per cent glucose at 100 mg/kg/24 hr).
- Septicemia: bacterial and fungal.

Hyperglycemia can cause at least two serious secondary problems. Osmotic changes (glucose 450 mg/dl equivalent to additional 24 mOsm/1) can cause brain volume change because of fluid shifts and may cause intraventricular hemorrhage. Glycosuria may increase renal water and electrolyte losses.

Treatment and prevention are effected by adjusting the glucose infusion rate to that tolerated by each individual infant. Rates of 4–8 mg/kg/min, previously suggested, are *usually* tolerated. Five per cent or DW2½ may be needed. Occasionally insulin infusion of 0.001–0.01 U/kg/min is indicated.[23] Monitoring (Dextrostix, urine glucose) is crucial.

It is important to stress the use of glucose calculations expressed as mg/kg/min since variations in either volume or sugar content result in variations in actual delivery of glucose to the infant. Many iatric effects of hyperglycemia and hypoglycemia in small infants have been caused by alterations in fluid volume delivery or glucose content without realizing the impact on actual glucose delivery to the infant.

If one is to use DW2½ per cent, one has to be very careful about osmolarity, since this solution is hypoosmolar and newborn red cells may be more fragile and susceptible to hemolysis. Use of this solution, therefore, requires the use of concomitant saline correction for osmolar defects. Because of concern for hypoosmolar hemolysis, I prefer to avoid the use of this solution and either reduce the volume of delivery or, in unusual circumstances of intractable hyperglycemia, institute concomitant insulin infusion. However, with infusion rates described above and careful monitoring of serum glucose measurements, fortunately the incidence of hyperglycemia is markedly reduced. **R. Tsang**

Transient Neonatal Diabetes[30, 33]

This is a rare disorder. Most infants are at or near term, with marked intrauterine malnutrition. Weight loss, dehydration, hyperglycemia, and occasional ketosis appear at a few days of age. Treatment is with insulin, usual daily dose 2–6 units. The diabetic state resolves in a few days to weeks, glucose metabolism is subsequently normal, and prognosis is good.

CALCIUM AND HYPOCALCEMIA

FETAL AND NEONATAL CALCIUM METABOLISM[6, 18, 39, 41, 43, 47]

The placenta actively transports calcium to the fetus and maintains fetal total and ionized calcium levels about 1 mg/dl above the respective maternal levels. Between 28 weeks' gestation and term, fetal weight triples, but calcium content quadruples as bone mineral density progressively increases (Figure 10–4). Fetal acquisition of calcium averages 150 mg/kg/day throughout this period.

Placental active transport allows fetal calcification to proceed normally. The calcium drain causes a modest drop in maternal calcium levels near term. Maternal parathyroid activity, 1,25-dihydroxyvitamin D, calcium absorption, and calcium mobilization from bone are all increased. Parathyroid hormone and calcitonin do not cross the placenta while 25-hydroxyvitamin D crosses.[47]

At birth, the rapid calcium supply is interrupted. Although the premature baby has skeletal reserves of calcium, the maintenance of serum calcium requires rapid changes in endocrine function and in the equilibrium between serum and bone. The factors affect-

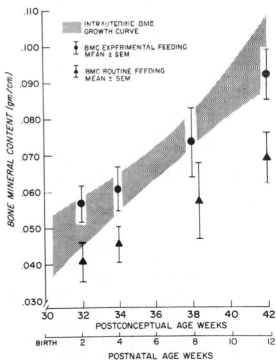

Figure 10–4. Hatched area is in utero rate of bone mineral content, depicting progressive bone mineralization during gestation until term. The symbol (▲) represents premature infants fed Similac 20 who have diminished bone mineral accumulation in contrast to (●) infants fed formula with calcium (1260 mg/l), phosphorus (630 mg/l), and vitamin D (1000 U/l) who have intrauterine rates of bone mineralization. These latter infants received 220–250 mg of calcium/kg/day and 110–125 mg of phosphorus/kg/day. The calcium intake exceeds the in utero rate of calcium accumulation (150 mg/kg/day), possibly as a result of fecal losses.[43]

ing calcium in the neonate can be summarized as follows.

1. Parathyroid hormone mobilizes calcium from bone, promotes calcium absorption from the gut, and increases renal phosphate excretion. Levels are low in cord blood, suppressed by the mild hypercalcemia caused by placental transport. Postnatally, even with hypocalcemia as a stimulus, parathyroid hormone remains low for the first 2 days, longer in prematures. Parathyroid response usually becomes effective by about 3–4 days.

2. Vitamin D is required for effective parathyroid hormone action on both bone and gut. Newborn stores are adequate, except in late winter and early spring or with maternal dietary inadequacy. Levels of 25-hydroxyvitamin D vary directly with gestational age, while its conversion to 1,25-dihydroxyvitamin D may be slow in prematures.[47]

3. Calcitonin inhibits calcium mobilization from bone. Levels are high in neonates and are further raised by asphyxia and prematurity. Unusually elevated calcitonin levels may relate directly to the incidence of hypocalcemia.

4. Serum phosphate rises after birth, even more so after birth asphyxia.

5. "Stress" factors introduced by perinatal illness are discussed later in relation to early neonatal hypocalcemia.

There is normally a fall in serum calcium in the first hours after birth, continuing for 24–48 hours and then stabilizing. Levels of total and ionized calcium are then about 8.0–9.0 and 3.5–4.0 mg/dl, respectively, and

subsequently rise gradually. By 1 week of age, breast-fed infants achieve a total calcium of 10.0 ± 1.0 mg/dl and phosphorus of 6.5 ± 1.0 mg/dl. In contrast, infants fed commercial formulae show calcium levels 1 mg/dl lower, phosphorus 1–2 mg/dl higher, and a greater variability in both values than the breast-fed group.

Studies of placental involvement in fetal calcium metabolism are intriguing. Homogenates of human placental villus (fetal tissue) synthesize 1,25-dihydroxyvitamin D from 25-hydroxyvitamin D. Calcium pump activity also has been studied in vesicles prepared from the microvillus brush border of the human placental syncytiotrophoblast. It is always a source of amazement to observe the complex functions that the placenta undertakes during a critical period of fetal life, and calcium and vitamin D metabolism appear to be no exception to this rule.

The ability of preterm infants to convert vitamin D to 25-hydroxyvitamin D and 1,25-dihydroxyvitamin D has been demonstrated in preterm infants of 32–37 weeks' gestation.

Tsang, R. C.: The quandary of vitamin D in the newborn infant. Lancet *1*:1370, 1983.

R. Tsang

METHODOLOGY[7, 42]

Serum total calcium, as routinely reported by clinical laboratories, represents the sum of protein-bound calcium, diffusable but complexed calcium (e.g., citrate-bound), and free ionized calcium. Only the ionized calcium fraction, normally 4.0–4.5 mg/dl, is physio-

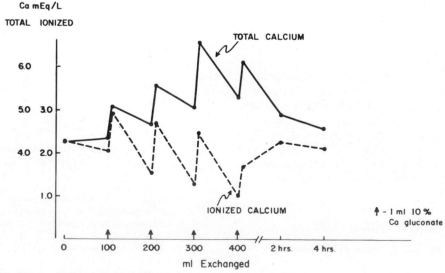

Figure 10–5. Effect of added calcium gluconate on total and ionized calcium during exchange transfusion with ACD blood.[26]

logically active, transported across membranes, or regulated homeostatically. When ionized calcium is determined directly with a calcium electrode,* values show reliable clinical correlation, with symptoms appearing at levels below 2.5–3.0 mg/dl.[42]

Variations in the two inert calcium fractions occur commonly with such conditions as alteration in serum protein, pH change, and citrate load postexchange (Figure 10–5) and make correlation of total and ionized calcium difficult. Use of the McLean-Hastings nomogram to estimate "ionized calcium" has not correlated well with direct measurements. The Q-oTc interval, derived from the electrocardiogram, has been shown to correlate with low ionized calcium.[7]

Direct determination of ionized calcium is now available, but when not possible, ionized calcium usually follows values for total calcium.

Ionized calcium electrodes have finally come of age, and it is now possible to determine ionized calcium accurately and reproducibly using fairly small volumes of blood. At present there are insufficient norms based on ionized calcium in the neonatal period, but these data should be forthcoming soon and will provide reference points for management of infant calcium-related problems.

R. Tsang

SYMPTOMS AND DEFINITION[3, 6, 45]

Hypocalcemia is often asymptomatic but causes twitching, "hyperalertness," increased tone, jitteriness, and convulsions. Cyanosis, vomiting or intolerance of feedings, and high-pitched cry have also been noted. None of these symptoms is specific for hypocalcemia, and all are common in high-risk infants generally. Chvostek's sign occurs in 20 per cent of hypocalcemic infants but is frequently seen also in normal infants. Hypocalcemia, therefore, can only be suspected and must be confirmed both by the laboratory and by response to specific treatment.

It is often erroneously assumed that unilateral or focal convulsions must be due to an intrinsic central nervous system lesion and are not the result of either hypoglycemia or hypocalcemia. This is quite incorrect, and we have seen unilateral and focal seizures as a result of both conditions, more specifically in hypocalcemic states. Some parts of the central nervous system are more subject to seizure stimulation than others given the identical stimulus. **L. Stern**

Serum calcium should be determined daily for all infants at risk for hypocalcemia and

*Orion Research Corp., Cambridge, Massachusetts. Not generally in use.

supportive treatment considered when low levels are encountered.

Early Neonatal Hypocalcemia[3, 38, 39, 45, 46]

Early neonatal hypocalcemia represents an exaggeration of the physiologic fall in serum calcium during the first 2 days of life. Thirty to forty per cent of all low-birth-weight infants develop chemical hypocalcemia, below 7 mg/dl less than 3.0–3.5 ionized, at this time. A smaller number become symptomatic. The following factors identify infants at high risk:
- Male sex; delivery in early spring (low maternal vitamin D)
- Prematurity
- Obstetric trauma, fetal distress, or abnormal presentation
- Neonatal asphyxia, metabolic acidosis requiring intravenous bicarbonate
- Neonatal illness—respiratory distress syndrome, cerebral injury, hypoglycemia, and sepsis
- Maternal diabetes, which exaggerates neonatal parathyroid immaturity.

The pathogenesis is a failure of homeostatic control of calcium partition between bone and serum. Interruption of calcium supply, parathyroid hypofunction, calcitonin excess, and unknown effects of acid-base balance shifts and cerebral injury all may contribute. The serum phosphorus is usually normal but may be elevated. Magnesium may be low.

In anticipation of hypocalcemia, serum calcium should be determined daily for high-risk infants. Hypocalcemia may be prevented by 24 mg/kg/day of elemental calcium IV or 75 mg/kg/day by enteric routes.[3, 31] Calcium and bicarbonate cannot be mixed in infusion solutions.[31]

Classic Neonatal Tetany[39, 41]

Less commonly, hypocalcemia occurs at 5–7 days of age in association with hyperphosphatemia. Three factors are important in the pathogenesis.

1. Formula with a high phosphorus content and a low calcium/phosphorus ratio. Breast milk contains 150 mg phosphorus per liter and has a Ca/P ratio of 2.3. In contrast, some formulae have 310–600 mg phosphorus per liter and Ca/P ratios of 1.3–1.4. Butterfat in some formulae can cause calcium malabsorption.

2. Immaturity of parathyroid vitamin D and renal function, causing phosphorus retention, hyperphosphatemia, and inability to support calcium levels. Factors associated with "early" hypocalcemia are present in 50 per cent of infants with classic tetany and include high parity, Asian mothers, male sex, low socioeconomic status, and borderline maternal vitamin D deficiency.

3. With current commercial formulae, classic neonatal tetany has become quite rare. With breast milk feeding, it should not occur at all. At present, therefore, infants presenting with hypocalcemia after 5 days of age must be followed for possible parathyroid disease.

In contrast, there are continued reports from the United Kingdom of neonatal tetany associated with the use of evaporated milks. An additional pathogenetic mechanism for hypocalcemia in the very low-birth-weight infant (less than 1250 gm) appears to be resistance to 1,25-dihydroxyvitamin D action. 1,25-Dihydroxyvitamin D is necessary for mobilization of calcium from bone, but even when extremely large doses of 1,25-dihydroxyvitamin D_3 are given to very low-birth-weight infants, serum calcium is not raised, in contrast to the positive response in larger preterm infants.

Very recently we have discovered that infants fed "humanized" commercial cow milk formula with phosphate content intermediate between cow and human milk can still have neonatal tetany, often dismissed by housestaff as "idiopathic seizures" that need to be controlled with phenobarbital. In following a group of such infants we have found that the serum parathyroid hormone concentrations remain significantly elevated for 6 months beyond the levels in breast-fed infants. This sequence would support the contention that even a moderate increase in phosphate load to term infants results in a "metabolic stress," and infants compensate for this stress by increasing parathyroid hormone production.

Venkataraman, P. S., Buckley, D., Neumann, V., et al: Profound neonatal hypocalcemia in very low birth weight infants with unresponsive parathyroid glands, refractory to 1,25-dihydroxyvitamin D_3. Pediatr Res 17:340A, 1983.

Venkataraman, P. S., Greer, F. R., Noguchi, A., et al: "Late" infantile tetany and secondary hyperparathyroidism in infants fed "humanized" cow milk formula. J Am Coll Nutr 1:123, 1982.

R. Tsang

Hypoparathyroidism [20, 39]

Maternal Hyperparathyroidism. Exposure to hypercalcemia in utero can cause persisting neonatal parathyroid suppression. Vague maternal symptoms, or a history of a previous infant with neonatal tetany, may be present.

The mother's disease is frequently clinically silent. Calcium and phosphorus determinations should be obtained for the mother whenever neonatal hypocalcemia is prolonged or resistant to treatment.

Although the mother's disease may be clinically silent, a careful search for renal stones and/or osteodystrophic changes (osteitis fibrosa cystica) may reveal the evidence of maternal disease that one is looking for with benefits for the child and likewise the mother. **L. Stern**

Transient Congenital Idiopathic Hypoparathyroidism. This is a benign, self-limited hypoparathyroid state persisting from 1–14 months, responding to calcium and/or moderate vitamin D supplements. The mother is euparathyroid.

Permanent Hypoparathyroidism. Hereditary and sporadic forms are described. It may be accompanied by absent thymus, immunodeficiency, micrognathia, and aortic arch anomalies (DiGeorge's syndrome).

Other Hypocalcemic Syndromes

Following exchange transfusion with citrated blood, ionized calcium is depressed owing to complexing with citrate (see Figure 10–5).

Severe maternal calcium and vitamin D deficiency can cause neonatal rickets and hypocalcemia.

Hypocalcemia can occur with uremia, hypoproteinemia (ionized calcium normal; no tetany), furosemide treatment, and magnesium deficiency (see below).

TREATMENT OF HYPOCALCEMIA

If desired supportive treatment may be given to asymptomatic infants at risk. Calcium, 24–35 mg/kg/24 hours, is added to intravenous infusion solution. Calcium Gluceptate Injection (Lilly), 18 mg calcium per ml, or 10 per cent calcium gluconate U.S.P., 9 mg calcium per ml, may be used. Infusion rate should be regulated by pump. Calcium may not be mixed with bicarbonate. Calcium has also been given by slow intravenous bolus injection every 6–8 hours, but this is more difficult.[3, 37]

In situations where calcium and an alkali need to be administered simultaneously one can substitute lactate for bicarbonate and permit the simultaneous infusion of the two to occur. **L. Stern**

FOR SYMPTOMATIC HYPOCALCEMIA

STAT TREATMENT. A calcium push is hazardous but indicated with seizures or extreme irritability as a therapeutic trial while awaiting laboratory confirmation. Use established intravenous line and monitor pulse or electrocardiogram continuously for bradycardia. Ten per cent calcium gluconate is injected over 10 minutes to a maximum dose of 3 ml/kg, stopping when clinical response is obtained.

CONTINUED TREATMENT

Parenteral. Calcium infusion, as just described, but with a dose of 75 mg calcium/kg/24 hours. Pulse must be checked frequently, serum calcium at least daily, and extravasation avoided. Calcium infusion is hazardous and is rarely required longer than 3 days.

Enteral. Dietary calcium therapy is indicated in prolonged or late-onset ("classic") hypocalcemia. Low phosphorus formula (Special Care [Ross], phosphorus 600 mg/l, Ca/P of 2.0, PM 60/40 [Ross], phosphorus 172 mg/l, Ca/P of 2.0) or breast milk is used. Calcium supplement as calcium lactate (13 per cent calcium), calcium gluconate (9 per cent calcium), or calcium glubionate (Neo-Calglucon [Dorsey], 23 mg calcium per ml) is added to raise the fed Ca/P ratio to between 4.0 and 6.0. This requires 35–70 mg supplemental calcium per dl of feeding. Enteric supplementation should not increase gastric tonicity and thus should be mixed with appropriate volumes of formula to avoid necrotizing enterocolitis.

Enteral treatment can usually be tapered after 2–4 weeks. With severely depressed parathyroid function, however, treatment may need to be prolonged beyond this period, and therapy with dihydrotachysterol or 1,25-dihydroxyvitamin D may be necessary.[39, 47]

The hazards of intravenous calcium injection include bradycardia, cardiac arrest, cutaneous necrosis, and intestinal gangrene. Care should be employed to insure patency to intravenous lines, with labels to avoid inadvertent flushing. Intraarterial calcium should be avoided.

Enteric calcium salts can be used to treat or prevent neonatal hypocalcemia at 75 mg/kg/day, divided into 6 equal doses. Enteric calcium salts are much safer than intravenous calcium salts and can be given to large numbers of sick neonates. The preferred approach at the Cincinnati Neonatal ICUs is early detection of neonatal hypocalcemia followed by prompt enteric calcium supplementation for 2–3 days (2 days full supplementation, or 1 day full dose followed by stepwise tapering doses for 2 days). This approach has drastically reduced the need for intravenous calcium therapy. Neo-Calglucon has a syrup base and high osmolality; apart from frequent stools its use might be a disadvantage in infants prone to necrotizing enterocolitis.   **R. Tsang**

PROGNOSIS

Hypocalcemia with seizures may present an immediate threat to life in an infant who frequently has other problems with which to contend. However, unlike with hypoglycemia, there seems to be no structural damage to the central nervous system. Thus, hypocalcemia alone has a good prognosis. If hypocalcemia is complicating other serious conditions such as asphyxia, the prognosis is determined by the other problems.

MAGNESIUM AND HYPOMAGNESEMIA

FETAL AND NEONATAL MAGNESIUM METABOLISM[6, 29, 39, 41, 44, 48]

Magnesium is actively transported from mother to fetus. Unlike calcium, this transfer is adversely affected both by placental insufficiency and by maternal magnesium deficiency due to poor diet or disease. Fifty per cent of total body magnesium (versus 1 per cent of calcium) is in soft tissue and plasma. Hypomagnesemia consequently reflects a true magnesium deficiency in the newborn rather than a disturbance in homeostasis with bone.

Parathyroid function has a small direct effect on serum magnesium levels. Magnesium, on the other hand, is critically necessary for normal parathyroid function.

Normal newborn serum magnesium is 1.5–2.8 mg/dl and relates directly to the mother's level. Through the first week of life, magnesium levels show small variations, correlating directly with changes in serum calcium and inversely with phosphorus.

Hypomagnesemia

Magnesium levels below 1.5 mg/dl are encountered:

- In fetal growth retardation of any cause, including multiple birth, or with malnourished or hypomagnesemic mothers

- In infants of diabetic mothers,[48] correlating with the severity of the mother's disease
- With hyperphosphatemia and following exchange transfusion. Magnesium, like calcium, is subject to citrate complexing
- In hypoparathyroidism
- In older infants secondary to diarrhea or malabsorption states
- Rarely, with a specific magnesium malabsorption syndrome in male infants.[44]

Hypomagnesemia can cause symptoms similar to those caused by hypocalcemia but is unresponsive to calcium therapy.

COEXISTENCE OF HYPOMAGNESEMIA AND HYPOCALCEMIA

These two metabolic problems frequently coexist.

1. They have common antecedents, such as maternal diabetes, hypoparathyroidism, malabsorption, exchange transfusion, and excess dietary phosphorus.

2. Magnesium deficiency causes failure of parathyroid hormone release and of parathyroid hormone effect on serum calcium. Magnesium appears crucial for normal bone-serum calcium homeostasis. Magnesium therapy alone can raise serum calcium in classic neonatal tetany.[6]

Occurrences of hypomagnesemia without hypocalcemia are so rare as to be of almost no clinical importance to the newborn. There have been one or possibly two isolated cases of familial hypomagnesemia occurring under these circumstances, but this represents an entirely different disease. Moreover, prolonged therapy with diuretics in adults can result in renal tubular magnesium losses and magnesium depletion, but this effect is unlikely in the newborn. Therefore, hypocalcemia, usually intractable to calcium therapy alone, needs to exist before hypomagnesemia as a possibility should be entertained.

L. Stern

THERAPY[6, 44]

Hypomagnesemia with tetany is treated with magnesium sulfate, 50 per cent, 0.2 ml/kg IM every 8–12 hours. Serum magnesium should be checked every 24 hours. Hypermagnesemia with hypotonia may occur with overtreatment. Alternatively, magnesium may be given with feedings. The sulfate, gluconate, chloride, or citrate salt may be used in an initial dose of 20–40 mg magnesium/kg/day. Excessive doses have a laxative effect.

Hypomagnesemic seizures are much more severe than hypocalcemic ones alone and are totally unaffected by regular anticonvulsive medication and/or infusions of calcium, even those that will raise serum calcium levels to normal. We would caution against any attempt to utilize oral therapy under these circumstances, as it is both ineffective clinically and likely, as has been pointed out, to result in diarrhea long before sufficient concentrations have been administered.

L. Stern

Hypermagnesemia [29]

Magnesium crossing the placenta following treatment for toxemia may produce hypotonia, flaccidity, respiratory depression, poor suck, and decreased gastrointestinal motility. Treatment is expectant, as magnesium levels decline by 48 hours.[29] If severe symptoms are present, calcium may reverse these effects, while forced diuresis may speed magnesium excretion.[29]

Hypermagnesemia may also occur in the neonatal ICU from overdosage during hyperalimentation and is often overlooked because serum magnesium measurements are not routinely made. Preterm infants are less able to excrete any magnesium excess. Curiously, magnesium treatment in mothers, which is associated with neonatal hypermagnesemia, results in elevation of neonatal serum calcium concentrations in spite of suppression of neonatal parathyroid function.

Donovan, E. F., Tsang, R. C., Steichen, J. J., et al: Neonatal hypermagnesemia: effect on parathyroid hormone and calcium homeostasis. J Pediatr 96:305, 1980.

R. Tsang

OSTEOPENIA–RICKETS OF PREMATURITY[43]

Bone mineralization in utero increases to term (see Figure 10–4). In contrast, prematurely born infants demonstrate diminished rates of bone mineralization. These infants are usually very low birth weight (less than 1.0 kg), have chronic problems (BPD, NEC, cholestasis, acidosis), require calciuric drugs (Lasix) or bicarbonate, and have diminished calcium, phosphorus, or vitamin D intake, are fed a soy-based formula or receive excess aluminum.

Osteopenia may be asymptomatic or show classic rickets at 1–4 months of age with undermineralized bone, pathologic fractures, craniotabes, rachitic rosary, hypocalcemia, hypophosphatemia, elevated parathyroid hormone, increased alkaline phosphatase, and increased 1,25-dihydroxyvitamin D levels (if not due to vitamin D deficiency). Copper deficiency must be ruled out. Treatment is usually effective with 1000–4000 U of vitamin D or lesser amounts of 1,25-dihydroxyvitamin D. In utero rates of bone mineralization may be achieved with formula containing calcium (1200–1400 mg/l), phosphorus (630–750 mg/l), and vitamin D (1000–1200 U/l) (see Figure 10–4). The fat-lactose-calcium interaction is also important in intestinal absorption since older formula resulted in only 40 per cent calcium absorption, while newer formula and breast milk result in 70 per cent or greater absorption.

For the latest discussion on osteopenia, see the study by Sedman et al (1985).

Sedman, A. B., Klein, G. L., Merritt, R. J., et al: Evidence of aluminum loading in infants receiving intravenous therapy. N Engl J Med 312:1337, 1985.

Hypercalcemia

Often, hypercalcemia is iatrogenic, but it may be due to (1) primary hyperparathyroidism, (2) maternal hypoparathyroidism, (3) massive idiopathic fat necrosis, (4) vitamin D toxicity, or (5) aluminum toxicity. Specific treatment is directed to the underlying disorder, while calcium excretion may be enhanced with fluids and diuretics.

Questions

True or False

The likelihood of hypoglycemia in a diabetic's offspring can be estimated before delivery.

Hypoglycemia in infants of diabetic mothers varies in incidence. The most important predictor is the severity of the mother's diabetic state.[19] Hyperglycemia at delivery should be avoided and is related to the incidence of hypoglycemia in the newborn. The statement is true.

We have seen instances in both directions when mothers with well-controlled diabetes have given birth to profoundly hypoglycemic infants and vice versa.
                                                                    L. Stern

In an asymptomatic infant of a diabetic mother, a blood sugar below 20 mg/dl is unusual yet requires no treatment.

Many IDMs have blood glucose below this value in the first 1–2 hours of life that spontaneously returns to normal. Careful observation, monitoring of glucose, and treatment with early feeding are indicated. If enteric feeding is not possible, intravenous glucose, 4–8 mg/kg/min, should begin. The statement is false.

In infants of insulin-dependent diabetic mothers I have taken a much more aggressive approach, in view of the fact that hypoglycemia occurs frequently. Serum glucose concentrations are determined every 30 minutes after birth for 2 hours, then hourly for 6 hours, and again at approximately 12 and 24 hours of age. If blood glucose levels are less than 40 mg/dl at any time, dextrose by constant infusion is given. The infusion is tapered to 75 per cent, and 50 per cent on succeeding days as enteric intake, which may be low in some IDMs, is increased. With this approach, intractable hypoglycemia does not occur.   **R. Tsang**

There is no particular evidence that hypoglycemia, whether asymptomatic or symptomatic, is particularly good for anyone. In the absence of evidence supporting the statement that asymptomatic hypoglycemia is not dangerous, we would urge treatment of all hypoglycemic infants of diabetic mothers.   **L. Stern**

Maternal beta blockers and sympathomimetic agents may cause neonatal hypoglycemia.[14, 23]

Both propranolol and various tocolytic beta mimetic drugs have been reported to result in neonatal hypoglycemia. Propranolol may inhibit glycogenolysis and lipolysis, while beta mimetic agents may produce hyperinsulinism.[14] The statement is true.

Infants of diabetic mothers have a high incidence of later developing diabetes.

The incidence of juvenile or adult onset diabetes is no greater for infants of diabetic mothers than it is for those born to diabetic fathers. Aside from the obvious direct genetic factors, fetal existence in a diabetic environment adds no further risks. This is always an important concern of the pregnant mother. The statement is true in that the risk is greater than in the general population but false when related to the abnormal maternal-fetal metabolic environment.

A 2.2 kg infant, 38 weeks by dates and 16 hours old, has become suddenly lethargic. The nurse, confidently, reports a Dextrostix of 45 mg/dl. Good news!

No news—The true glucose of this infant may be well below 30 mg/dl. Dextrostix are particularly unreliable when used in poor light and by inexperienced personnel. A quantitative glucose is needed. Furthermore, a true glucose above the "definition" value for hypoglycemia may result in hypoglycemic symptoms in some infants. Response to glucose therapy determines Rx of these patients. The statement is false.

A symptomatic infant with transient neonatal hypoglycemia may be treated orally.

Oral treatment has been shown to be ineffective in symptomatic hypoglycemia. Parenteral treatment is required. Many infants with glucose levels between 25 and 40 mg/dl will be asymptomatic and can be managed by early, frequent oral glucose feeding and careful monitoring. The statement is false.

Even with effective therapy, symptoms due to hypoglycemia may not respond promptly.

With severe or prolonged hypoglycemia, there may be a protracted recovery period. The statement is true.

In a convulsing neonate, a response to intravenous calcium gluconate does NOT prove that the seizure was due to hypocalcemia.

Intravenous calcium gluconate has a nonspecific anticonvulsant action. It is necessary to prove hypocalcemia chemically in pretreatment serum. The statement is true.

Early onset refractory hypocalcemia may respond to magnesium.

Assuming that 75 mg/kg/day of elemental calcium is adequate therapy, marked hyperphosphatemia is not present, and magnesium is essential for parathyroid hormone release/function, the statement is true.

Asymptomatic premature infants with hypocalcemia (6–7 mg/dl) may be managed with oral calcium supplements.

Such infants, if hypoproteinemic, may actually have no deficiency of ionized calcium. Assuming that actual hypocalcemia is present, oral treatment is preferable, when feasible, to parenteral treatment. The statement is true.

Match the remaining statements with the following conditions and state reasons:
A. Hypoglycemia
B. Hypocalcemia
C. Both
D. Neither

A maternal history of three miscarriages.

A history of excessive fetal wastage can mean maternal gestational diabetes with a risk of neonatal hypoglycemia and hypocalcemia. Fetal wastage is also seen with hyperparathyroidism. Therefore the answer is C.

An infant, 22 hours old, birth weight 1200 gm, 29 weeks' gestation, type I respiratory distress with mixed acidosis treated with intravenous bicarbonate.

This infant has multiple risk factors for hypocalcemia. His risk of hypoglycemia is not great, especially if he is receiving intravenous fluid and caloric support, as he should be with prematurity and respiratory distress. The answer is, therefore, B.

If under these circumstances the intravenous infusion is suddenly stopped, there is a risk of hypoglycemia occurring as a result of the previously infusion-induced hyperinsulinemia. This is a common cause of sudden hypogly-

cemia in infants under intravenous therapy and a good reason for not suddenly purposely discontinuing an infusion but slowing it down and discontinuing it slowly.

L. Stern

Following exchange transfusion for erythroblastosis.

Hypoglycemia may occur following exchange transfusion as a rebound effect precipitated by the glucose added to the donor unit. Citrate complexes calcium and causes a severe drop in the ionized fraction, which may in turn cause symptoms. The answer is C.

Since the decrease in calcium during "exchange" blood transfusion is in the ionized fraction, the total calcium may not be decreased. In fact, if calcium supplementation is given during the exchange transfusion, it is possible that total calcium concentrations might appear elevated, especially if the last calcium supplement has been given shortly before the determination of serum calcium was made. **R. Tsang**

Irritability, jitteriness, and seizures.

These symptoms may mean either hypoglycemia or hypocalcemia. The answer is C. Drug withdrawal should also be considered.

May be a clue to significant undiagnosed disease in the mother.

In a large-for-dates infant, early hypoglycemia should be sought (Dextrostix at 2 hours) and may indicate unsuspected maternal diabetes. Neonatal hypocalcemia may be a clue to a maternal parathyroid adenoma. The answer is C.

May be precipitated by medication taken during pregnancy.

Hypoglycemia of the newborn may be severe and prolonged if a mother is treated with oral hypoglycemics. Exchange transfusion may be necessary to remove the drug from the infant. Although much less likely, a mother with milk-alkali syndrome or vitamin D intoxication with hypercalcemia could have a hypocalcemic infant. The answer is C.

A 2600 gm newborn with a hemoglobin of 26 gm/dl.

Hypoglycemia is frequent in plethoric infants. A high hemoglobin level may be a factor in hypoglycemia in infants of diabetic mothers and with Beckwith's syndrome. A pair of parabiotic twins has been described in which the larger and more plethoric twin had hypoglycemia while his sibling did not. The answer is A.

A 3400 gm, 53 cm long infant with desquamation and meconium-stained nails and cord, estimated gestation 43 weeks, Apgar scores 9 and 9.

Postmaturity *per se* is not associated with hypocalcemia. When postmaturity is associated with placental insufficiency and signs of intrauterine malnutrition, hypoglycemia may be a problem after birth. The answer, in this infant, would be A. He should be fed early and watched closely.

A jittery and twitchy 4200 gm infant 2 hours old.

This infant is too young to be hypocalcemic. He is at a typical age for the early hypoglycemia of an infant of a diabetic mother. Of course, the problem might also be an anoxic insult at birth or CNS injury. The answer is A.

CASE PROBLEMS

Case One

You are called to see a 5 day old infant because of irritability and jerking movements of the left arm and leg. He was the product of a full-term pregnancy, birth weight 2.8 kg. Pregnancy was complicated by third trimester bleeding. Delivery was by cesarean section because of placenta previa. One minute Apgar score was 6; 5 minute Apgar was 9. Evaporated milk formula was begun at 16 hours of age, and he did very well until a few hours ago when he became tremulous and fed poorly. Intermittent convulsions were noted. Examination reveals irritability but no other abnormalities. However, as the examination ends, the child convulses.

What diagnostic tests and procedures would you perform Initially?

The symptoms shown by this baby are nonspecific. CNS injury or infection is possible, and a lumbar puncture must be done. There is nothing in the case history to suggest hypoglycemia as a *probable* cause of the seizures, but some less common hypoglycemic syndromes (tumor) may present this way, and Dextrostix should be performed. Serum should be drawn for electrolytes, calcium, BUN, and glucose.

Several features of this case suggest the possibility of hypocalcemia, notably: stormy obstetric course, formula feedings, the age of onset of symptoms after the initially benign course, and irritability and tremulousness as cardinal symptoms. These features would justify a trial with parenteral calcium after initial studies are done.

The therapeutic infusion is 2 ml/kg of 10 per cent calcium gluconate at 1 ml/minute into an established intravenous line with ECG monitoring.

I would just like to emphasize the importance of drawing initial blood studies *prior* to administration of parenteral calcium, because the calcium-regulating hormones are directly affected by calcium status in the blood. Hence, if one is trying to determine the cause of the condition, it is extremely important to be able to draw the sample prior to any intervention, presumably at the time of low calcium concentrations. Subsequent to the intervention, when the serum calcium concentrations have returned to normal, another blood sample should be drawn. The relationship between calcium-regulating hormones and calcium status is dynamic. For example, if parathyroid hormone concentration is measured at the time of severe hypocalcemia and found to be low, this would support the contention that the parathyroids of the infant are not able to mount an adequate response to the hypocalcemia and imply a parathyroid insufficient state. If serum parathyroid hormone concentrations are markedly elevated at the time when serum calcium concentrations are low, this would imply an appropriate response of the parathyroids and would suggest that the low calcium is related to some other disturbance; in this circumstance when the calcium concentrations are restored to normal, the parathyroid hormone concentrations in blood should then fall to the normal range too.   **R. Tsang**

Subsequent to immediate evaluation and treatment, the laboratory reports a calcium of 5.8 mg/dl and phosphorus of 11.5 mg/dl.

What factors may be important in pathogenesis of the hypocalcemia?

The high serum phosphorus indicates that dietary phosphorus load, relative hypoparathyroidism, and renal immaturity with retention of phosphate are important factors in the hypocalcemia. Maternal vitamin D status and/or neonatal vitamin D metabolism may be the cause.

What further tests are indicated?

Calcium and phosphorus should be determined in the mother. If hypocalcemia proves resistant to treatment, serum magnesium should be determined in the infant.

What management should be instituted?

Low phosphorus formula or formula with a favorable Ca/P ratio: special care, PM 60/40, or breast milk. Calcium supplementation: 62 mg calcium added to each 4 oz bottle of formula (10 per cent calcium gluconate, 7 ml; Neo-Calglucon syrup, 2.7 ml; calcium lactate, 470 mg). This will make the fed Ca/P ratio 5.0.

What is the prognosis?

Excellent. Supplemental calcium may be tapered and withdrawn at 3–4 weeks of age. Serum calcium should be monitored at this time to be sure hypocalcemia does not recur. There should be no long-term sequelae.

In my experience, acute treatment of hypocalcemia with 2 ml/kg of 10 per cent calcium gluconate is generally sufficient for any hypocalcemic seizure, preferably given diluted and slowly over 10 minutes. Only a few days of calcium supplementation may be needed. In this situation, when serum Ca levels have returned to normal for 2 days, I will generally start tapering the calcium supplements (50 per cent, 25 per cent) over a few days. This "trial" will often demonstrate that the infant now has enough "parathyroid reserve." If the infant "fails" the test, a work-up for hypoparathyroidism (radioimmunoassay, parathyroid response) will be in order. Since hypomagnesemic hypocalcemia may be a problem, serum magnesium levels should also be followed.   **L. Stern**

Case Two

You attend the delivery, at 36 weeks by cesarean section, of a 24 year old juvenile-onset diabetic. The infant boy weighs 3.8 kg, is plethoric, appears cushingoid, and has moderate hepatomegaly and splenomegaly and a respiratory rate of 60 without retractions or grunting. His Dextrostix at 15 minutes of age reads 90 mg/dl. At 2 hours of age, all seems well. A capillary blood glucose is obtained. An hour later, the laboratory reports a value of 12 mg/dl.

How would you proceed at this point?

Many infants of diabetic mothers will reach glucose levels as low as 12 mg/dl in the first 2 hours, and most will rebound satisfactorily (see Figure 10–1). Check the baby. If he is symptomatic, treat after drawing another sample. If symptoms are absent, draw a sample and feed milk immediately. If he is tachypneic, begin intravenous glucose at 4–8 mg/kg/min.

The laboratory reported the second sample as 27 mg/dl. At 4 hours, blood glucose was 34 mg/dl. What next?

Early feeding may be continued if clinical condition is good. Also repeat glucose values until stable and above 40 mg/dl.

At 24 hours of age, the baby is reported as irritable. Feedings have been started and are taken very slowly. Examination reveals that Moro's reflex and tone are reduced. Color is good, pulse 120/minute, and respirations 65/minute without retractions. Chvostek's sign is elicited. Blood glucose is 35 mg/dl. Serum calcium is 7.8 mg/dl.

Management?

This behavior calls for careful evaluation and observation for complications (venous thromboses, anomalies) found in these babies. Blood glucose is borderline low and more persistently depressed in the presence of symptoms; 2 ml/kg of 10 per cent dextrose followed by intravenous infusions of 8 mg/kg/min is now indicated. Furthermore, since calcium may continue to decline over the next 24 hours, calcium supplementation should begin.

Case Three

A 2 month old has increasing respiratory distress and an "incidental" finding on chest x-ray. He was a 27 week, 0.8 kg infant and has had RDS necessitating 1 month of respirator and 1 month of continuous positive airway pressure care. Multiple episodes of cor pulmonale requiring chronic diuretics and failure to establish enteral alimentation necessitated total parenteral alimentation. Direct reacting hyperbilirubinemia was evident at 1 month.

Figure 10–6 demonstrates what important observations?

In addition to chronic lung disease and cardiomegaly, metabolic bone disease is evident. Poorly mineralized bone, in addition to rachitic rosary and pathologic fractures, is present.

What common deficiency may be present?

Congenital rickets in the neonate is almost always due to severe maternal vitamin D deficiency. This patient has acquired nutritional rickets and may be deficient in calcium, phosphorus, or vitamin D.

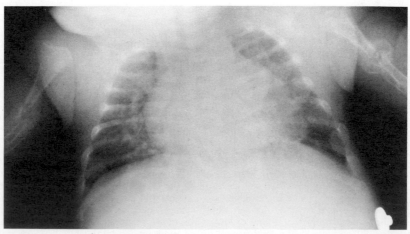

Figure 10–6. Respiratory distress and incidental radiographic findings in a 2 month old, 800 gm infant (Case Three).

What therapy should be started?

Vitamin D dose should be increased to 1000–4000 U per day. With hepatic dysfunction, 10,000 U may be needed. Occasionally, 1,25-dihydroxyvitamin D or 1α-hydroxyvitamin D may be indicated.

Why did this patient have pulmonary deterioration?

Rachitic muscle weakness or rib cage dysfunction may result in pulmonary insufficiency. Alternative approaches employ supplementation with calcium and phosphorus to enhance postnatal bone mineralization. Calcium, 250 mg/kg/day (elemental), and phosphorus, 125 mg/kg/day, may prevent this osteopenia and may be easily obtained from newer formulae containing calcium (1400 mg/l), phosphorus (750 mg/l), and vitamin D (1200 U/l).

A similar patient also demonstrates periosteal bone elevation, anemia, and neutropenia. What rarer nutritional deficiency is present?

In infants on prolonged hyperalimentation, trace mineral deficiency may occur. In this particular infant, copper intake was deficient.

REFERENCES

1. Battaglia, F., and Meschia, G.: Principal substrates of fetal metabolism. Physiol Rev 58:499, 1978.
2. Beard, A., Cornblath, M., Gentz, J., et al: Neonatal hypoglycemia—a discussion. J Pediatr 79:314, 1971.
3. Brown, D., Steranka, B., and Taylor, F.: Treatment of early onset neonatal hypocalcemia. Effects on serum calcium and ionized calcium. Am J Dis Child 135:24, 1981.
4. Brown, D., Woodbridge, P., and Ulstrom, R.: Methods to increase the reliability of blood glucose by the Dextrostix system. Pediatr Res (Abstract) 9:348, 1975.
5. Cahill, G.: Starvation in man. N Engl J Med 282:668, 1970.
6. Cockburn, F., Brown, J., Belton, N., et al: Neonatal convulsions associated with a primary disturbance of calcium, phosphorus, and magnesium metabolism. Arch Dis Child 48:99, 1973.
7. Colletti, R., Pan, M., Smith, E., et al: Detection of hypocalcemia in susceptible neonates. N Engl J Med 290:931, 1974.
8. Combs, J., Grunt, J., and Brandt, I.: New syndrome of neonatal hypoglycemia. N Engl J Med 275:236, 1966.
9. Cornblath, M., and Schwartz, R.: Disorders of Carbohydrate Metabolism in Infancy. 2nd ed. Philadelphia, W. B. Saunders Co., 1976.
10. Cornblath, M., Pildes, R., Schwartz, R., et al: Hypoglycemia in infancy and childhood. J Pediatr 83:692, 1973.
11. Cornblath, M., Segal, S., and Smith, C. (eds.): Energy metabolism in the newborn—an international exploration. Pediatrics 39:582, 1967.
12. Crowder, W., MacLaren, N., Gutberlet, R., et al: Neonatal pancreatic beta-cell hyperplasia: report of a case with failure of diazoxide and benefit of early subtotal pancreatectomy. Pediatrics 57:897, 1976.
13. Dweck, H., and Cassady, G.: Glucose intolerance in infants of very low birth weight. Pediatrics 53:189, 1974.
14. Epstein, M., Nicholls, E., and Stobblefield, P.: Neonatal hypoglycemia after beta sympathomimetic tocolytic therapy. J Pediatr 94:449, 1979.
15. Farquhar, J.: Metabolic changes in the infant of the diabetic mother. Pediatr Clin North Am 12:743, 1965.
16. Frantz, I., Medina, G., and Taeusch, H.: Correlation of Dextrostix values with true glucose in the range less than 50 mg per dl. J Pediatr 87:417, 1975.
17. Frazer, T., Karl, I., Hillman, L., et al.: Direct measurement of gluconeogenesis from [2,3-^{13}C$_2$] alanine in the human neonate. Am J Physiol 240:E 615, 1981.
18. Harvey, D., Cooper, L., and Stevens, J.: Plasma calcium and magnesium in newborn babies. Arch Dis Child 45:506, 1970.
19. Haworth, J., and Dilling, L.: Relationships between maternal glucose intolerance and neonatal blood glucose. J Pediatr 89:810, 1976.
20. Hertenstein, H., and Gardner, L.: Tetany of the newborn associated with maternal parathyroid adenoma. N Engl J Med 274:266, 1966.
21. Hirsch, H., Loo, S., Evans, N., et al: Hypoglycemia of infancy and nesidioblastosis: studies with somatostatin. N Engl J Med 296:1323, 1977.
22. Kalhan, S., Savin, S., and Adam, P.: Attenuated glucose production rate in newborn infants of insulin dependent diabetic mothers. N Engl J Med 296:375, 1977.
23. Kliegman, R., and Fanaroff, A.: Developmental metabolism and nutrition. In Gregory G. (ed.): Pediatric Anesthesiology. Churchill Livingstone, New York, 1983.
24. Landau, H., Perlman, M., Meyers, S., et al: Persistent neonatal hypoglycemia due to hyperinsulinism: medical aspects. Pediatrics 70:440, 1982.
25. Lilien, L., Pildes, R., Srinivasan, G., et al: Treatment of neonatal hypoglycemia with minibolus and intravenous glucose infusion. J Pediatr 97:295, 1980.
26. Maisels, M., Li, T.-K., Piechocki, J., et al: Effect of exchange transfusion on serum ionized calcium. Pediatrics 53:683, 1974.
27. Mamunes, P., Baden, M., Bass, J., et al: Early intravenous feeding of the low birth weight neonate. Pediatrics 43:241, 1969.
28. Martin, F., Dahlenburg, G., Russell, J., et al: Neonatal hypoglycemia in infants of insulin-dependent diabetic mothers. Arch Dis Child 50:472, 1975.
29. McGuinness, G., Weinstein, M., Cruikshank, D., et al: Effect of magnesium sulfate treatment on perinatal calcium metabolism. II. Neonatal responses. Obstet Gynecol 56:595, 1980.

30. Milner, R., Ferguson, A., Naidu, S.: Aetiology of transient neonatal diabetes. Arch Dis Child 46:724, 1971.
31. Nerves, C., Shott, R., Bergstrom, W., et al: Prophylaxis against hypocalcemia in low birth weight infants requiring bicarbonate infusion. J Pediatr 87:439, 1975.
32. Pagliara, A., Karl, I., Haymond, M., et al: Hypoglycemia in infancy and childhood. J Pediatr 82:365, 1973.
33. Pagliara, A., Karl, I., and Kipnis, D.: Transient neonatal diabetes: delayed maturation of the pancreatic beta cell. J. Pediatr 82:97, 1973.
34. Persson, B., Gentz, J., Kellum, M., et al: Metabolic observations in infants of strictly controlled diabetic mothers. II. Plasma insulin, FFA, glycerol, beta-hydroxybutyrate during intravenous glucose tolerance test. Acta Paediatr Scand 65:1, 1976.
35. Pildes, R.: Infants of diabetic mothers. N Engl J Med 289:902, 1973.
36. Raivio, K., and Osterlund, K., Hypoglycemia and hyperinsulinemia associated with erythroblastosis fetalis. Pediatrics 43:217, 1969.
37. Ramamurthy, R., Harris, V., and Pildes, R.: Subcutaneous calcium deposition in the neonate associated with intravenous administration of calcium gluconate. Pediatrics 55:802, 1975.
38. Robertson, N., and Smith, M.: Early neonatal hypocalcemia. Arch Dis Child 50:604, 1975.
39. Root, A., and Harrison, H.: Recent advances in calcium metabolism. J Pediatr 88:1, 177, 1976.
40. Sinclair, J., Driscoll, J., Heird, W., et al: Supportive management of the sick neonate—parenteral calories, water, and electrolytes. Pediatr Clin North Am 17:863, 1970.
41. Snodgrass, G., Stimmler, L., Went, J., et al: Interrelations of plasma calcium, inorganic phosphate, magnesium, and protein over the first week of life. Arch Dis Child 48:279, 1973.
42. Sorel, M., and Rosen, J.: Ionized calcium: serum levels during symptomatic hypocalcemia. J Pediatr 87:67, 1975.
43. Steichen, J., Gratton, T., and Tsang, R.: Osteopenia of prematurity: the cause and possible treatment. J Pediatr 96:528, 1980.
44. Tsang, R.: Neonatal magnesium disturbances. Am J Dis Child 124:282, 1972.
45. Tsang, R., and Oh, W.: Neonatal hypocalcemia in low-birth-weight infants. Pediatrics 45:773, 1970.
46. Tsang, R., Chen, I., Friedman, M., et al: Parathyroid function in infants of diabetic mothers. J Pediatr 86:399, 1975.
47. Tsang, R., Greer, F., and Steichen, J.: Perinatal metabolism of vitamin D. Clin Perinatol 8:287, 1981.
48. Tsang, R., Strub, R., Brown, D., et al: Hypomagnesemia in infants of diabetic mothers: perinatal studies. J Pediatr 89:115, 1976.
49. Zucker, P., and Simon, G.: Prolonged symptomatic neonatal hypoglycemia associated with maternal chlorpropamide therapy. Pediatrics 42:824, 1968.

11

Neonatal Hyperbilirubinemia

RONALD L. POLAND
ENRIQUE M. OSTREA, JR.

Generally speaking, [icterus neonatorum] is an affection of very little importance. In some cases, it has appeared to us to be connected with the want of a free evacuation of the meconium.

D. FRANCIS CONDIE
A PRACTICAL TREATISE OF THE DISEASES OF CHILDREN (1854)

INTRODUCTION

Neonatal hyperbilirubinemia received very little attention in the mid-nineteenth century, as Dr. Condie's statement indicates. The problems of newborn infants interested few physicians of that period. Early in this century, many more physicians (mainly obstetricians) began to focus their attention on the newborn infant, and the great value of neonatal jaundice as a clue to diagnosis became evident. As we approached the middle of this century, we recognized that bilirubin was not simply an indicator of illness in the newborn infant but it was also a toxin. By 1950, exchange transfusion was widely used for the prevention of the permanent damage to the central nervous system caused by bilirubin. In the early 1960s, the binding of bilirubin to albumin was described as a protective mechanism against bilirubin toxicity. The potential of other substances (including drugs) for interfering with this protective protein binding became evident then and is still under intensive investigation. Data on the potential usefulness of tests for reserve albumin-binding capacity became available over the next 10 years. We still have much to learn about mechanisms of bilirubin toxicity, appropriate alternatives for the treatment of neonatal hyperbilirubinemia, and when such treatment is really needed.

This chapter presents an approach to finding the cause of hyperbilirubinemia in a newborn infant and to the management of neonatal jaundice.

Neonatal hyperbilirubinemia occurs when the normal pathways of bilirubin metabolism and excretion in the newborn infant are impeded. One must consider these pathways to understand neonatal jaundice (Figure 11–1). Bilirubin is formed mainly (75–80 per cent) from the catabolism of hemoglobin. In addition, bilirubin is derived from other heme-containing compounds such as myoglobin, cytochromes, tryptophan pyrrolase, and peroxidases,[82] and from ineffective erythropoiesis.[5] Bilirubin formed from these secondary sources has been called shunt bilirubin. The major sites of bilirubin production are the spleen and the liver. However, all tissues of the body have macrophages that can produce bilirubin from hemoglobin. Macrophages contain microsomal heme oxygenase and biliverdin reductase, the two enzymes necessary for the degradation of heme to bilirubin.[73] The catabolism of 1 gm of hemoglobin results in the formation of approximately 35 mg of bilirubin.

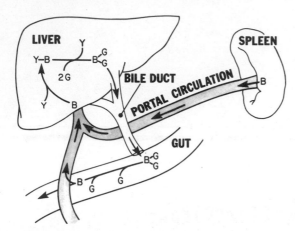

Figure 11–1. Pathways of bilirubin metabolism and excretion. B—bilirubin; G—glucuronide; and Y—ligand protein.

The Chemical Structure of Bilirubin

The structure of a compound controls its behavior in chemical and biologic systems. Bilirubin has a structure that allows for considerable variation in spatial arrangement (stereoisomerism). Therefore, the effects of bilirubin on tissues and those of the tissues on bilirubin depend upon the stereoisomer of bilirubin in question. For years, the basic chemical properties of bilirubin have been the subject of academic debates, partly because of our lack of understanding about the ability of this compound to change its properties as it changes its shape. Our understanding of these principles has increased greatly in recent times.

Bilirubin is a tetrapyrrole compound with specific substitutions in the side chains of the four pyrrole rings. The outer pyrrole rings are linked to the inner ones by methene bridges (containing one double bond each), but the two central rings are joined by a saturated methane bridge (no double bond). Thus, the bilirubin molecule can twist freely only about its central carbon atom. The sequence of pyrrole sidechains in bilirubin is dependent upon the site of oxidation of one of the one-carbon bridges in heme, a derivative of protoporphyrin IX. Normally, the methene bridge oxidized in heme is in the alpha position, and the resultant isomer is bilirubin IX-alpha (Figure 11–2). This is the predominant isomer of bilirubin in the body. Oxidation of heme in the beta position would result in bilirubin IX-beta, etc.

Bilirubin IX-alpha differs remarkably from the other bilirubin isomers in that it is poorly soluble in water. X-ray crystallographic studies have been used to explain this characteristic.[9] Bilirubin IX-alpha can rotate freely around the central methane bridge, and the double bonds in the methene bridges (C5 and C15) are most often in the cis or Z configuration. At acid pH, intramolecular hydrogen bonding (stippled lines) occurs between the hydrophilic groups of the molecule, leaving no sites for the attachment of water. At alkaline pH, however, the hydrogen bonds are opened, and the two propionic acid side chains make bilirubin a divalent anion that is water soluble (Figures 11–3 and 11–4). In addition, four pyrrolenitrogens and two carboxyl groups become available for bonding with water. Therefore, bilirubin IX-alpha (Z,Z) is soluble in water only at alkaline pH.

When one or both of the methene bridges at C5 and C15 of bilirubin IX-alpha are not cis (Z) but trans (E) in configuration, the compound becomes water soluble, also. These isomers are formed predominantly

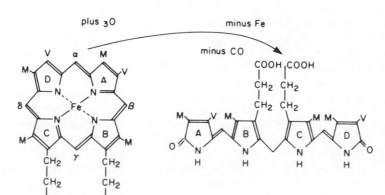

Ferroprotoporphyrin IX
(Protoheme)

Bilirubin IX α

Figure 11–2. Conversion of protoheme to bilirubin IX-α by cleavage at the α-methene bridge.

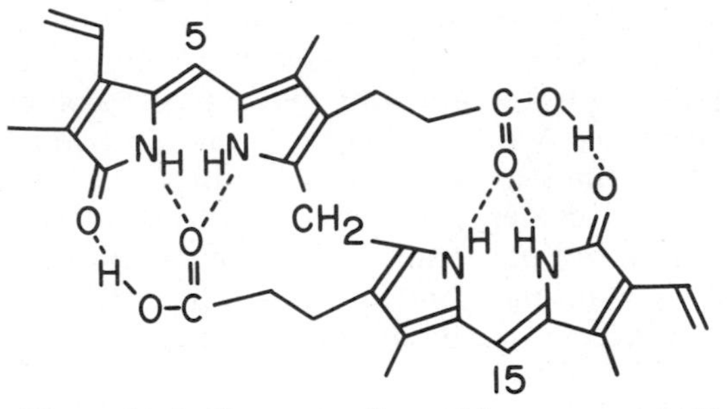

Figure 11–3. X-ray crystallographic structure of bilirubin IX-α. Dashed lines indicate hydrogen bonding.

during phototherapy and will be discussed in that context below (see p. 253).[40, 41]

Bilirubin Metabolism and Excretion

The unconjugated bilirubin (indirect-reacting in the van den Bergh reaction) that is formed by the catabolism of hemoglobin can dissolve readily in lipid[40, 41] and is poorly soluble in water at physiologic pH. It is transported in plasma bound to albumin. Bilirubin enters the hepatocyte by dissociation from its albumin carrier in the sinusoids of the liver and diffusion through the cell membrane. This diffusion process is facilitated by receptor-carrier proteins (Y and Z anion-binding proteins) that transport bilirubin within the cytoplasm of the hepatocyte.[37] Inside the hepatocyte, bilirubin is conjugated principally with glucuronic acid in a reaction that is catalyzed by the microsomal enzyme bilirubin-uridine diphosphate (UDP) glucuronyl transferase. The glucuronic acid moiety donated by uridine diphosphoglucuronic acid (UDPGA) is derived from the oxidation of uridine diphosphoglucose (UDPG) by UDPG-dehydrogenase (see Figure 11–1).

Conjugated (direct-reacting) bilirubin is water soluble and cannot diffuse through the lipid membranes of the cell. Therefore, an active transport mechanism exists to secrete the conjugated pigment into the biliary tree.[2] Conjugated bilirubin then appears in the duodenum as a component of bile.

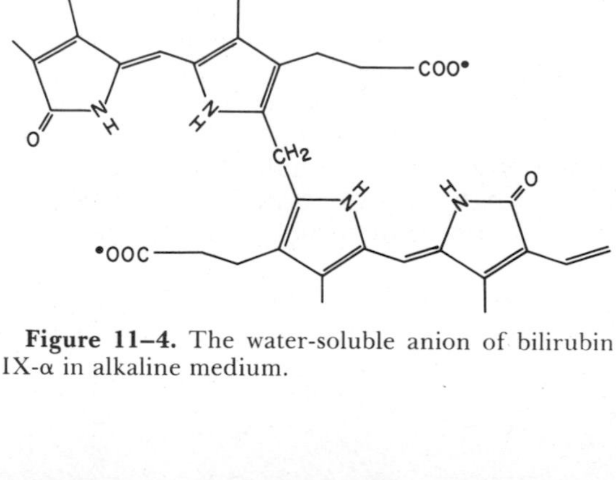

Much of the bilirubin found in the meconium and subsequent feces of newborn infants is not conjugated however.[8, 12] Beta-glucuronidase in the fetal and neonatal small bowel hydrolyzes bilirubin diglucuronide to yield lipid-soluble bilirubin and glucuronic acid.[33] This unconjugated bilirubin in the upper small bowel can be reabsorbed into the circulation of the fetus and newborn. Thus, in utero, bilirubin can be conjugated and excreted by the fetal liver, reabsorbed into the circulation, and excreted once again by the placenta. After birth, the bilirubin reabsorbed from the intestine contributes to the overall load of bilirubin that must be metabolized by the neonatal liver.[61]

PHYSIOLOGIC JAUNDICE

Serum bilirubin concentration rises from near-maternal levels at birth to an average of 7.0–7.5 mg/dl by the third day of life and gradually falls to less than 1.5 mg/dl by the tenth day in normal newborn infants. This rise and fall in serum bilirubin concentration is called physiologic jaundice. Visible jaundice (serum concentrations greater than 8 mg/dl in the full-term infant) in the first 36 hours or a serum bilirubin concentration exceeding 12.5 mg/dl at any time is considered abnormal (not "physiologic") and warrants a diagnostic investigation. The causes of physiologic jaundice during neonatal life are controversial and multiple.[47] Almost every phase of bilirubin disposition has been implicated.

The definition of what constitutes a normal serum bilirubin level in a healthy term infant is of more than passing interest. Our litigious brethren seem poised to pounce should we fail to initiate some investigation in an infant whose bilirubin level strays beyond the appointed norms (as listed by one or another expert) and who later turns up with a developmental problem. When we attempt to be precise about defining the limits of "physiologic" jaundice, however, we run into certain snags. The first is that measurements of serum bilirubin concentrations may vary drastically among different laboratories (Schreiner and Glick, 1982). Composite data from 11 large studies reviewed recently revealed a mean serum bilirubin level of 6.3 mg/dl on day two, 6.7 mg/dl on day three, and 6.0 mg/dl on days four to six (Maisels, 1981). Two standard deviations above the mean, on the third day of life, was a bilirubin of 12.7 mg/dl. These values are remarkably similar to those obtained from the collaborative perinatal project. In that study of approximately 32,000 infants with birth weights over 2500 gm, 6.2 per cent of white infants and 4.5 per cent of black infants had maximum serum bilirubin levels in excess of 12.9 mg/dl.

Figure 11–4. The water-soluble anion of bilirubin IX-α in alkaline medium.

In a sample of 2421 infants admitted to our well baby nursery, the mean serum bilirubin level on the second to third day of life was 6.2 ± 3.7 mg/dl (SD). Interestingly, our incidence of infants with serum bilirubin levels >12.9 mg/dl is 6.1 per cent—virtually identical with the white infants in the collaborative study (99% of our population is white). This suggests, contrary to some opinion, that the incidence of nonphysiologic jaundice has not increased.

When is jaundice visible? Certainly the interobserver variability in the detection of jaundice in the newborn must be considered. Some seem able consistently to detect a yellow tinge at bilirubin levels substantially below 8 mg/dl, and I believe the traditional teaching that jaundice is not visible below that level requires reevaluation.

Maisels, M. J.: Neonatal jaundice. *In* Avery, G. B. (ed.): Neonatology, Pathophysiology and Management of the Newborn. 2nd ed. Philadelphia, J. B. Lippincott Co., 1981, p. 473.

Schreiner, R. L., and Glick, M. R.: Interlaboratory bilirubin variability. Pediatrics *69*:273, 1982.

J. Maisels

The normal newborn infant produces 6–8 mg of bilirubin/kg of body weight/24 hours. This is 2.5 times the rate of bilirubin production in adults.[43] The greater production of bilirubin in newborns is partially explained by an average red cell life span of only 80–90 days in neonates, compared with 120 days for adult erythrocytes.[58, 69] Shunt bilirubin production has also been found to be greater in newborn infants.[76] Persistent postnatal flow of portal venous blood through the ductus venosus may impair hepatic clearance of bilirubin, too.[51] The facilitated diffusion of bilirubin into hepatocytes may be less efficient also because of low concentrations of intracellular anion-binding proteins in newborn infants. No direct evidence for this latter mechanism exists, but these carrier proteins are reduced in concentration in the livers of neonatal monkeys.[38]

Deficiency of bilirubin-UDP-glucuronyl transferase had been considered for many years to be central to the production of physiologic jaundice. Clinical and laboratory studies of this enzyme, however, have shown that its activity is closer to adult levels than previously suspected. In fact, the activity of the transferase enzyme is not low enough to account for most physiologic jaundice.[24, 70] The synthesis of UDPGA, the donor of glucuronic acid for conjugation with bilirubin, has been suggested also as a rate-limiting step in bilirubin elimination in the newborn. Indeed, the activity of UDPG-dehydrogenase appears to be low in the neonatal liver of some experimental animals.[14]

Finally, enterohepatic circulation of bilirubin following the hydrolysis of the conjugated pigment in the gut contributes to physiologic jaundice. A gram of meconium can contain more than a milligram of bilirubin. Many lines of evidence have led to the conclusion that intestinal reabsorption of bilirubin in normal infants contributes significantly to the production of physiologic jaundice.[61]

PATHOLOGIC JAUNDICE

Pathologic jaundice is an important clue in the early diagnosis of many diseases in the newborn period. Without the ability to recognize elevated bilirubin levels on physical examination, the clinician would have a more difficult time detecting many of these conditions in their early stages. These diseases produce hyperbilirubinemia either by increasing bilirubin production or by reducing its excretion (Table 11–1).

Pathologic jaundice within the first 36 hours of life is usually due to excessive production of bilirubin, since the hepatic clearance rate of bilirubin is not often reduced enough to cause the serum bilirubin concentration to rise above 10 mg/dl by this age. The reabsorption of bilirubin from the intestinal tract and the conversion of extravasated blood to bilirubin are categorized as overproduction, but they are both gradual processes that rarely lead to obvious jaundice in the first 36 hours of life. Thus, early icterus neonatorum is almost always due to a hemolytic disease.

Diagnosis of Hyperbilirubinemia

Overproduction

Hyperbilirubinemia due to overproduction should be suspected from the clinical appearance of jaundice before 36–48 hours of life. Rh-hemolytic disease (Table 11–1, A,1), once a very common cause of neonatal hyperbilirubinemia, is usually accompanied by both hepatic and splenic enlargement. Splenomegaly is rare in ABO disease. Pertinent laboratory tests include blood typing of mother and infant and direct and indirect Coombs' tests. A very high anti-A or anti-B antibody titer is often found in maternal serum in ABO disease, but it is not necessarily diagnostic. Specific anti-A or anti-B antibody eluted from the infant's red cells or low red cell acetyl-

TABLE 11–1 CAUSES OF NEONATAL HYPERBILIRUBINEMIA

Overproduction	Undersecretion	Mixed

A. Hemolytic disorders
  1. Fetomaternal blood group incompatibility ABO, Rh, others
  2. Genetic causes of hemolysis
    a. hereditary spherocytosis
    b. Enzyme defects—G6PD, pyruvate kinase, others
    c. Hemoglobinopathies—α-Thalassemia, β-δ-Thalassemia, others
    d. Galactosemia
  3. Drug-induced hemolysis—vitamin K
 	
B. Extravascular blood—petechiae, hematoma, pulmonary and cerebral hemorrhage, swallowed blood
 	
C. Polycythemia
  1. Chronic fetal hypoxia
  2. Maternal-fetal or fetofetal transfusion
  3. Placental transfusion (cord stripping)
 	
D. Exaggerated enterohepatic circulation
  1. Mechanical obstruction
    a. Atresia and stenosis
    b. Hirschsprung's disease
    c. Meconium ileus
    d. Meconium plug syndrome
  2. Reduced peristalsis
    a. Fasting or underfeeding
    b. Drugs (hexamethoniums, atropine)
    c. Pyloric stenosis
	E. Decreased hepatic uptake of bilirubin
	  1. Persistent ductus venosus shunt
	  2. Cytosol receptor protein (y) blocked by:
	    a. Drugs
	    b. Abnormal human milk inhibitor (? NEFA, ? may belong in D. or F.)
	
	F. Decreased bilirubin conjugation
	  1. Congenital reduction in glucuronyl transferase activity
	    a. Familial nonhemolytic jaundice (types I and II)
	    b. Gilbert's syndrome*
	  2. Enzyme inhibitor
	    a. Drugs and hormones—novobiocin, ? pregnanediol
	    b. Galactosemia (early)
	    c. Lucey-Driscoll syndrome
	    d. Abnormal human milk
	
	G. Impaired transport of conjugated bilirubin out of hepatocyte
	  1. Congenital transport defect—Dubin-Johnson and Rotor's syndromes
	  2. Hepatocellular damage secondary to metabolic disorders
	    a. Galactosemia (late)
	    b. α-1-Antitrypsin deficiency*
	    c. Tyrosinemia
	    d. Hypermethioninemia
	    e. Hereditary fructose intolerance*
	  3. Toxic obstruction (IV alimentation)
	
	H. Obstruction to bile flow
	  1. Biliary atresia
	  2. Choledochal cyst*
	  3. Cystic fibrosis*
	  4. Extrinsic obstruction (tumor or band)
		I. Prenatal Infection
		  1. Toxoplasmosis
		  2. Rubella
		  3. Cytomegalovirus (CMV)
		  4. Herpesvirus hominis
		  5. Syphilis
		  6. Hepatitis
		  7. Others
		
		J. Postnatal infections (sepsis)
		
		K. Multisystems disorders
		  1. Prematurity ± RDS
		  2. Infants of diabetic mothers
		  3. Severe erythroblastosis

*Not seen early in the neonatal period.

cholinesterase activity is a better index of ABO disease.[34] In Rh disease, anti-Rh antibody (most commonly anti-D) can be eluted from the cells of the infant.

Laboratory studies should include reticulocyte counts in addition to serial hematocrits and a blood smear. A reticulocyte count greater than 6 per cent after the third day of life usually signifies the presence of a hemolytic process. The blood smear is most useful in differentiating among the common hemolytic disorders. The presence of spherocytes, polychromatophilia, acanthocytes, and anisocytosis are all suggestive of a hemolytic disturbance. Bizarre-shaped cells, clumped hemoglobin within cells, and Heinz bodies are each seen in some form of hereditary anemia (Table 11–1, A,2). Examination of the parents' red cells may help in these cases as well as testing for the appropriate erythrocyte enzyme or hemoglobin variant.

Infants with extravasated blood (Table 11–1, B) rarely show significant anemia or reticulocytosis even though the blood is lost to the circulation and is destroyed by macrophages outside the circulation. In these cases, physical examination will reveal the presence of multiple ecchymoses or a large hematoma.

Maternal blood swallowed during the birth process can also contribute to neonatal jaundice. This blood can be catabolized in the intestinal mucosa to form an additional load of bilirubin.

Polycythemia has the potential to contribute to neonatal jaundice since it is associated with a larger than normal mass of red blood cells (Table 11–1, C). This condition may lead to impaired perfusion of the liver sinusoids secondary to hyperviscosity. In addition, the larger mass of red cells may lead to an increased rate of bilirubin production even at normal rates of destruction (approximately 1% daily).[65] However, a recent study of neonatal polycythemia did not find an increased incidence of hyperbilirubinemia in polycythemic infants over that of matched controls.[7]

In the study by Black et al[7] (1982), 37 per cent of the infants with hyperviscosity were treated with partial exchange transfusion at a mean age of 14 hours. Since the potential cause for hyperbilirubinemia was thus eliminated on the first day of life, it is not surprising that there was no increase in the incidence of hyperbilirubinemia in the polycythemic infants. In another study from the same institution, however, a serum bilirubin level of greater than 12 mg/dl was found in 9 of 18 infants with documented hyperbilirubinemia. This 50 per cent incidence (clearly higher than the expected 8–10%) occurred even though some infants were treated with exchange transfusion. (Unfortunately, the authors do not indicate at what age this procedure was performed.) Others have demonstrated a clear relationship between an increase in red cell volume and the severity of neonatal hyperbilirubinemia (Saigal et al, 1972).[65] If chronic fetal hypoxia is the cause of polycythemia, it may mitigate the hyperbilirubinemia. Presumably, chronic stress can produce an increase in glucuronyl transferase and enhance the liver's ability to clear bilirubin.   **J. Maisels**

For further discussion of polycythemia, see Chapter 15.

Chronic fetal hypoxia is often the underlying cause of polycythemia, although a maternal-fetal transplacental hemorrhage may be suspected. In the latter case, the infant's blood has more than 30 per cent adult hemoglobin or the infant's serum contains an elevated level of IgA. Differential agglutination will demonstrate two cell types in the infant's circulation if the blood types of the baby and mother differ. Fetofetal transfusion in twins should be suspected when the infants are discordant in size; the larger twin usually exhibits polycythemia, and the smaller is often anemic.

Jaundice due primarily to exaggerated enterohepatic circulation is relatively common (Table 11–1, D) and should be suspected in an infant with delayed passage of meconium.[64] It is important to review the nurses' observations concerning the initial passage of meconium and the frequency of stooling thereafter. If a meconium plug is present, a small saline enema may suffice. The meconium should then be tested for protein content or for enzymes (trypsin or disaccharidases) to identify the presence of cystic fibrosis.

Some physicians might be tempted to encourage the passage of meconium by inserting a glycerin suppository. The effect of early evacuation of meconium on serum bilirubin levels was studied in a prospective randomized fashion by Weisman et al (1983). The infants who received a suppository passed the first meconium stool earlier than the control group but did not have a significantly lower incidence of hyperbilirubinemia. Nevertheless, the suppository group consistently showed lower bilirubin levels at all intervals measured over the first 3 days (though these differences were not significant). Since there were only 40 babies in each group, it seems quite likely that if a larger population had been studied, these differences would have become statistically significant. It is unlikely, however, that they would be clinically important.

Weisman, L. E., Merenstein, G. B., Digirol, M., et al: The effect of early meconium evacuation on early onset hyperbilirubinemia. Am J Dis Child *137*:666, 1983.

                J. Maisels

Abdominal distension with bowel loops visible on the abdominal wall and bile-stained vomitus are hallmarks of intestinal obstruction (Table 11–1, D,1). See Chapter 6.

Undersecretion

Disease states leading to undersecretion of bilirubin must be considered in those patients with hyperbilirubinemia in whom no cause of bilirubin overproduction can be identified. These states can be divided into (1) those with decreased hepatic uptake, (2) those involving impaired bilirubin conjugation, (3) those in which transport of conjugated bilirubin into the biliary tree is defective, and (4) those with mechanical obstruction to biliary passages. The first two mechanisms lead to unconjugated hyperbilirubinemia and the latter two lead to conjugated hyperbilirubinemia (elevated direct-reacting bilirubin).

DECREASED HEPATIC UPTAKE OF BILIRUBIN. Hepatocellular uptake of bilirubin can be impeded in two ways (Table 11–1, E). First, the circulation of portal blood through the liver sinusoids may be reduced by the persistence of flow through the ductus venosus. This has been shown to occur in hypoxic infants with cardiorespiratory problems and in premature infants in general.[51] Hyperviscosity and hypovolemia may lead to reduced hepatic perfusion also. Second, the diffusion of bilirubin into the hepatocytes may be slowed by either a relative deficiency of intracellular bilirubin-binding proteins (so-called Y and Z proteins) or a saturation of these binding proteins with alternative ligands. Among the compounds known to compete with bilirubin for binding on these proteins are sulfobromophthalein (BSP) dye, chloramphenicol, thyroxine, steroid hormones, and free fatty acids.[29, 38]

DECREASED BILIRUBIN CONJUGATION. Familial nonhemolytic jaundice of infancy is caused by a lack of bilirubin-UDP-glucuronyl transferase activity in the endoplasmic reticulum of liver cells (Table 11–1, F,1). This condition is characterized by life-long unconjugated hyperbilirubinemia. Type I (Crigler-Najjar syndrome) is the more serious form, since the enzyme deficiency is complete and the hyperbilirubinemia more severe (concentrations exceeding 25 mg/dl). Type I is transmitted as an autosomal recessive disorder. The type II disorder represents a partial deficiency of the same enzyme activity. The hyperbilirubinemia is less severe in type II (serum bilirubin less than 25 mg/dl), and the inheritance is consistent with an autosomal dominant pattern. Patients with this milder disorder respond to inducers of hepatic enzyme activity such as phenobarbital.[1]

Hypothyroidism is also a cause of prolonged unconjugated hyperbilirubinemia,[77] although the mechanism has not been clearly defined. The absence of the distal femoral epiphysis on a roentgenograph in a term infant is indicative of hypothyroidism. A low serum thyroxine concentration and an elevated thyroid-stimulating hormone (TSH) level confirm the diagnosis. Because congenital hypothyroidism is difficult to diagnose early on clinical grounds and because it is a cause of mental retardation, many state health departments are now screening for this disorder routinely. The jaundice of hypopituitarism and that of anencephaly are most likely related to secondary hypothyroidism.

Drugs, hormones, and other chemicals (Table 11–1, F,2) associated with neonatal hyperbilirubinemia may interfere with the conjugation of bilirubin. They may also interfere with the hepatic uptake of bilirubin by competitive binding in the liver cytosol (see above).

Persistent jaundice in some breast-fed infants is associated with increased amounts of nonesterified fatty acids (NEFA) in the milk.

NEFA appear because of an unusual lipolytic activity found in the milk of certain women.[62] These fatty acids are in vitro inhibitors of the transferase that conjugates bilirubin, and they also bind to the Z protein in competition with bilirubin.[29] The exact mechanism leading to prolonged neonatal hyperbilirubinemia has not been clarified. Infants with this condition develop jaundice in the middle of the first week of life. The jaundice becomes exaggerated and persistent thereafter. If the bilirubin level is not a danger to the infant, no treatment is needed. The hyperbilirubinemia will subside gradually (often over a period of weeks). If the level is approaching that requiring intervention, then a temporary (1–4 day) cessation of breast feeding and substitution of formula should accelerate the fall in serum bilirubin concentration.[30, 60]

Gartner and coworkers found that normal milk inhibits intestinal bilirubin absorption in rats, whereas absorption is enhanced significantly by milk from mothers and infants with breast milk jaundice. These authors suggest that the exaggerated enterohepatic circulation of bilirubin may be related to the increased concentration of NEFA found in these milks.

Gartner, L. M., Lee, K. S., and Moscione, A.: Effect of milk feeding on intestinal bilirubin absorption in the rat. J Pediatr 103:464, 1983.

J. Maisels

Many clinicians have observed an increased incidence of neonatal hyperbilirubinemia among breast-fed infants when compared with bottle-fed controls; others have not. A review of the published data does not resolve this issue. Most studies have shown no significant differences in peak bilirubin concentrations between bottle-fed and breast-fed cohorts.[19, 45] The differences in experience reported may be related to local institutional practices such as the timing of the first feeding,[81] frequency of feeding,[21] variations in maternal support, and types of intrapartum and postpartum medications used.[22] Supplementing breast feeding with water or formula in the first few days of life does not appear to reduce the incidence of neonatal jaundice.[19, 20]

In an earlier analysis of 8 studies comparing serum bilirubin levels in breast-fed and bottle-fed babies (Maisels, 1981), mean serum bilirubin levels in the first 6 days of life in breast-fed babies were, on average, 0.8 mg/dl higher than those in bottle-fed infants. In only two of the eight studies were bilirubin levels significantly increased in breast-fed babies on the fifth and sixth days of life, and in only one study was there an increased incidence of hyperbilirubinemia at 72 hours in these infants. Although

I (and others) had concluded previously that there was little evidence to support an association between breast feeding and hyperbilirubinemia in the first 3 days of life, my own recent data and those of several other studies suggest that this conclusion is wrong. In almost all of the earlier surveys, small sample size prevented the study from having sufficient power to allow the investigator to accept the null hypothesis of no difference between the two populations. More recently, we analyzed serum bilirubin measurements on 2241 infants in our well-baby nursery. On the third hospital day we identified 57 infants who had no obvious cause for hyperbilirubinemia (serum bilirubin >12.9 mg/dl). Of these infants, 46 were breast fed, 3 were breast and bottle fed, and only 8 were bottle fed (p < 0.0001 versus those with bilirubins ≤12.9 mg/dl). Four other recent studies confirm these observations (Butler and MacMillan, Kuhr and Paneth, Osborn et al, and Saigal et al). The evidence now is compelling that there *is* a significant association between breast feeding and the incidence of nonphysiologic jaundice in a normal newborn population as early as the third day of life. This does not, of course, necessarily imply that breast feeding is the *cause* of the jaundice. There are many causes of neonatal hyperbilirubinemia, and breast feeding may be just one of many contributing factors. It is known, for example, that breast-feeding mothers are far less likely to smoke during pregnancy than are bottle-feeding mothers. Dr. Richard Naeye at our institution has examined this question using the data base of the collaborative perinatal project. His preliminary data suggest that one of the most powerful factors lowering serum bilirubin levels in the first few days of life is the number of cigarettes smoked daily by the mother during pregnancy. These observations clearly confound any documented association between breast-feeding and jaundice. It is unlikely, however, that this mechanism can explain the relationship between breast feeding and jaundice that appears at the end of the first week of life and persists thereafter. It is said that "true breast milk jaundice" occurs in only 1–2 per cent of breast-fed infants, but this has never been studied systematically. Using the transcutaneous bilirubinometer to follow babies for the first 6 weeks of life, we found that, when compared with bottle-fed infants, breast-fed infants had a significantly higher transcutaneous bilirubin (TCB) index from day 7 through day 42. At 3 weeks of life, about 30 per cent of breast-fed infants had an elevated TCB index. It is possible that these infants represent a mild form of the spectrum of "true breast milk jaundice." In fact, it would be strange if such a spectrum did not exist, and these data suggest that this condition may well be far more common than previously believed.

Butler, D. A., and MacMillan, J. P.: Relationship of breastfeeding and weight loss to jaundice in the newborn: Review of the literature and results of a study. Cleve Clin Quarterly 50:263, 1983.

Kuhr, M., and Paneth, N.: Feeding practices and early neonatal jaundice. J Pediatr Gastroenterol Nutr 1:485, 1982.

Maisels, M. J.: Neonatal jaundice. *In* Avery, G. B. (ed.): Neonatology, Pathophysiology and Management of the Newborn. 2nd ed. Philadelphia, J. B. Lippincott Co., 1981, p. 473.

Osborn, L. M., Rieff, M. I., and Bolus, R.: Jaundice in the full term neonate. Pediatrics 73:520, 1984.

Saigal, S., Lunyk, O., Bennett, K. J., et al: Serum bilirubin levels in breast and formula fed infants in the first 5 days of life. Can Med Assoc J 127:985, 1982.

J. Maisels

Patients with galactosemia may exhibit unconjugated hyperbilirubinemia during the first week of life. The accumulation of UDP-galactose in the liver cells may interfere with the production of UDP-glucuronic acid, although no convincing evidence of this mechanism exists.[67]

Arias and his associates[3] found that the sera of a group of infants described by Lucey and Driscoll were markedly inhibitory to the conjugation of bilirubin in an in vitro assay. Maternal sera in these cases were also inhibitory. Some of the infants had bilirubin encephalopathy. The inhibitor has not been identified, but it appears to be in the circulation of both mother and infant during the postnatal period. Diagnosis can be suspected from the family history, but only a special assay for inhibitor will confirm it.

IMPAIRED TRANSPORT OF CONJUGATED BILIRUBIN OUT OF HEPATOCYTES. Two genetic syndromes have been described in which the primary defect is in the active transport of conjugated bilirubin out of the hepatocyte (Table 11–1, G,1). These diseases are known as the Dubin-Johnson and Rotor's syndromes. The former is inherited as an autosomal recessive disorder and the latter as an autosomal dominant.[25] A special liver function test and a liver biopsy are needed for diagnosis of these syndromes.

Transport of conjugated bilirubin out of the hepatocyte into the biliary system is the rate limiting step in bilirubin excretion for infants with generalized hepatocellular destruction (Table 11–1, G,2).

Genetic-metabolic diseases such as galactosemia, hereditary fructose intolerance, tyrosinemia, and cystic fibrosis cause hepatocellular injury and hepatic fibrosis. Hereditary fructose intolerance does not usually cause problems early in a newborn's existence, since fructose-containing foods are usually introduced later. Patients with these diseases fail to thrive and have gastrointestinal symptoms such as vomiting and diarrhea. Diagnosis depends on tests of the urine and/or the serum for specific sugars or amino acids.[74] A sweat test will identify the patient with cystic fibrosis.

Alpha-1-antitrypsin deficiency and Neimann-Pick disease (types A and B) are also causes of conjugated hyperbilirubinemia in early infancy. The former is identified by a low alpha-1-globulin on serum protein electrophoresis and a low level of alpha-1-antitrypsin (protein or activity) in the serum. Patients with Neimann-Pick disease have massive hepatosplenomegaly, failure to thrive, and cherry red spots in their retinae.

Patients treated with total parenteral nutrition have been reported to develop conjugated hyperbilirubinemia.[5] These patients have little evidence of hepatic inflammation or destruction on liver biopsy, and most of them improve with time (whether the intravenous alimentation is discontinued or not). The mechanism for this problem is not known.

OBSTRUCTION TO BILE FLOW. Last under the category of bilirubin undersecretion, we have patients with mechanical obstruction to the flow of bile (Table 11–1, H). Biliary atresia occurs most frequently in full-term female infants of normal birth weight. These patients are not likely to have splenomegaly or evidence of hemolysis. Infants with giant cell hepatitis, on the other hand, are most often male, with signs of fetal infection such as splenomegaly, hemolysis, and intrauterine growth retardation. Patients with cystic fibrosis can have inspissation of the biliary tree with thick secretions.[72] Tumors, fibrous bands, and choledochal cysts can obstruct the biliary tree, also. Biliary atresia and choledochal cysts are usually diagnosed beyond the first few weeks of life. The latter may be palpable in the right upper quadrant of the abdomen and can be detected by ultrasonography.

Biliary obstruction is characterized by an elevated direct-reacting bilirubin level in the serum, bile in the urine, and acholic stools. Urine urobilinogen is not elevated in the neonate since the intestinal flora necessary for the conversion of bilirubin to urobilinogen takes about 6 weeks to develop.

Our usual diagnostic work-up of a relatively healthy infant with conjugated hyperbilirubinemia is outlined in Table 11–2. In the infant whose findings are limited to the liver, this scheme will lead to a satisfactory diagnosis in over 95 per cent of cases.[13] The history and physical examination may provide clues that lead to the use of other diagnostic tests, however. Although many laboratory tests designed to distinguish biliary

obstruction from hepatocellular diseases have been proposed, liver biopsy remains our most reliable diagnostic procedure.

Before proceeding to liver biopsy, it has been our practice to perform scintigraphic imaging following the administration of one of the N-substituted iminodiacetic acid agents. These agents are rapidly extracted by hepatocytes and excreted into the biliary tree. When labeled with ^{99m}Tc, they allow clear gamma camera imaging. Although some infants with severe intrahepatic cholestasis will show no significant excretion within 24 hours after injection, if excretion is shown, extrahepatic biliary atresia is ruled out. Another simple technique that is useful is the visual analysis of a 24 hour collection of duodenal fluid. The appearance of bilirubin-stained fluid is reassuring. A refinement of this technique involves the administration of technetium labeled DESIDA and quantification of the radioactivity in the duodenal fluid. Alternatively, bile acids can be measured in the duodenal aspirate. None should be detected in biliary atresia, whereas varying amounts will be detected in infants with neonatal hepatitis (Yamashiro et al 1983).

The initial evaluation of all infants with cholestasis should now involve ultrasonography. The appearance of a normal gallbladder by ultrasound (1.5 cm or greater in length) is good evidence against biliary atresia (Abrahamson et al, 1982). In some patients, the common bile duct also may be visualized.

Abrahamson, S. J., Treves, S., and Teele, R. L.: The infant with possible biliary atresia, evaluation by ultrasound or nuclear medicine. Pediatr Radiol 12:1, 1982.
Yamashiro, Y., Robinson, P. G., Lari, J., et al: Duodenal bile acids in diagnosis of congenital biliary atresia. J Pediatr Surg 80:278, 1983.

J. Maisels

Combined Overproduction and Undersecretion

Under this heading are prenatal infections (Table 11–1, I), including toxoplasmosis, ru-

---

TABLE 11–2 CONJUGATED HYPERBILIRUBINEMIA OF EARLY INFANCY

Suggested Work-Up
1. History and physical examination*
2. CBC and reticulocyte count
3. Coombs' test
4. Urinalysis, including reducing substances
5. Serum bilirubin concentration, total and direct-reacting
6. Total serum protein and protein electrophoresis
7. Serum transaminases
8. Alpha-1-antitrypsin concentration
9. Hepatitis-associated antigen and titers
10. Sweat chloride concentration
11. Serologic titers for rubella, CMV, etc.
12. Clotting factors, platelet count
13. Liver biopsy

---

*May lead one to order other diagnostic tests not listed.

bella, cytomegalovirus disease, herpes simplex, syphilis, and hepatitis. All of these infections can be transmitted through the placenta, and some of them are acquired by the newborn during parturition. Prenatal infection can elevate the cord blood IgM level and retard the growth of the fetus. Many infants with these infections have hepatosplenomegaly, hemolytic anemia, thrombocytopenia, and evidence of hepatocellular injury. The long bones may have a "celery stalk" appearance on x-ray in infants with toxoplasmosis, rubella, cytomegalovirus, and herpes simplex infection. Metaphyseal periostitis is seen in infants with syphilis. Microcephaly or hydrocephalus may be found in newborns with these diseases.[66] See Chapter 12.

Newborn infants with sepsis (Table 11–1, J) often become lethargic and feed poorly. They frequently show anemia that may be related to hemolysins elaborated by pathogenic bacteria. Septicemia may cause bone marrow depression, too. Intrahepatic bile stasis resulting in an elevation of the direct-reacting bilirubin fraction can also occur with sepsis. Even in the presence of bile stasis, however, there may be little evidence of hepatic inflammation by histologic or biochemical criteria. The white blood cell count may rise above 20,000/mm,[3] but more often it falls below 10,000, and the proportion of unsegmented neutrophils increases. A microsedimentation rate or measurement of the serum C-reactive protein level may help to confirm the presence of sepsis.[59] Culture of blood, spinal fluid, and perhaps urine should be performed before antibiotic therapy is begun. The selection of antibiotics will depend on the organism isolated, but a combination of a penicillin and an aminoglycoside is generally used until culture results are available.

The jaundice of prematurity (infants less than 38 weeks' gestation) occurs through complex mechanisms. All of the factors leading to "physiologic jaundice" have been invoked to explain the jaundice of premature infants by assuming that the hepatic clearance mechanisms are even further deficient in this group. Excessive production of bilirubin by extravascular hemolysis is often contributory because petechiae and ecchymoses of the skin and subcutaneous tissues are common in premature infants. Conjugated hyperbilirubinemia is rare in these patients, and a more specific diagnosis must be sought if it appears.

The etiology of jaundice frequently encountered in infants of diabetic mothers is also multifactorial. Enterohepatic circulation is prominent in some, and early or frequent feeding may be helpful. In others, polycythemia and hypovolemia may play a role in the production of jaundice.

Conjugated hyperbilirubinemia and bilirubinuria have been seen in severe hemolytic diseases. There may be no other evidence of intrinsic liver disease in these cases. The uptake and conjugation of bilirubin appear to exceed the capacity of the liver to excrete conjugated bilirubin because of the very high rates of bilirubin production.[2] Occasionally, infants with severe Rh or ABO hemolytic disease have some evidence of hepatic injury, also.[23]

Last, oxytocin and diazepam administered to mothers in labor have been associated with higher neonatal bilirubin levels. The mechanisms have not been defined.[22]

BILIRUBIN TOXICITY AND ITS PREVENTION

Bilirubin Toxicity

Bilirubin is toxic to all tissues, but its toxicity to the central nervous system is most important clinically. The recognition of bilirubin neurotoxicity early in this century has led to an extensive body of knowledge about the causes and treatment of neonatal hyperbilirubinemia. The term *kernicterus* (derived from Greek, meaning "yellow nucleus") represents a pathologist's description of gross yellow staining of the basal ganglia, hippocampus, and certain brainstem nuclei associated with histologic changes of neuronal degeneration and necrosis.[16, 31] Clinically, severe hyperbilirubinemia has been associated with certain acute and long-term signs and symptoms. These consist early of lethargy, poor suck, high pitched cry, and hypotonia. Later, irritability, hypertonia, opisthotonos, and seizures may occur. Fatalities, too, have been attributed to bilirubin neurotoxicity. Survivors may manifest severe neurologic sequelae characterized by an athetoid type of cerebral palsy, hearing loss, and mental retardation.[15] It is likely that bilirubin neurotoxicity may produce a spectrum of neurologic dysfunctions ranging from the severe manifestations described above to less severe forms, such as mild cognitive dysfunction, hyperkinesis and learning disability.[50]

In the past 10 years, a considerable amount of attention has been directed to assessing the risk of infants with low level of serum bilirubin for so-called "kernicterus" based essentially on gross pathologic observations of yellow staining of the brain.[35, 36, 57] Recently, evidence has emerged that not all yellow staining of the brain is accompanied by the characteristic neurohistopathologic changes of kernicterus.[75] We are no longer certain that criteria based on gross yellow staining are relevant to the task of preventing bilirubin neurotoxicity. Thus an ideal solution to the problem of determining the risk to a given infant of bilirubin neurotoxicity eludes us. To approach an answer to this problem, we need reliable criteria to define kernicterus at autopsy, and we also need more information about long-term neurologic outcome.

Bilirubin encephalopathy occurs secondary to the toxic effects of so-called free bilirubin (unconjugated bilirubin not bound to serum albumin). This hypothesis is based on tissue culture and whole animal studies, which have demonstrated that bilirubin is not toxic if it is protein-bound and relatively unable to traverse cell membranes. The free or unbound bilirubin, therefore, is the form of the compound that is able to traverse cell membranes, to bind with tissues, and to damage cells of the central nervous system.[10, 11, 80] Even in instances when the integrity of the "blood-brain barrier" may be disrupted, allowing protein-bound bilirubin to penetrate brain capillaries,[39] the cells of the brain are very likely protected by the protein binding.

The relationship of free to bound bilirubin is described by the reaction:

Bilirubin + Albumin $\longleftrightarrow$

Bilirubin − Albumin

The above formula is an extreme simplification of the conditions found in nature, however. It implies that the concentrations of bilirubin and albumin are the dominant factors in determining the concentration of "free" bilirubin. In reality, albumin has several binding sites for small molecules, and more than one of these bind bilirubin. Albumin probably has no binding site that binds bilirubin exclusively, and therefore many other compounds, drugs and naturally occurring products can compete for bilirubin-binding sites and reduce the effective concentration of albumin in the simple formula given above. The concentration of free bilirubin is determined by a number of factors, such as the rate of formation of bilirubin from its precursors, the concentration of albumin, and the degree of saturation of the binding sites of albumin with bilirubin and its competitors.

The affinity of bilirubin for albumin is high (association constant around 10^7 moles/l). In the presence of normal amounts of albumin and relative unsaturation of its binding sites, the concentration of free bilirubin is extremely small (circa 0.12 nmol/l or 7.0 ng/dl). However, in the presence of competitors for albumin binding sites, such as sulfonamides, diuretics, salicylate, and nonesterified fatty acids, the albumin carrier becomes saturated. Then, more bilirubin exists in the free state and can therefore diffuse into the cells and interfere with cellular respiration.

Free bilirubin is found in the serum in concentrations too small to be measured accurately by standard laboratory methods. The standard colorimetric tests for bilirubin, such as the van den Bergh reaction, measure bilirubin that is albumin-bound or conjugated (i.e., those forms of bilirubin that are nontoxic). However, an enzymatic reaction using horseradish peroxidase has been used as an assay for free bilirubin, based on the ability of the enzyme to catalyze indirectly the oxidation of free bilirubin but not protein-bound bilirubin. The clinical value of this test remains in question because of some mixed results obtained in animal and human studies of acute toxicity[53, 63, 79] and the lack of a long-term follow-up study verifying its usefulness. Nonetheless, since the equation above is in dynamic equilibrium, it follows that the higher the level of albumin-bound bilirubin, the greater the corresponding concentration of dissociated free bilirubin. Thus there is reason to infer clinically that the higher the serum bilirubin concentration, the greater the risk of kernicterus.[50]

Other laboratory methods have been used to estimate the danger of bilirubin toxicity. Since bilirubin has a high affinity for albumin, the concentration of free bilirubin will be insignificantly low as long as an adequate amount of albumin with free and open binding sites is present. On this basis, the tests for reserve albumin-binding capacity have evolved. Among these, the HBABA dye binding test and the salicylate saturation index have had the most study. Both of these have been validated to some extent with longitudinal studies,[32, 50] and they therefore deserve consideration as adjuncts to clinical decision-making.

CLINICAL MANAGEMENT

Every effort should be made to identify the cause of the jaundice in an infant before treatment is initiated. Jaundice can be an early sign of serious neonatal disease. Routine evaluation for the etiology of neonatal jaundice can lead to early diagnosis and specific treatment.

A minimal evaluation for jaundice includes:

- Review of maternal and infant history, including medications, feeding, and defecation.
- Blood type and Coombs' test. If the Coombs' test is positive, antibody should be eluted from the infant's cells for further identification.
- Hematocrit, hemoglobin concentration, white blood cell count, differential count, and reticulocyte count.
- Examination of the peripheral blood smear for red cell morphology and the presence of adequate numbers of platelets.
- Urinalysis for protein, cells, and reducing substances.
- Appropriate cultures, if infection is suspected.
- Serum T_4, especially for prolonged hyperbilirubinemia (done as part of state-sponsored genetic screening in many states).
- Storage of some serum for unanticipated tests (e.g., antibody titer).

Exchange Transfusion

Indications

The primary aim of exchange transfusion is to prevent the toxic effects of bilirubin by the removal of bilirubin from the body. Since the assessment of risk to the infant for kernicterus has changed substantially through the years, the indications for exchange transfusion have become less well established. However, the basic guidelines for exchange transfusion remain dependent on the level of serum bilirubin, the rate of rise of serum bilirubin concentration, and, in some institutions, an estimation of reserve albumin-binding capacity. It is important to emphasize that these criteria are based on laboratory tests; the clinical condition of the infant must also play an important role in the formulation of therapeutic decisions. In the presence of overt complications, such as gross prematur-

ity, asphyxia, acidosis, or sepsis, the cellular susceptibility to bilirubin toxicity may be modified significantly, and the risk of kernicterus cannot be predicted with certainty by any available laboratory test. Given the state of our knowledge, recommendations for exchange transfusion are still based on empiricism. Therefore, a striking set of conflicting guidelines has been proposed from various sources over the years.

Table 11–3 represents our view of a reasonable set of guidelines one could use to make difficult decisions about the use of exchange transfusion. Many of the guidelines are based upon laboratory tests, but judgments about clinical condition must be taken into account to complete the evaluation of an individual infant.

In infants with hemolytic disease, an exchange transfusion is performed to replace sensitized erythrocytes with those of a donor whose blood is compatible with both the mother's and the infant's serum. The percentage of infant's cells replaced is a function of the volume of the donor blood used, not its hematocrit. An 85 per cent replacement of the infant's circulating erythrocytes can be expected if the volume of the donor unit is twice that of the infant's blood. Bilirubin production, however, may remain quite high in infants with hemolytic disease even after

---

TABLE 11–3 INDICATIONS FOR EXCHANGE TRANSFUSION

Infants with Hemolytic Disease (otherwise uncomplicated)
1. Anemia (hematocrit <45%), positive Coombs' test, *and* a rate of rise in serum bilirubin >0.5 mg/dl/hour
2. In ABO disease, a rate of rise in serum bilirubin >1.0 mg/dl/hour
3. Reduced bilirubin binding capacity as indicated by tests such as the salicylate saturation index or HBABA dye binding capacity, if available
4. Serum bilirubin concentration ≥20 mg/dl at any time
5. Serum bilirubin concentration >15 mg/dl for more than 36 hours and binding capacity not available

Infants With or Without Hemolytic Disease
1. Serm bilirubin concentration >20 mg/dl
2. Clinical factors that may suggest exchange transfusion at lower serum bilirubin concentrations include:
   - Prematurity
   - Sepsis
   - Hypoxia and acidosis (present or past)
   - Hypoproteinemia or use of drug that competes for bilirubin binding sites
   - Evidence of reduced binding capacity (using binding tests noted above)
   - Bilirubin concentration close to exchange level for more than 36 hours

exchange transfusion, since sensitized cells may have already been sequestered in the reticuloendothelial system prior to the exchange transfusion.[44] Thus, more than one or two exchange transfusions may be needed in such infants.

The choice of donor blood type depends on the cause of the hemolytic disease. ABO-compatible Rh-negative cells are used in Rh incompatibility. Type O Rh-specific cells are used in ABO incompatibility along with a low titer of anti A and anti-B antibody (or type AB) plasma. Fresh blood is always desirable. However, CPD-preserved bank blood that is less than 4 days old can be used.

We have always recommended using blood less than 4 days old because of previous data indicating that serum potassium levels may reach 20 mEq/l by 7 days in ACD-preserved and 10 mEq/l in CPD-preserved blood (Gibson et al, 1961). It seems, however, that substantially higher plasma potassium levels may be found (Scanlon and Krakaur, 1980; Batton et al, 1983). We were surprised to find a mean plasma potassium concentration of 16.2 ± 4.3 mEq/l in blood only 24–48 hours old that was being used for exchange transfusion. This situation can be ameliorated by using washed red cells reconstituted to the desired hematocrit with fresh frozen plasma.

Batton, D. G., Maisels, M. J., and Schulman, G.: Serum potassium changes following packed cell transfusions in newborn infants. Transfusion 23:163, 1983.

Gibson, J., Gregory, C., and Button, L.: Citrate-phosphate-dextrose solution for the preservation of human blood. Transfusion 1:280, 1961.

Scanlon, J. W., and Krakaur, R.: Hyperkalemia following exchange transfusion. J Pediatr 96:108, 1980.

J. Maisels

Types

PACKED RED CELLS. A packed red cell exchange transfusion is used for severely sensitized infants who require immediate correction of anemia and anoxia at birth. With prior notice of the imminent delivery of an infant at risk for erythroblastosis, fresh O-negative blood is obtained and cross-matched against the mother's serum. The red cells are sedimented and brought to the delivery room area. Anemia is immediately assessed in the infant by his color, condition, and cord hematocrit. Immediate exchange transfusion with the packed erythrocytes is indicated if anemia (hemoglobin less than 12 gm/dl), edema, and hepatosplenomegaly are present.

The term *immediate exchange transfusion* suggests that this procedure should be performed in an emergency fashion, perhaps even in the delivery room. With the exception of an infant who is suffering profound cardio-respiratory decompensation, we feel this is almost never necessary. We have seen many infants with cord hemoglobin values of less than 12 gm/dl who show virtually no evidence of clinical distress, even if they are slightly edematous and have hepatosplenomegaly. Under these circumstances, although it is certainly likely that an exchange transfusion will be needed, there are good reasons not to perform it immediately after delivery. We like to wait until the infant is warm, in stable condition, and has normal blood gases before performing the exchange transfusion in the controlled environment of the neonatal intensive care unit.   **J. Maisels**

A catheter is inserted through the umbilical vein and the central venous pressure recorded. Systemic blood pressure is also measured by ultrasonic or direct (intraarterial) means. The exchange transfusion is carried out very slowly (using 5–10 ml increments) until a final hematocrit of 45 volumes per cent is achieved. Infants with severe Rh disease frequently have low blood volume, and any deficit created by the exchange transfusion may cause a significant fall in the systemic blood pressure. Therefore, it is important to monitor the infant's venous and arterial blood pressures frequently. Since the purpose of this sort of exchange transfusion is the correction of anemia, we do not attempt to complete a two-volume exchange in this situation because these infants are unstable. Rather, we transfer the infant to intensive care after correcting the hematocrit to 45 volumes per cent to allow the infant to reach a more stable condition. A vigorous approach to the correction of anemia, hypoxemia, and acidosis is required, often with the use of assisted ventilation. Only then do we complete a two-volume exchange transfusion (see Chapters 8 and 9).

WHOLE BLOOD EXCHANGE TRANSFUSION. Whole blood exchange transfusions are employed (1) to replace the infant's sensitized erythrocytes, (2) to remove circulating antibodies (a less efficient process), and (3) to remove bilirubin. Albumin may be used to facilitate the removal of bilirubin. Forty per cent more bilirubin can be removed by administration of 1 gm/kg of salt-poor albumin to the infant 1 hour before the start of the exchange transfusion.[49] This technique can increase the efficiency of an exchange transfusion when a significant pool of bilirubin exists outside the plasma space (i.e., when reserve albumin-binding capacity is low). When one is trying to remove sensitized red cells or when there is little bilirubin outside the plasma space, albumin priming is not indicated. Cardiac failure is another contraindication to the administration of albumin.

Technique

A properly identified donor unit is removed from the blood bank and allowed to warm to room temperature over a 1 hour period. Alternatively, a warming coil with proper safeguards against overheating (above 37°C) is used. Other forms of heat should not be applied since red cells near the surface of the unit may be destroyed, leading to dangerous extracellular concentrations of potassium.

We allow our patients to be fed up to the time of exchange transfusion because starvation may induce a rise in serum nonesterified fatty acids, competitors for bilirubin binding sites on albumin. We then insert a nasogastric tube to evacuate the infant's stomach. Hydration is maintained by intravenous infusion if the infant is not being fed.

Restrain the infant's arms and legs and provide for a warm environment. Monitor the skin temperature, heart rate (preferably with an oscilloscope), and blood pressure. A source of oxygen, suction apparatus, and equipment for neonatal resuscitation should be readily available.

We prefer to have three people involved in the exchange transfusion: two physicians to carry out the procedure and any necessary resuscitation and a circulating nurse who observes the oscilloscope and records vital signs, volumes of blood exchanged, venous pressures, etc.

We use a disposable exchange transfusion set together with a surgical prep and cutdown set. The size of the catheter used is French 5 or 8, and it is placed in the umbilical vein to a depth that allows for blood return (usually the first mark on the catheter).

If the catheter cannot be inserted, a supraumbilical cutdown or one using the anterior tibial or saphenous vein may be performed. The latter two sites are preferred if the infant's umbilical area is infected. We have had little experience in using the umbilical artery for exchange transfusion; this route may be considered when the above routes are not feasible and with caution, since serious complications such as paraplegia have been known to occur.

Once blood return is obtained from the venous catheter, infuse a small amount of isotonic saline to clear the catheter and measure venous pressure with a ruler. The pressure should remain between 4 and 9 cm H_2O during the procedure. Save the first 10 ml

drawn for bilirubin, hematologic, and miscellaneous studies as indicated. Passes of approximately 5 ml/kg are done (up to 20 ml in the largest infants), and the bag is gently mixed after every 50 ml of blood infused to prevent sedimentation of the cells.

The volume of blood used is twice the blood volume of the infant (about 170 ml/kg, up to one full unit of blood), and the exchange should not be performed in less than 1 hour from the first withdrawal to the last. After each 100 ml of blood exchanged, measure the venous pressure and evaluate the patient for hypocalcemia. If there is tachycardia or prolongation of the Q-T segment on the electrocardiogram, then infuse 1 ml of 10 per cent calcium gluconate slowly. Observe the infant for bradycardia during the calcium infusion and use saline to flush the catheter before and after the calcium infusion. Irritability has been attributed to low concentrations of ionized calcium in these infants, but this assertion has not been confirmed when studied systematically.[42] The hazards of the calcium infusion outweigh its theoretic usefulness in the absence of signs and symptoms of hypocalcemia.

Measure the venous pressure after each 50 ml of blood exchanged when dealing with a hydropic infant. The plasma protein concentration of this infant is initially low but gradually rises as the plasma from the donor unit is infused, causing edema fluid to shift into the intravascular space. Cardiac overload and failure of a compromised heart may result. These infants often need ventilatory support, and they may need to have their blood volume reduced more than once during the exchange transfusion.

Use the final aliquot of blood withdrawn for determination of bilirubin, hematocrit, electrolytes, and calcium and for future crossmatching. The postexchange serum bilirubin is usually half the preexchange value after a two-volume exchange transfusion.

After the procedure, monitor the infant's vital signs every 15 minutes for 1 hour and every 30 minutes for the next 3 hours. Resume feedings by 4 hours if the infant's condition is stable. Check the blood glucose at 30 minutes, 1 hour, and 2 hours after the exchange transfusion (earlier if heparinized blood was used). See Chapter 10.

Other complications to watch for during and after exchange transfusion are listed in Table 11–4. The mortality has been reported to be less than 1 per cent when one includes

TABLE 11–4 COMPLICATIONS OF EXCHANGE TRANSFUSIONS

Vascular
Embolization with air or thrombi
Thrombosis

Cardiac
Arrhythmias
Volume overload
Arrest

Electrolyte
Hyperkalemia
Hypernatremia
Hypocalcemia
Acidosis

Coagulation
Overheparinization
Thrombocytopenia

Infectious
Bacteremia
Hepatitis
Cytomegalovirus

Other
Mechanical injury to donor cells
Necrotizing enterocolitis
Hypothermia
Hypoglycemia

all causes of death 6 hours after exchange transfusion.[78] There is no need for antibiotic prophylaxis after this procedure.

Phototherapy

Since the original observation of Cremer et al[18] that serum bilirubin concentrations decreased faster in infants exposed to sunlight or blue fluorescent light, phototherapy has been used extensively for the treatment of neonatal hyperbilirubinemia.

Light reduces serum bilirubin levels by two basic mechanisms: photoisomerization and photosensitized oxidation. During photoisomerization, bilirubin is transformed from a relatively insoluble state (bilirubin IX-alpha Z,Z), into water-soluble photoisomers (photobilirubin).[17, 40, 41] These are bilirubin IX-alpha E,Z, bilirubin IX-alpha E,E, and bilirubin IX-alpha Z,E. The Z,E form is the predominant photoisomer. In its natural state, bilirubin IX-alpha Z,Z is insoluble in water at physiologic pH. Intramolecular hydrogen bonding prevents the access of water molecules to the polar sites. X-ray crystallography has shown that the Z,Z configuration

at the C4–C5 and C15–C16 double bonds allows optimum intramolecular hydrogen bonding. However, light energy of the proper wavelength can transform the Z or cis configuration into the E or trans form in one or both of the methene bridges, forming the alternative combinations seen in Figure 11–5. Such rearrangements interrupt the internal hydrogen bonding and expose the polar sites to water molecules, thereby making bilirubin water soluble. As a consequence, phototherapy converts poorly soluble natural bilirubin into a water-soluble isomer, allowing for its excretion without conjugation into the bile.

Since bilirubin is a photosensitizer, albeit a weak one, it can also capture light energy and become energized to its triplet state (asterisk in Figure 11–6). The photon-excited molecule can either return to the ground state, covalently bind to a substrate (usually one containing a hydroxyl or sulfhydryl group) to form a bilirubin adduct, or transfer its energy to molecular oxygen, which becomes the highly reactive oxygen radical, singlet oxygen. In turn, singlet oxygen can oxidize many important chemicals in the body as well as bilirubin itself. The photooxidation of bilirubin leads to its hydrolysis into water-soluble mono-, di-, and tripyrroles, which in turn can be excreted into the bile or urine. Many other biochemicals are similarly affected.

Thus, phototherapy reduces serum bilirubin concentrations by enhancing the water solubility of the compound through a process of photoisomerization or photooxidation. Either way, bilirubin or its degradation products are then excreted through the bile or urine.

The initial guidelines for the use of phototherapy were set by an ad hoc committee established by the National Academy of Sciences.[4] Their recommendations were as follows: (1) phototherapy can be used for infants at risk (e.g., premature infants) who have attained serum bilirubin levels of 10 mg/dl to prevent a further rise of the bilirubin to 15 mg/dl or greater, and (2) phototherapy may be used in mature infants with bilirubin concentrations between 15 and 20 mg/dl as an alternative means of limiting the degree of bilirubin accumulation. Modifications of these initial guidelines have been made in various neonatal centers and tailored to meet their individual needs. Suffice it to say, there is general agreement that photo-

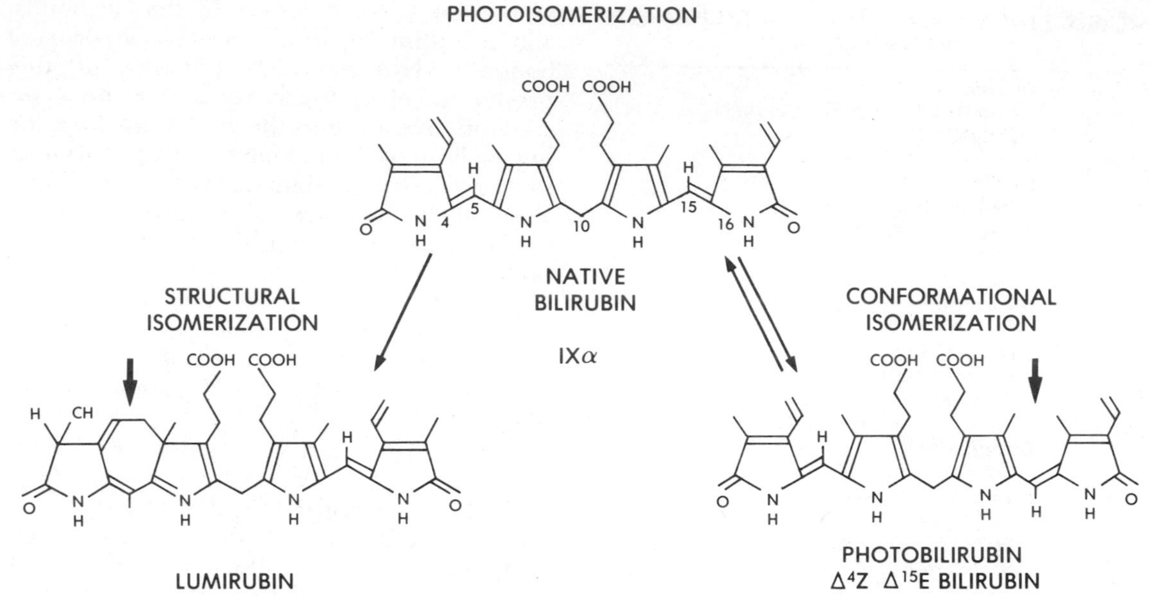

PHOTOISOMERIZATION

Figure 11–5. The photoisomerized conversion of bilirubin IX-α (Z,Z) to water-soluble bilirubin IX-α (Z,E) and lumirubin.

therapy cannot be used as a substitute for exchange transfusion if the latter is indicated and that phototherapy may not be effective in hemolytic diseases of the newborn if the level of serum bilirubin rises at a rate of 0.5–2.0 mg/dl/hour.

This caveat may no longer apply, depending on the indications for exchange transfusion. In some institutions, infants weighing 1 kg or less are subjected to exchange transfusions if their serum bilirubin concentrations exceed 10 mg/dl. In such cases we would opt for phototherapy or increase the dose of light by adding an extra lamp before we would consider exchange transfusion. Phototherapy has been shown to be more effective than exchange transfusion in achieving prolonged reduction of bilirubin levels in nonhemolytic jaundice.[70]

J. Maisels

Figure 11–6. Pathways of reaction of excited (triplet) bilirubin. The asterisk (*) represents the triplet state.

Likewise, *it is fundamentally important that any infant undergoing phototherapy should be investigated adequately for the cause of the bilirubin problem.*

Certainly, if it is to be used in a full-term infant, a full investigation of the cause of the jaundice must be undertaken before phototherapy is instituted. However, in many low-birth-weight infants, phototherapy is used almost prophylactically. It seems somewhat stringent to demand a full set of investigations into the cause of a serum bilirubin of 8 mg/dl in a 600 gm infant on a ventilator. In these circumstances we are prepared to accept the diagnosis of physiologic jaundice and to put the infant under the lights. **J. Maisels**

Editorial Comment: Cost containment policies have resulted in increased pressure for earlier discharge of neonates. This together with the desire to avoid prolonged separation of mother and infant has resulted in the use of *home phototherapy units.* Clearly it is imperative to select the patients carefully, establish the cause of the jaundice, and closely supervise such therapy. Initial reports in this regard are encouraging.

Slater, L., and Brewer, M. F.: Home versus hospital phototherapy for term infants with hyperbilirubinemia: a comparative study. Pediatrics 73:515, 1984.

The efficacy of phototherapy in reducing the serum bilirubin concentration depends on the spectral irradiance or flux of the light source in the 420–475 nm range. Thus, blue light is more effective than white light in view of the higher irradiance at these wavelengths. A disadvantage of blue light is that it makes infants appear blue and reduces our ability to recognize the onset of true cyanosis. The log of the energy output in the blue range (up to 1200 $\mu w/cm^2$ in the 400–480 nm range) correlates positively with rate of fall in the serum bilirubin concentration.[71]

The following guidelines apply when an infant is placed under phototherapy:

1. Monitor the temperature of the infant every 4 hours. For infants in incubators, the thermistor probe should be appropriately shielded from the light.

2. Weigh the infant every 8–12 hours and watch for significant weight loss secondary to increased evaporative water loss or diarrhea, especially in the premature infant. Provide for adequate fluid intake.

The requirement for weighing an infant every 8–12 hours seems excessive. Weighing tiny babies who are being ventilated is certainly a stressful event, and we question the utility of the information derived from this measurement in the first few days of life when arm boards, IV tubes, U bags, etc., are changed frequently.

J. Maisels

3. Shield the eyes and gonads of the infant from the light source.

4. Change the position of the infant every 6 hours.

5. Measure serum bilirubin levels every 6–8 hours. Do not rely on the color of the infant to assess the degree of jaundice.

6. Discontinue phototherapy whenever a parent visits the infant and remove eye shields to allow a natural interaction to occur between parent and infant.

7. Monitor the bilirubin levels every 8–12 hours for a day after the phototherapy is discontinued to detect any rebound rise in serum bilirubin concentration.

Infants undergoing phototherapy may manifest certain side effects (Table 11–5). Thus, close observation of the infant is necessary to judge when to discontinue phototherapy or when to institute corrective measures.

Much concern has been expressed over the safety of phototherapy in relation either to irradiation damage or more realistically to complications of photodynamic oxidation. Studies done in vitro and in animals have demonstrated that phototherapy can have an adverse effect on cell growth,[28] damage cell membranes,[48, 54] and produce breaks in strands of DNA.[26, 68] It can also oxidize essential fatty acids[55] and vitamins[26, 27] and disrupt biologic rhythms.[56] The thermal byproduct

TABLE 11–5 COMPLICATIONS OF PHOTOTHERAPY

Abnormality	Proposed Mechanism
1. Tanning	Induction of melanin synthesis and/or dispersion by ultraviolet light
2. Bronze baby syndrome	Reduced hepatic excretion of bilirubin photoproduct(s)
3. Diarrhea	Bilirubin-induced bowel secretion
4. Lactose intolerance	Mucosal injury of villous epithelium
5. Hemolysis	Photosensitized injury to circulating erythrocytes
6. Skin burns	Excessive exposure to short-wave emissions from fluorescent lamps
7. Dehydration	Increased insensible water losses from absorbed photon energy
8. Skin rashes	Photosensitized injury to skin mast cells with release of histamine

Adapted from Odell, G.: Neonatal Hyperbilirubinemia. New York, Grune & Stratton, 1980, p. 131.

of phototherapy lamps can also add to the thermal stress of infants, especially very small premature ones.[52] Although no lasting side effects of phototherapy have yet been documented in the human, the potential hazards dictate that phototherapy should be used with appropriate caution and balance with regard to its risks and benefits.

In the NIH collaborative study of phototherapy in infants weighing < 2 kg, 24.4 per cent of the control group (no phototherapy) received exchange transfusions versus 4.1 per cent of infants in the phototherapy group. Of the 48 infants dying in the phototherapy group who were autopsied, none had "kernicterus," whereas 3 of 52 infants in the control group had evidence of "kernicterus" at autopsy. For infants with birthweights < 1500 gm, 0/40 autopsied infants in the phototherapy group had kernicterus versus 3/29 infants in the control group. These differences approached, but did not achieve, statistical significance (p = 0.07) (Brown et al, 1983).[14, 46] The primary purpose of this study was to test the safety and efficacy of phototherapy. The results of the developmental outcome of these infants are not yet available.

In most intensive care nurseries, phototherapy is used quite liberally in very low-birth-weight infants. Although it has been difficult to document that this is beneficial to the infants concerned, several studies prior to the NIH collaborative study showed that its use dramatically reduced the necessity for exchange transfusion. In our intensive care unit (where we do use phototherapy liberally) we have not performed an exchange transfusion for uncomplicated hyperbilirubinemia in a low-birth-weight infant in over 10 years. We have yet to see our first case of kernicterus.   **J. Maisels**

Editorial Comment: *Where does the bilirubin go when you turn on the lights?* The mechanism whereby phototherapy reduces the serum bilirubin is unfolding at last. Both in vivo and in vitro studies have shown that there are two types of isomers formed (configurational E bilirubins and structural isomer lumirubin—see Figures 11–5 and 11–6) when bilirubin is exposed to light. In a series of studies, Ennever et al documented that although the E bilirubins are formed more rapidly, their excretion is too slow to account for the decline in serum bilirubin. Lumirubin on the other hand appears to be the principal route of pigment elimination during phototherapy (Knox et al, 1985). There have been a number of recent publications delineating the effects of phototherapy on bilirubin, as well as clinical studies indicating that there is little benefit from the early introduction of phototherapy. Furthermore, the long awaited NIH collaborative study has finally been published, so there is a plethora of reading for the "biliphile."

Costarino, A. T., Ennever, J. F., Baumgart, S., et al: Bilirubin photoisomerization in premature neonates under low and high dose phototherapy. Pediatrics 75:519, 1985.

Ennever, J. F., Knox, I., Denne, S., et al: Phototherapy for neonatal jaundice: in vivo clearance of bilirubin photoproducts. Pediatr Res 19:205, 1985.

Kivlahan, C., and James, E. J. P.: The natural history of jaundice. Pediatrics 74:364, 1984.

Knox, I., Ennever, J. F., and Speck, W. T.: Urinary excretion of an isomer of bilirubin during phototherapy. Pediatr Res 19:198, 1985.

McDonagh, A. F., and Lightner, D. A.: Bilirubin jaundice and phototherapy. Pediatrics 75:443, 1985.

NIH Special Study Group, National Institute of Child Health and Human Development: Randomized, controlled trial of phototherapy for neonatal hyperbilirubinemia. Pediatrics 75 (Suppl 2):385, 1985.

Osborn, L. M., Lenarsky, C., Oakes, R. C., et al: Phototherapy in full-term infants with hemolytic disease secondary to ABO incompatibility. Pediatrics 74:371, 1984.

Osborn, L. M., Reiff, M. I., and Bolus, R.: Jaundice in the full-term neonate. Pediatrics 73:520, 1983.

Questions

True or False

Bilirubin is produced from the degradation of hemoglobin in the liver and spleen only.

All tissues of the body have macrophages with the enzymes necessary for the conversion of heme to bilirubin. The statement is false.

Bilirubin must be conjugated in the liver before it is excreted into the biliary tree.

This is true only for the Z,Z isomer of bilirubin IX-alpha. Photoisomers of bilirubin can be excreted without conjugation. The statement is false.

Once bilirubin is conjugated in the liver and excreted into the bile, it is still possible for it to return to the infant's circulation.

The statement is true. Beta-glucuronidase in the infant's gut lumen hydrolyzes conjugated bilirubin, and the resultant unconjugated bilirubin can be reabsorbed into the infant's circulation.

Visible jaundice in the first 36 hours of life can be a normal finding.

False. Visible jaundice is relatively common in infants by the end of the third day of life, but jaundice before 36 hours is always abnormal and is usually related to a hemolytic process.

Jaundice will subside in cases of breast milk jaundice even if the infant is maintained on breast feeding.

This is true. The serum bilirubin concentrations will fall very slowly under these circumstances, but if the infant is not in danger from bilirubin toxicity, breast feeding can be continued.

One assumes that the jaundice will subside *eventually*, but when will this occur? In certain infants serum bilirubin rises with remarkable rapidity and may reach levels of 25 or even 30 mg/dl. Under these circumstances, it is a brave soul who will not interrupt nursing pending the decline in serum bilirubin. Thus, it is hard to know whether or not the bilirubin would, in fact, have continued to increase if breast feeding had continued.
                    J. Maisels

Yellow staining of the brain at autopsy represents a failure to treat neonatal hyperbilirubinemia adequately.

The brain may be stained yellow at autopsy in the absence of evidence of bilirubin toxicity. Capillary integrity can be lost through a number of unrelated factors (anoxia, trauma, etc.), and bilirubin bound to albumin can produce diffuse yellow coloration even if the concentration of bilirubin remains below 10 mg/dl. The statement is false.

The eyes of the infant should be covered when phototherapy is used because fluorescent light of that intensity can damage the retina.

Animal studies have confirmed that the retina can be damaged by the usual intensities of light used for phototherapy. The statement is true.

The administration of 1 gm/kg of albumin 1 hour prior to an exchange transfusion influences the amount of bilirubin removed.

The administration of albumin just before the exchange will result in the removal of about 40 per cent more bilirubin if there is a significant extravascular pool of bilirubin. In this case, the infusion of unsaturated albumin increases the concentration of bilirubin in the plasma by attracting bilirubin from the extravascular pool. If the infant's own albumin is not saturated, administration of albumin may actually decrease the efficiency of the exchange transfusion slightly, since the serum bilirubin concentration is likely to be diluted. In either case the statement is true. Albumin must be given cautiously since it acutely increases blood volume.

Phenobarbital appears to be a safe drug for lowering serum indirect-reacting bilirubin; therefore it is prudent to use it as a prophylactic given to either the mother or the infant.

Although phenobarbital does lower the serum bilirubin, a very large number of infants would have to receive this prophylactic to reduce a potential problem in a few. Phenobarbital does have measurable effects on infant behavior and may have other effects that may only be discovered with more widespread use. We do not feel that the potential benefit clearly outweighs the risk in this instance and do not recommend phenobarbital prophylaxis.

It does seem reasonable, however, to administer phenobarbital for 1–2 weeks prior to delivery to a mother with documented Rh sensitization and to her newborn infant. This has been shown to reduce bilirubin levels in the affected neonate.   **J. Maisels**

Hypoglycemia is a complication that is sometimes noted following an exchange transfusion for erythroblastosis.

Hypoglycemia has been seen after exchange transfusion done for any reason. It may be more likely to occur with Rh-erythroblastosis, since many infants in that group exhibit excessive insulin secretion early in life. The statement is true.

Infants without hemolytic disease are generally safe from bilirubin encephalopathy even when their serum indirect bilirubin concentrations reach 20 mg/dl.

If there are no other factors predisposing the infant to bilirubin toxicity, such as a competing drug (furosemide, for example), prematurity, hypoproteinemia, or sepsis, the statement is true. For an amusing exposition of this concept, read Watchko, F., and Oski, F.; Bilirubin 20 mg/dl = Viginitiphobia. Pediatrics 71:660, 1983.

Watchko and Oski's exposition was amusing but naughty. Absence of evidence is not, necessarily, evidence of absence.   **J. Maisels**

Some infants become gray-black following the use of bilirubin lights.

The statement is true. This discoloration appears to be due to the accumulation of some product(s) of the photodegradation of bilirubin. Infants with elevated direct-reacting bilirubin concentrations before therapy are more likely to exhibit this "bronze baby" appearance. No long-term sequelae to this phenomenon are known, but we do not use phototherapy when the direct-reacting fraction is elevated.

If an infant does not appear jaundiced in the newborn period, it is not necessary to measure the serum bilirubin level routinely.

The statement is true. Jaundice appears as a reliable sign of hyperbilirubinemia in the newborn; it is not necessary to obtain a serum concentration in an infant who does not appear jaundiced. The exception to this rule is an infant under phototherapy. In the latter case, the serum may contain a high concentration of bilirubin while the skin appears anicteric.

A mother with group O Rh-negative blood has an infant, also with group O Rh-negative blood type but with a positive Coombs' test. The blood smear confirms the diagnosis of erythroblastosis fetalis. How is this possible?

The maternal Rh antibody may occupy all of the Rh-positive antigenic sites on the infant's cells, and therefore the typing serum cannot reach these sites. Thus, the infant is mislabeled Rh-negative. An alternative explanation is that the blood group incompatibility involves a less common antigen such as Cc, Ee, Kell, Duffy, etc.

CASE PROBLEMS

Case One

Baby G. is a full-term male infant, the product of a normal first pregnancy and easy delivery. The infant cried and breathed spontaneously. On physical examination, at 1 hour of life, he was completely normal. Jaundice was noted on the first day of life. The mother was O Rh-positive, and the infant was A Rh-positive and Coombs' positive. The hemoglobin concentration was 19.8 gm/dl.

What is the likely diagnosis?

The most likely diagnosis is an ABO blood group incompatibility in which the baby's A cells have traversed the placenta and the mother has developed a hyperimmune anti-A antibody, which in turn sensitized the red cells in the infant's circulation. An O mother with a B baby is much more likely to produce clinical disease than an O mother with an A baby, but the B-O combination is less common.

How could you confirm the diagnosis?

Look at the infant's blood smear for microspherocytes in the first 24 hours of life. Test an eluate of the infant's cells for anti-A antibody. Red cell cholinesterase activity is low in ABO hemolytic disease. The mother's serum will have an unusually high IgG titer to type A red cells, but this is less specific than the previous tests.

At 36 hours of life, the bilirubin reaches 12 mg/dl. Should the infant now be given a replacement transfusion or albumin, or should he be placed under bilirubin lights?

We would continue to observe the infant without therapy for jaundice. When the bilirubin reaches 12 mg/dl, we would perform a test for albumin saturation or reserve albumin binding. If the test indicates that there is little or no reserve for bilirubin binding, then we would perform an exchange transfusion. Otherwise, we would follow the course of the serum bilirubin and the saturation test.

Even if a reduced reserve binding capacity is of relevance in this situation, I do not know why an exchange transfusion would be preferable to a trial of phototherapy, particularly when phototherapy is frequently effective in reducing serum bilirubin levels in these circumstances. Bilirubin levels could be monitored frequently and exchange transfusion performed if they continued to rise.

J. Maisels

At 48 hours, the bilirubin reaches 13.5 mg/dl with 2.0 mg/dl direct-reacting. At this time, should we perform an exchange transfusion, continue phototherapy, give albumin, or none of the above?

The conversion of some of the infant's serum bilirubin to the direct-reacting fraction in the absence of phototherapy is usually a good prognostic sign. It means that the rate of conjugation now exceeds the rate of excretion. This usually means that bilirubin is likely to fall significantly in the next 24 hours. However, if this infant has been treated with bilirubin lights, the rise in conjugated bilirubin could be secondary to the phototherapy. The answer is none of the above.

On the seventh day, the bilirubin level drops to 4 mg/dl. The infant is discharged. Three weeks after discharge, what should be looked for in this infant?

We would check this infant every 2 or 3 weeks because hemolysis will continue, the hemoglobin concentration will fall, and a small transfusion may be required. The hemoglobin concentration will reach a nadir in the sixth to twelfth week of life.

Case Two

Baby T. is the product of a 21 year old mother who has had diabetes mellitus for the past 8 years.

She was moderately well controlled on insulin through this pregnancy and had no ketosis or hypoglycemia. At delivery, the infant weighed 4.1 kg and was estimated to be in the thirty-eighth week of gestation. Apgar scores were good, and the infant experienced transient tachypnea requiring oxygen therapy. On the third day, the serum bilirubin concentration reached 12.2 mg/dl.

At this time should the infant be treated for the hyperbilirubinemia? How?

The infant of a diabetic mother with some respiratory distress may have a reduced hepatic clearance of bilirubin due to a persistent flow through the ductus venosus or a reduced body water content. These infants need to be watched carefully for hypoglycemia, and they need help to maintain adequate hydration. No specific therapy for jaundice is needed at the moment, since the bilirubin concentration is still within normal limits.

At 6 days of age, the bilirubin rises to 15.3 mg/dl. At this time, which of the following should be done?
A. Exchange transfusion
B. Phototherapy
C. Albumin infusion
D. Continued feeding

Some clinicians would choose B. However, the elevation in bilirubin concentration is modestly above normal, and infants of diabetic mothers tend not to mobilize nonesterified fatty acids well. This latter characteristic leads to larger than usual binding capacities. This can be confirmed by the use of a binding test. We would follow the bilirubin concentration, perform a binding test, and maintain hydration and nutrition. Therefore, the answer is D.

Case Three

Baby M. is a 1200 gm premature infant, the product of a 30 week gestation complicated by some bleeding during the early weeks of pregnancy. On physical examination, the infant was normal except for increasing respiratory distress requiring assisted ventilation at 14 hours of age. At 60 hours the infant began to improve significantly. The infant was about to be weaned from the ventilator when a total bilirubin concentration of 12 mg/dl was noted.

At this time, the infant should:
A. Be placed under the lights
B. Receive an exchange transfusion
C. Be left alone
D. Receive an albumin transfusion
E. Any of the above

The answer could very well be E. The small premature infant with respiratory distress and hyperbilirubinemia is at increased risk of bilirubin encephalopathy, but we get very little help from the collected experience in the literature to know how to manage the problem. Since the serum albumin is usually low in these infants, it might be helpful to give them small transfusions of plasma or albumin. If the infant's saturation test showed little reserve binding capacity, we would perform an exchange transfusion. In the absence of an abnormal binding test, we might still perform exchange transfusion in the infant at a bilirubin concentration less than 20 mg/dl because of all of the added risk factors (prematurity, asphyxia, acidosis, hypoproteinemia, etc.). In that case we might perform the exchange transfusion when the bilirubin concentration reached 15 mg/dl. The latter value, however, has no particular support from relevant clinical studies.

Case Four

An otherwise healthy infant is seen as an outpatient because of persistent jaundice. She is the product of a normal 40 week gestation, and she had no complications at birth. Her birth weight was 3200 gm, and she weighs 3200 gm at 14 days. She is being breast-fed exclusively, and she is vigorous and healthy on physical examination. Her serum bilirubin concentration is 13.8 mg/dl, with 0.2 mg/dl direct-reacting.

The most likely cause of persistent jaundice in this case is:
  A. Sepsis
  B. Hereditary fructose intolerance

C. Breast milk jaundice
D. Isoimmune hemolytic disease
E. None of the above

The correct answer is C. This infant may be slightly behind in weight gain, but lack of intake would not cause this degree of jaundice this late. Persistent unconjugated hyperbilirubinemia can also be caused by galactosemia, hypothyroidism, or familial nonhemolytic jaundice (type I or II). The first two of these diagnoses should be ruled out before one assumes that the breast feeding is the cause.

Assuming the work-up for other diseases was negative, how would you manage this case of breast milk jaundice?

No treatment at all is necessary in this case. The present bilirubin concentration is not a danger to the infant and will fall eventually. One may elect to substitute formula for 1–4 days to help confirm the diagnosis, but this maneuver is not a necessity. If the bilirubin level rose above 15 mg/dl, we might elect to substitute formula for breast milk until the concentration fell significantly. If the binding capacity was found to be low in an infant with uncertain intake, we would give the infant a glucose infusion (1 gm/kg/hour for 2–3 hours) and repeat the saturation test. This is done because nonesterified fatty acids are important competitors for bilirubin binding, and these infants may not be receiving all the calories they need. Therefore, NEFA may be elevated in their circulation and can be reduced by the infusion of glucose.

REFERENCES

1. Arias, I., Gartner, L., Cohen, M., et al: Chronic nonhemolytic unconjugated hyperbilirubinemia with glucuronyl transferase deficiency. Am J Med 47:395, 1969.
2. Arias, I., Johnson, L., and Wolfson, S.: Biliary excretion of injected conjugated and unconjugated bilirubin by normal and Gunn rats. Am J Physiol 200:1091, 1961.
3. Arias, I., Wolfson, S., Lucey, J., et al: Transient familial neonatal hyperbilirubinemia. J Clin Invest 44:1442, 1956.
4. Behrman, R., Brown, A., Currie, M., et al: Preliminary report of the committee on phototherapy in the newborn infant. J Pediatr 84:135, 1974.
5. Berk, P., Blaschke, T., Scharschmidt, B., et al: A new approach to quantitation of the various sources of bilirubin in man. J Lab Clin Med 87:767, 1976.
6. Bernstein, J., Chang, C.-H., Brough, A., et al: Conjugated hyperbilirubinemia in infants associated with parenteral alimentation. J Pediatr 90:361, 1977.
7. Black, V., Lubchenco, L., Lucky, D., et al: Developmental and neurologic sequelae of neonatal hyperviscosity syndrome. Pediatrics 69:426, 1982.
8. Blumenthal, S., Ikeda, R., and Ruebner, B.: Bile pigments in humans and in nonhuman primates during the perinatal period: composition of meconium and gallbladder bile of newborns and adults. Pediatr Res 10:664, 1976.
9. Bonnett, R., Davis, J., Hursthouse, M., et al: The structure of bilirubin. Proc R Soc Lond (Biol) 202:249, 1978.
10. Brodersen, R.: Bilirubin solubility and interaction with albumin and phospholipid. J Biol Chem 254:2364, 1979.
11. Brodersen, R.: Binding of bilirubin to albumin: implications for prevention of bilirubin encephalopathy in the newborn. CRC Crit Rev Clin Lab Sci 11:305, 1979.
12. Brodersen, R., and Hermann, L.: Intestinal reabsorption of unconjugated bilirubin: a possible contributing factor in neonatal jaundice. Lancet 1:1242, 1963.
13. Brough, A., and Bernstein, J.: Conjugated hyperbilirubinemia. Hum Pathol 5:507, 1974.
14. Brown, A. K., Kim, M. H., and Bryla, D.: Report on the NIH cooperative study of phototherapy: efficacy of phototherapy in controlling hyperbilirubinemia and preventing kernicterus. Report of the 85th Ross Conference on Pediatric Research. Columbus, Ohio, Ross Laboratories, 1983.

15. Byers, R., Paine, R., and Crothers, B.: Extrapyramidal cerebral palsy with hearing loss following erythroblastosis. Pediatrics 15:248, 1955.

16. Claireaux, A.: Pathology of human kernicterus. In Sass-Kortsak, A. (ed.): Kernicterus. Toronto, University of Toronto Press, 1959, pp. 140–149.

17. Cohen, A., and Ostrow, J.: New concepts in phototherapy: photoisomerization of bilirubin IX-alpha and the potential toxic effect of light. Pediatrics 65:740, 1980.

18. Cremer, R., Perryman, P., and Richards, D.: Influence of light on the hyperbilirubinemia of infants. Lancet 1:1094, 1958.

19. Dahms, B., Krauss, A., Gartner, L., et al: Breast feeding and serum bilirubin values during the first 4 days of life. J Pediatr 83:1049, 1973.

20. De Carvalho, M., Hall, M., and Harvey, D.: Effects of water supplementation on physiological jaundice in breast-fed babies. Arch Dis Child 56:568, 1981.

21. De Carvalho, M., Klaus, M., and Merkatz, R.: Frequency of breast feeding and serum bilirubin concentration. Am J Dis Child 136:737, 1982.

22. Drew, J., and Kitchen, W.: The effect of maternally administered drugs on bilirubin concentrations in the newborn infant. J Pediatr 89:657, 1976.

23. Dunn, P., and Chir, D.: Obstructive jaundice, liver damage and Rh haemolytic disease of the newborn. Jewish Mem Hosp Bull 10:94, 1965.

24. Dutton, G., Langelan, D., and Ross, P.: High glucuronide synthesis in newborn liver: choice of species and substrate. Biochem J 93:4P, 1964.

25. Edwards, R.; Inheritance of the Dubin-Johnson-Sprinz syndrome. Gastroenterology 68:734, 1976.

26. Ennever, J., and Speck, W.: Photochemical reactions of riboflavin; covalent binding to DNA and to poly(dA)-poly(dT). Pediatr Res 17:234, 1983.

27. Ennever, J., Carr, H., and Speck, W.: Potential genetic damage from multivitamin solutions exposed to phototherapy illumination. Pediatr Res 17:192, 1983.

28. Epel, B., and Krauss, R.: The inhibitory effect of light on growth of prototheca sopfi. Biochem Biophys Acta (Amsterdam) 120:73, 1966.

29. Foliot, A., Ploussard, J., Housset, E., et al: Breast milk jaundice: in vitro inhibition of rat liver bilirubin–uridine diphosphate glucuronyltransferase activity and Z protein-bromosulfophthalein binding by human breast milk. Pediatr Res 10:594, 1976.

30. Gartner, L., and Arias, I.: Studies of prolonged neonatal jaundice in the breast-fed infant. J Pediatr 68:54, 1966.

31. Haymaker, W., Margolis, C., Pentshchew, A., et al: Pathology of kernicterus and posticeteric encephalopathy. In: Kernicterus in Cerebral Palsy. American Academy for Cerebral Palsy Meeting. Springfield, Charles C Thomas, 1961, pp. 21–229.

32. Johnson, L., and Boggs, T., Jr.: Bilirubin-dependent brain damage: incidence and indications for treatment. In Odell, G., Schaffer, R., and Simopoulos, A. (eds.): Phototherapy in the Newborn: An Overview. Washington, National Academy of Sciences, 1974, p. 122.

33. Kandall, S., Thaler, M., and Erickson, R.: Intestinal development of lysosomal and microsomal beta glucuronidase and bilirubin uridine diphosphogluronyl transferase in normal and jaundiced rats. J Pediatr 82:1013, 1973.

34. Kaplan, E., Herz, F., and Hsu, J.: Erythrocyte acetylcholinesterase activity in ABO hemolytic disease of the newborn. Pediatrics 33:205, 1964.

35. Keenan, W., Perlstein, P., Light, I., et al: Kernicterus in small sick premature infants receiving phototherapy. Pediatrics 49:652, 1972.

36. Kim, H., Yoon, J., Sher, J., et al: Lack of predictive indices in kernicterus: a comparison of clinical and pathologic factors in infants with or without kernicterus. Pediatrics 66:852, 1980.

37. Levi, A., Gatmaitan, Z., and Arias, I.: Two hepatic cytoplasmic protein fractions, Y and Z, and their possible role in the hepatic uptake of bilirubin, sulfobromophthalein, and other anions. J Clin Invest 48:2156, 1969.

38. Levi, A., Gatmaitan, Z., and Arias, I.: Deficiency of hepatic organic anion-binding protein, impaired organic anion uptake by liver and "physiologic" jaundice in newborn monkeys. N Engl J Med 283:1136, 1970.

39. Levine, R., Fredericks, W., and Rapoport, S.: Entry of bilirubin into the brain due to opening of the blood-brain barrier. Pediatrics 69:255, 1982.

40. Lightner, D., Wooldridge, T., and McDonagh, A.: Configurational isomerization of bilirubin and the mechanism of jaundice phototherapy. Biochem Biophys Res Comm 86:235, 1979.

41. Lightner, D., Wooldridge, T., and McDonagh, A.: Photobilirubin: an early bilirubin photoproduct detected by absorbance difference spectroscopy. Proc Natl Acad Sci 76:29, 1979.

42. Maisels, M., Li, T-K., Piechocki, J., et al: The effect of exchange transfusion on serum ionized calcium. Pediatrics 53:683, 1974.

43. Maisels, M., Pathak, A., Nelson, N., et al: Endogenous production of carbon monoxide in normal and erythroblastotic newborn infants. J Clin Invest 50:1, 1971.

44. Maisels, M., Pathak, A., and Nelson, N.: The effect of exchange transfusion on endogenous carbon monoxide production in erythroblastotic infants. J Pediatr 81:705, 1972.

45. McConnell, J., Glasgow, J., and McNair, R.: Effect on neonatal jaundice of oestrogens and progestogens taken before and after conception. Br Med J 3:605, 1973.

46. NIH Special Study Group, National Institute of Child Health and Human Development: Randomized, controlled trial of phototherapy for neonatal hyperbilirubinemia. Pediatrics 75 (Suppl 2):385, 1985.

47. Odell, G.: Neonatal Hyperbilirubinemia. New York, Grune & Stratton, 1980, p. 35.

48. Odell, G., Brown, R., and Kopelman, A.: The photodynamic action of bilirubin on erythrocytes. J Pediatr 81:473, 1972.

49. Odell, G., Cohen, S., and Gordes, E.: Administration of albumin in the management of hyperbilirubinemia by exchange transfusion. Pediatrics 30:613, 1962.

50. Odell, G., Storey, G., and Rosenberg, L.: Studies in kernicterus. III. The saturation of serum proteins with bilirubin during neonatal life and its relationship to brain damage at five years. J Pediatr 6:12, 1970.

51. Ogawa, J.: Post-natal circulatory observations of liver and intestine in newborn infants. In: Proceedings of the XI International Congress of Pediatrics. 1965, p. 87.

52. Oh, W., Hanson, J., and Lind, J.: Peripheral circulatory response to phototherapy in newborn infants. Acta Paediatr Scand 62:49, 1973.

53. Oie, S., and Levy, G.: Effect of sulfisoxazole on pharmacokinetics of free and plasma protein-bound bilirubin in experimental unconjugated hyperbilirubinemia. J Pharm Sci 68:6, 1979.

54. Ostrea, E., Jr., and Odell, G.: Photosensitized shift in the O_2 dissociation curve of fetal blood. Acta Paediatr Scand 63:341, 1974.

55. Ostrea, E., Jr., Fleury, C., Balun, J., et al: Degradation of essential fatty acids by phototherapy. J Pediatr 102:617, 1983.

56. Park, T., Padget, S., Root, A., et al: Effect of phototherapy and nursery light on neonatal biorhythms. Pediatr Res 10:429, 1976.

57. Pearlman, M., Gartner, L., Lee, K.-S., et al: Absence of kernicterus in low-birth-weight infants from 1971 through 1976: comparison with findings in 1966 and 1967. Pediatrics 62:460, 1978.

58. Pearson, H.: Life span of the fetal red blood cell. J Pediatr 10:166, 1967.

59. Phillip, A., and Hewitt, J.: Early diagnosis of neonatal sepsis. Pediatrics 65:1036, 1980.

60. Poland, R.: Breast-milk jaundice. J Pediatr 99:86, 1981.

61. Poland, R., and Odell, G.: Physiologic jaundice: the enterohepatic circulation of bilirubin. N Engl J Med 284:1, 1971.

62. Poland, R., Schultz, G., and Garg, G.: High milk lipase activity associated with breast milk jaundice. Pediatr Res 14:1328, 1980.

63. Ritter, D., Kenny, J., Norton, J., et al: A prospective study of free bilirubin and other risk factors in the development of kernicterus in premature infants. Pediatrics 69:260, 1982.

64. Rosta, J., Makoi, Z., and Kertesz, A.: Delayed meconium passage and hyperbilirubinaemia. Lancet 2:1138, 1968.

65. Saigal, S., O'Neill, A., Yeldandi, S., et al.: Placental transfusion and hyperbilirubinemia in the premature. Pediatrics 49:406, 1972.

66. Sever, J., Larsen, J., and Grossman, J.: Handbook of Perinatal Infections. Boston, Little, Brown and Company, 1979.

67. Sidbury, J., Jr.: Investigations and speculations on the pathogenesis of galactosemia. In Hsia, D. (ed.): Galactosemia. Springfield, Charles C Thomas, 1969, p. 13.

68. Speck, W., and Rosenkranz, H.: Phototherapy for neonatal hyperbilirubinemia—a potential environmental health hazard to newborn infants: a review. Environ Mutagen 1:321, 1979.

69. Stevenson, D., Bartoletti, A., Ostrander, C., et al: Pulmonary excretion of carbon monoxide in the human newborn infant as an index of bilirubin production: III. Measurement of pulmonary excretion of carbon monoxide after the first postnatal week in premature infants. Pediatrics 64:598, 1979.

70. Tan, K.: Comparison of the effectiveness of phototherapy and exchange transfusion in the management of non-hemolytic hyperbilirubinemia. J Pediatr 87:609, 1975.

71. Tan, K.: The nature of the dose-response relationship of phototherapy for neonatal hyperbilirubinemia. J Pediatr 90:448, 1977.

72. Taylor, W., and Qaqundah, B.: Neonatal jaundice associated with cystic fibrosis. Am J Dis Child 123:161, 1972.

73. Tenhunen, R., Marver, H., and Schmid, R.: Microsomal heme oxygenase. J Biol Chem 244:6388, 1969.

74. Thomas, G., and Howell, R.: Selected Screening Tests for Genetic Metabolic Diseases. Chicago, Year Book Medical Publishers, 1973.

75. Turkel, S., Miller, C., Gittenberg, M., et al: A clinical pathologic reappraisal of kernicterus. Pediatrics 69:267, 1982.

76. Vest, M.: Studies on haemoglobin breakdown and incorporation of [15N] glycine into haem and bile pigment in the newborn. In Bouchier, I., and Billings, B. (eds.): Bilirubin Metabolism. Philadelphia, F. A. Davis Co., 1967, p. 47.

77. Weldon, A., and Danks, D.: Congenital hypothyroidism and neonatal jaundice. Arch Dis Child 47:469, 1972.

78. Weldon, V., and Odell, G.: Mortality risk of exchange transfusion. Pediatrics 41:797, 1968.

79. Wennberg, R., Ahlfors, C., Bickers, L., et al: Abnormal auditory brainstem response in a newborn infant with hyperbilirubinemia: improvement with exchange transfusion. J Pediatr 100:624, 1982.

80. Wennberg, R., Ahlfors, C., and Rasmussen, L.: The pathochemistry of kernicterus. Early Hum Devel 3:353, 1979.

81. Wennberg, R., Schwartz, R., and Sweet, A.: Early versus delayed feeding of low birth weight infants: effects on physiologic jaundice. J Pediatr 68:800, 1966.

82. Yamamoto, T., Skanderberg, J., Zipursky, A., et al: The early appearing bilirubin: evidence for two components. J Clin Invest 44:31, 1965.

12

Neonatal Infections

WILLIAM T. SPECK
STEPHEN C. ARONOFF
AVROY A. FANAROFF

Neonatal sepsis, a generalized bacterial infection accompanied by a positive blood culture during the first month of life, is a significant cause of mortality and morbidity. Prior to the 1940s, the hemolytic streptococcus *S. pyogenes* was most often responsible for life-threatening perinatal infection. The introduction and widespread use of penicillin were accompanied by a decline in the incidence of streptococcal disease and, in the 1950s, the emergence of the hemolytic staphylococcus *S. aureus* as the predominant neonatal pathogen. Alterations in infant care practices (rooming in, ultraviolet lighting, nasal creams, antiseptic bathing, artificial colonization, barrier nursing, etc.), the development of antimicrobial agents active against penicillinase-producing staphylococci, and the improved survival of low-birth-weight infants coincided in the late 1950s with the appearance of gram-negative enteric microorganisms, primarily *Escherichia coli*, as major neonatal pathogens. The 1960s were noteworthy for an improved understanding of the epidemiology of gram-negative bacterial colonization and disease, the introduction of antimicrobial agents active against enteric microorganisms, and the emergence of the group B streptococcus, *S. agalactiae*, as the principal cause of neonatal septicemia and meningitis. The past decade has witnessed a decrease in the incidence of neonatal group B streptococcal disease and the occurrence of non–group D alpha-hemolytic streptococci, *Haemophilus influenzae*, *Staphylococcus epi-*

dermidis, and *Streptococcus pneumoniae* as important neonatal pathogens. This changing epidemiology emphasizes the opportunistic nature of neonatal bacterial infection; any bacterial species is capable of causing life-threatening illness in this patient population.

The clinical manifestations and pathophysiology of most intrauterine and postnatally acquired viral infections have been detailed recently in review articles, monographs, and textbooks. The goal of this chapter is to present a working approach to the problem of bacterial sepsis in the neonatal period, emphasizing the predisposing factors, laboratory evaluation, and appropriate antimicrobial therapy.

INCIDENCE AND MORTALITY RATE

The incidence of neonatal septicemia is inversely related to gestational age. Thus, 1 in 250 premature infants and 1 in 15,000 term infants experience a systemic bacterial infection in the first month of life. Prior to the introduction of effective antibiotic therapy, the mortality rate for neonatal septicemia approached 100 per cent. Despite the availability of effective chemotherapy, the mortality rate remains between 20 and 30 per cent.[28] The mortality rate from neonatal sepsis is dependent on a number of related factors. More specifically, mortality is increased in the premature infant in the presence of the noninfectious complications of

262

prematurity (respiratory distress syndrome, intraventricular hemorrhage, necrotizing enterocolitis), with simultaneous infection of the central nervous system (meningitis is present in 30% of neonates with septicemia), and when signs and symptoms appear within the first few days of life ("early onset septicemia"). Recent data suggest a slight increase in the mortality rate for neonatal sepsis, presumably reflecting the availability of sophisticated life support systems that enable extremely low-birth-weight infants to survive for extended periods of time before succumbing to nosocomial infection.

There are few data available on the morbidity of neonatal septicemia in the absence of meningitis. Estimates are that approximately 25 per cent of infants surviving bacterial sepsis are left with residual handicaps; however, these are often the result of the noninfectious complications of prematurity.[1] In the presence of meningitis, sequelae are more common (learning disabilities, seizures, hydrocephalus, and hearing loss) and may approach 50 per cent.

FACTORS IN NEONATAL SEPTICEMIA

Host Factors

The single most important risk factor for neonatal septicemia is *prematurity*. Accordingly, those perinatal events that promote prematurity predispose to postnatal bacterial infections. The increased susceptibility of *male infants* to bacterial infection is not completely understood; however, this male predominance has not been described for intrauterine infection or postnatal infections due to the group B streptococci.[74] *Twin pregnancy* also predisposes to neonatal septicemia even when controlled for prematurity and low-birth-weight.[52] *Galactosemic* neonates and infants receiving *intramuscular administration of iron-dextran* appear unusually susceptible to life-threatening septicemia and meningitis due to *E. coli.*[9, 12, 35] *Congenital abnormalities* that disrupt the skin and/or mucous membranes or interfere with the immunologic response to infection (e.g., congenital absence of the spleen) increase the risk of bacterial infection.

The immune system of the newborn differs from that of the infant and older child, and this difference predisposes to infections due to a wide variety of pathogens.[3, 20, 27, 43, 44, 61, 68]

Abnormalities in the neonate's *nonspecific defense mechanisms* include defective granulocyte function (abnormal chemotaxis, phagocytosis, and bactericidal activity), abnormal serum opsonic activity (due to low concentrations of specific antibody, complement, and/or nonspecific opsonins, including fibronectin), and deficiencies in the classical complement pathway (C1q, C3, C5) and the properdin pathway for complement activation. Abnormalities in the neonate's *specific host defense mechanisms* include defective primary (IgM) and secondary (IgG) antibody response and qualitative and quantitative abnormalities in circulating immunoglobulins. More specifically, neonatal IgG is acquired transplacentally and is dependent on the gestational age of the infant and to a lesser extent the level of maternal IgG. Thus, fetal concentrations of IgG remain low until the seventeenth week of gestation, at which time levels increase such that at term the neonatal IgG level is equal to or greater than the maternal level. Thus, in the preterm infant the serum IgG level is less than the maternal level and directly related to gestational age. (The levels of the four IgG subclasses in cord serum are equivalent to maternal levels, indicating that transplacental passage of all IgG immunoglobulins is equivalent.[46]) (See Table 12–1.) IgA does not cross the placenta, and fetal synthesis, which begins at approximately 30 weeks of gestation, is deficient. Thus, cord blood rarely contains detectable levels of IgA (cord levels of IgA may increase following congenital infection and maternal-fetal hemorrhage). IgM antibodies are not transplacentally transported; however synthesis begins by the thirtieth week of gestation, and trace amounts are detected in cord blood. Elevated concentrations of IgM in cord serum (greater than 20 mg/dl) indicate intrauterine antigenic stimulation, often the result of infection.

TABLE 12–1 IgG ANTIBODIES PASSIVELY ACQUIRED BY THE FETUS

Protective	Diagnostically Confusing
Tetanus antitoxin	VDRL
Diphtheria antitoxin	FTA-ABS
Poliovirus	Toxoplasma
Streptococcus (groups A and B)	Cytomegalovirus
Haemophilus influenzae	Herpes simplex
Anti–hepatitis B surface antigen	
Varicella-Zoster	
Rubella	

However, this finding is nonspecific, and infants with congenital infections may have normal levels of IgM at birth. Significant synthesis of IgM begins in the immediate postnatal period regardless of gestational age, presumably secondary to exposure to gastrointestinal antigens.[2] IgM is the principal immunoglobulin synthesized by the neonate during the first few months of life.

Maternal Factors

Maternal race, health, and vaginal flora are important factors that predispose to neonatal septicemia. Studies from New York suggest that neonatal infection is more common in black than nonblack populations of comparable economic status.[43] Some have suggested that this association reflects the lack of antenatal care available to our urban nonwhite population. Although less well studied, *ethnic background* may affect the incidence of neonatal septicemia. Thus, Anthony et al and Collado et al demonstrated that group B streptococcal colonization and presumably neonatal disease were less common among Mexican-American women than whites and blacks of comparable age and economic status.[5, 21]

Investigations have suggested that *antenatal coitus* predisposes to neonatal infection.[48] However, this observation has been criticized because infection was defined on the basis of histologic abnormalities in the subchorionic plate of the placenta. *Maternal illness* increases the risk of neonatal septicemia. Thus, symptomatic bacteriuria during pregnancy predisposes to premature birth and so indirectly to neonatal sepsis. (A similar association has not been established between asymptomatic bacteriuria and prematurity.[51]) *Maternal bacteremia or viremia* may result in transplacentally transmitted infection (Tables 12–2 and 12–3). *Maternal fever* in the perinatal period, even in the absence of an identifiable focus, is also associated with an increased risk of neonatal sepsis. Additional maternal factors that predispose to neonatal septicemia include *prolonged rupture of membranes* (greater than 24 hours), *maternal amnionitis* (characterized clinically by suprapubic pain and discharge with or without fever), *endometritis*, *excessive bleeding*, and a *prolonged second stage of labor*, particularly when associated with fetal distress.

The importance of prolonged ruptured membranes in the pathogenesis of neonatal bacterial disease is uncertain. Assuming that approximately 10–15 per cent of women have ruptured membranes of 12 hours or longer and that the rate of neonatal bacterial diseases is 1–5 cases/1000 live births, then from <1–5 per cent of babies born to mothers with prolonged ruptured membranes may become septic. The actual rate is probably closer to 1–2 per cent. **G. McCracken**

The effect of *maternal genitourinary colonization* on perinatal mortality (prematurity and neonatal septicemia) has not been satisfactorily investigated. Many of the early studies demonstrating an association between mater-

TABLE 12–2 INTRAUTERINE AND PERINATALLY ACQUIRED BACTERIAL INFECTIONS IN THE NEONATE

Organism	Clinical Manifestations	Prognosis	Treatment
Escherichia coli	Poor feeding, respiratory distress, seizures, meningitis	Meningitis—poor	Ampicillin or moxalactam
Listeria monocytogenes	Intrauterine—chronic abortions; perinatal—sepsis, meningitis	10–15% mortality	Ampicillin
Mycobacterium tuberculosis	Asymptomatic (majority), perinatal acquisition, dissemination	Usually excellent; disseminated infection—poor	Isoniazid
Neisseria gonorrhoeae	Sepsis, ophthalmia neonatorum	Blindness if untreated	Eye prophylaxis, penicillin
Treponema pallidum	Asymptomatic; skin rash, chorioretinitis, meningitis, periostitis, hepatosplenomegaly	Excellent if treated	Non-CNS—benzathine penicillin × 1; CNS—penicillin G × 10 days
Ureaplasma urealyticum	Sepsis (rare), afebrile pneumonitis	Excellent	Erythromycin

TABLE 12–3 EFFECTS OF MATERNAL VIRAL INFECTIONS ON THE FETUS

| Virus | Clinical Manifestations | | Prognosis | Treatment |
	Intrauterine Infection	Perinatal Infection		
Coxsackie	Rare; meningitis	Meningitis, pancarditis	Meningitis — excellent; pancarditis — lethal	None
Cytomegalovirus	Rare; thrombocytopenia, hepatosplenomegaly, chorioretinitis, SGA, cerebral calcifications, "blueberry muffin" spots	Asymptomatic; acquired from blood products, afebrile pneumonitis	Intrauterine — mental retardation; perinatal — excellent	None
Hepatitis B	Rare; chronic carrier, neonatal hepatitis	Typically asymptomatic carrier	Public health problem	HBIG at birth and 3 mos; HB vaccine at 3, 4, 10 mos
Herpes simplex	Rare; prematurity or perinatal-type of infection	Cutaneous vesicles, CNS infection, hepatitis, pneumonitis	50–70% mortality; survivors often mentally retarded	Vidarabine ?Acyclovir
Rubella	Rare; anomalies of eyes, heart, ears; cerebral calcifications, periostitis	Unusual	Mental retardation, deafness	None
Varicella-zoster	Rare; skin scarring, developmental delay, encephalitis; asymptomatic	Cutaneous vesicles, pneumonitis	Perinatal infection may be lethal	V-ZIG at birth

nal colonization with sexually transmitted pathogens (group B streptococci, *Neisseria gonorrhoeae, Chlamydia trachomatis, Ureaplasma urealyticum, Mycoplasma hominis,* and *Treponema pallidum)* and prematurity have limitations that include (1) poor study design and failure to control for maternal factors associated with prematurity—including young age, low socioeconomic status, black race, and primigravidity (all of which are associated with increased risk of sexually transmitted infections); (2) investigation of single pathogens and elimination of the contributions of other, more fastidious microorganisms, acting alone or in combination with the study microorganism; and (3) failure to differentiate between primary and recurrent infection. Nevertheless, recent studies have demonstrated an increased risk of low-birth-weight infants and premature rupture of membranes among IgM-seropositive women with *C. trachomatis* infection (presumably a primary infection) and a correlation between antepartum *M. hominis* colonization and postpartum endometritis.[29, 31] Investigators have also confirmed an association between maternal colonization with the group B streptococci and postnatal infection when

associated with a maternal deficiency of type-specific antibody, heavy colonization, premature labor, prolonged rupture of membranes, and intrapartum fever.[6, 15-17, 25] Thus, in evaluating neonates for septicemia, it is important to identify risk factors and to appreciate that such factors do not act independently but rather combine in individual circumstances to place the infant more or less at risk for life-threatening infection.

Environmental Factors

In utero, the normal infant is in a "germ-free" environment surrounded by sterile amniotic fluid, which inhibits the growth of most microorganisms.[33] Bacterial pathogens that result in intrauterine contamination, colonization, or infection gain access to the newborn infant by a number of routes. The principal mechanism for intrauterine colonization and infection is the ascending route, whereby the normal vaginal flora gain access to the amniotic fluid and the uterine cavity (Table 12–4). *Ascending infection* can occur through intact fetal membranes (amniotic infection syndrome); however, colonization

TABLE 12—4 INTRAUTERINE AND PERINATALLY-ACQUIRED PROTOZOAN INFECTIONS IN THE NEONATE

Infection	Clinical Manifestations	Prognosis	Treatment
Chlamydia vaginalis	Conjunctivitis, afebrile pneumonitis, eosinophilia	Usually excellent	Erythromycin
Malaria	Intrauterine—rare; transfusion-acquired—jaundice, hemolytic anemia, hepatosplenomegaly	Usually excellent	Chloroquine phosphate
Toxoplasma gondii	Intrauterine—SGA, hepatosplenomegaly, cerebral calcifications	Mental retardation	None

and infection are more common following rupture of fetal membranes, particularly when the duration of rupture exceeds 24 hours.[13] Aspiration of contaminated amniotic fluid into the lungs or gastrointestinal tract, which commonly occurs during fetal distress and/or asphyxia, predisposes to bacterial colonization, invasion, and systemic infection. *Transplacental transmission* and intrauterine infection due to bacterial pathogens are uncommon but have been reported with *Listeria monocytogenes, Mycobacterium tuberculosis*, Haemophilus spp., Streptococcus spp., and Salmonella spp.

All newborns become contaminated with vaginal flora during labor and delivery except when delivery follows cesarean section. Under normal circumstances, the skin and mucous membranes of the neonate permit postnatal colonization and resist bacterial invasion. Infection occurs when a compromised newborn (asphyxia, prematurity, etc.) is heavily colonized with virulent microorganisms (group B streptococci) for extended periods of time (premature rupture of membranes) and when alterations of the normal mucocutaneous barriers of the newborn are compromised (congenital anomalies, fetal monitoring, obstetric manipulation, vigorous resuscitative efforts), thereby favoring tissue invasion.

The presence of leukocytes in the external ear or gastric aspirate of the newly born infant is of maternal origin and reflects the status of the amniotic fluid at birth. The gastric aspirate leukocyte count is elevated in direct relationship to the duration of ruptured membranes and in babies born to mothers with amnionitis. The significance of leukocytes in these sites is uncertain, but their presence certainly does not uniformly signify sepsis in the baby. There is too great a tendency to overinterpret gastric aspirate and external ear smears and cultures; the results of these studies must be considered in the total context of the clinical and other laboratory findings of each infant. **G. McCracken**

Following delivery, the newborn infant is transported from the microbial world of the mother to the hostile microbial world of the nursery or intensive care unit. Following a ritual bath, which removes maternal genitourinary microorganisms along with the vernix caseosa, bacterial contamination with nursery pathogens begins after contact with the contaminated and/or colonized hands of nursing attendants. Accordingly, within 3 days the anterior nares, throat, and skin of the neonate are colonized with gram-positive microorganisms (alpha-hemolytic streptococci, *S. aureus*, and *S. epidermidis*). Within 1 week anaerobic microorganisms and the *Enterobacteriaceae* family colonize the gastrointestinal tract (*E. coli* is the predominant aerobic species in the stools of formula-fed infants, and mixtures of *E. coli* and Lactobacillus spp. predominate in the stools of breast-fed infants).[7] The bacterial flora of infants maintained in an intensive care unit differs from that observed in the normal newborn infant. More specifically, the skin, respiratory tract, and gastrointestinal tract of intensive care infants, many of whom receive treatment with broad-spectrum antibiotics, are colonized with multiple drug-resistant gram-positive (e.g., *S. epidermidis*) and gram-negative (e.g., *E. coli*, Klebsiella spp., Pseudomonas spp.) microorganisms. Opportunities for bacterial invasion and resultant infection increase in direct proportion to the number of invasive diagnostic and therapeutic procedures performed during hospitalization.

SIGNS AND SYMPTOMS OF NEONATAL SEPSIS

The newborn infant's ability to respond to stress is limited. Thus, poor feeding, weak suck, weak cry, lethargy, and irritability are often the initial manifestations of sepsis in the newborn infant. Temperature instability is also an early manifestation of bacterial infection since hypothermia and hyperthermia occur with equal frequency in septic neonates.

Additional signs and symptoms are also nonspecific and may be indicative of neonatal septicemia and/or manifestations of noninfectious disease processes (Table 12–5). Thus, *respiratory distress* with tachypnea, apnea, intercostal and subcostal retractions, grunting, and clinical or radiographic findings of alveolar disease suggests neonatal septicemia and pneumonia. However, in premature infants, such findings must be differentiated from the more common idiopathic respiratory distress syndrome due to a surfactant deficiency. Congenital heart disease, hypocalcemia, hypoglycemia, and congenital anomalies of the thorax and diaphragm must also be included in the differential diagnosis. *Gastrointestinal abnormalities* are common in newborns with sepsis and must be differentiated from similar manifestations occurring as a result of a noninfectious illness. Thus, decreased oral intake, abdominal distension, vomiting, and diarrhea may be signs of a systemic bacterial infection. However, these signs and symptoms are also compatible with a number of noninfectious diseases. *Neurologic findings*, such as lethargy and irritability, may herald the onset of bacterial infection even in the absence of central nervous system involvement. Seizures, hypotonia, tremors, and a full fontanelle may be observed in neonatal septicemia in the absence of meningitis. Thus, septicemia must be included in

the differential diagnosis when evaluating a neonate with nervous system abnormalities. *Cardiovascular changes*, including cyanosis, tachycardia, and bradycardia, may be observed in septic neonates. When evaluating a child for congenital heart disease, the possibility of neonatal sepsis must be considered.

Inspection of Table 12–6, with its clinical data and features of neonatal septicemia, reveals that many conditions can masquerade as infection.

Early Versus Late Onset Illness

Two patterns of illness based on the time of onset of clinical manifestations have been recognized in newborns with systemic bacterial infection (Table 12–7). These two syndromes differ with respect to clinical presentation, epidemiology, pathogenesis, and prognosis. More specifically, the more common "early onset" disease tends to occur in high-risk infants (premature onset of labor, premature rupture of membranes, intrapartum fever) and presents within the first few days of life (mean age at onset of 20 hours) as an overwhelming multisystem illness associated with a high mortality rate (approximately 50%). The microorganisms responsible for early onset illness are part of the "normal" vaginal flora encountered at the time of labor and delivery (e.g., group B streptococcus, *H. influenzae*, *L. monocytogenes*, *S. pneumoniae*, *E. coli*, and Klebsiella spp.). "Late onset" sepsis occurs after the first week of life (mean age of 3 weeks) in infants without perinatal complications. Central nervous system involvement (meningitis) is common, and the mortality rate approaches 20 per cent. The microorganisms responsible for late onset disease are diverse and often nosocomially acquired. *S. aureus*, *S. epidermidis*, and Pseudomonas spp. in addition to microorganisms that usually constitute part of the vaginal flora (group B streptococci, *L. monocytogenes*, and *E. coli*) have been implicated in late onset infections.

MICROORGANISMS CAUSING NEONATAL SEPTICEMIA

The changing pattern of microorganisms responsible for neonatal septicemia and meningitis is reflected in the recent report from the Yale–New Haven Hospital covering the

TABLE 12–5 CLINICAL FEATURES OF NEONATAL SEPSIS

General	**Gastrointestinal**
Poor feeding	Diarrhea
Irritability	Hematochezia
Lethargy	Abdominal distension
Temperature instability	
	Hematopoietic
Respiratory	Thrombocytopenia
Grunting	Leukocytosis,
Nasal flaring	leukopenia
Intercostal retractions	
Tachypnea/apnea	**Cardiovascular**
	Bradycardia/tachycardia
CNS	Hypotension
Hypotonia	Cyanosis
Seizures	
Poor spontaneous	
movement	
Skin	
Petechiae	
Pustulosis	
Sclerema	
Hyperemia	

TABLE 12–6. DIAGNOSTIC FEATURES OF SOME TRANSPLACENTALLY ACQUIRED INFECTIONS COMPARED WITH ERYTHROBLASTOSIS FETALIS*

Finding	Septicemia	Congenital Syphilis	Toxoplasmosis (generalized form)	Cytomegalic Inclusion Disease	Rubella Syndrome	Erythroblastosis Fetalis
Jaundice	+++	+++	+++	+++	+	+++
Anemia	+++	++++	+++	++	+	+++
Thrombocytopenia	+	++	+	++	+++	+
Hepatomegaly	++	++++	+++	++++	++	+++
Splenomegaly	+	+++	++++	++++	++	+++
Purpura	+	+	+	+++	+++	+
Skin rash	+	++	+	+	+	0
Chorioretinitis	0	+	+++	++	+	0
Intracranial calcifications	0	0	+	+	0	0
Generalized edema	+	++		+	0	+
Small-for-dates	+	++	++	+++	+++	−
Special features	Temperature Pustules Red hands and feet with gram-negative septicemia Convulsions	Mucocutaneous lesions Periostitis Snuffles Positive serology	Convulsions Microcephaly Hydrocephaly Positive dye test	Pneumonia Cytomegalic inclusion cells in urine	Cataract Glaucoma Heart defects Deafness Microcephaly Hydrocephaly Bone lesions Rubella virus recoverable	Positive Coombs' test Evidence of blood group incompatibility between mother and child

0 not described

+ present in approximately 1–25% of cases

++ present in approximately 26–50% of cases

+++ present in approximately 51–75% of cases

++++ present in approximately 76–100% of cases

*Adapted from Oski, F. A., and Naiman, J. L.: *Hematologic Problems in the Newborn.* 3rd ed. Philadelphia, W. B. Saunders Co., 1982.

TABLE 12–7 CHARACTERISTICS OF "EARLY ONSET" AND "LATE ONSET" INFECTIONS

Characteristic	Early Onset (<5 days)	Late Onset (≥5 days)
Mean age at onset	20 hours	20 days
Prematurity	Increased	Uncommon
Obstetric complications	Increased	Uncommon
Clinical presentation	Severe, fulminant	Moderate, slowly progressive, usually focal
Mortality	10–50%	20%

period 1933–1978 (Table 12–8). Similar changes have been recognized at other centers.

Group B Streptococci (GBS)

The group B streptococci (*S. agalactiae* or GBS) are the principal gram-positive microorganisms responsible for neonatal septicemia and meningitis. (Recent evidence suggests a decrease in the incidence of neonatal GBS disease.[7]) This pathogen can be differentiated from other streptococci based on its biochemical profile and colony morphology. A type-specific cell wall carbohydrate permits subclassification of the GBS into five serotypes: IA, IB, IC, II, and III. Animal studies suggest that antibodies to type-specific cell wall polysaccharide are protective.[7]

Two "distinct" clinical syndromes have been recognized in infants infected with GBS; however, exceptions are common. The syndromes relate to perinatal events, age at onset, clinical presentation, and morbidity and mortality. Epidemiologic studies have confirmed that in early onset disease the infant acquires GBS from the mother at the time of labor and delivery. Maternal colonization rates vary between 4 and 30 per cent, depending on the technique utilized to recover the colonizing microorganisms and the population under investigation. Vertical transmission occurs in 60–70 per cent of neonates delivered to colonized women, and the attack rate for invasive disease in culture-positive infants is less than 1 per cent. One explanation for the disparity between maternal colonization and neonatal disease relates to the observation that colonized women have higher concentrations of serum antibody against the colonizing serotype than noncolonized women.[8] Accordingly, the offspring of colonized women are passively immunized via transplacentally transmitted type-specific protective antibody. However, infants delivered prior to the thirty-fourth week of ges-

TABLE 12–8 BACTERIA CAUSING NEONATAL SEPSIS AT YALE–NEW HAVEN HOSPITAL (1933–1978)

Organism	1933–43	1944–57	1958–65	1966–78
Beta-hemolytic streptococcus	18	11	8	86*
Group A	16	5	0	0
Group B	2	4	1	76
Group D	0	1	7	9†
Group F	0	1	0	0
Staphylococcus aureus	4	8	2	12
Streptococcus pneumoniae	5	3	2	2
Haemophilus spp.	0	0	1	9‡
Escherichia coli	11	23	33	76
Klebsiella-Enterobacter spp.	0	0	8	28
Pseudomonas aeruginosa	0	13	11	5
Proteus spp.	0	0	0	4
Mixed	3	1	0	11
Other	3	3	8	6
Total	44	62	73	239
Mortality	90% (1933–36)	67% (1937–57)	45%	26%

Adapted from Freedman, R. M., Ingram, D. L., Gross, I., et al: A half century of neonatal sepsis at Yale. Am J Dis Child *135*:140, 1981.

*One case of nongroupable.

†Six cases of enterococcus, three cases of *Streptococcus bovis*.

‡One type B; one type D; two type F; four nontypable; one *H. parainfluenzae*.

tation receive low concentrations of transplacentally transmitted IgG, and this may explain the high attack rate of GBS in small premature infants delivered to culture-positive women. In contrast to early onset disease, which presents acutely as a multisystem illness characterized clinically by apnea, respiratory distress, and hypotension, late onset illness presents insidiously after the first week of life (mean age 3 weeks). The most common presentation for the late onset disease is meningitis (80%); however, other presentations are common and include bacteremia without a recognized focus, bone and joint infection, skin and soft tissue involvement, and conjunctivitis. Type III GBS is most frequently isolated from infants with a late onset presentation (90%), regardless of the focus of infection, in contrast with an equal distribution of serotypes among asymptomatically colonized infants and neonates with early onset illness in the absence of meningitis.[7] Circumstantial evidence suggests that infants with late onset disease acquire their GBS nosocomially; however, evidence of posthospitalization acquisition has been reported.

Group A Streptococci

Common prior to the availability and widespread use of penicillin, group A streptococcal disease is now uncommon. Although sporadic reports of early onset septicemia and/or meningitis appear in the literature, most neonatal infections with this microorganism occur as an epidemic following exposure to a colonized adult(s).[50, 53] Neonatal infection is typically confined to the skin and mucous membranes (blood stream invasion is uncommon), and the mortality rate is low. Nursery epidemics due to this microorganism are easily controlled following identification, isolation, and treatment of carrier infected individuals.

Group C Streptococci

These have been recognized in asymptomatically colonized infants, as pathogens in mild, nonfatal puerperal sepsis following normal delivery and septic abortion, and uncommonly as agents for early onset septicemia and meningitis.[23, 67] Since group C streptococci can be bacitracin sensitive, it is conceivable that infections with this microorganism have been attributed to the Group A streptococcus.[39]

Group D Streptococci

A common cause of neonatal sepsis,[10, 65] this group of microorganisms includes the enterococci (S. faecalis and S. faecium), which are uniformly resistant to the penicillins and the cephalosporins, and the nonenterococcal strains (S. bovis and S. equinus), which are uniformly sensitive to the penicillins and cephalosporins. The clinical presentation is similar to early onset GBS disease, with most infants presenting with respiratory distress and hypotension.

Group G Streptococci

These are part of the normal flora of the female genitourinary tract and are an uncommon cause of early onset sepsis.[4] This microorganism is beta hemolytic on blood agar plates and bacitracin resistant and cross-reacts serologically with GBS.

A recent increase in the incidence of non–group D alpha-hemolytic streptococcal infections has been observed in a number of neonatal units.[18] Infected neonates present with early onset illness in the absence of obstetric complications. Meningitis, shock, pneumonia, and death are uncommon (mortality of 8.8%) when compared with other microorganisms causing early onset disease, suggesting that this pathogen is less virulent for newborn infants.

Several reports suggest an increase in the incidence of neonatal septicemia and meningitis due to S. pneumoniae.[14, 45, 59] Although not part of the "normal" vaginal flora (puerperal infections are uncommon), this microorganism can be transmitted vertically to the neonate at the time of labor and delivery and result in clinical findings indistinguishable from early onset septicemia due to GBS. High-risk infants (premature onset of labor, premature rupture of membranes, intrapartum fever) present within the first few hours of life with overwhelming septicemia characterized by apnea, respiratory distress, cyanosis, and cardiovascular instability. The mortality rate for neonatal pneumococcal disease approaches 50 per cent.

Coagulase-Negative Staphylococci

Part of the normal skin flora, these staphylococci were traditionally classified as "nonpathogens," and accordingly, their isolation from clinical specimens was attributed to faulty technique and resultant "contamination." Over the past 2 decades it has become apparent that these microorganisms cause infection in orthopedic devices, intravenous catheters, prosthetic heart valves, central nervous system shunts, and peritoneal dialysis catheters.[37] Infection with this group of microorganisms has also been recognized in patients with malignancy and/or granulocytopenia.[72] More recently, coagulase-negative staphylococci have been identified as an important cause of neonatal mortality and morbidity.[26, 47] Of the many species identified, *S. epidermidis* is the principal human pathogen, due in part to its unique ability to adhere to and modify the surfaces of polyethylene in travenous catheters.[11, 54] Accordingly, infection is more common in infants receiving parenteral hyperalimentation. Infected neonates are often premature and present, after the first week of life ("late onset infection"), with recurrent apnea, bradycardia, and temperature instability in the absence of an obvious focus. Therapy requires removal and/or replacement of all infected intravenous catheters (if present) and parenteral administration of appropriate chemotherapeutic agents. The choice of antibiotics is complicated by the fact that many isolates of *S. epidermidis* are resistant to the semisynthetic penicillinase-resistant penicillins (methicillin, nafcillin, and oxacillin) and cross-resistant to the cephalosporins. Accordingly, most authorities recommend treating infections due to methicillin-resistant *S. epidermidis* with parenteral vancomycin. Concomitant therapy with rifampin or gentamicin has been recommended for adults with deep-seated infections involving prosthetic devices.[72]

Escherichia Coli

Escherichia coli is the principal gram-negative microorganism causing neonatal septicemia and meningitis. A number of investigators have confirmed that a majority of the *E. coli* strains causing early onset septicemia and meningitis contain a unique capsular (K) antigen.[60, 75] This K1 antigen is an acidic polysaccharide similar immunologically to the capsular antigen of group B *Neisseria meningitidis*. Epidemiologic studies have established that vertical transmission from mother to infant is the principal means of neonatal acquisition; however, nosocomial transmission has been documented. Thus, one investigation of K1-positive infants delivered to K1-negative mothers revealed that the neonatal strains were identical to K1-bearing strains isolated from nursery attendants.[63] Laboratory studies have demonstrated that K1-positive strains have enhanced virulence in animal models and that mortality and morbidity in neonates with meningitis are related to the amount of K1 antigen detected in serum and/or CSF.

The identification of enteropathogenic *E. coli* (EEC) in a stool culture from a single infant in a nursery is cause for alarm because of its epidemiologic consequences. Although there are many who recommend that these strains no longer be routinely identified by bacteriology laboratories, I am not certain that this would be wise. Infants with enteropathogenic serotypes of *E. coli* in their stool represent a source for spread of these agents to other babies and for the development of epidemic diarrhea in a nursery. Thus, it is important to identify and treat all positive babies irrespective of their clinical status. The carrier rate of EEC in the open population is approximately 5 per cent; this rate would be obviously higher during nursery outbreaks. My colleague John Nelson has recently shown that oral neomycin therapy significantly shortens the period of diarrhea and excretion of the organisms when compared with placebo therapy. Although the mechanism of diarrhea in EEC disease is unknown, these nonenterotoxigenic and noninvasive strains, when fed to healthy adult volunteers, produce diarrhea (Levine et al, 1978). These facts certainly argue against the discontinuation of routine serotyping of *E. coli*.

Levine, M., Berquist, E., Nalin, D., et al: *Escherichia coli* strains that cause diarrhoea but do not produce heat-labile or heat-stable enterotoxins and are non-invasive. Lancet 1:1119, 1978.

G. McCracken

Anaerobic Bacteria

With the development of sophisticated laboratory techniques for the isolation and identification of fastidious microorganisms, *anaerobic bacteria* are being recognized with increasing frequency in a variety of infections. Although well established as pathogens in adults, the exact role of anaerobes in neonatal sepsis has not been established. The proportion of neonatal infections due to anaerobic microorganisms may be as high as 20 per cent. Acquisition of anaerobic bacteria occurs by vertical transmission at the time of labor and delivery. The clinical manifestations of neonatal anaerobic septicemia are similar to those described for other bacterial pathogens. Chow and coworkers analyzed systemic neonatal infections due to anaerobic organisms and classified them into four groups: (1) transient bacteremia following premature rupture of membranes and amnionitis, (2) septicemia (often polymicrobial) following surgical manipulation of the gastrointestinal tract, (3) fulminant septicemia due to Clostridium spp., and (4) those causing intrauterine death and septic abortion.[19] The mortality rate in anaerobic septicemia (excluding clostridial sepsis, which has a high fatality rate) is low and rarely exceeds 10 per cent.

Listeria Monocytogenes

A ubiquitous, short gram-positive non–spore-forming motile rod, L. monocytogenes is capable of causing disease in a wide variety of animals and humans. Listeriae have been isolated from the genital tract of both sexes and may be responsible for repeated abortion. Transplacental transmission can occur and typically follows a nonspecific maternal illness characterized by fever, chills, and headache several days or weeks prior to abortion, stillbirth, or neonatal death. Infants infected transplacentally are typically premature with diffuse hepatosplenomegaly and evidence of multisystem disease characterized by respiratory distress, cardiovascular instability, hypotension, and a salmon-colored rash on the skin (cutaneous granulomas) and mucous membranes. Vertical transmission is more common, and infected neonates present with early onset septicemia indistinguishable from that seen with the GBS. A late onset form of listeriosis has been described and invariably involves the meninges; patients present with lethargy, fever, vomiting, and seizures.

Haemophilus Influenzae

H. influenzae is an increasingly common neonatal pathogen, with the majority of reports appearing since 1975.[22, 30, 36, 56] One explanation for the emergence of this microorganism as a neonatal pathogen relates to improvements in microbiologic techniques, including routine Gram stain and subculture of all blood culture broths on chocolate agar. (Haemophilus spp. often produce no turbidity in blood culture systems.) The addition of anticomplement and antiantibody substances to blood culture broth to block the inhibitory activity of human serum on nontypable H. influenzae may increase the yield of these microorganisms. A recent review by Wallace and coworkers describes 11 cases of neonatal septicemia and meningitis observed during a

6 year period.[73] In contrast with previous reports, a majority of these isolates were nontypable. (The spontaneous agglutinin reaction characteristic of nontypable Haemophilus spp. and responsible for many typing errors can be eliminated by confirming all positive slide agglutination reactions with counterimmunoelectrophoresis.) The prevalence of beta-lactamase–producing stains is low (3%). The major clinical presentation of septicemia due to H. influenzae is early onset disease indistinguishable from early onset GBS sepsis, with a mortality rate of approximately 50 per cent. Localized Haemophilus infections (abscess, cellulitis, and/or vesicular eruptions) are not uncommon and are associated with an excellent prognosis.

Detection of antigen in body fluids is very helpful in distinguishing between bacterial and nonbacterial infections and in identifying the specific etiologic agent. Using a special high-titered antiserum, we have detected polysaccharide antigen in cerebrospinal fluid from 90 per cent of infants with group B streptococcal meningitis and from approximately 70 per cent of infants with disease caused by E. coli K1. The limulus lysate assay will measure endotoxin in cerebrospinal fluid of 75 per cent of neonates with gram-negative bacillary meningitis. These and other screening tests should be considered adjuncts to diagnosing bacterial disease rather than as a substitute for careful examination of gram-stained smears of the body fluids. In the Cooperative Meningitis project, stained smears of spinal fluid were correctly interpreted in 80 per cent of the neonates with disease caused by coliform bacteria. There is no substitute for the microscopic examination of cerebrospinal fluid.   **G. McCracken**

LABORATORY DIAGNOSIS

Direct Techniques

The diagnosis of neonatal septicemia is ultimately dependent upon a positive blood culture in a symptomatic infant. Thus, every effort should be made to recover the responsible pathogen by obtaining an appropriate amount of blood from a peripheral vein under aseptic conditions. There is little information on the number of blood cultures required or the volume of blood necessary before initiation of antimicrobial therapy. Several authors have suggested obtaining two simultaneous blood cultures to increase the yield of pathogenic microorganisms and to avoid confusion after recovery of "nonpathogens." Our policy has always been to obtain a single culture with at least 2 ml of blood from a peripheral vein. Blood cultures obtained from cord blood or through intravascular catheters are unsatisfactory because of the high yield of false-positive results. Alternative techniques for blood sampling include aseptic removal of blood from a double-clamped section of the umbilical cord and the use of the heel stick blood cultures.[32, 58]

In addition to blood cultures, cerebrospinal fluid (CSF) cultures should be obtained in all infants with suspected sepsis, since meningitis is common in septic newborns (30%). Neonates with meningitis can have negative blood cultures (10%), and the choice and duration of antimicrobial therapy are different in the presence of central nervous system infection. In evaluating the cerebrospinal fluid, it is important to recall that the cellular and chemical content of the spinal fluid of the newborn infant differs from those of the older infant and the adult and that "normal" cerebrospinal fluid does not exclude the diagnosis of meningitis.[71] Obviously contraindicated is cerebrospinal fluid examination in the critically ill neonate, in whom performance of a lumbar puncture may further compromise cardiovascular and/or pulmonary function or unnecessarily delay initiation of treatment. Under these circumstances, treatment is initiated, and a lumbar puncture is deferred until the infant's condition is stable. Appropriate therapy for meningitis should be continued if the delayed cerebrospinal fluid examination suggests partially treated meningitis.

Urine cultures should be performed in all newborn infants with presumed septicemia because the genitourinary tract may serve as both a portal of entry for bacterial pathogens and a site of deposit for bacteria disseminated by the blood stream. Several authors have commented on the value of clean catch and midstream urine collections in newborn infants;[24] however, the timing and reliability of these techniques are limiting. Accordingly, we perform a suprapubic bladder aspiration prior to initiating antimicrobial therapy in all neonates with presumed sepsis. However, in view of the low yield of urine cultures in early onset infection (positive urine cultures with negative blood cultures are uncommon in neonates less than 72 hours of age), we avoid bladder aspiration when evaluating the unstable infant and will not delay treatment to obtain a satisfactory urine specimen.[70]

Bacterial cultures of the skin, external auditory canal, umbilicus, and gastric aspirate are of little or no value in the diagnosis and treatment of neonatal septicemia. More specifically, these "surface cultures" only provide information on bacterial contamination at the time of labor and delivery and accordingly reflect the bacterial flora of the maternal genitourinary tract. Treatment decisions are not based on the information obtained from such cultures.

The recently developed techniques of counterimmunoelectrophoresis (CIE), latex agglutination, staphylococcal agglutination, and enzyme-linked immunosorbent assay provide simple, rapid, and accurate means of detecting bacterial antigens in blood, urine, and cerebrospinal fluid. Limitations of these laboratory procedures include a lack of available antisera for all bacterial pathogens (resulting in false-negative results) and cross-reactions between related bacterial species (with false-positive reactions).

Histologic examination and selective staining of material obtained from needle aspiration of an infected site or tissue biopsy may assist in the diagnostic evaluation of the neonate with presumed sepsis.

Indirect Techniques

Indirect techniques for the diagnosis of neonatal septicemia are numerous and of differing sensitivity. A white blood cell count should be obtained in all neonates with presumed sepsis. An abnormally elevated (>24,000 cells/mm^3) or depressed (<3,000 cells/mm^3) white blood cell count at the onset of symptoms is suggestive of bacterial infection. The differential white blood cell count, however, is a better indicator of bacterial infection, particularly when the absolute number of immature neutrophils (bands and metamyelocytes) is increased, the ratio of immature neutrophils to total neutrophils is increased, or the absolute neutrophil count is decreased because of exhaustion of the bone marrow reserves.[38] Manroe and coworkers have established criteria for neonatal bacterial infection utilizing these three values (Table 12–9). Thrombocytopenia (<100,000 cells/mm^3 during the first 10 days of life), toxic granulations, and/or Döhle inclusion bodies in the blood smear are insensitive indicators of systemic bacterial infection. Examination of a gram-stained, methylene blue–stained, and/or acridine orange–stained buffy coat or blood smear represents additional indirect techniques for diagnosing bacteremia. Recent studies suggest a correlation between positive buffy coat smears and

TABLE 12–9 NEONATAL NEUTROPHIL VALUES AS PREDICTORS OF SEPSIS*

	Value (granulocytes/mm³)	Age (hours)
Neutropenia	<1800	Birth
	<7200	<12
	<3600	12–48
	<1800	48–60
Increased band forms	>1100	Birth
	>1400	<12
	> 800	12–60
Increased band/neutrophil ratio	> 0.20	

*From Manroe et al.[38]

the severity of bacterial infection. Gastric acid smears have also been suggested as an indirect technique for diagnosing bacterial infection.[57] The presence of an abnormal number of gastric leukocytes (more than five per high power field) is used as an indirect indication of amnionitis and supports the diagnosis of septicemia in a symptomatic neonate. Similarly, the demonstration of granulocytes in fluid recovered from the external auditory canal is indirect evidence for exposure to an infected intrauterine environment (amnionitis) and may identify the neonate at risk for early onset septicemia.[64] Cultures of these areas are of little value and simply reflect the bacterial flora of the maternal genitourinary tract.

Numerous studies have determined that the erythrocyte sedimentation rate (ESR) is elevated in neonates with bacterial infection and normal in most newborns with noninfectious illnesses, such as respiratory distress syndrome, meconium aspiration, and transient tachypnea of the newborn. The ESR does not vary with gestational age, birth weight, or sex, and normal values range from less than 1 mm/hour on the first day of life to 17 mm/hour in 2 week old infants. Falsely elevated ESR values are common in neonates with severe hemolytic disease, since the ESR is inversely related to the hematocrit and abnormally low values are not uncommon in septic infants with disseminated intravascular coagulation.

Abnormal values for the C-reactive protein (over 2 mg/dl) are found in 80 per cent of newborn infants with bacterial infection.[62] False-positive elevations from noninfectious causes are uncommon. The Limulus lysate assay, used to detect endotoxin in body fluids of patients with gram-negative infection, is another indirect technique for diagnosing bacterial infection in newborn infants. Despite the high frequency of false-positive results in serum, the assay has proved useful in detecting minute quantities of endotoxin in the cerebrospinal fluid and urine of neonates with gram-negative bacillary meningitis and/or septicemia. Additional screening tests include determination of serum haptoglobin, serum fibrinogen, and alpha$_1$-acid glycoprotein concentrations. More specifically, these proteins are acute-phase reactants and thus increase in the presence of inflammation. Cerebrospinal fluid concentration of lactic dehydrogenase and lactate (elevated in bacterial meningitis), CSF pH (depressed in bacterial meningitis), and gas chromatographic analysis of body fluids to detect bacterial metabolites have also been utilized as indirect techniques for diagnosing neonatal bacterial infection.

The large number of indirect techniques available for diagnosing neonatal septicemia is testimony to the fact that no single laboratory test can reliably identify all neonates with bacterial infection. Accordingly, several investigators have recommended a panel of screening tests as a means of improving predictability.[55] Such "sepsis screens" lack sensitivity, and accordingly, a number of false-positive results continue to occur in patients without proven infection.

Table 12–10 outlines the laboratory criteria for the diagnosis of bacterial sepsis in newborn infants.

TREATMENT (See Appendix A–2)

Treatment of neonatal septicemia must begin following appropriate diagnostic studies and prior to identification and antibiotic sensitivity testing of the responsible pathogen(s). The initial choice of antibiotics requires an understanding of the microorganisms most often responsible for neonatal bacterial infection, the antibiotic sensitivity pattern(s) of the most likely pathogen(s), the location of the infection, the likelihood of obtaining bactericidal concentrations of antibiotics at the infected focus, and the toxicity of the available antimicrobial agent(s).

Expectant therapy for early onset septicemia must provide coverage against the gram-positive cocci, particularly GBS and gram-negative enteric bacilli. Although other microorganisms, such as *L. monocytogenes, H.*

TABLE 12–10 LABORATORY DIAGNOSTIC CRITERIA FOR SEPSIS IN THE NEONATE

Definitive
Positive culture of blood, cerebrospinal fluid, or urine

Highly probable
Demonstration of bacterial antigen in blood, CSF, or urine by counterimmunoelectrophoresis, latex fixation, or ELISA

Probable
Absolute granulocytopenia, elevated band/PMN ratio, C-reactive protein over 3 μg/ml, elevated erythrocyte sedimentation rate, elevated serum IgM, thrombocytopenia

Possible
Pulmonary infiltrates on chest x-ray, elevated C-reactive protein or sedimentation rate 3 days into antimicrobial therapy

influenzae, and *S. pneumoniae*, may be responsible for early onset infection, it is possible to administer a combination of antimicrobial agents with activity against all or the most likely pathogens. Thus, initial expectant therapy for early onset infection usually includes a broad spectrum semisynthetic penicillin (e.g., ampicillin) and an aminoglycoside (e.g., kanamycin, tobramycin, gentamicin, or amikacin).

Expectant antibiotic therapy for late onset infection must also provide coverage against the staphylococcus as well as hospital-acquired gram-negative microorganisms, including Pseudomonas spp. and Serratia spp. Thus, expectant therapy for late onset illness traditionally includes an antistaphylococcal penicillinase-resistant penicillin (nafcillin or oxacillin) and an aminoglycoside. In nurseries where methicillin-resistant *S. aureus* and *S. epidermidis* are common nosocomial pathogens, vancomycin should be substituted for the penicillinase-resistant penicillin. (Although many methicillin-resistant strains of *S. aureus* and *S. epidermidis* are inhibited in vitro by the cephalosporins, bactericidal concentrations of this group of antibiotics are not uniformly achieved in vivo, thereby precluding their use in the treatment of neonatal staphylococcal infection.)

Following identification of the responsible pathogen and determination of the antibiotic sensitivity pattern, we recommend continuation of therapy with the single most effective agent. Exceptions to this single agent recommendation include enterococcal sepsis (in which a combination of ampicillin and gentamicin, which is synergistic against most en-

terococci, is utilized throughout the treatment period) and infections caused by Klebsiella spp. and Pseudomonas spp. More specifically, some authorities would recommend combination chemotherapy with a broad-spectrum penicillin (ticarcillin or piperacillin) and an aminoglycoside in infections due to Klebsiella spp. and Pseudomonas spp. Following the initiation of antibiotic treatment in the absence of a pathogen, a clinical decision must be made regarding the advisability of continuing antimicrobial therapy. Obviously, many infants are treated empirically for presumed septicemia, although few have culture-proven sepsis. Most physicians reevaluate the culture-negative patients following 48–72 hours of antibiotic therapy. If this reevaluation demonstrates an infant who is clinically well and in whom the diagnosis of bacterial sepsis seems unlikely retrospectively, most would discontinue antibiotic therapy and observe the child for an additional 24 hours. If the child continues to appear ill and/or the initial signs and symptoms cannot be explained by a noninfectious illness, we would continue therapy with both agents despite negative cultures, since bacterial infection may occur in the absence of bacteremia.[66]

The duration of antimicrobial therapy in documented bacterial infection depends on the clinical response of the patient, the identity of the responsible pathogen, and the location of the infection. We routinely treat nonstaphylococcal septicemia, pneumonia, urinary tract infection, and skin and soft tissue infections for 7–10 days with the appropriate antimicrobial agent(s). Deep-seated staphylococcal infections tend to metastasize and/or recur following abbreviated therapeutic courses and accordingly should be treated for a minimum of 21 days. Meningitis is treated for 14–21 days.

Neonatal meningitis occurs in approximately 30 per cent of newborns with culture-proven sepsis. The microorganisms responsible for meningitis are the same as those causing neonatal septicemia. As a result, initial antimicrobial therapy for meningitis is similar to the expectant therapy recommended for septicemia. However, unlike septicemia, the treatment of meningitis is complicated by the fact that many of the agents utilized to treat septicemia, especially the aminoglycosides, fail to achieve bactericidal concentrations in the cerebrospinal fluid, even when injected directly into the lumbar subarachnoid space. This low level of antimicrobial activity—combined with the immunologic inadequacy of the cerebrospinal fluid (decreased concentration of immunoglobulins and complement and defective opsonization, phagocytosis, and chemotaxis by neutrophils in the cerebrospinal fluid)—is responsible for the delayed clinical and microbiologic response characteristic of neonatal meningitis.

Although the optimal therapy for neonatal meningitis remains uncertain, the high mortality and morbidity of this entity mandate an aggressive therapeutic approach. Whatever the regimen, it must result in bactericidal concentrations of antibiotic(s) in the cerebrospinal fluid for gram-positive cocci and gram-negative microorganisms. (Bacteriostatic activity as measured by the standard minimal inhibitory concentration [MIC] is not sufficient.) Accordingly, treatment of neonatal meningitis should be initiated with a combination of antibiotics, including ampicillin (active against most gram-positive microorganisms including GBS and *L. monocytogenes* and many gram-negative pathogens) and a third generation cephalosporin. Two of the latter group of antibiotics, moxalactam and cefotaxime, are approved for use in children with meningitis. The third generation cephalosporins have a number of advantages, which include a spectrum of activity not too dissimilar from that of the aminoglycosides, an ability to achieve bacterial concentrations in the cerebrospinal fluid for most gram-negative microorganisms (Pseudomonas spp. are important exceptions), and a relative lack of toxicity. (Ceftriaxone is a new third generation cephalosporin with unique pharmacologic properties that include a long serum half-life and cerebrospinal fluid accumulation. This agent may replace moxalactam and cefotaxime as the third generation cephalosporin of choice in neonatal gram-negative meningitis.)

Thus, if initial diagnostic studies fail to identify the responsible microorganism (negative Gram stain and/or assays for antigen detection), we initiate treatment of neonatal meningitis with parenteral ampicillin and moxalactam. A repeat lumbar puncture is performed 24 hours after the start of treatment in culture-proven meningitis to determine sterility, antibiotic concentration(s), and bactericidal activity of the cerebrospinal fluid (the latter should exceed a dilution of 1:8). Once the offending microorganism has been identified, we continue treatment with the single most effective agent and monitor bacteriologic response with repeated lumbar punctures until the CSF is sterile. Reexaminations of the cerebrospinal fluid to determine sterility should occur following completion of therapy (21 days).

Failure to sterilize the cerebrospinal fluid following 24 hours of therapy is common in neonatal meningitis and in the absence of clinical deterioration rarely calls for alterations in the choice or route of antibiotic administration. However, failure to sterilize the spinal fluid following 72 hours of appropriate parenteral therapy or clinical deterioration constitutes treatment failure and suggests the presence of ventriculitis. Ventriculitis is the most common cause of treatment failure in neonatal meningitis, can be diagnosed by CT scan or ultrasound, rarely responds to treatment with parenteral therapy, and is a recognized indication for intrathecal administration of antimicrobial agents, especially by the ventricular route. McCracken and Mize, in a collaborative study of neonatal gram-negative meningitis, compared the efficacy of parenteral gentamicin alone and parenteral gentamicin plus lumbar intrathecal gentamicin in two groups of patients receiving ampicillin.[40] The mortality was similar in both treatment groups. Failure of the administered gentamicin to reach the ventricles was considered to be a possible reason for the results of this study. Accordingly, a second collaborative study was undertaken to investigate the value of direct instillation of gentamicin into the ventricular system in neonates with gram-negative meningitis.[42] This study was terminated prematurely because of the higher mortality in the systemic and intraventricular therapy group. This latter study has been criticized by a number of investigators and contrasts with the good results obtained by other investigators treating neonatal meningitis with aminoglycosides administered directly into the ventricles through a subcutaneous reservoir.[34, 69] Thus, in neonates with positive cerebrospinal fluid cultures following 72 hours of appropriate antimicrobial therapy, a deteriorating clinical course, and radiographic evidence of ventriculitis, we begin intraventricular aminoglycoside therapy through a subcutaneous reservoir. Treatment of gram-negative meningitis should be continued for 21 days and is followed by a repeat posttreatment lumbar puncture to determine sterility. Abnormal spinal fluid cytology and/or chemistries may persist for months following discontinuation of therapy and are not an indication for continued treatment.

Shock, seizures, respiratory failure, and fluid and electrolyte disturbances are some of the more common complications of neonatal septicemia and meningitis and must be treated appropriately. Adjunct therapy with granulocyte transfusions, exchange transfusions, and/or intravenous use of plasma or immunoglobulin has recently been utilized for neonates with septicemia. Investigations documenting the efficacy of these new therapeutic approaches are inconclusive, but preliminary results appear promising.

Septicemia, particularly when associated with neutropenia, continues to be a significant cause of neonatal morbidity and mortality, despite the early use of broad-spectrum antibiotics and improvements in supportive care. Thus, attention has recently focused on granulocyte transfusions as a potential adjunct treatment modality.

The normal range for the total neutrophil count (TNC) was defined by Manroe el al[38] for the first 28 days of life and is markedly different from the accepted definition of neutropenia in adults as 500 neutrophils/mm³ or less. In neonates, the TNC peaks at 12–14 hours of life at 7000–14,500 neutrophils/mm³. Thereafter, the TNC stabilizes at 1750–5400 neutrophils/mm³. The ratio of immature/total neutrophils (I/T) remains 0.16 or less for the first 60 hours of life.

After the early reports from Laurenti et al of improved survival of infants with gram-negative sepsis who received granulocyte transfusions, Christensen and colleagues did a controlled, randomized study of septic, neutropenic neonates. These infants all had a clinical diagnosis of sepsis and a positive blood or CSF culture or Gram stain. In addition, bone marrow aspiration demonstrated marked neutrophil storage pool depletion (less than 7% neutrophil precursors). All seven of the transfused infants survived, compared with only one survivor from the nine nontransfused infants. Christensen et al have now shown in a small number of infants that an I/T ratio of 0.8 or more peripherally is associated with bone marrow storage pool depletion.

The efficacy of granulocyte transfusions in septic neonates still remains to be proved. The number of infants studied is very small. Bone marrow examinations, which may result in hematoma, infection, or fracture, require an expertise that makes them difficult to obtain quickly. Acquiring fresh granulocytes rapidly is also difficult. Potential adverse reactions include fluid overload, graft versus host disease, transfusion reactions, pulmonary sequestration, blood group sensitization, and transmission of cytomegalovirus (CMV), hepatitis, or AIDS. Although adverse reactions have not been reported, we have observed respiratory decompensation in one infant during two successive transfusions. Further prospective, controlled studies of septic neonates are needed before granulocyte transfusions can be considered a clinically useful therapeutic modality.   **J. Baley**

Stork, E., Baley, J., and Shurin, S.: A controlled trial of granulocyte transfusion in neutropenic neonates. Pediatr Res *19*:366A, 1985.

Questions

Match the following

A. Skin pustule
B. Ecthyma gangrenosum
C. Nikolsky's sign
D. Ritter's disease
E. Intranuclear inclusions
F. Snuffles
G. Kernicterus
H. Abortion/stillbirth
I. Gray baby syndrome
J. Sabin-Feldman dye test
K. Galactosemia
L. Intramuscular iron

1. L. monocytogenes
2. Pseudomonas aeruginosa
3. S. aureus
4. Chloramphenicol
5. Sulfonamides
6. T. pallidum
7. Cytomegalovirus
8. Toxoplasmosis
9. E. coli

A–3, B–2, C–3, D–3, E–7, F–6, G–5, H–1, I–4, J–8, K–9, L–9.

True or False

T. pallidum cannot cross the placenta during the first trimester of pregnancy. Thus, treatment of the mother during early pregnancy does not require follow-up and treatment of the infant.

Recent reports have demonstrated that *T. pallidum* can cross the placenta during the first trimester. Adequate maternal therapy during pregnancy is curative in the infant. In the absence of adequate maternal therapy, neonatal treatment with either benzathine penicillin (for non-CNS infections) or parenteral penicillin would be indicated. The statement, therefore, is false.

Asymptomatic bacteriuria during pregnancy is associated with premature births.

Symptomatic bacteriuria has been associated with prematurity, but asymptomatic bacteriuria has not. Therefore, the statement is false.

Cytomegalovirus:
A. Occasionally causes an intrauterine infection characterized by hepatosplenomegaly, "blueberry muffin" spots, and microcephaly.
B. Is a cause of the afebrile infant pneumonia syndrome.
C. Is highly contagious and may spread rapidly through a nursery and to nursing and medical staff.
D. Typically causes an asymptomatic carrier state in infected infants.
E. May be acquired from blood products.

Cytomegalovirus, one of the five known herpes-viruses in humans (herpes simplex I and II, Epstein-Barr virus, varicella-zoster virus, and cytomegalovirus), is capable of causing symptomatic and asymptomatic infection in neonates, infants, older children, and adults. Symptomatic congenital infection most often follows primary maternal infection (the maternal illness may be inapparent or accompanied by a nonspecific symptom) and may be accompanied by premature labor and delivery. Affected neonates can present with a number of clinical findings, including microcephaly, hepatosplenomegaly, "blueberry muffin" spots (sites of extramedullary hematopoiesis) and jaundice. Cerebral calcifications, pneumonia, and chorioretinitis are noted less frequently. Asymptomatic congenital infection is more common and may be acquired transplacentally, vertically at the time of labor and delivery, or postnatally following close contact with infected neonates or infected maternal secretions or transfusion with infected blood products. (The use of seronegative donors reduces viral shedding in hospitalized neonates and eliminates CMV infection in infants born to seronegative mothers.) Asymptomatic neonates may present with an afebrile respiratory illness during the first few months of life. (This afebrile pneumonia syndrome may also be observed in infants infected with *C. trachomatis*, *U. urealyticum*, and *Pneumocystis carinii*.) Infected children may excrete the virus in their urine or saliva for months or even years. Although cytomegalovirus has not been associated with nursery epidemics, the theoretic possibility exists that the infected neonate may transmit virus to a susceptible individual. Accordingly most nurseries try to limit contact between seronegative women and infected neonates by means of isolation, handwashing, and careful handling of body secretions (urine and stool). The correct answers are A, B, D, and E.

CASE PROBLEMS

Case One

A 23 year old primigravida is admitted to the delivery suite. Cultures taken from the cervix at her last prenatal visit were positive for *Neisseria gonorrhoeae*. She goes on to deliver a normal, healthy infant.

Which would be the appropriate treatment for the infant?
A. *Observation.*
B. *Cultures of blood, urine, and cerebrospinal fluid and treatment for presumed sepsis.*
C. *Cultures of throat and rectum.*
D. *Prophylactic treatment with a single dose of 50,000 units/kg of penicillin G.*

The correct answers are A, C, and D. Infants delivered vaginally to women with gonorrheal infections are at increased risk for developing ophthalmia neonatorum and gonococcal septicemia. In the absence of symptoms, a single intramuscular dose of penicillin G provides adequate prophylaxis. However, if during the period of observation the infant develops symptoms of sepsis, a complete sepsis evaluation and a parenteral course of antimicrobial therapy are indicated. The infant should be followed prospectively for the development of ophthalmia neonatorum, which typically occurs after the first week of life.

Case Two

An infant is noted to have bilateral purulent conjunctivitis on the second day of life.

A reasonable approach would be:
A. *Observation.*
B. *Gram stain and culture.*
C. *Obtain conjunctival epithelial scrapings and look for intracytoplasmic inclusions.*
D. *Culture for sepsis and begin antimicrobial treatment.*

The most common cause of neonatal conjunctivitis is chemical conjunctivitis, which typically occurs within the first 6–8 hours of life and may persist for 24 hours. Silver nitrate drops, used for prophylaxis of gonococcal conjunctivitis, are usually the cause, and no treatment is needed. Gonococcal conjunctivitis may appear at any time during the first 1–2 weeks of life but usually occurs after 24 hours of age. Gram stains of the conjunctival exudate often show gram-negative diplococci, and cultures yield *N. gonorrhoeae*. A 10 day course of parenteral penicillin G is required for treatment. Nongonococcal bacterial conjunctivitis is usually caused by *S. aureus* and develops after the third day of life. The diagnosis is also made by a Gram stain and culture. Treatment with topical antimicrobial agents is usually adequate. Conjunctivitis due to *C. trachomatis* begins after 7 days of life, typically between the second and fourth weeks of life. This diagnosis is established by demonstration of intracytoplasmic inclusions in the conjunctival scrapings. Treatment with oral erythromycin is recommended. Over half of the children with *C. trachomatis* conjunctivitis subsequently develop an afebrile pneumonia and eosinophilia. The correct answers are A, B, and C.

Case Three

During a routine prenatal history, a 20 weeks' pregnant woman is found to have been exposed to tuberculosis. A 5 unit purified protein derivative (PPD) is placed on her forearm and is subsequently positive.

Which of the following constitutes the correct management of the mother?

A. *Begin isoniazid therapy.*
B. *Repeat the skin test in 3 months.*
C. *Obtain a chest x-ray and, if it is negative, observe the mother.*
D. *Immunize the mother with bacille Calmette-Guérin (BCG) vaccine.*

Answer C is correct. A chest x-ray is obtained with proper shielding of the abdomen to identify evidence of active pulmonary tuberculosis. In the absence of a positive chest x-ray or evidence of extrapulmonary infection, observation is recommended for asymptomatic individuals. Although isoniazid has not been shown to be teratogenic, most authorities withhold chemoprophylaxis in the asymptomatic pregnant woman with a normal chest x-ray. Isoniazid chemoprophylaxis for a positive skin test reaction in the absence of active disease is started following delivery.

The mother previously described develops night sweats, fever, and a purulent cough at 8 months' gestation. A chest x-ray obtained at this time shows hilar lymphadenopathy and a left upper lobe cavity.

Correct management of the mother would include which of the following?
A. *Repeat skin test with a 5 unit PPD.*
B. *BCG vaccination.*
C. *Begin therapy with isoniazid and rifampin.*
D. *Begin therapy with isoniazid and ethambutol.*

The correct answer is D. Although many consider isoniazid and rifampin the drugs of choice for progressive pulmonary tuberculosis, rifampin toxicity (teratogenic in animals) precludes its use as a first line drug in this situation. Rifampin may be added if a third agent is needed or if the organism is considered resistant to isoniazid. Pyridoxine (50 mg/day) should be included in any treatment regimen to prevent isoniazid-associated neurotoxicity in the fetus or newborn. BCG is not approved currently in the United States and is only used prophylactically in areas of high risk. Repeating the PPD is of little or no efficacy.

What is your approach to the infant?

Neonates acquiring *M. tuberculosis* infection are at an increased risk for disseminated disease. It is important to recall that the most common source of neonatal infection is from parents or close family contacts with undiagnosed disease. If significant exposure is avoided by aggressive treatment of the mother, skin testing and observation are required. If the mother is actively shedding the tubercle bacillus (culture or smear) at the time of birth, chemoprophylaxis of the neonate with isoniazid (10 mg/kg/day) is recommended. While BCG may be used successfully to vaccinate these infants (if the skin test and chest radiograph are negative), it is usually reserved for infants exposed to isoniazid-resistant bacilli or in cases in which medical follow-up and compliance are suspect.

Case Four

Mrs. G. W. is a 28 year old gravida II parity I mother whose first pregnancy resulted in a normal term male infant who died at 2 days of age of group B streptococcal sepsis and meningitis. The family consults you during the last trimester of pregnancy and is concerned about the new infant developing the same disease.

The most appropriate approach is:
A. *Reassure the mother not to worry.*
B. *Culture the mother's cervix and rectum for group B streptococcus.*
C. *Empirically treat the mother with broad-spectrum antibiotics.*
D. *Immunize the mother with Pneumovax.*

The correct answer is B. Although 15–40 per cent of women may be colonized with group B streptococcus, a recent study suggests that the density of intrapartum vaginal colonization directly affects the rate of neonatal colonization and subsequent invasive disease.[16] Empiric antimicrobial therapy of the high-risk mother prior to the intrapartum period is variably effective since recolonization occurs following cessation of prophylaxis (Merenstein et al, 1980). The cross reactivity between the antibodies produced by Pneumovax and the IgG antibodies against *S. agalactiae* has been investigated and does not provide protection against neonatal streptococcal disease.

Although this infant seems to be at risk of neonatal sepsis by history, maternal factors associated with early onset group B streptococcal disease occur perinatally. Boyer and others identified these factors, and they include prematurity, prolonged rupture of the amniotic membranes (over 19 hours), and maternal intrapartum fever.[15]

Merenstein, G. B., Todd, W. A., Brown, G., et al.: Group B beta-hemolytic streptococcus: randomized controlled treatment study at term. Obstet Gynecol 55:315, 1980.

The mother is cultured, and group B streptococci type II are recovered. An appropriate response would be:
A. *Reassure the mother that she has normal vaginal flora.*
B. *Treat the mother and the father with antimicrobial therapy.*
C. *Treat the mother with local therapy.*
D. *Treat the mother with ampicillin within 24 hours of delivery.*

The correct answer is D. Oral antimicrobial therapy for the mother and the father prior to the immediate peripartum period has not been demonstrated to be effective in eliminating group B streptococcus from the vaginal flora. The use of local therapy is without clinical efficacy. A recent study by Boyer et al[17] has demonstrated that intravenous administration of ampicillin to culture-positive women given 12–24 hours prior to delivery markedly decreases neonatal colonization and the incidence of invasive disease.

The mother delivered at home and did not receive the ampicillin prophylaxis that you had recommended. The infant is transported to the nursery at half an hour of age. The infant is vigorous and alert at this time.

The most appropriate management of the infant at this time would be:
A. Perform surface cultures and treat the child prospectively with ampicillin and gentamicin.
B. Perform cultures of blood, urine, and cerebrospinal fluid and begin broad-spectrum antimicrobial therapy.
C. Give the infant a single dose of 50,000 units/kg of penicillin G.
D. Have the infant bathed in an antiseptic solution.

The correct answer is C. Since 61 per cent of the infants developing early onset disease are bacteremic at birth or within the first hour of life, intrapartum administration of ampicillin is preferred in high-risk situations. A large randomized study demonstrated a reduction in early onset streptococcal disease in term infants receiving a single intramuscular dose of penicillin at the time of birth. While surface cultures may demonstrate colonization with the group B streptococcus, they are not an effective predictor of invasive disease. In the absence of clinical signs of septicemia, it is not necessary to perform a full sepsis evaluation. This infant should be closely observed during the nursery stay. Parenteral therapy and a complete sepsis evaluation should be performed if signs of sepsis develop.

Case Five

A 19 year old primigravida delivers a healthy full-term male infant vaginally. Additional history obtained postpartum reveals that the mother has had herpes genitalis in the past year. She denies any recurrences during the pregnancy.

A reasonable approach would be:
A. Immediately treat the infant with systemic vidarabine or acyclovir.
B. Culture the mother for herpes simplex virus and treat the infant if she is positive.
C. Observe the mother for the development of genital vesicles and treat the infant if they develop.
D. Culture the infant's nasopharynx, eyes, and stool for herpes simplex virus and observe him for cutaneous lesions, changes in liver function, or seizures.

Although neonatal infections with herpes simplex virus (HSV) may occur in utero, HSV is usually acquired at the time of labor and delivery. The majority of women giving birth to infected neonates deny a history of herpes genitalis, herpes orolabialis, or herpetic whitlow. In women with recurrent herpes genitalis, viral shedding may precede the development of genital vesicles by as long as 1 week. Prospective viral cultures of the cervix are recommended in these cases and should be performed weekly during the last month of pregnancy; if positive within 2 weeks of the anticipated delivery, cesarean section is recommended.

Although the onset of clinically apparent neonatal HSV infection may occur as early as 2 days of age, most cases develop between the first and second week of life. Seventy per cent of the affected neonates will develop cutaneous vesicles. The remainder may present with disseminated disease (shock, abnormal liver function tests, thrombocytopenia, and coma) or localized CNS disease (seizures, lethargy, or irritability).

The early use of vidarabine has greatly reduced the morbidity and mortality of neonatal HSV infections and should be started at the earliest sign of cutaneous or systemic involvement. Therapy may be started if the infant is found to be colonized with the virus. Although data are sparse, antiviral therapy may be started if the mother is culture positive. Ophthalmic use of the drug is employed in our institution to prevent herpes keratoconjunctivitis. To date there are no data on the prophylactic use of parenteral vidarabine nor are there published data comparing acyclovir with vidarabine in newborn infants. The correct answers are B and D.

Recent studies have demonstrated that infants may acquire HSV from sources other than the mother. Parents or hospital personnel with herpetic whitlow or herpes orolabialis should avoid contact with newborn infants.

Case Six

A 22 year old gravida I parity I mother develops clinically apparent varicella 24 hours after delivering a healthy full-term male infant.

The infant should be:
A. Isolated from other infants.
B. Isolated from his mother and from other infants.
C. Passively immunized with gamma globulin.
D. Passively immunized with varicella-zoster hyperimmune globulin (V-ZIG).
E. Treated with vidarabine.

The correct answers are B and D. Varicella-zoster infections during pregnancy may affect the fetus or neonate in one of three ways, depending on when the illness occurs during pregnancy. Congenital varicella is rare and follows maternal varicella during the period of fetal organogenesis. In this situation, varicella-zoster virus acts as a teratogen. Cicatricial scarring of the skin, extremity hypoplasia, encephalitis, ocular anomalies, cortical atrophy, and low birth weight have been associated with the congenital varicella syndrome. Maternal varicella in the perinatal period (4 days antepartum to 1 week postpartum) may result in neonatal varicella. Failure of the neonate to acquire protective IgG antibody passively against varicella-zoster virus places the infant at risk for disseminated infection. As a result, the prophylactic use of V-ZIG is recommended in this situation. Since both mother and father are potentially infectious to others, isolation of the pair from other parents and susceptible hospital personnel is imperative. If the infant has not acquired varicella-zoster virus in utero, infection may follow repeated contact with the mother. Thus, the infant should be isolated from his mother until all of her lesions have crusted and from the other infants in the nursery until discharge. Maternal varicella occurring after fetal organogenesis and before the peripartum period may result in an asymptomatic infection in the fetus. Fetal acquisition of maternal IgG to varicella-zoster virus is protective. No precautions or treatment of the infant is required in this situation.

Case Seven

A 19 year old primigravida delivers a term female infant. A VDRL (Venereal Disease Research Laboratory) test and an FTA-ABS (fluorescent treponemal antibody absorption) test obtained prior to delivery are positive.

How would you proceed?

T. pallidum can cross the placenta and cause intrauterine infection. Congenitally infected, nontreated neonates may present with diffuse periostitis in infancy, which gives rise to the well-described stigmata of this disease (saddle nose, saber shins, frontal bossing, and meningoencephalitis).

The questions of when and how to treat exposed infants is frequently raised in our institution. In general, the infants of mothers who have completed adequate therapy during pregnancy require only close monitoring of the VDRL. The infant in this case requires therapy. In the absence of CSF findings (pleocytosis, elevated protein, or a positive CSF VDRL), a single intramuscular dose of benzathine penicillin (50,000 U/Kg) is adequate. CNS infections require prolonged therapy with penicillin (100,000 U/kg/day for 10 days). In both instances, serial VDRL titers are obtained to document the efficacy of therapy. FTA-ABS conversion is lifelong and is therefore not helpful in determining the outcome of therapy. Recent developments in determining IgM–FTA-ABS are promising in the rapid diagnosis of congenitally infected infants; to date, these techniques are still under investigation.

Case Eight

A 24 year old gravida II parity II mother gives birth to a 4200 gm term infant. At 6 hours of age, the infant is noted to have central cyanosis. A chest x-ray is unremarkable. An arterial blood gas obtained while the child is breathing 100 per cent oxygen is remarkable for a PaO_2 of 35 mm Hg. Cardiac catheterization demonstrates transposition of the great vessels and a balloon septostomy is performed. The infant does well postoperatively but on the sixth day of life develops lethargy, vomiting, abdominal distension, and bloody stools.

Evaluation of this problem should include:
A. An abdominal flat plate and cross-table lateral x-ray.
B. Blood culture, urine culture, stool culture, and CSF culture.
C. CBC with differential and platelet count.
D. Guaiac and reducing substances of the stool.
E. D-xylose tolerance test.

Answers A, B, C, and D are correct. Acquired neonatal sepsis may present in a variety of ways. Presentation with gastrointestinal symptoms is not unusual. Meningitis and bacterial enteritis need to be eliminated from the differential diagnosis. A D-xylose tolerance test is of little efficacy in this evaluation.

Laboratory results return and are remarkable for thrombocytopenia (50,000 platelets/mm³), leukopenia (WBC of 2500 cells/mm³ with 10% polys), positive stool guaiac and reducing substances, and thickening of the bowel wall.

What is your diagnosis? How would you proceed?

Necrotizing enterocolitis (NEC) is a well-described entity in the neonate, yet the etiology is poorly understood. In general, three groups of neonates are at risk for NEC: premature infants, term infants with asphyxia neonatorum, and term infants with cyanotic heart disease. Epidemiologically, the onset of symptoms correlates inversely with gestational age. The sine qua non for NEC is interstitial air in the bowel wall, although benign cases of pneumatosis coli have been described. Hematochezia, stool-reducing substances, leukopenia, and thrombocytopenia have been described with NEC.

The initial management of the neonate with NEC consists of support and observation. Gastric decompression and discontinuation of oral feeds are routinely employed. Broad-spectrum antimicrobial therapy is utilized in our institution because of the risk of polymicrobial sepsis in this disease. Serial abdominal films are obtained to determine the progression of the disease and to observe for bowel perforation. Frequent physical examinations and monitoring of white blood cell counts, platelet counts, and acid-base status are also necessary. Finally, isolation of the infant is helpful since epidemics of NEC have been reported in high-risk nurseries.

What are the indications for surgery in NEC?

We use the following criteria in assessing the need for surgical intervention:

A. Progression of the disease and clinical deterioration in spite of optimal medical management.

B. Free intraperitoneal air.

C. Cellulitis or erythema of the abdominal wall.

D. Persistent acidosis, thrombocytopenia, or leukopenia. For further discussion, see pages 137 to 139.

Case Nine

An 18 year old heroin-addicted mother develops jaundice during the last trimester of her pregnancy. Her serum is positive for hepatitis B surface antigen (Hb_s Ag).

Which of the following is appropriate for the subsequent management of the infant?

A. Intravenous administration of adenosine arabinoside or acyclovir for 10 days.

B. Administration of gamma globulin.

C. Separation of the infant from the mother at the time of birth.

D. Discourage breast feeding.

E. Administration of high titer hepatitis B immunoglobulin and initiation of vaccination with hepatitis B vaccine.

The correct answers are D and E. Infants born to mothers who either have active hepatitis B infections or are chronic carriers of the virus are at high risk for becoming chronic carriers or developing overt disease. Although intrauterine infection has been reported, acquisition of the virus usually occurs in the immediate postpartum period. Hepatitis B hyperimmune globulin (HBIG), 0.5 ml intramuscularly, is administered to high-risk infants within the first 48 hours of life. Gamma globulin (0.06 ml/kg) may be used if HBIG is unavailable. The same dosage of HBIG is repeated at 3 months of age, at which time active immunization with hepatitis B vaccine (HBV) is begun. HBV is given at 3, 4, and 10 months of age. Serum for Hb_sAg, antibody to Hb_sAg, and anti-core antigen antibody should be obtained at 1 year of age. If the patient has responded to vaccination, only the anti-Hb_sAg antibody should be positive. Both antibody titers will be positive if the patient has been actively infected. Persistence of Hb_sAg with absent antibody titers represents chronic carriage of the virus.

Since the virus may be transmitted in breast milk, many authors recommend avoidance of breast feeding in cases of chronic maternal viral carriage. No antiviral agent has been proved effective against the hepatitis B virus.

Case Ten

An 8 day old infant delivered of an uncomplicated pregnancy and labor develops seizures and hypotonia. A lumbar puncture demonstrates: total cell count—8000 cells/mm³; differential—94% polys; protein—110 mg/dl; glucose—5 mg/dl. A Gram stain shows numerous polymorphonuclear neutrophils (PMNs) and no discernible organisms.

Appropriate antimicrobial therapy would be:

A. Ampicillin and gentamicin.

B. Ampicillin and chloramphenicol.

C. Moxalactam or cefotaxime.

D. Ampicillin and either moxalactam or cefotaxime.

Group B streptococci (*S. agalactiae*), members of the Enterobacteriaceae, and *L. monocytogenes* are the principal CSF pathogens in the newborn. Ampicillin is effective as initial drug therapy against both the streptococci and Listeria. Ampicillin is variably effective against *E. coli*, the most frequently encountered member of the Enterobacteriaceae causing neonatal meningitis, and ineffective against most Klebsiella. The addition of an aminoglycoside to the initial drug regimen would provide adequate antibacterial activity against the ampicillin-resistant pathogens; however, CSF penetration of parenterally administered aminoglycosides is poor and usually does not achieve bactericidal concentrations. Intrathecal administration of gentamicin is not effective in the treatment of neonatal gram-negative meningitis. The use of intraventricular gentamicin is controversial, but it may be used if parenteral therapy fails to sterilize the CSF. Chloramphenicol does not eliminate enteric bacilli in the CSF, and its use in gram-negative meningitis has been associated with an increased mortality.

Moxalactam and cefotaxime are beta-lactam antibiotics related to the cephalosporin family. Unlike earlier cephalosporin derivatives, both of these agents are effective against the Enterobacteriaceae and achieve bactericidal concentrations in the CSF. The correct answer is D.

Forty-eight hours after admission, a gram-negative rod is recovered from the cerebrospinal fluid and identified as *E. coli*. Sensitivity testing reveals that the organism is killed by moxalactam or cefotaxime at concentrations of 0.1 µg/ml and by ampicillin at a concentration of 2 µg/ml.

The appropriate response is to:

A. Continue moxalactam or cefotaxime for 3—4 weeks of therapy.

B. Continue moxalactam or cefotaxime for 3–4 weeks and reculture the CSF every 48 hours until sterile.

C. Continue ampicillin therapy and reexamine the CSF.

D. Begin therapy with trimethoprim-sulfamethoxazole.

Ampicillin and moxalactam (or cefotaxime) achieve approximately the same concentration in CSF (3–5 μg/ml). Sande (1981) has noted that to treat bacterial meningitis effectively, concentrations of drug in the CSF need to exceed the minimum bactericidal concentration (MBC) of the pathogen by at least ten-fold. Since the MBC of moxalactam and cefotaxime against the patient's organism is ten-fold less than the MBC of ampicillin, continued therapy with moxalactam or cefotaxime is recommended. Trimethoprim-sulfa-methoxazole has been used successfully in the treatment of gram-negative meningitis, however, sulfa agents increase unbound bilirubin and therefore place the neonate at increased risk for kernicterus.

Sande, M. A.: Antibiotic therapy of bacterial meningitis: lessons we've learned. Am J Med 71:507, 1981.

Repeat CSF examinations and cultures are necessary in enteric meningitis. Unlike childhood bacterial meningitis, sterilization of the CSF in gram-negative infections occurs more slowly, frequently requiring 4–5 days of adequate therapy. In our institution, CSF is also examined for bactericidal activity against the patient's organism. This provides definitive evidence of adequate therapy. The correct answer is B.

REFERENCES

1. Alfven, G., Bergvist, G., Bolme, P., et al: Long term follow-up of neonatal septicemia. Acta Paediatr Scand 67:769, 1978.
2. Allansmith, M., McClennan, B. H., Butterworth, M., et al: The development of immunoglobulin levels in man. J Pediatr 72:276, 1968.
3. Altemeier, W., and Smith, R.: Immunologic aspects of resistance in early life. Pediatr Clin North Am 12:663, 1965.
4. Ancona, R. J., Thompson, J. R., and Ferrieri, P.: Group G streptococcal pneumonia and sepsis in a newborn infant. J Clin Microbiol 10:758, 1979.
5. Anthony, B. F., Okada, D. M. and Hobel, C. J.: Epidemiology of group B streptococcus: longitudinal observations during pregnancy. J Infect Dis 1337:524, 1978.
6. Baker, C. J.: Summary of the workshop on perinatal infections due to group B streptococci. J Infect Dis 136:137, 1977.
7. Baker, C. J.: Group B streptococcal infections. Adv Intern Med 25:475, 1980.
8. Baker, C. J., and Kasper, D. L.: Correlation of maternal antibody deficiency with susceptibility to neonatal group B streptococcal infection. N Engl J Med 294:753, 1976.
9. Barry, D. M. J., and Reeve, A. W.: Iron injections and serious gram negative infections in polynesian newborns. NZ Med J 78:376, 1973.
10. Bavikahe, K., Schreiner, R. L., Lemons, J. A., et al: Group D streptococcal septicemia in the neonate. Am J Dis Child 133:1149, 1979.
11. Bayston, R., and Penny, S. R.: Excessive production of mucoid substance in staphylococcus S(II)A: a possible factor in colonization of holter shunts. Dev Med Child Neurol 27 (suppl):25, 1972.
12. Becroft, D. M. O., Dix, M. R., and Farmer, K.: Intramuscular iron-dextran and susceptibility of neonates to bacterial infections. Arch Dis Child 52:778, 1977.
13. Blanc, W. A.: Amniotic infection syndrome. Pathogenesis, morphology and significance in circumnatal mortality. Clin Obstet Gynecol 2:705, 1959.
14. Bortolussi, R., Thompson, T. R., and Ferrieri, P.: Early-onset pneumococcal sepsis in newborn infants. Pediatrics 60:352, 1977.
15. Boyer, K. M., Gadzala, C. A., Burd, L. I., et al: Selective intrapartum chemoprophylaxis of neonatal group B streptococcal early-onset disease. I. Epidemiologic rationale. J Infect Dis 148:795, 1983.
16. Boyer, K. M., Gadzala, C. A., Kelly, P. D., et al: Selective intrapartum chemoprophylaxis of neonatal group B streptococcol early-onset disease. II. Predictive value of prenatal cultures. J Infect Dis 148:802, 1983.
17. Boyer, K. M., Gadzala, C. A., Kelly P. D., et al: Selective intrapartum chemoprophylaxis of neonatal group B streptococcal early-onset disease. III. Interruption of mother-to-infant transmission. J Infect Dis 148:810, 1983.
18. Broughton, R. A., Kratka, R., and Baker, C. J.: Non–group D alpha-hemolytic streptococci: new neonatal pathogens. J Pediatr 99:450, 1981.
19. Chow, A. W., Leake, R. D., Yamauchi, T., et al: The significance of anaerobes in neonatal bacteremia: analysis of 23 cases and review of the literature. Pediatrics 54:736, 1974.
20. Coen, R., Grush, O., and Kander, E.: Studies of the bactericidal activity and metabolism of the leukocyte in full term neonates. J Pediatr 75:400, 1969.
21. Collado, M. D., Kretshmer, R. R., Becker, I., et al: Colonization of Mexican pregnant women with group B streptococcus. J Infect Dis 143:134, 1984.
22. Courtney, S. E., and Hall, R. T.: *Haemophilus influenzae* sepsis in the premature infant. Am J Dis Child 132:1039, 1978.
23. Drusin, L. M., Ribble, J. C., and Topf, B.: Group C streptococcal colonization in a newborn nursery. Am J Dis Child 125:820, 1973.
24. Edelmann, C. M., Ogwo, J. E., Fine, B. P., et al: The prevalence of bacteriuria in full-term and premature newborn infants. J Pediatr 82:125, 1973.
25. Fischer, G., Horton, R. E., and Edelman, R.: Summary of the national institutes of health workshop

on group B streptococcal infection. J Infect Dis *148*:163, 1983.

26. Fleer, A., Senders, R. C., Visser, M. R., et al: Septicemia due to coagulase-negative staphylococci in a neonatal intensive care unit: clinical and bacteriological features and contaminated parenteral fluids as a source of sepsis. Pediatr Infect Dis *2*:426, 1983.

27. Gotoff, S. P.: Neonatal immunity. J Pediatr *85*:149, 1974.

28. Gotoff, S., and Behrman, R.: Neonatal septicemia. J Pediatr *76*:142, 1970.

29. Gravett, M. G., and Holmes, K. K.: Pregnancy outcome and maternal infection: the need for comprehensive studies. JAMA *150*:1751, 1983.

30. Halal, F., Delorme, L. Brazeau, M., et al: Congenital vesicular eruption caused by *Haemophilus influenzae* type B. Pediatrics *62*:494, 1978.

31. Harrison, H. R., Alexander, E. R., Weinstein, L., et al: Cervical *Chlamydia trachomatis* and Mycoplasma infections in pregnancy: epidemiology and outcomes. JAMA *150*:1721, 1983.

32. Knudson, R. P., and Alden, E. R.: Neonatal heelstick blood culture. Pediatr Ann *65*:505, 1980.

33. Larsen, B, Snider, I. S., and Galask, R. P.: Bacterial growth inhibition by amniotic fluid. I. *In vitro* evidence for bacterial growth-inhibiting activity. Am J Obstet Gynecol *119*:492, 1974.

34. Lee, E. L., Robinson, M. J., Thong, M. L., et al: Intraventricular chemotherapy in neonatal meningitis. J Pediatr *99*:911, 1977.

35. Levy, H. L., Sepe, S. J., Shin, V. E., et al: Sepsis due to *Escherichia coli* in neonates with galactosemia. N Engl J Med *297*:823, 1977.

36. Lilien, L. D., Yeh, T. F., Novak, G. M., et al: Early-onset Haemophilus sepsis in newborn infants: clinical, roentgenographic and pathologic features. Pediatrics *62*:299, 1978.

37. Lowy, F. D., and Hammer, S. M.: *Staphylococcus epidermidis* infections. Ann Intern Med *99*:834, 1983.

38. Manroe, B. L., Weinberg, A. G., Rosenfeld, C. R., et al: The neonatal blood count in health and disease. I. Reference values for neutrophilic cells. J Pediatr *95*:89, 1979.

39. Maxted, W. R.: The use of bacitracin for identifying group A haemolytic streptococci. J Clin Pathol *6*:224, 1953.

40. McCracken, G. H., Jr., and Mize, S. G.: A controlled study of intrathecal antibiotic therapy in gram-negative enteric meningitis of infancy. Report of the neonatal meningitis cooperative study group. J Pediatr *89*:66, 1976.

41. McCracken, G. H., Jr., and Shinefield, H.: Changes in the pattern of neonatal septicemia and meningitis. Am J Dis Child *112*:33, 1966.

42. McCracken, G. H., Jr., Mize, S. G., and Threlkeld, N.: Intraventricular gentamicin therapy in gram-negative bacillary meningitis of infancy. Lancet *1*:787, 1980.

43. Miller, E. M.: Chemotactic function in the human neonate: humoral and cellular aspects. Pediatr Res *5*:487, 1971.

44. Miller, E. M., and Stiehm, E. R.: Phagocytic opsonic and immunoglobulin in newborns. Calif Med *119*:43, 1973.

45. Moriartey, R. R., and Finer, N. F.: Pneumococcal sepsis and pneumonia in the neonate. Am J Dis Child *133*:601, 1979.

46. Morrell, A., Skvaril, F., Hitzig, W. H., et al: IgG subclasses: development of the serum concentrations in "normal" infants and children. J Pediatr *80*:960, 1972.

47. Munson, D. P., Thompson, T. R., Johnson, D. E., et al: Coagulase-negative staphylococcal septicemia: experience in a newborn intensive care unit. J Pediatr *101*:602, 1982.

48. Naeye, R. L.: Coitus and associated amniotic-fluid infection. N Engl J Med *300*:819, 1979.

49. Naeye, R., and Banc, W.: Relation of poverty and race to antenatal infection. N Engl J Med *283*:555, 1970.

50. Nelson, J. D., Dillon, N. C., Jr., and Howard, J. B.: A prolonged nursery epidemic associated with a newly recognized type of group A streptococcus. J Pediatr *89*:792, 1976.

51. Norden, C. W., and Kass, E. H.: Bacteriuria of pregnancy—a critical appraisal. Ann Rev Med *19*:431, 1968.

52. Pass, M. A., Khare, S., and Dillon, H. C., Jr.: Twin pregnancies: incidence of group B streptococcal colonization and disease. J Pediatr *97*:635, 1980.

53. Peter, G., and Hazard J.: Neonatal group A streptococcal disease. J Pediatr *87*:454, 1975.

54. Peters, G., Locci, R., and Pulverer, G.: Adherence and growth of coagulase-negative staphylococci on surfaces of intravenous catheters. J Infect Dis *146*:479, 1982.

55. Philip, A. G., and Hewitt, J. R.: Early diagnosis of neonatal sepsis. Pediatrics *65*:1036, 1980.

56. Pickering, L. K., and Simon, F. A.: Reevaluation of neonatal *Haemophilus influenzae* infections. South Med J *70*:205, 1977.

57. Pole, J. R. G., and McAllister, J. A.: Gastric aspirate analysis in the newborn. Acta Paediatr Scand *64*:109, 1975.

58. Polin, R. D., Know, L. Baumgard, S., et al: Use of umbilical cord blood culture for detection of neonatal bacteremia. Obstet Gynecol *57*:233, 1981.

59. Rhodes, P. G., Burry, V. F., Hall, R. T., et al: Pneumococcal septicemia and meningitis in the neonate. J Pediatr *86*:593, 1975.

60. Robbins, J. B., McCracken, G. H., Jr., Gotschlich, E. C., et al: *Escherichia coli* K1 capsular polysaccharide associated with neonatal meningitis. N Engl J Med *290*:1216, 1974.

61. Rothberg, R.: Immunoglobulin and specific antibody synthesis during the first weeks of life of premature infants. J Pediatr *75*:391, 1969.

62. Sabel, K. G., and Hanson, L. A.: The clinical usefulness of C-reactive protein (CRP) determination in bacterial meningitis and septicemia in infancy. Acta Paediatr Scand *63*:381, 1974.

63. Sarff, L. D., McCracken, G. H. Jr., Schiffer, M. S., et al: Epidemiology of *Escherichia coli* K1 in healthy and diseased newborns. Lancet *2*:1099, 1975.

64. Scanlon, J.: The early detection of neonatal sepsis by examination of liquid obtained from the external ear canal. J Pediatr *79*:241, 1971.

65. Siegel, J. D., and McCracken, G. H., Jr.: Group D streptococcal infections. J Pediatr *93*:542, 1978.

66. Squire, E., Favara, B., and Todd, J.: Diagnosis of neonatal bacterial infection: hematologic and pathologic findings in fatal and nonfatal cases. Pediatrics *64*:60, 1979.

67. Stewardson-Krieger, P., and Gotoff, S.: Neonatal meningitis due to group C beta hemolytic streptococcus. J Pediatr *90*(1):103, 1977.

68. Stossel, T. P., Alper, C. A., and Rosen, F. S.: Opsonic activity in the newborn: role of properdin. Pediatrics 52:134, 1973.
69. Swartz, M. N.: Intraventricular use of aminoglycosides in the treatment of gram-negative bacillary meningitis: conflicting views. J Infect Dis 143:293, 1981.
70. Visser, V. E., and Hall, R. T.: Urine culture in the evaluation of suspected neonatal sepsis. J Pediatr 94:635, 1979.
71. Visser, V. E., and Hall, R. T.: Lumbar puncture in the evaluation of suspected neonatal sepsis. J Pediatr 96:1063, 1980.
72. Wade, J. C., Schimpff, S. C., Newman, K. A., et al: Staphylococcus epidermidis: an increasing cause of infection in patients with granulocytopenia. Ann Intern Med 97:503, 1982.
73. Wallace, R. J., Jr., Baker, C. J., Quinones, F. J., et al: Nontypable Haemophilus influenzae (biotype 4) as a neonatal, maternal and genital pathogen. Rev Infect Dis 5:123, 1983.
74. Washburn, T. C., Medearis, D. N., Jr., and Childs, B.: Sex differences in susceptibility to infections. Pediatrics 35:57, 1965.
75. Wilfert, C. M.: E. Coli meningitis: K₁ antigen and virulence. Ann Rev Med 291:129, 1978.

13

The Heart

DAVID TEITEL
MICHAEL A. HEYMANN
JEROME T. LIEBMAN

Congenital heart disease is one of the most common causes of morbidity and mortality in a pediatric referral hospital. Most children with serious heart disease present early in the first month of life. Care for these newborns dictates an awareness of the cardiac defects most likely to occur. In this regard, the data from the New England Regional Infant Cardiac Program concerning the diagnostic distribution of critically ill infants in the first month of life are helpful (Table 13–1), as are the composite autopsy data of Rowe. Together these studies stress that 70 per cent of neonates with potentially fatal cardiac malformations will have one of the following five types of defects: the hypoplastic left heart syndrome; aortic arch anomalies, including interruption or hypoplasia of the aortic arch and coarctation of the aorta; complete transposition of the great arteries; the hypoplastic right heart syndrome; or severe tetralogy of Fallot.*

From the standpoint of clinical presentation, these break down into problems of systemic perfusion (hypoplastic left heart and aortic arch anomalies and coarctation) and

hypoxemia (transposition of the great arteries, hypoplastic right heart, and severe tetralogy of Fallot).

N. Talner

Careful evaluation of the history, physical examination, laboratory data (including the response of blood gases and arterial oxygen saturation in an enriched oxygen environment), x-ray, electrocardiogram, echocardiogram, and sometimes cardiac catheterization will help to delineate the specific congenital cardiac defect. In addition, noncardiac disorders, such as parenchymal lung disease or disorders associated with persistent pulmonary hypertension, may be confused with heart disease. Recently, two-dimensional echocardiography (with Doppler) has eliminated much of the clinical guesswork by providing detailed functional and anatomic data. To make a complete cardiac evaluation, the physician must be familiar with relevant cardiovascular physiology and pathophysiology.

This is an exceedingly important point. If the clinician is familiar with the physiologic effects of the various pathologic states that can alter cardiovascular function in the newborn, then the approach to diagnosis and management sits on a firm foundation. Specifically, this would include an appreciation of (1) the factors that affect cardiac output and oxygen transport in the newborn, (2) changes in the pulmonary and systemic circulations following delivery, and (3) the role of the fetal pathways that can modulate the clinical picture. **N. Talner**

This chapter will consider the physiology and pathophysiology of the fetal and neonatal cardiovascular systems; the low-risk newborn with heart disease; and the high-risk newborn with heart disease.

---

*Classifications of congenital heart disease do not usually include persistent patency of the ductus arteriosus (PDA) in infants born prematurely. A large majority of these infants, particularly very low-birth-weight (<1250 gm) preterm infants, have a PDA of varying hemodynamic severity and therefore require specific care. It is estimated that these infants represent about 1 per cent of all live births, a number approximately equal to that proposed for the incidence of congenital heart disease.

TABLE 13–1 DIAGNOSTIC DISTRIBUTION OF
CRITICALLY ILL CARDIAC INFANTS 0–30 DAYS
OF AGE, 1968–1971*

Diagnosis (In Rank Order)	Number	Per Cent
Transposition of the great arteries	81	14
Hypoplastic left ventricle	76	13
Coarctation of the aorta (includes simple and complicated)	51	9
Hypoplastic right ventricle (includes pulmonary atresia and tricuspid atresia group)	49	9
Tetralogy of Fallot	44	8
Ventricular septal defect	44	8
Other malpositions	31	5
Single ventricle	21	4
Patent ductus arteriosus	19	3
Atrioventricularis communis	15	3
Pure pulmonary stenosis	14	2
Myocardiopathy	12	2
Total anomalous pulmonary venous return	12	2
Truncus arteriosus	9	2
Others	108	18
Total	586	

*Adapted from Fyler, D., Buckley, L., Hellenbrand, W., et al: Report of the New England Regional Infant Cardiac Program. Pediatrics 65 (Suppl):375, 1980.

It is important to note that these are babies who were critically ill but did not necessarily die or need surgery to live. The table is also not broken down as to day of onset of illness. Thus, a child with a ventricular septal defect who became ill at 30 days is included and is likely to survive with medical therapy.

PHYSIOLOGY AND PATHOPHYSIOLOGY

Fetal and Neonatal Circulations

In the adult, the pulmonary and systemic circulations are arranged in series so that oxygenated blood returns from the lungs and is ejected by the left side of the heart to the systemic circulation; in turn the deoxygenated blood returns from the systemic circulation to the right side of the heart, where it is ejected to the pulmonary circulation. In the fetus, circulation of the blood is more complex (Figure 13–1). Oxygenated blood returns from the placenta to both the left and the right ventricles. The major portion of the right ventricular output does not perfuse the lungs but bypasses the pulmonary circulation through the ductus arteriosus and is thereby directed toward the body, returning to the placenta for oxygenation. Because of this parallel circulation, individual organs may receive blood from both ventricles. It has therefore become customary to express the output of the fetal heart as *combined*

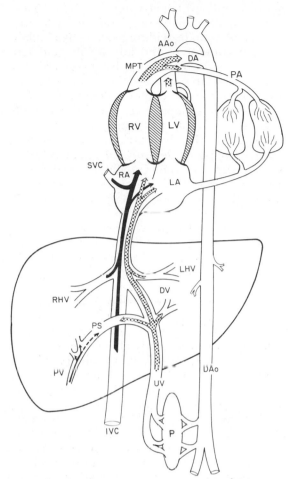

Figure 13–1. Diagrammatic representation of the normal fetal circulation. QP, pulmonary flow; QS, systemic flow.

ventricular output (CVO). In the normal fetus, combined ventricular output is approximately 450 ml/kg of fetal body weight/minute.*

About 200 ml of oxygenated blood/kg of fetal body weight/minute returns from the placenta via the umbilical veins (40% of CVO). Approximately 50 per cent of this blood enters the inferior vena cava directly through the ductus venosus, thereby bypassing the hepatic microcirculation; the remainder passes through the liver and enters the inferior vena cava through the hepatic veins. Although venous return from the lower body, ductus venosus, and hepatic veins passes through the thoracic inferior vena cava, these streams do not mix completely, and there is preferential streaming within the inferior vena cava. Blood from the ductus

---

*In this chapter, all of the data on the fetal circulation are derived from studies on fetal sheep.

venosus and left hepatic veins tends to stream preferentially across the foramen ovale into the left atrium, providing blood with a higher oxygen content to the left atrium and left ventricle and thereby supplying cerebral and myocardial circulations with blood of a relatively high oxygen content. Venous drainage from the right hepatic veins and the abdominal inferior vena cava tends to stream preferentially to the right atrium and right ventricle. Similarly, desaturated superior vena caval return is preferentially directed to the right ventricle through the tricuspid valve, although some blood may enter the left atrium.

The left and right ventricles do not eject similar volumes in the fetus. The right ventricle is dominant and ejects approximately 65 per cent of the CVO, whereas the left ventricle ejects approximately 35 per cent (the difference is probably smaller in the human because of the larger brain and greater cerebral blood flow). Of the right ventricular output, only about 12.5 per cent (approximately 30–35 ml/kg/min or 8% of CVO) passes to the pulmonary circulation. Left ventricular output is distributed mainly to the upper body, including the brain (approximately 20% of CVO) and the myocardium (3%); the remainder (about 10%) crosses the aortic isthmus to the lower body.

In the fetus, the ductus arteriosus had long been considered a passive conduit that allowed blood to bypass the pulmonary circulation. However, recent studies have shown that vasoactive products of arachidonic acid cause active dilatation of the ductus arteriosus during fetal life; prostaglandin E_2 almost certainly is the most important of these substances. The oxygen tension of blood in the fetus (20–25 mm Hg) is significantly lower than that in the adult. This lowered oxygen tension may cause the active constriction of the muscular resistance vessels in the lungs, which in turn permits only a very small flow through the pulmonary circulation. In the presence of the low oxygen environment, other vasoactive substances, which actively constrict the pulmonary circulation, may be released and may also actively control flow through the lungs; products of arachidonic acid metabolism that cause vasoconstriction, such as the leukotrienes, might be involved.

There is an exploding body of knowledge concerning the role of pharmacologic mediators in the maturation of the pulmonary vascular bed during the newborn period. While there certainly appears to be a direct oxygen effect on the ductus arteriosus and pulmonary resistance vessels, the release of mediators, particularly the prostaglandins that may involve either vasoconstriction or vasodilatation, may also influence the local control of vascular beds. At the present time there appears to be no agent that is specific for the pulmonary circulation in terms of vasodilatation with the exception of oxygen. The exact mechanism whereby hypoxia induces pulmonary vasoconstriction is still controversial. Uncertainty as to why oxygen under certain circumstances appears to increase pulmonary blood flow, while in other situations does not, contributes to the management problems encountered in the clinical arena.   **N. Talner**

CIRCULATORY CHANGES AFTER BIRTH

The onset of breathing produces a dramatic increase in pulmonary blood flow (from 30–35 ml/kg/min to 350–400 ml/kg/min) and decrease in pulmonary vascular resistance. Although the air that replaces the intraalveolar fluid may contribute slightly to the fall in pulmonary vascular resistance, the major factor is relaxation of the constricted resistance vessels in the lungs. With the onset of ventilation, the oxygen environment to which the vessels are exposed increases markedly. In contrast to the fetal condition, the higher oxygen concentration that occurs immediately after birth may directly dilate the pulmonary vascular smooth muscle and/or cause the release of vasodilating substances. Bradykinin, a potent pulmonary vasodilator, is released when the lungs are exposed to oxygen; prostacyclin (prostaglandin I_2), a pulmonary vasodilator derived from the metabolism of arachidonic acid, is released when the lung is mechanically ventilated or exposed to other vasoactive substances, such as bradykinin or angiotensin II. Inhibiting prostaglandin production by the administration of a cyclooxygenase inhibitor (such as indomethacin) attenuates the normal ventilation-induced fall in pulmonary vascular resistance, further supporting the role of these vasoactive substances in the establishment of a normal pulmonary circulation after birth.

The initial dramatic fall in pulmonary vascular resistance is secondary to relaxation of the resistance vessels. There is then a slow progressive fall over the next 2–6 weeks of life, as these pulmonary arterioles remodel from their fetal pattern, which has a large amount of smooth muscle in the medial layer, to the adult pattern, with very little muscle in the media. The development of the "physiologic anemia" that normally occurs during this time decreases the viscosity of blood perfusing the lungs and also contributes to the overall fall in the pulmonary vascular resistance.

The postnatal changes in pulmonary vascular resistance can be divided into those factors that influence the remodeling of the pulmonary vascular bed, which include lung inflation, removal of lung liquids, and maturational changes in the pulmonary resistance vessels, and alterations in blood viscosity. The exact site of the pulmonary resistance vessels is a debatable point and in the fetus and newborn may involve larger vessels than in the adult, where the pulmonary arterioles constitute the major site for resistance changes. The postnatal decrease in viscosity is consequent to the fall in hemoglobin concentration, which takes place over the first 2 to 3 months of life.

N. Talner

Closure of the Foramen Ovale

After the placenta is removed from the circulation, blood flow through the inferior vena cava to the right atrium decreases dramatically; when breathing begins, blood flow through the pulmonary bed to the left atrium increases. Associated with these changes in flow patterns into the heart are changes in left and right atrial pressures: left atrial pressure, which is lower in the fetus than pressure in the right atrium, now exceeds right atrial pressure, thereby causing the valvelike flap of the foramen ovale to close. Although functional closure of the foramen ovale occurs in most infants, anatomic closure is not always complete, and the foramen may remain probe patent for many years, occasionally into adult life.

It is important to point out that any pathologic state that raises pulmonary vascular resistance can permit right-to-left shunting through the foramen ovale as right atrial pressure rises and exceeds left atrial pressure. Under certain circumstances, however, a left-to-right shunt can occur through the foramen ovale as a consequence of an elevation of left atrial pressure and resulting incompetence of the foramen ovale. This has been demonstrated in patients with large-volume left-to-right shunts and obstructive lesions involving the left heart, as well as in any process such as asphyxia or inflammatory disease that could impair myocardial contractility and thereby result in an elevated left atrial pressure. **N. Talner**

Closure of the Ductus Arteriosus

Much like the rapid pulmonary vasodilatation that occurs after birth, closure of the ductus arteriosus is a complex phenomenon that is not yet fully understood. The fetal ductus arteriosus contains medial smooth muscle that is maintained in a relaxed state, probably by the action of prostaglandins, specifically circulating prostaglandin E_2. Closure after birth reflects removal of the stimuli that maintain relaxation and the addition of factors that produce active constriction. Prostaglandin E_2 is almost completely metabolized as it passes through the pulmonary circulation. Circulating concentrations in the fetus are high because of the very low pulmonary blood flow. After delivery, the placental source of prostaglandin E_2 is removed, and there is a dramatic increase in pulmonary blood flow, which increases the metabolism of any circulating prostaglandin E_2. As a result, serum levels of prostaglandin E_2 fall, and active constriction of the ductus arteriosus will be unopposed. This active constriction is caused by an increase in environmental PO_2 as well as in several vasoactive substances. Bradykinin is released from the lungs with the initial oxygenation and has a constrictor effect on the ductus arteriosus; similarly, other vasoactive substances such as catecholamines and histamine may be involved. The ductus arteriosus constricts rapidly after birth; in mature infants functional closure generally occurs within the first 12 hours. Permanent closure by intimal proliferation, fibrosis, and thrombosis may take several weeks.

Persistent patency of the ductus arteriosus occurs relatively frequently in premature infants as compared with full-term infants. The exact mechanisms are not clear. The ductus arteriosus in premature animals is certainly less responsive to the constricting effects of oxygen. The relaxing effects of prostaglandin E_2 as well as prostacyclin are greater in the immature ductus arteriosus, and the metabolism of prostaglandin E_2 is not efficient. As a result of these phenomena, even small circulating concentrations of prostaglandin E_2 that may be present in the immature infant can cause the ductus arteriosus to remain in a partially relaxed state. Constriction of the ductus arteriosus in premature infants has been achieved by pharmacologic manipulation with inhibitors of prostaglandin synthesis.

Persistent patency of the ductus arteriosus allowing a left-to-right shunt into the pulmonary circulation constitutes one of the many life-threatening problems facing the preterm infant. The ability to manipulate the ductus arteriosus by pharmacologic means or by surgical ligation if necessary permits the clinician to remove the effects of increased pulmonary blood flow on cardiopulmonary function in the premature infant. This allows earlier weaning from ventilatory support and administration of adequate fluids and calories. **N. Talner**

Myocardial Performance and Cardiac Output

Fetal myocardium develops less tension for a given stretch than does adult myocardium. Therefore, ventricular output can be increased only modestly by volume loading and only at relatively low atrial pressures; unlike the adult, output increases only slightly at levels above 10 mm Hg. Inotropic stimulation of the fetal myocardium also increases cardiac output relatively little. This inability to respond to changes in preload and in inotropic state is related in part to immaturity of muscle structure. At early gestational ages, there are relatively few contractile elements, and considerable interstitial tissue is present; toward term, more contractile elements are present, and these are arranged in a more orderly fashion. Another factor limiting fetal myocardial performance is incomplete sympathetic innervation, which limits response to inotropic stimulation. The fetus is best able to increase ventricular output by increasing its heart rate. There is a linear relationship between ventricular output and heart rate up to about 250 beats/minute; thereafter ventricular output reaches a plateau and even starts to decline. As heart rate falls below the normal range, ventricular output falls dramatically because of the limited ability to increase stroke volume. As a result of all these limitations, the stressed fetus responds by redistributing rather than increasing cardiac output.

It should be emphasized that the neonatal myocardium operates under a high-volume load as compared with the adult myocardium and responds poorly to any increase in ventricular afterload. While adrenergic support can be supplied either by circulating catecholamines or through neural pathways, the overall quantitative response may be less than in the adult. The control of cardiac rate and the distribution of cardiac output are the major mechanisms for maintenance of circulatory function. In the face of asphyxia with alterations in pH, P_{O_2}, and P_{CO_2}, the net effect is to compromise myocardial performance, and these are factors that must be addressed in an attempt to restore cardiac output and thus improve oxygen transport.   **N. Talner**

After birth, however, left ventricular output increases dramatically, from about 150 ml/kg/minute to 350–400 ml/kg/minute. Right ventricular output does not change significantly. Over the ensuing 6–8 weeks, right and left ventricular outputs fall to less than half this value. Because of the high resting values in the immediate newborn period, ventricular output can be increased only modestly by volume loading or inotropic

stimulation; as resting values drop progressively over the next month, ventricular output can be increased much more. Studies on myocardial contractility have also shown that in the first weeks after birth, resting contractility is high; it decreases progressively over the following month. Thus, isoproterenol produces little change in contractility in the newborn but has a much greater effect in the older infant.

While this has been observed in the experimental animal when the heart is performing normally, in certain clinical states such as that associated with asphyxia, myocardial contractility may be impaired, whereupon inotropic agents may very well be able to restore contractility toward normal. The newborn heart responds in a positive fashion to inotropic agents such as isoproterenol, dopamine, and dobutamine as well as to the administration of calcium ion.   **N. Talner**

NORMAL PHYSIOLOGIC DATA IN THE NEWBORN

A box diagram is useful in evaluating the hemodynamic data of the heart and great vessels of children with heart defects. Such diagrams are used as illustrations in this chapter.

The normal physiologic values in the heart and great vessels appear in Figure 13–2. Pulmonary arterial pressures in the newborn are quite variable but generally fall to half of systemic pressure within 8–12 hours and to one third of systemic pressure within a day or so. Over the next 4 weeks, there is a further slow progressive fall to adult levels.

The oxygen saturation on the right side of the heart is approximately 60–70 per cent; that on the left side of the heart is 92–95 per cent. The oxygen saturations may be used to determine the direction of shunting within the heart or great vessels. For example, an increased saturation in the right atrium suggests a left-to-right shunt at the atrial level; a decreased saturation in the left atrium indicates a right-to-left shunt at the atrial level, if pulmonary venous blood is not also desaturated because of pulmonary disease with intrapulmonary right-to-left shunting.

PHYSICAL FACTORS THAT CONTROL BLOOD FLOW

Flow (Q) through a vascular bed is governed by the resistance to flow (R) and the pressure fall across the bed (ΔP) (Ohm's law).

$$Q = \frac{\Delta P}{R}$$

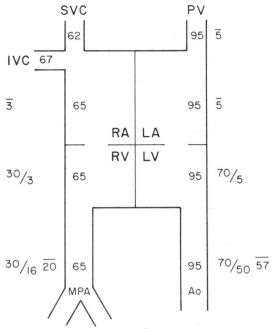

Figure 13–2. Representative blood oxygen saturation (per cent) and pressure (mm Hg) in various cardiac chambers and vessels in a normal newborn infant. SVC = superior vena cava; IVC = inferior vena cava; PV = pulmonary vein; RA = right atrium; LA = left atrium; RV = right ventricle; LV = left ventricle; MPA = main pulmonary artery; Ao = aorta.

Further, by applying Poiseuille's law, resistance to flow is directly related to viscosity of the blood and inversely related to the cross-sectional area of the bed (radius).

An appreciation of the general relationship of pressure, resistance, and flow is important in understanding the pathophysiology and natural history of various congenital heart defects. *Blood flows where resistance is least.*

Vascular resistance is calculated from the formula:

$$R = \frac{\Delta P}{Q}$$

For the systemic circulation, the ΔP (pressure drop) is systemic arterial pressure (SAP) minus systemic venous pressure (SVP); for the pulmonary circulation, the ΔP is pulmonary arterial pressure (PAP) minus pulmonary venous pressure (PVP).

Pulmonary vascular resistance (PVR) =
$$\frac{PAP - PVP}{Pulmonary\ flow}$$

Systemic vascular resistance (SVR) =
$$\frac{SAP - SVP}{Systemic\ flow}$$

If the pressure drop is measured in mm Hg and the flow is measured in l/min/m² then the calculated vascular resistance is considered in *resistance units*. The maximum normal PVR is 2.5–3 units, and the maximum normal SVR is 15–20 units.

The calculation of pulmonary and systemic vascular resistances represents an attempt to define alterations from the normal produced by certain disease states. There are a number of factors that influence pulmonary vascular resistance in addition to the pulmonary resistance vessels. These include the height of the pressure on the pulmonary venous side and the volume of blood in the pulmonary vascular bed. Furthermore, changes in blood viscosity may also influence the pulmonary vascular resistance. *It should not be inferred that because there is pulmonary hypertension there is necessarily pulmonary vasoconstriction.* In certain situations there may be fewer resistance vessels, pulmonary parenchymal alterations (e.g., diaphragmatic hernia), or structural alterations in the pulmonary resistance vessels. **N. Talner**

Peripheral vascular resistance is not the only type of resistance that will affect flow. For example, a narrowed valve provides more resistance to blood flow than does a wide open valve; a small ventricular septal defect provides more resistance to blood flow than does a large ventricular septal defect; and a thick, noncompliant ventricular chamber provides more resistance to blood flow than does a thinner, more compliant ventricular chamber.

If two similar cardiac chambers or arteries (one left-sided or systemic and the other right-sided or pulmonary) communicate with each other and the opening between them is so large that there is little or no resistance to blood flow, the defect is considered *nonrestrictive*. The pressures on each side of the opening will be fully transmitted and approximately equal. If the opening is small (*restrictive*), there will be resistance to blood flow, and the pressures will not be fully transmitted. In the presence of a nonrestrictive defect, the resistances to outflow from each of the two communicating chambers will determine the output of each chamber. For example, with a large ventricular septal defect (Figure 13–3) in which ventricular pressures are equal, pulmonary vascular resistance is usually lower than systemic vascular resistance, and pulmonary blood flow is greater than systemic blood flow; that is, a left-to-right shunt is present (Figure 13–3A). Since the flows and shunting pattern depend on the relationship of pulmonary to systemic vascular resistance, these are called *dependent shunts.* When the two resistances are equal, no shunt occurs (Figure 13–3B). When resistance to outflow of the right ventricle exceeds that of the left ventricle (Figure 13–3C)—as might occur with the development of pulmonary vascular disease or, more commonly, when there is an associated pulmonic stenosis (tetralogy of Fallot)—right-to-left shunting is present. In situations in which there is a communication between the two sides of the heart at different anatomic levels (e.g., arteriovenous malformation, left ventricular–right atrial communication), the pressure difference between the two will dictate the magnitude of the shunt; these are called *obligatory shunts*.

It is customary to relate the cardiac outputs and pressures in each side of the heart. Thus, if there is three times as much flow into the pulmonary artery as into the aorta, there is a 3:1 pulmonary/systemic flow ratio. If the pressure in the pulmonary artery is 60 mm Hg and that in the aorta is 90 mm Hg, we speak of pulmonary hypertension at two thirds systemic level.

The pulmonary to systemic blood flow relationship may be somewhat misleading. For example, if there is severe compromise of systemic perfusion, the pulmonary blood flow may be normal in the face of marked compromise of systemic blood flow. This can result in normalization of arterial oxygen tension, and the development of a metabolic acidemia is the result of the compromise in systemic blood flow. **N. Talner**

THE LOW-RISK NEWBORN

Statistically, the defects encountered most frequently in the newborn are the simple left-to-right shunt lesions. Isolated ventricular septal defect accounts for between 30 and 40 per cent of all congenital heart disease. Atrial septal defect and patent ductus arteriosus are less common but important. Occasionally, difficulty occurs late in the neonatal period (3–4 weeks of life) from a ventricular septal defect or patent ductus arteriosus, but this is extremely rare for a simple atrial septal defect.

From the standpoint of timing of presentation, the infant with the small ventricular septal defect may be recognized in the immediate newborn period by the presence of the typical murmur in the absence of symptomatology relating to left-to-right shunting into the pulmonary circulation. With the large ventricular septal defect, however, there is a lag period relating to the delay in the postnatal fall in pulmonary vascular resistance, so that the clinical findings of murmur and the alterations in respiratory function take between 2–3 weeks to present themselves. The exception to this situation is encountered in the preterm infant, in whom there may be significant left-to-right shunting via a patent ductus arteriosus or ventricular communication within a few days following delivery.

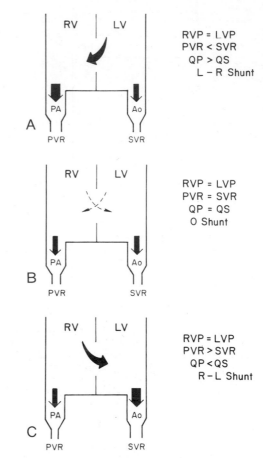

Figure 13–3. Diagrammatic representation of intracardiac shunting patterns as related to outflow resistances of the two sides of the heart.

Typically, however, the large left-to-right shunt lesion has a lag period before the onset of tachypnea, which represents the change in respiratory pattern attendant on the increase in pulmonary blood flow and alterations in lung compliance. **N. Talner**

Ventricular Septal Defect (VSD)

In the large, nonrestrictive VSD (Figure 13–3), the pressure in the right ventricle and pulmonary artery is at systemic levels. If the thick-walled pulmonary vessels matured normally, the vascular resistance would decrease rapidly, and there would be a large left-to-right shunt with left ventricular failure and pulmonary edema. Such a series of events is unusual. In fact, when a large VSD is present, a heart murmur is not usually heard, even in the newborn period. The left-to-right shunt does not develop rapidly because the pulmonary resistance vessels remain heavily muscular for a longer period than normal and the fall in pulmonary vascular resistance is delayed. The variation in pulmonary vascular resistance from one child to the next is considerable. Some infants decrease their resistance considerably; others hardly at all. When there is a large defect, the shunt is usually maximal by 2–3 weeks of age, so that congestive heart failure, when it occurs, is usually present by 4 weeks of age.

On the other hand, the majority of ventricular septal defects are very small and restrictive. In these children, the great resistance to flow between the left and right ventricles allows the pulmonary vessels to mature normally into adult-type vessels. With a rapid decrease in pulmonary vascular resistance, there is a rapid decrease in right ventricular pressure, and a left ventricular–right ventricular pressure gradient will be present. Therefore a left-to-right shunt can develop quickly, so with small defects, the systolic murmur is often present and quite loud (grades 3–4/6) even in the newborn period. The murmur also may have a crescendo-decrescendo character typical of a VSD (maladie de Roger). Despite the low pulmonary vascular resistance, the great resistance to flow at the ventricular septal defect prevents much left-to-right shunting; therefore congestive heart failure does not occur frequently. Pulmonary hypertension does not develop readily because the defect is very small. A large percentage of these small defects close spontaneously, and pulmonary hypertension does not develop even in those that remain the same size throughout life.

CASE PROBLEMS

Two cases are illustrated in which there are no symptoms in the newborn period, although a heart murmur is heard. The physiologic events during that time are directly related to the eventual course. The preceding discussion of pathophysiology not only helps to answer these questions but also should provide a basis for understanding the very complicated defects to be discussed later.

Case One

At the 2-week checkup, a murmur is heard for the first time in an acyanotic, well baby. The diagnosis of ventricular septal defect with left-to-right shunt is made. The family is very upset with the physician for not having heard the murmur in the newborn period.

Is the family justified? Why or why not?

Obviously the family is not justified. It is probable, although not definite, that this is a moderately large VSD. If so, then by definition the pressure in the right ventricle and pulmonary artery will be elevated. The high pulmonary artery pressure is believed to be one of the factors in delaying maturation of the pulmonary arterioles. The delayed maturation means that pulmonary vascular resistance comes down slowly. Consequently, the left-to-right shunt begins slowly, causing the murmur to develop after the early neonatal period.

The onset of symptomatology in the large left-to-right shunt occurs in a subtle fashion. The earliest finding is that of an increase in respiratory frequency without the presence of respiratory distress. The respiratory rate may be in the range of 60/minute without retractions, alar flaring, or wheezing. Tachypnea represents the accumulation of lung water and alterations in lung compliance and is sometimes accompanied by some difficulty in feeding and eventually by failure to thrive. The failure to thrive under these conditions is the result of the increased work of breathing, impaired caloric intake, and probably increased metabolic demands secondary to the release of catecholamines. It should be remembered that while there is a high output state in terms of systemic oxygen transport, there may be significant compromise of oxygen delivery to the tissues.   **N. Talner**

Is it at all possible that congestive heart failure will develop before the next regularly scheduled visit at 1 month?

The maximal left-to-right shunt is believed to develop by about 1 month of life, so that when congestive heart failure is recognized, it is usually by then. Occasionally, it is initially diagnosed a little later, but in those patients referred with congestive heart failure at 3–4 months, it has probably been present for a while.

Is pulmonary hypertension likely to be present at this time?

The larger the defect, the higher the right ventricular pressure. Thus, with large defects and no pulmonary stenosis, high pulmonary artery pressure must be present no matter what the shunt. With a moderate defect, the pressure is moderately elevated.

Case Two

On the first day of life, the physical examination of a full-term baby is normal, but at 48 hours, the house officer hears a murmur at the lower left sternal border. The child is acyanotic, and the murmur is typical of a VSD with left-to-right shunt.

Is a ventricular septal defect possible? Why?

The left ventricular pressure is not transmitted to the right side through the small restrictive VSD. Therefore there is nothing to impede the normal drop in pulmonary vascular resistance. As the pulmonary vascular resistance decreases, the right ventricular pressure decreases as it would normally. Therefore there is a large pressure gradient between the ventricles, and an early left-to-right shunt is possible.

Is whatever defect present likely to be small or large?

The shunt rarely becomes large because of the high resistance to flow through the small defect. The major key to suspecting that the defect is small is the early onset of the loud, typical murmur.

Is eventual congestive heart failure likely?

Heart failure is not likely when the left-to-right shunt is small.

Is pulmonary hypertension likely?

When ventricular septal defects are small, there is great resistance to flow from one ventricle to the other; thus, there is no transmission of the high left ventricular pressure to the pulmonary arterioles. Consequently, the pulmonary arterioles are not affected by the ventricular septal defect and mature normally. Pulmonary hypertension is thus unlikely.

One of the house officers argues that the physical examination suggests a large atrial septal defect, which must not be missed. The chief resident, however, counters that unless there is obstruction to flow into the left side of the heart, such as mitral stenosis or atresia, physiologic principles teach that atrial septal defect is not associated with left-to-right shunt in the early newborn period.

What are the important physiologic principles at work in impedance of left-to-right shunting through an atrial septal defect?

In the presence of a large atrial septal defect with equalization of right and left atrial pressures, the shunting is determined, at least in part, by the difference in resistance to flow out of the atria. In the newborn period, because the right ventricle is usually thicker than the left, the right ventricular compliance is less. Since blood flow goes where resistance is least, left atrial blood flows into the left ventricle rather than through the atrial septal defect to the right atrium and then the ventricle.

I would stress that a left-to-right shunt encountered in the immediate newborn period should point to the additional and more important presence of left heart obstructive disease or myocardial dysfunction. In both of these conditions, the foramen ovale may become incompetent with resultant left-to-right shunting.

N. Talner

Is it known that the largest simple left-to-right shunt lesions in childhood tend to be atrial septal defects? Are there not dire complications if the defect is not recognized early in life?

In the first several weeks after the newborn period, because systemic vascular resistance is higher than pulmonary vascular resistance, the left ventricle becomes more muscular and thicker than the right ventricle. Meanwhile, the pulmonary vascular resistance falls as the fetal vessels mature to adult-type vessels. During infancy, the left-to-right shunt at the atrial level increases gradually. By the time the left-to-right shunt is large, the pulmonary arterioles are mature, thin-walled, and able to dilate maximally. Therefore the pulmonary artery pressure is not elevated in childhood.

Consequently, atrial septal defects of the simple type are rarely recognized early in life. Pulmonary hypertension in childhood is virtually unknown, and eventual congestive heart failure in childhood is very uncommon.

Patent Ductus Arteriosus (PDA)
(Figure 13–4)

The principles discussed for ventricular septal defect also apply to patent ductus arteriosus. However, because there is length to the ductus arteriosus as well as caliber, resistance to flow is greater. A nonrestrictive PDA is less common, so that systemic level pulmonary hypertension is also less common.

Editorial Comment: The exception (see below) is the very low-birth-weight infant with a PDA often complicating RDS.

If there is a PDA in the full-term baby, the outcome depends on the size of the channel. With the gradual fall in postnatal PVR, a left-to-right shunt develops from aorta to pulmonary artery, which produces excessive pulmonary blood flow, increased pulmonary venous return, and left atrial and ventricular dilatation. A small PDA will produce only the typical murmur and full pulses. A moderate to large PDA may produce signs of congestive heart failure as well as a typical continuous murmur and wide pulse pressure (bounding pulse), often in the second month of life. Only very rarely does failure occur in the newborn period.

PDA IN PRETERM INFANTS

As discussed previously, preterm infants and particularly very low-birth-weight infants

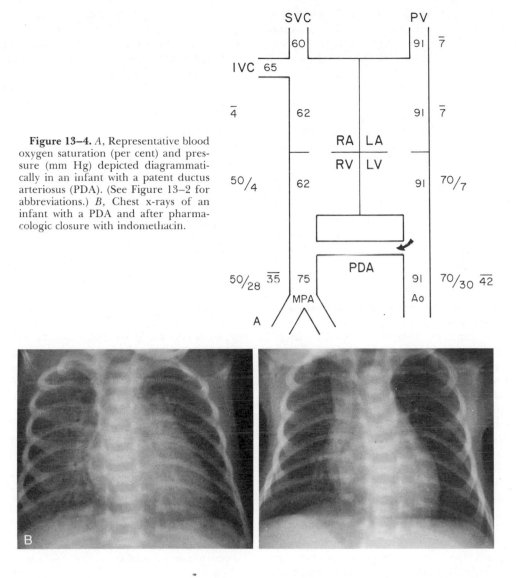

Figure 13–4. *A*, Representative blood oxygen saturation (per cent) and pressure (mm Hg) depicted diagrammatically in an infant with a patent ductus arteriosus (PDA). (See Figure 13–2 for abbreviations.) *B*, Chest x-rays of an infant with a PDA and after pharmacologic closure with indomethacin.

have a significant incidence of persistently patent ductus arteriosus. The PDA of the preterm infant with RDS provides special problems. Since the ill premature infant has a high oxygen consumption and cardiac output, the left ventricular myocardium—which, as mentioned above, is not optimally functional at this stage of development—is already working at near maximum ability. Consequently, even a small increase in volume from a left-to-right shunt may cause heart failure. With left ventricular failure, there may be pulmonary venous congestion that interferes with gas exchange and causes carbon dioxide retention and further hypoxemia. There is also a high pulmonary venous pressure, which together with the effect of

the large opening between the aorta and pulmonary artery will cause pulmonary hypertension. The high pulmonary artery pressure with increased pulmonary blood flow and pulmonary edema may cause a decrease in lung compliance, further compounding the primary pulmonary problem.

The diagnosis of a PDA may be difficult, since a continuous murmur is *not* usually present. A wide pulse pressure is often present, as is increased precordial activity. The diagnosis of heart failure may be very difficult. When the roentgenogram shows a large heart and pulmonary venous congestion in the presence of signs of a PDA and a large liver, there is no problem in diagnosis. However, for many reasons, the heart may not be very large, and severe RDS may obscure x-ray findings of cardiomegaly and pulmonary edema. As discussed below, current practice dictates intervention before this stage so that congestive heart failure does not occur.

In many instances, the typical clinical findings are not evident. A PDA may produce no murmur in some infants or intermittent murmurs in others. Ventilator therapy and continuous positive airway pressure may mask the findings of PDA. In all infants with severe respiratory distress syndrome, a PDA must be suspected when the illness is protracted, blood gases suddenly deteriorate and require manipulation of ventilation, or apneic episodes are intensified. Fluid balance must be closely monitored since excess fluid administration may produce a clinically significant PDA and congestive heart failure. See Chapter 6.

Infants must be auscultated for murmurs several times a day during the illness, for the murmur may be intermittent. The infant should be briefly removed from the ventilator to permit proper auscultation.

Echocardiography and Doppler have been particularly useful in indicating the presence of a left-to-right shunt through a PDA. A large left atrium and left ventricle suggest that the ductus is hemodynamically significant.

Similarly a hyperdynamic left ventricle or increased pulsation of the descending thoracic aorta suggests a significant shunt. Displacement of the interatrial septum into the right atrial cavity also suggests an increased left atrial volume load. Doppler evaluation of retrograde flow in the descending aorta, reduced diastolic forward flow in branches of the ascending aorta, and turbulent diastolic flow in the main pulmonary artery contributes to the diagnosis.

The approach to management of these infants, particularly those under 1250 gm birth weight, is not clearly established. First, the term "hemodynamic significance" is very broadly applied. To some physicians, any change from the standard, expected management of an infant without a patent ductus arteriosus constitutes significance; this includes the requirement for fluid and (hence) calorie restriction or the requirement for diuretic administration to prevent obvious clinical and echocardiographic evidence of volume overload. In many institutions, however, the shunt is deemed significant and requires more specific intervention only

when severe fluid restriction and diuresis together with aggressive ventilatory management fail. Furthermore, the type and the timing of the intervention are not standard. Whenever feasible, therapy should be aimed at the cause of the problem rather than the adverse effects. For patent ductus arteriosus, this is now possible in most situations; surgical closure can be offered with relatively low morbidity, and, more importantly, pharmacologic closure by inhibition of prostaglandin synthesis with indomethacin has an acceptably low failure rate as well as relatively few adverse effects. A major attempt to control the heart failure would therefore seem unacceptable as a primary approach, especially because digoxin, the drug used in term infants or older children to improve myocardial performance, has little positive effect in premature infants and a high risk of toxicity. We now recommend administering indomethacin on first diagnosis of a patent ductus arteriosus (usually by 2–3 days after birth) in infants under 1000 gm; in infants over 1000 gm birth weight, we only administer indomethacin when it is apparent that the PDA is stimulating changes in management or is "hemodynamically significant." Continued deterioration toward true heart failure in any of these situations prompts immediate ligation. See Appendix A–1.

In the overall management of the preterm infant, the clinician should attempt to eliminate all factors that would impair the ability of the premature infant to grow. Therefore, if the patent ductus arteriosus is contributing to an impairment of oxygen transport and is compromising lung function, it should be managed by either pharmacologic manipulation or surgical intervention so that adequate calories and fluids can be readily administered.

N. Talner

Combined or Complicated Shunts

Although an isolated ventricular septal defect, patent ductus arteriosus, or atrial septal defect very rarely causes problems in the newborn, combinations of these are more likely to do so. For example, if an infant with the clinical features of ventricular septal defect develops cardiac failure and respiratory distress (see next section) in the first week or two of life, an additional shunt or another cardiac or vascular abnormality might be present. Another situation in which an isolated shunt might produce signs of failure occurs when the lung, particularly the pulmonary vascular bed, is underdeveloped, such as with diaphragmatic hernia or omphalocele. In these infants, a small shunt seems much larger because of the reduced size of the pulmonary vascular bed.

With an endocardial cushion defect, left ventricular to right atrial shunting may occur; this is an *obligatory shunt* not dependent on pulmonary vascular resistance. Thus, this lesion may produce signs of cardiac failure early in life. Mitral or tricuspid insufficiency plus ventricular shunting aggravates the situation.

The importance of combined lesions, particularly the association of left heart obstructive disease such as coarctation with a ventricular septal defect, demands early intervention. It has become apparent that the major problem in most situations relates to the left heart obstructive disease, which must be relieved to maintain systemic perfusion. The removal of the left heart obstruction may then permit the infant to adapt to the shunt lesion, and, in fact, in many instances the shunt lesions may undergo spontaneous closure.   **N. Talner**

THE HIGH-RISK NEWBORN

Presentation

Severe forms of congenital heart disease usually present in one of three ways in the immediate newborn period, although there is some overlap. We will discuss these three types of presentation, the most common lesions in each, the diagnostic tests necessary to distinguish among the lesions, subsequent therapy, and the differential diagnosis of noncardiac disease. This section discusses only those lesions with symptoms that require diagnostic and therapeutic interventions. As described in the section The Low-Risk Newborn, some infants present in the first month of life with murmurs as the only sign of potential heart disease and are later found to have no heart disease or to have low risk, isolated lesions. Also, murmurs in the newborn are frequently nonspecific. We believe it is more prudent to reevaluate such infants at several weeks of age: at that time, the physical findings are more specific since adaptation to extrauterine life is complete. Thus, many infants with innocent murmurs or minor lesions would not undergo exhaustive and expensive diagnostic procedures.

During the neonatal period, infants with serious heart disease present either with persistent cyanosis, marked respiratory distress, a low systemic output state, or a combination of these. Although infants with complex heart disease usually present with more than one of these findings, we will classify each lesion according to its predominant feature.

I would have to disagree here. While persistent cyanosis and low systemic perfusion are certainly signs of serious heart disease, with a left-to-right shunt lesion there may not be marked respiratory distress. As mentioned previously, the earliest sign of increased blood flow into the pulmonary circulation, as might be encountered in a large patent ductus arteriosus and ventricular septal defect, is rapid, shallow breathing (tachypnea) without necessarily signs of grunting, retractions, and alar flaring. While respiratory distress can occur late, it would be important for the clinician to pick up the early signs so that appropriate interventions can be undertaken before the infant is in severe difficulty.   **N. Talner**

GENERALIZED CENTRAL CYANOSIS

Central cyanosis indicates a reduced arterial blood-oxygen saturation. The infant with cyanotic heart disease is usually cyanotic in the first few hours of life, although not in severe respiratory distress. This cyanosis may initially occur with crying or feeding only and then progress as the circulation adapts to postnatal life, particularly as the ductus arteriosus begins to close. The level of systemic arterial blood-oxygen saturation depends entirely on the effective pulmonary blood flow—that is, the amount of blood oxygenated by the lungs that subsequently passes into the systemic arterial circulation. Pulmonary function is generally normal, and therefore pulmonary venous blood returning to the heart is essentially fully saturated with oxygen. Admixture of deoxygenated systemic and oxygenated pulmonary venous return occurs in the heart; the resultant systemic arterial oxygen saturation depends on the relative volumes that mix and the oxygen content of each. There are two major subgroups of lesions that feature cyanosis as the primary finding (Table 13–2): (1) those lesions with decreased pulmonary blood flow, in which the inflow to or outflow from the right ventricle is compromised (e.g., pulmonary atresia—Figure 13–5), and (2) those lesions with normal or increased pulmonary blood flow but with lack of passage of this blood to the systemic circulation (the transposition complexes—Figure 13–6). In both subgroups, effective pulmonary blood flow is low.

In practice, the differential diagnosis of these infants is limited to mild pulmonary disease or persistent pulmonary hypertension of the newborn (PPHN). Methemoglobine-

TABLE 13–2 CARDIAC CAUSES OF CYANOSIS WITHOUT CONGESTIVE HEART FAILURE

Decreased Pulmonary Blood Flow
Critical pulmonary stenosis with intact ventricular septum
Ebstein's anomaly
Pulmonary atresia with intact ventricular septum
Severe pulmonary stenosis with ventricular septal defect (tetralogy of Fallot)
Tricuspid atresia with intact ventricular septum, pulmonary atresia, or small ventricular septal defect
Tricuspid insufficiency secondary to myocardial ischemia
Tricuspid stenosis
Univentricular hearts with severe pulmonic stenosis

Normal Pulmonary Blood Flow with Poor Mixing
Simple transposition of the great vessels
Taussig-Bing syndrome
Transposition of the great vessels with associated lesions (complex)

mia (rarely seen) should always be considered a possible cause. Infants with decreased lung volumes caused by external compression in utero and those with severe parenchymal lung disease presenting with cyanosis will invariably show severe respiratory distress; such cases do not enter into the differential diagnosis. (They will be discussed in the following section.)

Initial evaluation usually directs the physi-

cian to strongly suspect cardiac disease. The history of the cyanotic infant with heart disease is generally benign, the pregnancy and delivery uneventful. The infant with PPHN, however, often has a history of perinatal distress or meconium aspiration. An exception in the cardiac group is tricuspid insufficiency secondary to myocardial ischemia, in which a history of perinatal asphyxia is common. The physical examination rarely distinguishes between the cardiac and noncardiac patients: most are tachypneic, with some respiratory distress. (Infants with mild arterial oxygen desaturation can show hyperpnea with no distress, which is caused by chemoreceptor stimulation.) If the hypoxemia is severe and mild metabolic acidemia develops, this increased respiratory effort is accentuated, making it extremely difficult to differentiate from the respiratory distress associated with mild or moderate primary pulmonary disease. Most cyanotic infants have increased right ventricular impulses resulting from high right ventricular pressures (except in hypoplastic right heart syndrome), and murmurs are frequently present in noncardiac lesions (PPHN with secondary tricuspid insufficiency) or absent in heart disease (transposition with intact ventricular septum).

Other diagnostic procedures are needed in those infants. It helps to compare arterial

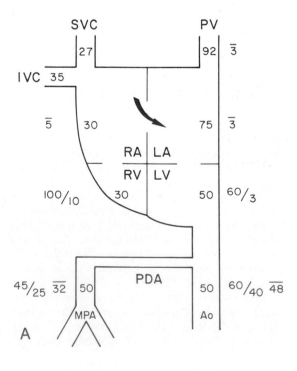

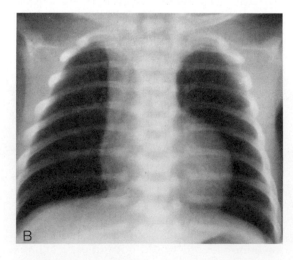

Figure 13–5. *A,* Representative blood oxygen saturation (per cent) and pressure (mm Hg) depicted diagrammatically in an infant with pulmonary atresia. (See Figure 13–2 for abbreviations.) *B,* Chest x-ray of an infant with pulmonary atresia.

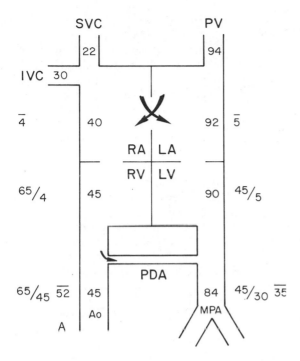

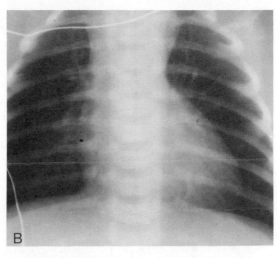

A

Figure 13–6. *A,* Representative blood oxygen saturation (per cent) and pressure (mm Hg) depicted diagrammatically in an infant with complete transposition of the great arteries. (See Figure 13–2 for abbreviations.) *B,* Chest x-ray of an infant with complete transposition of the great arteries.

blood-oxygen saturation and PO_2 in the right radial or temporal artery (and thus above the ductus arteriosus) with those in the umbilical artery (below the ductus arteriosus). In most forms of cyanotic heart disease, the two saturations or PO_2s are similar; in PPHN, pulmonary vascular resistance is very high, and the ductus arteriosus, if patent, shows right-to-left ductal shunting with subsequent lowering of the umbilical blood-oxygen saturation or PO_2 in the descending aorta. The "hyperoxia" test, or ventilation with a high inspired oxygen concentration, is frequently considered a valuable diagnostic tool. Although an increase greater than 20–30 torr in systemic arterial PO_2 is often seen in primary pulmonary problems (especially since high levels of oxygen tend to dilate the pulmonary arterioles and drop the pulmonary arterial pressures), the converse is not necessarily true. That is, one may encounter a significant increase in systemic arterial blood oxygen tension or saturation in cyanotic heart disease. As long as effective pulmonary blood flow is reasonable, there will be a fair increase in oxygen delivered to the systemic arterial bed. This in turn increases the systemic venous blood-oxygen saturation as oxygen delivery to the tissues increases, and systemic arterial blood-oxygen saturation will increase further.

Editorial Comment: A hyperoxia test can be accomplished noninvasively using a transcutaneous oxygen monitor. See Chapter 8.

Chest x-rays in the first few days of life usually show normal heart size in most lesions. (Exceptions may be those lesions such as Ebstein's anomaly, in which tricuspid insufficiency is a major problem and marked right atrial enlargement occurs.) Since thymic involution occurs quite early in cyanotic infants, it is helpful to examine the cardiac contour. Most cyanotic lesions are associated with either a diminutive pulmonary artery (e.g., pulmonary atresia) or one that is transposed to the right, and thus the normal pulmonary artery contour at the upper left region of the cardiac silhouette is absent. The aortic arch should be visualized; the aorta frequently descends to the right of the spine in right-sided obstructive lesions, particularly with an associated ventricular septal defect (tetralogy of Fallot). Examination of the lung fields may rule out pulmonary abnormalities secondary to displacement by abdominal organs. Vascularity may be low, normal, or even increased in cyanotic heart disease. (Consider transposition of the great arteries with ventricular septal defect in which pulmonary blood flow is high, although effective pulmonary blood flow—that blood then passing to the systemic circulation—may be very low.) Thus, vascularity may not be helpful in diagnosis.

An electrocardiogram (ECG) in the first few days of life is often nonspecific because the right ventricle is dominant in the normal fetus and in most forms of cyanotic heart disease. Over the next few weeks, as pulmonary resistance falls, the T wave normally inverts in the right precordial leads, and thus, after this time interval, the T wave in lesions associated with right ventricular hypertrophy can be distinguished. Unfortunately, cyanotic heart disease must be diagnosed much sooner. There are some lesions with specific ECG patterns—right atrial hypertrophy in Ebstein's anomaly, left axis deviation and right atrial hypertrophy with decreased right ventricular forces in tricuspid atresia with intact ventricular septum—but these are exceptions.

If the possibility of cyanotic heart disease is entertained after these initial studies, further procedures must be performed. A two-dimensional echocardiogram with Doppler studies can almost always accurately define the anatomy of the heart.

An exception is the diagnosis of total anomalous pulmonary venous return, which even with the most detailed two-dimensional and Doppler examination remains difficult at best without cardiac catheterization.

M. Miller

If the patient is not in a facility where an echocardiogram or cardiac catheterization can be performed, immediate transfer is mandatory. Stabilization prior to the transport is of utmost importance: metabolic requirements must be reduced to a minimum to provide adequate substrate delivery, and, if oxygen delivery is borderline (measured blood oxygen saturation $\leq 70\%$, $Po_2 \leq 30$–35 torr, or in the presence of metabolic acidosis), prostaglandin E_1 (Prostin VR) should be infused. See Appendix A–1 for dosage.

The use of prostaglandin E_1 is based on the physiologic information that prostaglandins dilate the ductus arteriosus. Initially, prostaglandin E_1 was used only in those infants with ductus-dependent lesions, such as hypoplastic right ventricle and pulmonary atresia. In most of these infants, pulmonary blood flow is provided entirely through the ductus arteriosus. When the ductus closes after birth, hypoxemia and acidemia progressively worsen unless a palliative surgical procedure is performed immediately. Prostaglandin E_1 effectively dilates the ductus to provide adequate pulmonary blood flow; the infant can then stabilize and be carefully evaluated. More recently, it became apparent that most infants with complete transposition of the great arteries also have better mixing between the pulmonary and systemic circulations when the ductus arteriosus is dilated with prostaglandin E_1. It is appropriate, therefore, to infuse prostaglandin E_1 into any cyanotic infant in whom the diagnosis of cyanotic congenital heart disease is strongly suspected, even before a complete evaluation. It should be remembered, however, that prostaglandin E_1 has definite side effects, such as apnea, hypotension with peripheral vasodilatation, and a possible increased risk of infection.

In certain patients, cardiac catheterization must be considered. It is necessary to catheterize the newborn when the diagnosis is uncertain, a therapeutic procedure is necessary (e.g., balloon atrial septostomy in transposition of the great arteries), or surgery is imminent and better definition of the anatomy is required (e.g., the right ventricular outflow tract and pulmonary arteries in pulmonary atresia when a pulmonary valvotomy or outflow patch is to be performed). In many infants, because two-dimensional echocardiography can accurately define the anatomy, immediate catheterization is not required and can be delayed beyond the neonatal period, after which time the risks are fewer and the angiographic detail is better.

In summary, an infant who presents with cyanosis and little respiratory distress usually has cardiac disease and requires prompt evaluation and stabilization. When the initial evaluation cannot exclude cardiac disease, it is important to proceed with a complete cardiovascular evaluation. With the dramatic improvements in echocardiography, Doppler technology, cardiac catheterization, and neonatal surgery and the advent of prostaglandin E_1 use to maintain ductal patency, we can offer a more normal life to infants with cyanotic heart disease.

RESPIRATORY DISTRESS

Infants with congenital heart disease who present with respiratory distress are the most difficult to diagnose: their symptoms are usually more insidious and less dramatic than cyanosis, the differential diagnosis is broader, and the yield of heart disease is much less, thus lowering one's index of suspicion. When a physician chances upon a newborn lying in a crib, blue and comfortable, the diagnosis is almost always cardiac disease; when the infant is tachypneic and shows marked retractions, it usually is not.

Infants with respiratory distress usually have varying degrees of systemic blood-oxygen desaturation, depending upon the type of circulatory derangement and the severity of pulmonary edema. The respiratory distress is related to decreased lung compliance in these patients, and there may be interstitial fluid present. Thus, even with a normal separation of circulations, some degree of hypoxemia is present. A more important source of hypoxemia in many of these infants is the redirection of systemic venous return to the aorta. In fact, infants with respiratory distress on a cardiac basis can be categorized into two major subgroups: (1) those with mixing of systemic and pulmonary venous blood in the heart with resultant desaturation of arterial blood, and (2) those with no mixing, in whom any desaturation is secondary to alveolar fluid and intrapulmonary shunting (Table 13–3). Once again, both groups may have elevated pulmonary venous pressures or pulmonary blood flow that causes interstitial edema, at which point respiratory distress becomes apparent.

The first subgroup of infants represents a wide spectrum of complex congenital heart diseases. Admixture of systemic and pulmonary venous blood may occur at the venous, atrial, ventricular, or arterial level. Admixture at the venous level occurs in total anomalous pulmonary venous connection. There is rarely respiratory distress in this lesion during the neonatal period, unless there is obstruction to pulmonary venous return. This is most commonly seen when the connection is below the diaphragm to the portal venous system. An example of admixture at the atrial level with respiratory distress is tricuspid atresia with a large ventricular septal defect: since there is no entrance of systemic venous blood to the right ventricle, the blood must cross an interatrial communication into the left atrium and left ventricle. Complete admixture at the ventricular level can be seen in double outlet right ventricle. At the ventriculoarterial level, truncus arteriosus is the classic example. When pulmonary venous obstruction is not present, congestive heart failure develops late as the pulmonary resistance drops and pulmonary blood flow increases. Even more systemic arterial desaturation occurs in lesions in which there is preferential return of systemic venous blood back to the aorta and pulmonary venous blood back to the pulmonary artery. Increased pulmonary blood flow causes congestive heart failure with marked cyanosis. This occurs in transposition of the great arteries with a large ventricular septal defect or occasionally a large patent ductus arteriosus and in certain forms of double outlet right ventricle.

In cases of an absent pulmonary valve, the hemodynamic pattern is similar to that in tetralogy of Fallot, but there often is severe respiratory distress. The massively dilated pulmonary arteries compress the airways and cause ventilatory embarrassment.

In the second subgroup, the blood entering the aorta has the same saturation as that in the pulmonary veins—that is, there is no right-to-left shunt. Atrial septal defects, atrioventricular septal defects (endocardial cushion defects), ventricular septal defects, aortopulmonary windows, patent ductus arteriosus, and arteriovenous malformations are examples of left-to-right shunts at each level in the circulation that can produce cardiac failure and thereby respiratory distress. As discussed previously, infants with these lesions rarely present in the neonatal period, except when the infant is premature (most typically with a patent ductus arteriosus, although we have seen several premature infants in heart failure with endocardial cushion defects or ventricular septal defects) or when there is an associated lesion. The latter is often an obstruction to left ventricular outflow (see the following section), such as coarctation or interruption of the aorta. This

TABLE 13–3 CARDIAC CAUSES OF RESPIRATORY DISTRESS

Usually with Systemic Arterial Hypoxemia
Absent pulmonary valve
Complex transposition of the great vessels (with ventricular septal defect ± pulmonary stenosis)
Double outlet right ventricle without severe pulmonary stenosis
Splenic syndromes (asplenia, polysplenia)
Taussig-Bing syndrome
Total anomalous pulmonary venous connection
Tricuspid atresia with large ventricular septal defect
Truncus arteriosus
Univentricular hearts without severe pulmonic stenosis

With No Significant Hypoxemia
Aortopulmonary window
Arteriovenous fistula
Endocardial cushion defect
Patent ductus arteriosus
Ventricular septal defect (usually with patent ductus arteriosus or atrial septal defect)

is seen most commonly with ventricular septal defects or aortopulmonary windows.

Interference with inflow to the left ventricle, as in congenital mitral stenosis or cor triatriatum, may lead to severe pulmonary venous congestion and respiratory distress but may not compromise systemic perfusion to any major degree. Infants with cor triatriatum have been diagnosed as having chronic lung disease and treated for many months before a congenital cardiac malformation was suspected.

The differential diagnosis of infants with respiratory distress secondary to heart disease is obviously any form of parenchymal lung disease or the more usual, severe forms of PPHN. The premature infant with resolving respiratory distress syndrome who requires increasing respiratory support may have either an increasing ductal shunt or the onset of interstitial lung disease. The full-term infant with total anomalous pulmonary venous connection is often first thought to have PPHN, an aspiration syndrome, or pneumonia. The infant with truncus arteriosus may first appear to have transient tachypnea until it is obviously no longer transient. Thus it may take several days of careful evaluation before the presence of heart disease is fully appreciated.

The initial evaluation of the infant with respiratory distress rarely points to cardiac problems. The perinatal history is usually benign, but this is also true for infants with early onset pneumonias. The physical examination reveals an infant with tachypnea and marked retractions, often with no detectable cyanosis, for it is only when blood-oxygen saturations reach quite low levels (probably 75%) that cyanosis is appreciated in the newborn. Examining the peripheral pulses is helpful when there is a large runoff of blood from the aorta into either the venous system (e.g., arteriovenous malformation) or the low resistance bed of the lungs (e.g., patent ductus arteriosus and truncus arteriosus). But when the shunt is proximal (thus maintaining a normal aortic diastolic pressure) or when there is an associated low output state, this does not occur. Hepatomegaly is common in both cardiac and lung disease. The assessment of liver size is complicated by the downward displacement of the diaphragm secondary to hyperinflation. The precordium is hyperactive because of increased volume load or pulmonary arterial pressures in most shunt lesions as well as in primary lung disease. The presence of a systolic ejection click suggests lesions in which a large volume of blood is crossing one usually abnormal valve, as in truncus arteriosus; this may also be found with the suprasystemic pressures in the pulmonary artery seen in total anomalous venous connection. A single second heart sound may suggest the absence of a pulmonary valve (e.g., truncus arteriosus) or its posterior displacement (e.g., transposition with ventricular septal defect). Murmurs are more frequent in these lesions than in cyanotic heart disease since there is a large flow of blood across an abnormal connection into the pulmonary artery. A peripheral murmur will indicate an arteriovenous malformation (e.g., over the cranium). An important exception is the absence of murmurs in total anomalous pulmonary venous connection.

As previously mentioned, values for arterial blood-oxygen saturation vary widely depending on the flow patterns and the amount of pulmonary edema. A hyperoxic test is unhelpful in infants with respiratory distress due to congenital heart disease, since a large portion of the desaturation is due to pulmonary edema and thus a significant improvement often occurs when oxygen is administered. The chest x-ray may show cardiomegaly because of the increased pulmonary blood flow in many of the lesions in this category. Similarly, pulmonary vascularity is often increased, although this may be difficult to interpret when parenchymal disease is present. Passive congestion is seen when the pulmonary venous pressures are markedly elevated. In the newborn, the presence of interstitial fluid and often some cardiac enlargement in pneumonia makes the above findings relatively nonspecific for cardiac disease. The ECG is helpful only when it is specific for particular lesions. For example, in total anomalous pulmonary venous connection, the suprasystemic pressures in the pulmonary artery are often reflected in the ECG by the presence of qR waves in the right precordial leads. Unfortunately, specific ECG patterns are the exception rather than the rule.

A high index of suspicion is required to consider the presence of heart disease in an infant with respiratory distress. When the course is not classic for pneumonia or another lung disorder, the history does not support lung disease, or there are signs that raise doubts about the diagnosis, it is necessary to consider heart disease. A two-dimensional echocardiogram with Doppler studies and saline contrast injection will enable primary lung and cardiac problems to be differentiated. (Shaken saline has "microbubbles" of air out of solution that are highly echoreflectant and thus can be followed as blood travels from the systemic veins throughout the circulation until a capillary bed is reached.) Even in total anomalous pulmonary venous connection, a careful study will usually demonstrate the abnormal vessel either above or below the diaphragm. The diagnosis can be confirmed by the absence of contrast (saline) in that vessel alone, since it is the only part of the circulation that is separated from the systemic veins by a capillary bed. It is necessary to consider the possibility of heart disease in any term (and occasionally preterm) infant with respiratory distress.

HYPOPERFUSION STATES

The last common manner of presentation of critical heart disease in the newborn is hypoperfusion. The course may be rapidly progressive over the first few hours of life or insidious in onset over the first few weeks. The differential diagnosis of noncardiac disease presenting as hypoperfusion covers a wide range of organ systems (Table 13–4). The physician must promptly assess the potential causes of the low output state and begin treatment prior to confirmatory studies.

Hypoperfusion is secondary to an inadequate ejection of blood by the left ventricle into the systemic arterial system, with subsequent hypotension and progressive metabolic acidosis. Heart disease that presents in this manner may be divided into two categories: those lesions in which flow through the left side of the heart or the systemic arterial tree is obstructed and thus even a normal ventricle cannot eject an adequate output; and those lesions in which flow is unobstructed, but the pump function of the heart is seriously impaired such that output is inadequate. Obstructive lesions are far more common, and the most common are coarctation of the aorta and hypoplastic left heart syndrome (Figure 13-7A, B). As mentioned above, hypoperfusion syndromes often have associated features. Many lesions have some degree of systemic arterial desaturation (e.g., in hypoplastic left heart syndrome the aorta is perfused by the pulmonary artery via the ductus arteriosus, and thus systemic venous blood returns to the arterial system), and most involve respiratory distress since pul-

TABLE 13–4 CAUSES OF HYPOPERFUSION

Cardiac	Noncardiac
Obstructive Lesions	
Left ventricular inflow obstruction	Adrenal insufficiency
Cor triatriatum	Anemia
Mitral stenosis	Hypovolemia
Supravalvular mitral ring	Inborn errors of metabolism
± Total anomalous pulmonary venous connection	Metabolic (decreased Ca^{2+}, Mg^{2+}, glucose, H^+)
Left ventricular outflow obstruction	Polycythemia
Coarctation of the aorta	Sepsis
Hypoplastic left heart syndrome	Severe neurologic dysfunction
Interrupted aortic arch	Pneumothorax
Severe aortic stenosis	Pneumopericardium
Nonobstructive Lesions	
Arrhythmia	
Complete heart block	
Supraventricular tachycardia	
Intrinsic myocardial abnormality	
Abnormal coronary arteries (arteritis, calcinosis)	
Anomalous left coronary artery	
Endocardial fibroelastosis	
Glycogen storage disease	
Infiltrative diseases of the myocardium (e.g., congenital leukemia)	
Myocardial ischemia/infarction with normal coronary arteries	
Myocarditis	
Primary cardiomyopathies	
Pericarditis	

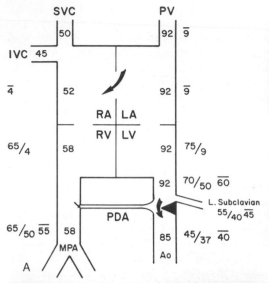

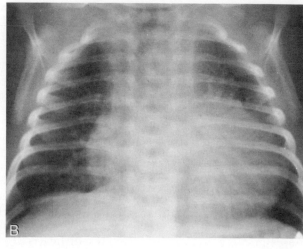

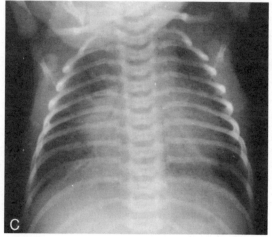

Figure 13–7. *A,* Representative blood oxygen saturation (per cent) and pressure (mm Hg) depicted diagrammatically in an infant with coarctation of the aorta. (See Figure 13–2 for abbreviations.) *B,* Chest x-rays of an infant with coarctation of the aorta *(B)* and hypoplastic left heart syndrome *(C).* The chest x-ray usually cannot differentiate between left-sided obstructive lesions.

monary venous pressures are elevated when the left ventricle fails to eject a normal stroke volume. However, infants with the most striking characteristics are lethargic and mottled with pallor and poor pulses.

The differential diagnosis of noncardiac disease is broad: sepsis, adrenal insufficiency, anemia, hypovolemia, inborn errors of metabolism, and neurologic instability all may present with hypoperfusion as the major finding. The most frequent misdiagnosis in an infant with heart disease and hypoperfusion is sepsis. Because overwhelming infection is life-threatening, it is reasonable to perform a septic workup and perhaps even begin therapy on any infant who presents with signs of low output, but it is important to consider cardiac disease as well.

The history can help distinguish between cardiac and noncardiac disease and among the specific cardiac lesions. An early presentation within the first few hours to first few days of life is more commonly associated with hypoplastic left heart syndrome in the obstructive group and congenital infection or arrhythmia in the nonobstructive group. Coarctation or interruption of the aorta presents later in the first few weeks of life, as do coronary artery abnormalities. There is sometimes a history of perinatal problems. A history of recent viral infection in the mother may be elicited in infants with myocarditis. Fetal hydrops occurs in intrauterine supraventricular tachycardia, cardiomyopathy, premature closure of the foramen ovale, and, on rare occasions, hypoplastic left heart syndrome. Maternal diabetes will suggest diabetic cardiomyopathy, and a familial history might suggest other forms of cardiomyopathy.

The physical examination uniformly shows a pale, tachypneic, and lethargic infant. The heart rate is markedly elevated (220–270 bpm) in supraventricular tachycardia, although it can be above 200 bpm in any stressed infant with a sinus tachycardia. Frank cyanosis is most often seen in hypoplastic left heart syndrome, but even then it is uncommon. Peripheral pulses are decreased in low output states generally, but a differential pulse or blood pressure between the upper and lower extremities can be revealing. In coarctation of the aorta, the lower limb pressures may be low (unless the ductus arteriosus is nonrestrictive); in hypoplastic left heart syndrome, the opposite may be true. It is important to realize that the left subclavian artery frequently arises at the origin of the coarctation and thus should not be used to represent ascending aortic pressures in coarctation (Figure 13–7A). Similarly, the right subclavian artery may arise aberrantly from the descending aorta, making it impossible to obtain ascending aortic blood pressures. The precordial impulse is often nonspecific, usually showing a right ventricular heave. The second heart sound is single in hypoplastic left heart syndrome but, because of the tachycardia in low output states, it is often difficult to appreciate a split sound in other lesions as well. Murmurs rarely help the diagnosis in this group: in the presence of severe failure, most lesions are not associated with murmurs or have nonspecific ones. Coarctation of the aorta in which a ventricular septal defect or subaortic stenosis is present is an exception, but critical aortic stenosis may have little or no murmur when the left ventricular output is low. Rales are heard in most low output states as a result of elevated pulmonary venous pressures.

Arterial blood gases often show a metabolic acidosis at the time of diagnosis. Differential blood-oxygen saturations between the right radial or temporal arterial sample and the umbilical arterial sample may be very helpful. In coarctation or interruption of the aorta, the saturation in the umbilical artery will be lower if the ductus is patent because there will be right-to-left shunting from the pulmonary artery to the descending aorta. Conversely, if the saturation is higher in the descending aorta, transposition with ventricular septal defect and coarctation should be considered. The chest x-ray often shows cardiomegaly and interstitial edema in both cardiac and noncardiac lesions once there is severe heart failure and thus is not useful for diagnosis. The electrocardiogram is helpful in several lesions. For example, left-sided forces are absent in hypoplastic left heart syndrome; the regular rapid heart rate of supraventricular tachycardia is diagnostic (Figure 13–8); there are signs of an anterolateral ischemia or infarction in anomalous left coronary artery; endocardial fibroelastosis has prominent q and R waves in the precordial leads; there usually is marked right ventricular hypertrophy in coarctation of the aorta or critical aortic stenosis; and ST-T wave abnormalities are present in myocarditis. The echocardiogram is diagnostic in most obstructive lesions; however, the entire aortic arch is sometimes difficult to see adequately in the newborn. The echocardiogram is also very useful in assessing ventricular performance and the response to therapeutic interventions. An immediate catheterization is best avoided in left-sided obstructive lesions unless absolutely necessary, because infants with such lesions are often barely compensated and even a small stress could cause rapid metabolic deterioration. Also, these infants do not tolerate large volumes of contrast because of its high osmolarity. Selective retrograde aortography via the umbilical ar-

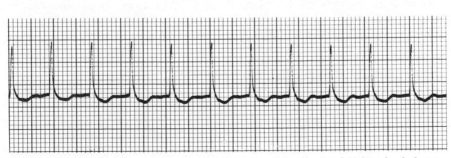

Figure 13–8. Electrocardiogram illustrating paroxysmal atrial tachycardia. Lead II Standard electrocardiogram at speed 50. Heart rate = 300 beats per minute. No P waves are seen.

tery to evaluate the presence of coarctation is often the only invasive procedure required initially.

Therapy must be prompt. Once deterioration begins, it is usually rapidly progressive. Initial measures must be directed to the metabolic derangements: partial correction of the metabolic acidosis, maintenance of adequate substrate, hemoglobin, and blood volume, and inotropic support with rapidly acting agents such as isoproterenol or dopamine should be undertaken promptly. Prostaglandin E_1 (PGE_1) is of utmost importance when obstructive lesions are considered—by maintaining ductal patency, the lower body may be perfused from the pulmonary artery in interruption or coarctation of the aorta. The entire body can be perfused by this route in critical aortic stenosis. Next, a specific diagnosis must be made and appropriate therapy instituted. For example, if the infant has supraventricular tachycardia and is severely decompensated, cardioversion at 0.25–1.0 watt-second should be performed. If the infant is relatively stable after the initial assessment, facial immersion in cold water or pharmacologic cardioversion may be attempted using digoxin, propranolol, or verapamil.

If verapamil is used, both calcium and isoproterenol should be ready at the bedside to be given immediately in the event of severe hypotension resulting from myocardial depression. In left ventricular obstructive lesions other than hypoplastic left heart syndrome, the infant should be maintained on PGE_1 prior to surgery. If the diagnosis is in doubt, antibiotics should be instituted after a septic workup, and high dose steroids should be considered if adrenal insufficiency is a possibility.

PRACTICAL HINTS

1. Heart sounds in most newborns with congenital heart disease of a serious nature are usually abnormal. A single second sound after the first 12 hours often indicates heart disease. A well-split second sound suggests total anomalous pulmonary venous connection. The presence of a pulmonary systolic ejection click may be normal in the first hours, but after that any systolic ejection click is abnormal, indicating a large pulmonary artery, large aorta, or true truncus arteriosus. If the patient has pulmonary disease without congenital heart disease and has a narrowly

split or single second sound, then a high pulmonary vascular resistance is expected.

The clinician should never depend on one finding alone to either rule in or rule out significant cardiac disease. Rather, the various findings should be added to see if they point toward a cardiac etiology. The most important findings relate to the level of arterial oxygen tension, heart size, respiratory pattern, and the adequacy of systemic perfusion. **N. Talner**

2. Visible central cyanosis in the early newborn period usually indicates a very low arterial oxygen tension. Even when the clinical judgment is that of only questionable cyanosis, the arterial PO_2 may be very low.

3. Peripheral cyanosis (acrocyanosis) is normal and must be differentiated from central cyanosis.

4. Systemic arterial blood gases may be helpful in differentiating pulmonary from cardiac cyanosis. A PaO_2 greater than 150 mm Hg in an enriched oxygen environment effectively eliminates severe heart disease with anatomic right-to-left shunt. In questionable cases, hypoxemia without significant hypercapnia (CO_2 retention) tends to suggest primary cardiac disease. However, pulmonary venous congestion, as in the hypoplastic left ventricle syndrome, may result in considerable CO_2 retention. It may also result in a somewhat low PO_2, which increases in a high oxygen environment.

A suspicion of hypoxemia must be verified by arterial blood gas determinations. While peripheral cyanosis may be normal, this is only in the face of adequate systemic perfusion as verified by the volume of the arterial pulsations, skin temperature, and capillary refill. Again, a single finding by itself does not rule in or rule out cardiac disease. It is possible to have a PaO_2 greater than 150 in the face of a basically cyanotic lesion such as truncus arteriosus. Furthermore, there may be hypercapnia in the face of pulmonary overcirculation, and, on the other hand, the PCO_2 may be extremely low with impaired systemic perfusion. **N. Talner**

5. Heel stick blood gases do not provide accurate measures of the arterial PO_2. However, the error is always on the low side, so that in cyanotic congenital heart disease a reasonably high heel stick PO_2 is reassuring.

6. Transcutaneous PO_2 measurements are inaccurate at low levels and in the presence of hypoperfusion. They are valuable for monitoring trends.

7. Femoral pulses must be carefully palpated in all newborn infants. The femoral pulse may be palpable even with significant coarctation of the aorta while the ductus is open, disappearing when the ductus closes.

8. A high index of suspicion is required to diagnose congenital heart disease early. Care-

ful history taking, physical examination, and laboratory measurements—including chest x-rays, electrocardiogram, and blood gas studies in an enriched oxygen environment—will often help establish the diagnosis. However, two-dimensional echocardiography permits accurate and definitive diagnosis, accomplished without delay.

9. Life-threatening congenital heart disease will sooner or later be associated with respiratory distress or frank cyanosis or both.

10. The presence of a large liver usually indicates systemic venous congestion, which may not necessarily indicate congestive heart failure. Many conditions in the neonatal period can produce an enlarged liver.

11. When a baby with a congenital heart defect is symptomatic early in the newborn period, death is likely unless a surgical procedure or balloon septostomy can be performed.

12. On occasion, in the presence of respiratory distress syndrome and a patent ductus arteriosus, congestive heart failure may be diagnosed without cardiomegaly.

CASE PROBLEMS

One must note the difficulty in recognizing cyanosis caused by right-to-left intracardiac shunting in the first days of life. The degree of desaturation is usually underestimated. It is also important to recognize two major forms of cyanotic congenital heart disease: (1) that associated with insufficient pulmonary blood flow, and (2) that in which there is increased pulmonary blood flow, since the oxygenated blood from the pulmonary veins does not reach the systemic circulation.

Case One

A baby girl is considered normal at birth, but on the second day of age cyanosis is noted. The heart is quiet. No murmur is heard, and there is no respiratory distress. On the third day, cyanosis is more obvious, and the respiratory rate is increased. The child's x-ray shows a small heart with decreased pulmonary vascularity. The electrocardiogram shows left ventricular hypertrophy.

Can a diagnosis be suggested?

When the heart is quiet and the child is blue, insufficient pulmonary blood flow is suggested. The x-ray is consistent. These findings and the electrocardiogram indicate that perhaps the right ventricle is hypoplastic.

A cardiac catheterization is performed. The right ventricle is entered with great difficulty.

	Pressure (mm Hg)	Per Cent Saturation
SVC and RA	m = 10	20
RV	160/10	20
LA	m = 5	50
PV	m = 5	95
LV	80/5	50
Femoral artery	80/50	50

Cineangiograms are done from the right and left ventricles.

Are the physiologic data consistent with the diagnosis?

At catheterization, there is no left-to-right shunt as far as the ventricle, while the saturation of 50 per cent in the LA indicates a large right-to-left shunt at the atrial level. The very high RV pressure indicates severe obstruction to outflow, while the large difference in pressure between the RV and LV reveals that there must be little or no ventricular communication. Although there is a large right-to-left shunt at the atrial level, the marked difference in pressure between the RA and LA indicates that there is small communication. Thus, the clinical diagnosis fits with the catheterization diagnosis of pulmonary atresia with a moderately hypoplastic right ventricle and an intact ventricular septum.

How does blood reach the pulmonary circulation?

All of the systemic venous return flows through the atrial septal defect into the left atrium and then through the left ventricle and aorta. Almost invariably there is a patent ductus arteriosus connected to the pulmonary arteries. A moderately hypoplastic main pulmonary artery extends to the atretic pulmonary valve, and the main branch arteries are somewhat small.

Is there some treatment that can be done before completing the catheterization?

If not already done, an infusion of PGE$_1$ (0.05 μg/kg/min) should be started.

Prostaglandin E$_1$ infusion should be started when the clinical evidence is that of impaired pulmonary or systemic blood flow so that the infant can be transported in an improved metabolic state consequent to either an increase in systemic perfusion or improved pulmonary blood flow and an increase in PaO$_2$. In terms of the transport, however, the transport team should be alerted to the possibility of apnea with a PGE$_1$ infusion and be prepared to ventilate if necessary.   **N. Talner**

Should the surgeon be called?

Yes, as soon as possible. However, because of the PGE₁ infusion, surgery can be delayed awhile as the infant is allowed to stabilize.

How can the surgeon help?

By making an anastomosis between the root of the aorta and the right pulmonary artery, thereby increasing pulmonary blood flow (aortopulmonary shunt). The surgeon should also attempt a pulmonary valvotomy and right ventricular outflow patch, if possible, which may help in promoting growth of the right ventricle.

What is the prognosis?

The prognosis is not known. Much depends on whether the hypoplastic right ventricle and pulmonary arteries will grow. In general, unless the right ventricle and tricuspid valve are well developed, the outlook is poor.

Case Two

A baby girl is considered normal at birth, but on the second day cyanosis is noted. The heart is quiet. A grade 4/6 holosystolic ejection murmur is heard at the lower left sternal border. There is no respiratory distress.

At this point, in comparison to Case One, is there any suggestion as to a different diagnosis?

As in Case One, the heart is quiet, suggesting that cyanosis is associated with decreased pulmonary blood flow. The x-ray reveals a small heart and decreased pulmonary vascularity. The most important difference is the long, loud murmur.

On the sixth day, cyanosis remains minimal. The chest x-ray still shows a small heart with questionable decreased pulmonary vascularity. The electrocardiogram shows right ventricular hypertrophy.

Can a diagnosis be suggested?

The most likely diagnosis from the above information is a ventricular septal defect with pulmonic stenosis and right-to-left shunt (tetralogy of Fallot) or valvular pulmonic stenosis with an atrial right-to-left shunt.

The presence of cyanosis has to be documented by determination of arterial oxygen tension. In the face of pulmonary valve stenosis with a right-to-left atrial shunt, it would seem imperative to perform diagnostic cardiac catheterization to document the severity of the obstruction that is the major hemodynamic problem and that may or may not be accompanied by atrial right-to-left shunting. If there is an atrial right-to-left shunt, this usually accompanies rather severe pulmonary valve obstruction and is of the type that usually requires surgical intervention. With the development of balloon catheter techniques, it may be possible to relieve obstruction in some of these infants and, therefore, prevent the development of hypoxemia. The cyanosis seen in the face of severe left heart obstructive disease, such as coarctation, is a reflection of markedly impaired systemic perfusion plus the additional factor of the presence of pulmonary edema. It is not unusual for these patients to have close to normal arterial oxygen tensions reflecting a high pulmonary to systemic blood flow ratio in the face of impaired systemic perfusion. My personal opinion is that there is no role for the administration of digitalis for the acute low output state secondary to coarctation. These patients should receive a prostaglandin E₁ infusion to dilate the ductus arteriosus if this is possible and thereby improve systemic perfusion. In the face of low output congestive heart failure, these children should be operated upon as soon as possible, and, therefore, time spent in assessing the response to digitalis should be eliminated. It is perfectly possible for an infant with severe isolated coarctation to be in acute low output failure and to require surgical intervention. Therefore, I would stress that time should not be lost looking for the response to digitalis. If an inotropic agent is to be used while the infant is readied for surgery, it should be a titratable agonist such as isoproterenol, dopamine, or dobutamine.   **N. Talner**

Should cardiac catheterization be performed?

Not yet. Eventually catheterization may be required to define the anatomy more clearly, but since the cyanosis is only minimal and no immediate surgery is contemplated, an echocardiographic diagnosis is sufficient. Because the cyanosis has not progressed over 6 days, this infant could be discharged and followed.

Case Three

A baby is considered normal at birth, but on the second day of life cyanosis is noted. The heart is hyperdynamic. A grade 2/6 systolic ejection murmur is heard at the upper left sternal border, and there is no respiratory distress. On the third day, the cyanosis is more obvious, and the respiratory rate is increased. The chest x-ray shows a normal-sized heart. However, there is a suggestion of increased pulmonary vascularity, despite which the pulmonary artery cannot be recognized. The electrocardiogram shows the normal right ventricular dominance of a newborn.

Can a diagnosis be suggested?

The most striking difference between this case and Cases One and Two is that the heart is hyperdynamic. In addition, pulmonary vascularity is shown by x-ray to be increased. Thus, the cyanosis is not likely to be caused by decreased pulmonary blood flow but rather by inadequate mixing. The oxygenated pulmonary venous return is not getting to the systemic circulation. This understanding, together with the fact that the pulmonary artery cannot be recognized despite increased pulmonary vascularity, suggests an abnormality of the great arteries.

A cardiac catheterization is performed.

	Pressure (mm Hg)	Per Cent Saturation
SVC	m = 5	20
RA	m = 5	40
RV	80/5	40
LA	m = 10	95
PV	m = 10	95
LV	40/10	95
Femoral artery	80/50	40

What is the likely pulmonary artery saturation?

With a femoral artery saturation of 40 per cent, it is likely that the aorta arises from the right ventricle. The fact that the two ventricles have such different pressures indicates that there is little or no communication between them. The pulmonary artery arises from the left ventricle, and its oxygen saturation will be less than 95 per cent, depending on how much aorta-to–pulmonary artery shunt there is through a patent ductus arteriosus.

What is the likely pulmonary artery pressure?

The pressure in the pulmonary artery can be no more than 40 mm Hg systolic and may be less if there is some mild pulmonic stenosis (pulmonary artery arises from the left ventricle).

Is there something therapeutic that can be done before completing the catheterization?

Clearly, more mixing is needed between the two sides. The safest way to accomplish this is to create an atrial septal defect using a balloon catheter. The catheter is placed into the left atrium, blown up with saline, and pulled back hard.

Is surgery resulting in normal systemic saturation possible?

Because the pulmonary artery pressure is low, pulmonary vascular disease does not develop as readily as when there is a large ventricular septal defect. Thus, the baby is an ideal candidate for corrective surgery at approximately 2–3 months of age. The surgical procedure allows the venous return to be redirected to the appropriate systemic circuit.

Case Four

A full-term baby boy (birth weight 4400 gm) was considered to be well at birth, although at examination there was a question of decrease in femoral pulses. The baby was discharged from the hospital at 5 days of age, feeding nicely. The femoral pulses were still difficult to palpate, but this finding was discounted as being common at this age, especially in chubby babies. At 3 weeks of age, the child was admitted to the hospital with respiratory difficulty. He was breathing very rapidly, was sweating profusely, and was moderately cyanotic. The liver was large, femoral pulses were absent, and the brachials were not strong. Flush pressures were 50 mm Hg in each arm and 40 mm Hg in the legs. A grade 2 short systolic ejection murmur was heard slightly better in the back than at the mid left sternal border. The x-ray showed a large heart with pulmonary venous congestion. The electrocardiogram showed right ventricular hypertrophy.

Can a diagnosis be suggested?

There are strong clues to the diagnosis of coarctation of the aorta, despite the lack of blood pressure gradient. The most important clues are that femoral pulses are absent and that the murmur is maximal in the back. (Femoral pulses can appear in the presence of coarctation of the aorta, but they are usually weaker and delayed in relation to the brachials. The murmur may also be louder anteriorly than posteriorly.)

Can you explain the lack of blood pressure gradient with the femoral pulse?

If the coarctation is severe, the blood pressure will essentially come from collaterals. However, the pulse pressure will be very narrow. For a pulse to be felt, a good pulse pressure must be present. Meanwhile, because of severe congestive heart failure, the cardiac output may be very low, and there may be insufficient ejectile force to create a high blood pressure even above the coarctation. Thus, there may be little or no systolic gradient across a severe coarctation of the aorta in the presence of congestive heart failure.

Can you explain the cyanosis?

The cyanosis is probably pulmonary caused by venous congestion secondary to left heart failure.

After digitalization and diuresis the pulses were strong in each brachial with flush pressures of 120 mm Hg. The femoral pulses remained absent with flush pressures of 60 mm Hg. The murmur in the back was louder (grade 3), and the cyanosis was no longer seen. The heart was not hyperdynamic.

Is cardiac catheterization necessary?

The diagnosis is now quite evident for simple coarctation of the aorta. There is much difference of opinion over the necessity of catheterization. The fact that the baby went into heart failure at 3 weeks of age, responded so readily, and had classic clinical findings suggests that the coarctation is likely to be isolated. However, there are some cardiologists who, knowing the poor prognosis when there is an additional lesion, insist on a cardiac catheterization to be absolutely certain. Two-dimensional echocardiography and Doppler studies can usually adequately delineate the anatomy. In view of this, and the good response to medical management that obviates immediate surgical intervention, cardiac catheterization is not indicated in this patient.

What is the prognosis with medical management?

If an isolated coarctation is present, the prognosis with medical therapy is good. Eventually, surgical correction will be required.

Case Five

A 4 day old, full-term baby boy is transferred to the intensive care nursery because of poor feeding for 2 days and recent respiratory difficulties. The child is dusky and sweating profusely and has very poor pulses. The liver is very large. The chest x-ray shows a large heart with pulmonary venous congestion. The electrocardiogram demonstrates no P waves and a ventricular rate of 300 beats/minute (see Figure 13–8). The diagnosis of supraventricular tachycardia is made.

Should a cardiology consultant be called in immediately?

A cardiac consultant cannot be depended upon exclusively for the knowledge necessary to diagnose and treat paroxysmal atrial tachycardia (PAT) of infancy. There is not likely to be time for such a luxury. When a child is admitted with congestive heart failure, it usually indicates that the supraventricular tachycardia has been constant for at least 48 hours. Death may be imminent.

Blood tests were drawn. Which test would you perform and why?

A radial arterial blood sample was obtained. The child may be quite acidotic. Furthermore, if the Po_2 is low, secondary to pulmonary venous congestion, the low Pao_2 and pH may significantly cause an increase in the pulmonary vascular resistance and depress myocardial function. Despite the congestive heart failure, it may be helpful to give sodium bicarbonate as well as oxygen.

The intern wished to start intramuscular digoxin immediately. Do you approve of this? If not, what would you do?

There is no dispute in this area. Intramuscular digoxin may be dangerous in this baby. First, this infant requires immediate conversion to sinus rhythm, and even if the digoxin was well absorbed the effects would not occur for at least 2 hours. Second, perfusion is poor, so that many hours after the dose, digoxin may still be entering the blood stream. Thus, it may be difficult to judge how much medication to give in succeeding doses. With intravenous digoxin, there is exact control as well as reliably fast action. Action begins in 10 minutes. If this is to be the initial approach (in a very ill infant, this is not our first approach—see below) half the calculated digitalizing dose (50 μg/kg) is given immediately, with the next quarter dose 1 hour later. If the rhythm has still not converted, the final quarter dose may be given in another hour. Thus, digitalization can be accomplished safely within 2 hours if necessary.

Are there other pharmacologic or manipulative avenues that should be considered first?

There are other avenues, but carotid pressure and eyeball massage are *not* included. They do not work and are dangerous. A satisfactory method of obtaining vagal action is to immerse the infant's face (holding the nose shut) in cold water for 10 seconds or, more appropriately, to apply an ice pack to the infant's face. If this is unsuccessful, intravenous verapamil might be considered as the next step. In the infant in severe distress, it is important not to prolong the duration of tachycardia unnecessarily and, if these two maneuvers are not successful, to consider cardioversion immediately. If the infant is not in severe distress, rapid intravenous digitalization is generally a prudent and successful approach.

If the baby is hypotensive, a sympathomimetic agent should be used. Isoproterenol, epinephrine, and levarterenol are contraindicated because of the high risk of ventricular fibrillation. Phenylephrine (which causes no cardiac stimulation) is preferable. Even if the baby is not hypotensive and if digitalization has not resulted in sinus rhythm, phenylephrine, to a level that raises blood pressure above normal, will usually convert the arrhythmia to sinus rhythm.

The use of other drugs, such as quinidine, procainamide (Pronestyl), or propranolol, is rarely necessary during the acute period. However, a baby will occasionally go in and out of the arrhythmia for many months. In such infants, another maintenance medication, especially propranolol, has been useful in controlling the arrhythmia.

Is there an alternative besides rapid digitalization?

The alternative treatment is that of direct current countershock (cardioversion). There are some who prefer to use this method as the one of choice, digitalizing the patient only after conversion. We prefer digitalization plus the other adjuncts as described because they are usually effective.

What chance is there that something is structurally wrong with the heart?

The vast majority of the children with supraventricular tachycardia (PAT) have nothing structurally wrong with the heart. One rule of thumb suggesting the prognosis is: when the child is a boy, there will almost invariably be nothing wrong with the heart; if the child is a girl, there is a greater chance of structural abnormality.

Is the patient likely to be prone to supraventricular arrhythmias in the future?

In the few weeks after the first episode of PAT, the rhythm may intermittently revert to abnormal in many children. In the majority of children on digoxin throughout the first year, another arrhythmia never occurs. After 1 year of age, when the digoxin is discontinued, repeat episodes of PAT are rare. It is of great interest that an occasional boy or girl with PAT will be seen to have the Wolff-Parkinson-White syndrome. We had usually expected that the prognosis in this situation was not good; however, we have been pleased to find that the Wolff-Parkinson-White syndrome also often disappears.

I would summarize the approach to the infant with supraventricular tachyarrhythmia by stating that the simple methods such as immersion in ice water be attempted first, with follow-up of cardioversion if the infant shows signs of impaired systemic perfusion. If the infant is not too ill, then one can choose between intravenous digoxin or verapamil as agents that have had a considerable degree of success in managing the arrhythmia. We have placed all of these infants on maintenance digoxin following conversion except those with the Wolff-Parkinson-White syndrome in whom we have used a beta receptor blocking agent such as propranolol. Additional points to keep in mind include correction of pH and hypothermia and having a syringe ready with a calcium ion solution to counter any deleterious effects of slow channel blocking agents (verapamil).

N. Talner

REFERENCES

General Fetal and Newborn Physiology and Pathophysiology

1. Adams, F., and Lind, J.: Physiologic studies on the cardiovascular status of normal newborn infants. with special reference to the ductus arteriosus. Pediatrics *19*:431, 1957.
2. Berman, W., Jr., and Musselman, J.: Myocardial performance in the newborn lamb. Am J Physiol *237*:H66, 1979.
3. Cassin, S.: Role of prostaglandins and thromboxanes in the control of the pulmonary circulation in the fetus and newborn. Semin Perinatol *4*:101, 1980.
4. Cassin, S.: Humoral factors affecting pulmonary blood flow in the fetus and newborn infant. *In* Peckham, G., and Heymann, M. (eds.): *Cardiovascular Sequelae of Asphyxia in the Newborn*. Report of the Eighty-third Ross Conference on Pediatric Research. Columbus, Ohio, Ross Laboratories, 1982, pp. 10–18.
5. Emery, J., and Mithal, A.: Weights of cardiac ventricles at and after birth. Br Heart J *23*:313, 1961.
6. Emmanouilides, G., and Baylen, B.: Neonatal cardiopulmonary distress without congenital heart disease. Curr Probl Pediatr IX 7:1, 1979.
7. Emmanouilides, G., Moss, A., Duffie, E., Jr., et al: Pulmonary arterial pressure changes in human newborn infants from birth to 3 days of age. J Pediatr *65*:327, 1964.
8. Friedman, W.: The intrinsic physiologic properties of the developing heart. Prog Cardiovasc Dis *15*:87, 1972.
9. Goetzman, B., and Riemenschneider, T.: Persistence of the fetal circulation. Pediatr Rev 2:37, 1980.
10. Haworth, S., and Reid, L.: Persistent fetal circulation: newly recognized structural features. J Pediatr *88*:614, 1976.
11. Heymann, M., and Rudolph, A.: Effects of congenital heart disease on the fetal and neonatal circulations. Prog Cardiovasc Dis *15*:115, 1972.
12. Klopfenstein, H., and Rudolph, A.: Postnatal changes in the circulation and responses to volume loading in sheep. Circ Res *42*:839, 1978.
13. Levin, D., Heymann, M., Kitterman, J., et al: Persistent pulmonary hypertension of the newborn infant. J Pediatr *89*:626, 1976.
14. Murphy, J., Rabinovitch, M., Goldstein, J., and Reid, L.: The structural basis of persistent pulmonary hypertension of the newborn infant. J Pediatr *98*:962, 1981.
15. Nacye, R.: Arterial changes during the perinatal period. Arch Pathol *71*:121, 1961.
16. Reid, L.: The development of the pulmonary circulation. *In* Peckham, G., and Heymann, M. (eds.): *Cardiovascular Sequelae of Asphyxia in the Newborn*. Report of the Eighty-third Ross Conference on Pediatric Research. Columbus, Ohio, Ross Laboratories, 1982, pp. 2–10.
17. Rudolph, A.: The changes in the circulation after birth: the importance in congenital heart disease. Circulation *41*:343, 1970.
18. Rudolph, A., Heymann, M., and Lewis, A.: Physiology and pharmacology of the pulmonary circulation in the fetus and newborn. *In* Hodson, W. (ed.): *Lung Biology in Health and Disease. Development of the Lung*. New York, Marcel Dekker, 1977, pp. 497–523.

General

1. Fyler, D., Buckley, L., Hellenbrand, W., et al: Report of the New England Regional Infant Cardiac Program. Pediatrics *65* (Suppl):375, 1980.
2. Fyler, D., Parisi, L., and Berman, L.: The regionalization of infant cardiac care in New England. Cardiovasc Clin *4*:339, 1972.
3. Gootman, N., Scarpelli, E., and Rudolph, A.: Metabolic acidosis in children with severe cyanotic congenital heart disease. Circulation *31*:251, 1963.
4. Krovetz, L., and Goldbloom, J.: Normal standards for cardiovascular data. II. Pressure and vascular resistances. Johns Hopkins Med J *130*:187, 1972.

5. Lambert, E., Tinglestad, J., and Hohn, A.: Diagnosis and management of congenital heart disease in the first week of life. Pediatr Clin North Am *13*:943, 1966.
6. Mitchell, S., Karones, S., and Berendes, H.: Congenital heart disease in 56,109 births: incidence and natural history. Circulation *3*:323, 1971.
7. Noonan, J.: Syndromes associated with cardiac defects. Cardiovasc Clin *11*:97, 1980.
8. Nora, J.: Etiologic factors in congenital heart disease. Pediatr Clin North Am *18*:1050, 1971.
9. Nora, J., and Nora, A.: The evolution of specific genetic and environmental counselling in congenital heart disease. Circulation *57*:205, 1978.
10. Rowe, R.: Severe congenital heart disease in the newborn infant. Diagnosis and management. Pediatr Clin North Am *17*:967, 1970.
11. Talner, N., and Ordway, N.: Acid-base balance in the newborn infant with congestive heart failure. Pediatr Clin North Am *13*:983, 1966.

Atrial Septal Defect

1. Hoffman, J., Rudolph, A., and Danilowicz, D.: Left-to-right shunts in infants. Am J Cardiol *30*:868, 1972.
2. Mody, M. R.: Serial hemodynamic observations in secundum ASD with special reference to spontaneous closure. Am J Cardiol *32*:978, 1973.
3. Wagenvoort, C., Newfeld, H., Dushane, J., et al: The pulmonary arterial tree in atrial septal defect: a quantitative study of anatomic features in fetuses, infants and children. Circulation *23*:733, 1961.
4. Weidman, W., Swan, H., Dushane, J., et al: A hemodynamic study of atrial septal defect and associated anomalies involving the atrial septum. J Lab Clin Med *50*:165, 1957.
5. Wyler, F., and Rutishauser, M.: Symptomatic atrial septal defect in the neonate and infant. Helv Paediatr Acta *30*:399, 1976.

Ventricular Septal Defect

1. Haworth, S., Sauer, U., Buhlmeyer, K., et al: Development of the pulmonary circulation in ventricular septal defect: a quantitative study. Am J Cardiol *40*:781, 1977.
2. Hoffman, J., and Rudolph, A.: Natural history of ventricular septal defects in infancy. Am J Cardiol *16*:634, 1965.
3. Sigman, J., Perry, B., Behrendt, D., et al: Ventricular septal defect: results after repair in infancy. Am J Cardiol *39*:66, 1977.
4. Wagenvoort, C., Newfeld, H., Dushane, J., et al: The pulmonary arterial tree in ventricular septal defect: a quantitative study of anatomic features in fetuses, infants and children. Circulation *23*:740, 1961.

Patent Ductus Arteriosus

1. Cassels, D.: *The Ductus Arteriosus.* Springfield, Ill. Charles C Thomas, 1973.
2. Clyman, R.: Ontogeny of the ductus arteriosus response to prostaglandins and inhibitors of their synthesis. Semin Perinatol *4*:115, 1980.
3. Clyman, R., and Heymann, M.: Pharmacology of the ductus arteriosus. Pediatr Clin North Am *28*:77, 1981.
4. Coceani, F., and Olley, P.: Role of prostaglandins, prostacyclin and thromboxanes in the control of prenatal patency and postnatal closure of the ductus arteriosus. Semin Perinatol *4*:109, 1980.

5. Danilowicz, D., Rudolph, A., and Hoffman, J.: Delayed closure of the ductus arteriosus in premature infants. Pediatrics *37*:74, 1966.
6. Heymann, M., Rudolph, A., and Silverman, N.: Closure of the ductus arteriosus in premature infants by inhibition of prostaglandin synthesis. N Engl J Med *295*:530, 1976.
7. Mahony, L., Carnero, V., Brett, C., et al: Prophylactic indomethacin therapy for patent arteriosus in very low-birth-weight infants. N Engl J Med *306*:506, 1982.
8. Siassi, B., Emmanouilides, G., Cleveland, R., et al: Patent ductus arteriosus complicating prolonged assisted ventilation in respiratory distress syndrome. J Pediatr *74*:11, 1969.
9. Siassi, B., Blanco, C., Cabal, L., et al: Incidence and clinical features of patent ductus arteriosus in low-birth-weight infants: a prospective analysis of 150 consecutively-born infants. Pediatrics *57*:347, 1976.
10. Zackman, R., Steinmetz, G., Botham, R., et al: Incidence and treatment of the patent ductus arteriosus in the ill premature neonate. Am Heart J *87*:697, 1974.

Hypoplastic Left Ventricle Syndrome

1. Deeley, W.: Hypoplastic left heart syndrome: anatomic, physiologic and therapeutic considerations. Am J Dis Child *121*:168, 1971.
2. Noonan, J., and Nadas, A.: The hypoplastic left ventricle syndrome: an analysis of 101 cases. Pediatr Clin North Am *5*:1029, 1958.
3. Saied, A., and Folger, G.: Hypoplastic left heart syndrome: clinicopathologic and hemodynamic correlation. Am J Cardiol *29*:190, 1972.
4. Strong, W., Liebman, J., and Perrin, E.: Hypoplastic left ventricle syndrome: electrocardiographic evidence of left ventricular hypertrophy. Am J Dis Child *120*:511, 1970.

Aortic Arch Anomalies

1. Becker, A., Becker, M., and Edwards, J.: Anomalies associated with coarctation of the aorta: particular reference to infancy. Circulation *441*:1067, 1970.
2. Moulaert, A., Bruins, C., and Oppenheimer-Dekker, A.: Anomalies of the aortic arch and ventricular septal defects. Circulation *53*:1011, 1976.
3. Rudolph, A., Heymann, M., and Spitznas, U.: Hemodynamic considerations in the development of narrowing of the aorta. Am J Cardiol *30*:514, 1972.
4. Sinha, S., Kardatzka, M., Cole, R., et al: Coarctation of the aorta in infancy. Circulation *40*:385, 1969.
5. Talner, N., and Berman, M.: Postnatal development of obstruction in coarctation of the aorta: role of the ductus arteriosus. Pediatrics *56*:562, 1975.

Aortic Stenosis

1. Hastreiter, A., Oshima, M., Miller, R., et al: Congenital aortic stenosis syndrome in infancy. Circulation *28*:1084, 1963.
2. Moller, J., Nakib, A., Eliot, R., et al: Symptomatic congenital aortic stenosis in the first year of life. J Pediatr *69*:728, 1968.

Hypoplastic Right Ventricle Syndrome

1. Bharati, S., McAllister, H., Tatooles, C., et al: Anatomic variations in underdeveloped right ventricle related to tricuspid atresia and stenosis. J Thorac Cardiovasc Surg *72*:383, 1976.
2. Cole, R., Muster, A., Lev, M., et al: Pulmonary

atresia with intact ventricular septum. Am J Cardiol *21*:23, 1968.

3. Freed, M., Heymann, M., Lewis, A., et al: Prostaglandin E in infants with ductus arteriosus–dependent congenital heart disease. Circulation *64*:899, 1981.

4. Lewis, A., Freed, M., Heymann, M., et al: Side effects of therapy of prostaglandin E in infants with critical congenital heart disease. Circulation *64*:893, 1981.

5. Luckstead, E., Mattioli, L., Crosby, I., et al: Two-stage palliative surgical approach for pulmonary atresia with intact ventricular septum (Type I). Am J Cardiol *29*:490, 1972.

6. Zuberbuhler, J., Allwork, S., and Anderson, R.: The spectrum of Ebstein's anomaly of the tricuspid valve. J Thorac Cardiovasc Surg *77*:202, 1979.

Transposition of the Great Arteries

1. Kawabori, I., Guntheroth, W., Morgan, B., et al: Surgical correction in infancy to reduce mortality in transposition of the great arteries. Pediatrics *60*:83, 1977.

2. Leibman, J., Cullum, L., and Belloc, N.: The natural history of transposition of the great arteries. Circulation *40*:237, 1969.

3. Levin, D., Paul, M., Master, A., et al. D-transposition of the great vessels in the neonate. Arch Int Med *137*:1421, 1977.

4. Mahony, L., Turley, K., Ebert, P., et al: Long-term results after atrial repair of transposition of the great arteries in early infancy. Circulation *66*:253, 1982.

5. Noonan, J., Nadas, A., Rudolph, A., et al: Transposition of the great arteries: a correlation of clinical, physiologic and autopsy data. N Engl J Med *263*:592, 1960.

6. Rashkind, W., and Miller, W.: Creation of an atrial septal defect without thoracotomy: a palliative approach to complete transposition of the great arteries. J Am Med Assoc *196*:991, 1966.

Total Anomalous Pulmonary Venous Return

1. Gathman, G., and Nadas, A.: Total anomalous pulmonary venous connection: clinical and physiologic observations of 75 pediatric patients. Circulation *42*:143, 1970.

2. Gersony, W., Bowman, F., Jr., Steeg, C., et al: Management of total anomalous pulmonary venous drainage in early infancy. Circulation *43* (Suppl I):19, 1971.

Truncus Arteriosus

1. Bharati, S., McAllister, H., Rosenquist, G., et al: The surgical anatomy of truncus arteriosus communis. J Thorac Cardiovasc Surg *67*:501, 1974.

2. Calder, L., van Praagh, R., van Praagh, S., et al: Truncus arteriosus communis: clinical, angiocardiographic and pathologic findings in 100 patients. Am Heart J *92*:23, 1976.

3. Crupi, G., Macartney, F., and Anderson, R.: Persistent truncus arteriosus. Am J Cardiol *40*:569, 1977.

4. Singh, A., DeLeval, M., Pincott, J., et al: Pulmonary artery banding for truncus arteriosus in the first year of life. Circulation *54* (Suppl III):17, 1976.

5. Sullivan, H., Sulayman, R., Replogle, R., et al: Surgical correction of truncus arteriosus in infancy. Am J Cardiol *38*:113, 1976.

Tetralogy of Fallot

1. Anderson, R., Allwork, S., Ho, S., et al: Surgical anatomy of tetralogy of Fallot. J Thorac Cardiovasc Surg *81*:887, 1981.

2. Ikeda, M., and Hirasawa, K.: Tetralogy of Fallot. Circulation *38* (Suppl 5):21, 1968.

Echocardiography

1. Alverson, D., Eldridge, M., Dillon, T., et al: Noninvasive pulsed Doppler determination of cardiac output in neonates and children. Pediatr *100*:46, 1982.

2. Foale, R., Stefanine, L., Rickards, A., et al: Left and right ventricular morphology in complex congenital heart disease defined by two-dimensional echocardiography. Am J Cardiol *49*:93, 1982.

3. Goldberg, S., Allen, H., and Sahn, D.: *Pediatric and Adolescent Echocardiography.* Chicago, Year Book Medical Publishers, 1980.

4. Hirschfeld, S., and Riggs, T.: Echocardiographic assessment of normal and abnormal postnatal cardiovascular adaptation. Perinatol/Neonatal *1*:35, 1977.

5. Hirschklau, M., DiSessa, T., Higgins, C., et al: Echocardiographic diagnosis: pitfalls in the premature infant with a large patent ductus arteriosus. J Pediatr *92*:474, 1978.

6. Kleinman, C., Hobbins, J., and Jaffe, C., et al: Echocardiographic studies of the human fetus. Prenatal diagnosis of congenital heart disease and cardiac dysrhythmias. Pediatrics *65*:1059, 1980.

7. Meyer, R. A.: Echocardiography in pediatric patients. Cardiovasc Clin *11*:187, 1982.

8. Rice, M., Seward, J., Hagler, D., et al: Impact of two-dimensional echocardiography on the management of distressed newborns in whom cardiac disease is suspected. Am J Cardiol *51*:288, 1983.

9. Riggs, T., Hirschfeld, S., Fanaroff, A., et al: Neonatal circulatory changes: an echo study. Pediatrics *59*:338, 1977.

10. Silverman, N., and Snider, A.: *Two-Dimensional Echocardiography in Congenital Heart Disease.* New York, Appleton-Century-Crofts, 1982.

14

The Kidney

WARREN E. GRUPE

The kidneys are commonly described as excretory organs, but the assignment of such a limited role scarcely does them justice.

R. F. PITTS
PHYSIOLOGY OF THE KIDNEY AND BODY FLUIDS
(PREFACE TO THE FIRST EDITION)

Whether or not the fetal kidney contributes any useful function prior to delivery is undetermined. Although fetal urine contributes to the formation of amniotic fluid and renal disease existing prenatally may influence development, the fetus with complete renal agenesis is not markedly altered metabolically, probably because the placenta assumes the regulatory functions in utero. All of this changes drastically postnatally, and the rapid onset of renal function, even in the premature infant, shows the functional potential of the immature kidney. The immature kidney, although capable of adjusting to normal variations, is less capable than the mature kidney of adjusting to the stresses imposed by disease, injudicious management, unrealistic expectations, or unreasonable demands.

Even if metabolically unimportant, fetal kidney function per se leads to prenatal damage of the renal parenchyma in the presence of obstruction to the urinary flow.

E. Gautier

BASIC CONSIDERATIONS[19, 28, 57, 71, 76]

Developmental Anatomy

Developmental anomalies of the genitourinary tract account for 3.5–10 per cent of

314

hospital admissions. The explanation for many lies in anomalies of embryonic development, for which the reader is referred to standard texts.

Defects during the time nephrons are forming have direct expression as developmental anomalies. For example, agenesis can result from any one of several developmental arrests. Absence of ureteric bud development leads to an absence of both kidney and ureter. If the ureteric duct fails to make contact with the metanephric blastema, a short, blind ureter with a normal bladder insertion results. If the ureteric bud enters the mesonephric tissue but there is a failure of induction and/or differentiation, the result is a nubbin of "aplastic," nonfunctioning tissue at the end of an otherwise normal ureter.

Nephrogenesis begins at 7–8 weeks of gestation and continues until the thirty-fourth to thirty-fifth week. Glomeruli form in situ from the metanephric blastema under stimulation from the dividing and invading ureteric bud. Renal growth and differentiation progress in concert with somatic growth with sufficient predictability to make examination of the glomerular zones one of the tools to measure the stage of gestation.

Developmental Physiology[2, 13, 20, 21, 38-40, 42, 47, 50, 66, 80, 88]

Renal blood flow, glomerular filtration, and tubular function do exist, but at low levels in the fetus. Urine is produced from about the twelfth gestational week through functioning but immature and developing nephrons. The loop of Henle functions by the fourteenth week, leading to a decrease in urine production despite a progressive increase in glomerular filtration rate (GFR).

Separation from the placenta, however, suddenly places increased demands on these essentially untried kidneys. Nevertheless, the immature kidney appears to function at a level that is appropriate to the infant's needs. Qualitatively, the kidneys at term appear able to perform all of the functions thus far measured. Quantitatively, especially when compared with the older child or adult, the kidneys are limited in their ability to respond promptly to abnormal stress. A marked improvement in function occurs within a few days, followed by a slower, progressive rise to essentially adult levels by the end of the first year. The pattern and rate of this postnatal improvement are similar to those of a fetus of the same conceptual age. The effective mediators of this improvement seem to be a decrease in renal vascular resistance leading to increased renal blood flow, increased glomerular filtration surface, and changes in intrarenal blood distribution. The relationship of these changes to the renin-angiotensin system, vascular response to catecholamines, and prostaglandins is inviting to surmise, though speculative. It is of interest and concern, in this regard, that drugs that interfere with renin-angiotensin (captopril), prostaglandins (indomethacin), and the adrenergic response (tolazoline) have been implicated in a decrease in renal blood flow and glomerular filtration or frank renal failure.[11, 17, 38, 98]

The progressive change in renal function is not linear.[2] Prior to 34 weeks' gestation, glomerular filtration is low, glycosuria common, and amino nitrogen excretion high. A sudden increase in glomerular filtration at 34 weeks coincides with the completion of nephrogenesis and heralds a dramatic rise in renal function. For example, the absolute glomerular filtration rate, which averaged only 0.45 ml/min before 34 weeks, doubles to 1.01 ml/min between 34 and 37 weeks, then doubles again to 2.24 ml/min after 37 weeks. During extrauterine life, functional demands may, at least in part, stimulate quantitative improvement in function. Certainly the level of function is related to both gestational age and the duration of postnatal existence.

When measured in the first 3 days of life, inulin clearance increases from 11 ml/min/1.73 m² in prematures born after 30 weeks of gestation to 20 ml/min/1.73 m² in babies born at term. In both groups, inulin clearance will double in the first 2 postnatal weeks. **E. Gautier**

GLOMERULAR FUNCTION

Premature infants fed a high protein diet increase GFR faster than controls. In the young rat, such an increase can also be stimulated with albumin, globulin, casein, and glycine, but not urea; the effect of salt is variable. Compensatory hypertrophy does not occur until after birth.

However, infants with a single kidney usually have enlargement of that kidney at birth. This must represent some kind of prenatal hypertrophy. **W. Weil, Jr.**

Previous studies have shown depressed reabsorption of amino acids, phosphate, and glucose and a decreased ability to excrete hydrogen ion and to secrete paraaminohippuric acid (PAH). Although designated as glomerulotubular imbalance, this may be more related to experimental conditions. For example, glomerulotubular balance for glucose is present in every infant, when appropriately studied, regardless of gestational age or the duration of extrauterine life. When appropriately controlled, studies have shown levels of glomerulotubular balance approaching adult levels for both solute and water. Recent anatomic and animal data would also suggest that concern over glomerulotubular imbalance deserves reexamination.

The relative immaturity of the neonatal nephron quantitatively limits its response to changing loads. An example is the infant's limited capacity to tolerate abrupt changes in *sodium* intake. Although the infant is limited in his response to either an increase or a decrease in sodium intake, his ability to handle excess is particularly limited. This quantitative response appears operative over a reasonably broad range; infants ordinarily muster enough to excrete the sodium in proprietary formulae that approach three times the load of human milk.[97] Challenged by practices of early feeding of solids, they can defend against a load ten times that of human milk. However, the renal response to a sodium load is slow, so that balance is achieved only after significant expansion of extracellular fluid volume, which is 45 per cent of body weight as compared with only 20 per cent in the adult. This suggests that the immature control system responds only to large changes in volume. The neonate has a reduced operating reserve with which to meet stresses in excess of normal; the "safety zone" is further reduced by both acute and chronic changes in exogenous sodium load.

Once stimulated, the direction of the qualitative response is normal. It is the reduced quantitative response that renders the infant more vulnerable to a sodium load, much like that seen in older patients with renal insufficiency. Conversely, the very immature nephron has a high fractional excretion of sodium with a limited capacity to retain sodium when faced with sodium deprivation.

This should be stressed: the greater the degree of prematurity, the higher the risk of a negative sodium balance in the first 10 days of life and sometimes for several weeks thereafter if sodium intake is less than 3–4 mEq/kg/24 hr. Because hyponatremia is mostly asymptomatic in the premature, one must closely monitor the sodium blood level and adapt the intake to the needs of each individual case. This high fractional excretion of sodium results from an incapacity of reabsorption in the proximal tubule in relation to a small surface of reabsorption, a low concentration of Na/K ATPase in the membrane, and possibly unresponsiveness to aldosterone.

E. Gautier

Functional limits also render the immature infant less capable of excreting water loads or of concentrating the urine to conserve *water*. There appears to be incomplete development of the control mechanism, since a young animal ceases to excrete a water load before it has all been eliminated. Recent evidence would suggest this limit rests more with the slower intestinal absorption of water than with the kidney's inability to excrete.

Faced with water deprivation, the maximum urine osmolality reached by the newborn is around 750 mOsm/l. The major limitation here seems not to be immaturity but the smaller number of osmoles (particularly urea) excreted in the urine, reflecting the powerful anabolic state that the demands of growth create.

Altering the rate of urea excretion by feeding urea or high protein diets to newborns increases their ability to concentrate the urine. This is not without some risk, since high protein diets are in some way irritating to the immature kidney, producing cylindruria, proteinuria, and acidosis in some infants.

The influence of renal immaturity on the *reabsorption of bicarbonate* or the excretion of hydrogen ion has also been noted. During the first few days of life, the normal newborn may not be able to attain a urine pH below 6.0. Infants in general maintain a normal blood pH and a lower concentration of plasma bicarbonate and have a reduced capacity to excrete a strongly acidic urine. Although several factors play a role, a renal threshold for bicarbonate as low as 20 mEq/l in young infants appears important: the bicarbonate reabsorptive tubular maximum is set at a lower threshold than in the older child and adult, due in part to nephron heterogeneity. During the first 4–6 weeks of life, infants also excrete less ammonium in their urine in response to an ammonium chloride load than do older children. When corrected for glomerular filtration rate, however, these differences become less apparent. Under usual circumstances, the lower blood bicarbonate is dependent not as much on the limitations of hydrogen ion excretion as on the limited ability to reabsorb bicarbonate.

In summary, the immature kidney has the capability to respond appropriately under stress. The control mechanisms for these homeostatic operations do exist and respond qualitatively but are sluggish and require greater stimuli to initiate a response that may be quantitatively limited. Current data suggest that glomerulotubular balance exists. Where functions do not appear up to adult standards, they are in general still appropriate to the infant's normal needs.

The process of growth, with its strong anabolic drive, assists the kidney by reducing the excretory load of sodium, water, phosphorus, hydrogen, and nitrogen. By the same token, however, the limited ability of the same kidney to concentrate urine is in part due to the small amount of urea available for excretion. It is worthwhile remembering that the anabolic state reverses promptly when growth is altered by acute illness, thereby increasing the demands to excrete at a time when the kidney is possibly less able to respond quantitatively.

Renal immaturity also limits the newborn's ability to excrete drugs. The bulk of most pharmacologic agents administered to the newborn is excreted by the kidney. Dosage schedules should take this into account. The plasma half-life of such commonly used drugs as the penicillins, aminoglycosides, polymyxins, barbiturates, and digoxin varies inversely with creatinine clearance.[59] The clearance of penicillin G is one fifth that of the adult, and blood levels persist three times as long.[60] Although tubular secretion is more important in excreting the penicillin analogues in the older child, glomerular filtration is more important in the neonate. The newborn's limited ability to elaborate an acid urine can also impede excretion of weak bases.

The more immature the infant, the more limited the excretory capacity for drugs. This is of particular importance for the infant between 25 and 34 conceptual weeks. The plasma half-life for ampicillin is 4.7–6.2 hours in the premature and 3.1–4.7 hours in the full-term infant in the first 3 days. For methicillin, the half-life is 3 times longer in the premature than in the term infant and twice as long for carbenicillin. The serum half-life of intravenous trimethoprim-sulfamethoxazole in normal newborn infants approaches that seen in uremic adults.[90] The serum level of digoxin, on the same maintenance dose per kg, is 4.4 times higher in an infant of < 1000 gm than in an infant of 2500 gm. The half-life for gentamicin, which is 5 hours in the term neonate, may be greater than 1 week in the premature. Knowledge of the renal clearance will not only dictate alteration of the dose but the frequency of administration for these drugs as well.

As renal function also varies with postnatal age, the same relationship exists in patterns of drug excretion, so that the capability increases with postnatal age, irrespective of gestational age. The plasma half-life for penicillin G is 2.3 times as great in the first 6 days of life as it is after 2 weeks; 2 times as great for ampicillin, gentamicin, and carbenicillin; 1.3 times as great for kanamycin; and 4 times as great for methicillin.

These neonatal differences in the renal handling of drugs have a number of important clinical implications. Penicillin G can thus be given as crystalline penicillin on a q/12 hr regimen in the newborn to obtain the same kind of long-acting effect as one gets with procaine penicillin in the older child and adult. The toxicity of chloramphenicol, however, is in part related to such poor renal handling, which provides one of the reasons (along with hepatic immaturity) for the toxicity of this agent in producing the "gray syndrome" in the neonate. **L. Stern**

These limits can be further altered by adverse conditions. Asphyxia can reduce GFR,[21, 22, 40] renal plasma flow, and hence drug excretion; for example, the plasma half-life for amikacin is doubled in hypoxia. Patients with reduced renal function should have the dosage schedule of renal-excreted drugs altered proportionally to the decrease in renal excretory capacity. The drugs themselves can be nephrotoxic, with methicillin, oxacillin, nafcillin, gentamicin, kanamycin, streptomycin, bacitracin, neomycin, cephalo-thin, and amphotericin B being commonly used antibiotics on the list.

VASOACTIVE SUBSTANCES[11, 17, 25, 35, 41, 48, 89, 94, 98]

The role of vasoactive substances in the modulation of glomerular function, renal blood flow, or intrarenal blood distribution is not clear. If, as some have shown,[42] vascular resistance rather than glomerular surface area or permeability is the factor limiting glomerular filtration in the neonate, changes or imbalances in vasoactive products could be important mediators. The renin-angiotensin system, for example, is very active in the newborn; plasma renin activity and renin substrate are regularly higher in the term newborn when compared with the older child or the normal adult. The fetus produces renin as early as 17 weeks' gestation. In the preterm infant, the plasma levels increase dramatically in the early postnatal days. Thereafter, levels fall gradually over the next 3–6 weeks to plasma levels that are still higher than those in the normal adult. The postnatal fall in renin activity does not appear to be directly related to an increasing sodium intake. However, other data show a close relationship between the renin-angiotensin system and sodium status in the low-birth-weight premature infant, to the extent that sodium supplementation prevents the postnatal increase in plasma renin activity, plasma aldosterone, and urinary aldosterone excretion. This may have therapeutic implications for preterm infants on breast milk or low solute formulae. Inhibition of the renin-angiotensin system may not improve glomerular function or renal plasma flow in the normal newborn. Yet saralasin, an inhibitor of angiotensin II, can prevent the fall in GFR produced by hypoxia in experimental animals, while captopril, an inhibitor of the converting enzyme, does not. Captopril, however, has been associated with fetal anuria when given to the mother.

Levels of prostaglandins and prostacyclin are elevated also in the neonate and gradually decline with postnatal age. These hormones may influence vascular resistance either directly or indirectly by stimulating renin production. Some animal data have implicated prostaglandins in the regulation of renal function and the control of sodium excretion. Interference of prostaglandin synthesis with indomethacin often decreases glomerular filtration, increases the filtration fraction, and lowers urine output. This effect is by no means universal, however—many studies show no effect on renal hemodynamics or function.

In situations characterized by increased vasoconstrictor activity—for example, sodium/volume depletion or congestive heart failure—renal function becomes more dependent upon vasodilator prostaglandins. Under these circumstances, indomethacin may depress renal function to a greater extent.   **J. Stork**

Some data have suggested an increased sensitivity of the neonatal vascular bed to catecholamines, and several studies have noted an increase in blood levels of epinephrine and norepinephrine in newborns. Experimental data demonstrate an increase in the number and the affinity of catecholamine receptors in the outer cortex of the immature kidney. Tolazoline, an alpha-adrenergic blocker that is a partial agonist, can produce oliguria and a fall in glomerular filtration.

The interacting mechanisms and mediators that physiologically modify renal vascular resistance in the neonate are not yet clear. Nevertheless, the general increase in the activity of vasomotor systems in the neonate has diagnostic and therapeutic implications for the physician.

ACUTE RENAL INSUFFICIENCY[20, 22, 56, 69, 79, 98]

Altered renal function can be quite common in an intensive care nursery; in one series in a children's hospital, it was detected in 23 per cent of admissions.[69] In most instances, renal insufficiency occurs within 48 hours of life and is associated with major perinatal complications. Hypoperfusion, associated with hypoxia and hypovolemia, is the most frequent cause in the nursery. In fact, reports since 1976 regularly emphasize the role of the respiratory distress syndrome, perinatal anoxia, hemorrhage, sepsis, shock, pneumonia, and meconium aspiration. Vascular accidents and incompletely corrected hypoperfusion are the most prevalent reasons for parenchymal injury, although nephrotoxic drugs are gaining in importance. Disseminated intravascular coagulation, usually secondary to sepsis or systemic disease, is another important cause. Congenital abnormalities of the genitourinary tract, with or without obstruction, also maintain an important etiologic position. Delayed micturition may be mistaken for anuria or oliguria.[18, 64]

Measurements of the electrolyte composition of the urine seem to be the most sensitive diagnostic tests to distinguish between hypoperfusion and parenchymal injury; these include urinary sodium concentration, urine/plasma sodium, urine/plasma creatinine, and fractional excretion of sodium. The fractional excretion of sodium offers the best discrimination, with sodium excretion in excess of 2.5–3 per cent most likely representing parenchymal injury and an excretion below 1 per cent almost always indicating hypoperfusion. Obstructive uropathy usually has indices suggestive of parenchymal injury; thus, radiologic investigation is important in almost all of these infants.

Ultrasound studies for renal size, shape, and position and cystography are generally more valuable than intravenous pyelography in the newly born infant.   **W. Weil, Jr.**

Infants in whom renal failure is the first sign of a congenital or obstructive uropathy often demonstrate congenital malformation of other organ systems.

Treatment is dictated by the degree, not the etiology, of the renal failure. Problems that require urgent attention are hyperkalemia, hypoxia, severe hypovolemia, circulatory collapse, metabolic acidosis, hypertension, hypocalcemia, and osmolar disequilibrium. Hypovolemia, if present, should be carefully corrected over a 1–3 hour period, usually intravenously. In one series, this alone improved function in 70 per cent of infants.[69] A lack of response to adequate fluid and electrolyte replacement is strong evidence of parenchymal injury. In these instances, fluid maintenance should be reduced to match urine output, insensible losses, gastrointestinal losses, losses through surgical drains, endogenous water of oxidation, and preformed water. Change in weight is still the most reliable measure of overall fluid balance. Sodium balance is usually maintained with less than 1 mEq/kg/day. Because of the risk of hyperkalemia, administered fluids should be potassium free until the infant's need for additional potassium is firmly established. Metabolic acidosis, unresponsive to improved peripheral perfusion and correction of anoxia, can be treated with a bicarbonate source; since this usually means sodium-containing agents, the amount of sodium must be included in calculations of sodium balance. Starvation increases protein catabolism and contributes to urea generation, endogenous water production, hyperkalemia, acidosis, and hyperphosphatemia;

this is thwarted only by the provision, orally or parenterally, of adequate calories as carbohydrate or fat. Medications that are metabolized or excreted by the kidneys should have dosage schedules modified proportional to the degree of renal failure. Dialysis therapy, both hemodialysis and peritoneal dialysis, is possible in the neonate. The indications for dialysis include irreversible hyperkalemia, intractable fluid overload, uncontrolled severe acidosis, unchecked hyper- or hyponatremia, and encephalopathy.

Peritoneal dialysis is generally to be preferred because it is effective, especially in fluid overload, and it is less likely to disturb precarious hemodynamic balance.

W. Weil, Jr.

Acute renal failure still has an unsatisfactory prognosis in the neonate, despite sophisticated technology. Only 23 per cent of infants recover completely. This is usually because the infants have more than one life-threatening clinical problem. Thus, therapeutic effort toward the primary conditions may be at least as valuable as management of the renal failure. In fact, early therapy of the primary clinical problem to prevent the development of renal insufficiency may have more life-saving potential.

PRACTICAL CONSIDERATIONS

The Physical Examination

Inspection and palpation of the abdomen of the newborn are more easily accomplished during the first 24 hours of life, since muscle tone is minimal. Two methods of palpation have become widely applied to the neonate.[65, 73] Each takes only 30 seconds. The first starts with the palpating hand in the upper quadrant while the other hand supports the flank. The palpating hand moves medially to encounter the lower pole of the kidney, then to the midline, then sweeps through the lower quadrant. The process is repeated on the opposite side. Finally, hands placed on each flank are compressed medially to allow the abdominal contents to pass between the opposing fingers to detect a freely movable mass. The second method differs mainly in the use of the thumb as the probing appendage. In this method, the flank is grasped by the palpating hand with the fingers behind, while the thumb explores all portions of the abdomen using gentle pressure to oppose thumb and fingers.

Normally, the lower pole of both kidneys can be palpated. The bladder is also normally percussed or palpated a few centimeters above the symphysis. It is often difficult to identify the newborn bladder because of its very thin wall, unless percussion is used. Persistent distention of the bladder may be due to congenital urinary tract obstruction. *The vast majority of all palpable abdominal masses in the newborn are renal in origin.*

The importance of considering the kidney in any palpable abdominal mass in the newborn cannot be overestimated. It has been our experience that between 90 and 95 per cent of such masses are either renal or renal-related. This figure is even higher than that given by the author in a later case discussion (see p. 325).   **L. Stern**

Congenital absence of the abdominal musculature (prune-belly syndrome)[71, 82] can be diagnosed at birth. The characteristic appearance is a wrinkling and atonicity of the abdominal wall (hence the name), with the abdomen usually bulged and the flanks flaccid and limp. This is associated with both abnormalities of testicular descent and a variety of underlying genitourinary defects, including hydroureter, hydronephrosis, megacystis, renal dysplasia, and patent urachus; other associated abnormalities include imperforate anus, malrotation of the colon, rib cage abnormalities, cardiovascular abnormalities, and lower limb defects. The presence of urethral obstruction evidently defines a particularly poor prognosis. The infant is invariably male, although rare case reports of females do exist.

Although the appearance of the umbilical cord at birth is often deceiving, the presence of remnants of the urachus in the cord should be determined. Any discharge from an otherwise normal-appearing cord should arouse suspicion of a patent urachus, particularly a moist cord that does not appear to be separating. The fluid discharge from such a cord may be present at birth, appear within the first few days, or be delayed several weeks. Examination of the fluid shows all the characteristics of urine, particularly an elevated specific gravity. Radiopaque dye injected into a urachus will outline the urachal tract and enter the bladder. Occasionally, a cystogram or ultrasonography will demonstrate the tract along the anterior abdominal wall. Surgical excision provides the most successful therapy.

Edema often indicates a cardiac or renal disorder, although an etiology is not always identified. Ascites[33] in the newborn is associated with urinary tract obstruction in a high percentage of cases. Obstruction is usually confined to the lower urinary tract and is often a posterior urethral obstruction. The ascites is usually due to rupture in the collecting system. Hydrometrocolpos and megacystis can be easily confused with ascites. The differential diagnosis of ascites in the neonatal period includes hemolytic disease of the newborn, peritonitis, severe congestive heart failure, thoracic duct obstruction, hepatoportal venous obstruction, and anomalies of the urinary tract. Infants with ascites may present with severe abdominal distension, producing respiratory distress that can be an immediate threat to life. Conditions producing severe abdominal distension that may mimic ascites include meconium peritonitis, intestinal obstruction, intraabdominal tumors, and ileus. Edema of the abdominal wall is often present with fluid in the peritoneal cavity. Ascites may also appear within a few days of birth in congenital nephrotic syndrome. Detailed investigation is important in the presence of ascites, including complete evaluation of the urinary tract.

The detection of congenital anomalies is a major concern, particularly those that may obstruct urine outflow. Associated physical abnormalities—such as imperforate anus, abnormal ears, aniridia, microcephaly, meningomyelocele, pneumomediastinum, unexplained pneumothorax, hemihypertrophy, absent abdominal muscles, persistent urachus, ascites, bony abnormalities, lower limb deformities, and hypertension—can alert the physician to underlying renal defects. In the male, if the meatus can be visualized, phimosis does not exist. An opening on the ventral surface of the penis denotes hypospadias; an opening on the dorsal surface is epispadias. Both can be associated with abnormalities of the upper urinary tract. It should be determined whether the testes are at the external inguinal ring or in the scrotum. Hypospadias[54, 58] and cryptorchidism, either alone or together, may be an expression of intersexuality as well as indicative of other major genitourinary malformations. An infant with cryptorchidism, ambiguous genitalia, or hypospadias should be investigated with chromosome karyotype, buccal smear, intravenous pyelogram, and estimations of urinary 17-ketosteroids and 17-hydroxycorticosteroids. Intersexuality tends to occur in those infants with the more severe degrees of hypospadias. First-degree hypo-

spadias, in which the meatus is at the base of the glans, is much less likely to have associated abnormalities. In hypospadias, the remnant hood of foreskin should not be removed, since it can be useful in later surgical procedures. Abnormal external genitalia have been reported in males as a presenting sign of hydantoin embryopathy syndrome.

Abnormalities of the female external genitalia should also be sought. Hydrometrocolpos, detected as a bulge of the perineum through which a bluish discoloration can be seen, occurs in the absence of the usual small openings in the hymen.[43] This can be associated with a lower abdominal cystic mass—the distended uterus—which can easily be confused with a distended bladder. A ureterocele can sometimes be detected protruding through the urethral meatus of a crying child. The presence of a urogenital sinus should raise questions of intersexuality. X-ray visualization with radiopaque dye in the sinus, urethroscopy, and ultrasonography may help distinguish the origins of a single perineal opening and the nature of the internal organs.

A composite of clinical characteristics that have come to be associated with a variety of severe, irreversible abnormalities of the kidney was recognized by Potter in association with bilateral renal agenesis.[76, 83] These anomalies, which include bilateral dysplasia, hypoplasia, multicystic dysplasia, and aplasia, are incompatible with life. Recognition of these characteristics at birth discourages the multitude of surgical and investigative procedures that may ensue. The appearance, usually in a male, is of widely spaced eyes flanking a depressed nasal bridge and retroussé nose with a very prominent fold arising from the epicanthus and progressing inferiorly then laterally beneath the eyes. The chin is receded, and the face is prematurely senile in appearance. The ears are posteriorly rotated, asymmetric, floppy, and low-set. Oligohydramnios is often present by history, and the placenta is abnormal. A report of twins, one of whom had bilateral agenesis, suggests that the facial, limb, pulmonary, and skin abnormalities in this syndrome are due to the oligohydramnios, which itself is a function of decreased or absent fetal urine output.[57] Associated abnormalities include imperforate anus, hydrocephalus, meningomyelocele, skeletal anomalies (including hypoplasia of the pelvis), abnormalities of the lower extremities, and hypoplasia of the lungs. The infants fail to pass urine. Not all die in uremia, as might be expected; many die with cyanosis and dyspnea or pneumothorax resulting from the lung abnormality before uremia can intercede. Recent family studies, using ultrasonography, disclosed that 11 per cent of parents and first-degree relatives of these infants had nonlethal malformations of either metanephric or müllerian duct derivatives.[83] Siblings with Potter's syndrome were noted on two occasions in this survey.

In her original descriptions Potter indicates an association in approximately 70 per cent of cases between pulmonary hypoplasia and renal agenesis. Two points are clinically important from this association. It has been our experience that virtually all of the cases of Potter's syndrome have presented initially as bilateral pneumothorax occurring at birth or shortly thereafter when resuscitation is attempted. Spontaneous pneumothorax, especially if bilateral, is unusual so early after birth, and its occurrence in the immediate postnatal period should always give rise to the suspicion of and the search for the other features that are characteristic of renal agenesis.

In addition, we have observed the occurrence of pneumothoraces, often unilateral and often only detected at autopsy if the chest is opened under water, associated with a variety of other renal malformations of varying degrees.

Mauer, S., Dobrin, R., and Vernier, R.: Unilateral and bilateral renal agenesis in monoamniotic twins. J Pediatr *84*:236, 1974.

L. Stern

URINALYSIS[2, 20, 29, 46, 63, 68, 78]

Evaluation of the urine must be considered part of the physical examination of a child who is suspected of having a urinary tract abnormality. It is also a useful tool in the evaluation of the general status of the infant. Twenty-five per cent of males and seven per cent of females void at birth. Although 98 per cent of infants void in the first 30 hours, a delay in urination for as long as 48 hours should not be a cause for immediate concern in the absence of palpable bladder, and manipulative or radiographic procedures are not necessary.[18, 64] Preterm infants and infants of diabetic mothers tend to void earlier (see Appendix G–5). Urinary retention has been associated with hypoxia, the use of ephedrine, and hypoperfusion of otherwise normal kidneys, followed by parenchymal disease such as agenesis, vascular accidents, nephrosis, or nephritis. Posterior urethral valves are the most common cause of obstruction in the male, with ureterocele the most common in the female (see Chapter 6).

Under normal circumstances, little urine is produced during the first few days of life, with as little as 30–60 ml during the first 48 hours considered normal. Urine output, however, may be diminished in infants with severe disease, such as cardiac failure, dehydration, respiratory distress syndrome, or asphyxia, and might be expected to increase coincident with clinical improvement. The normal newborn urine is usually quite pale in color, almost clear. However, clouds of urates may be present. Increasing amounts of conjugated bilirubin can produce a yellow-brown to deep olive-green color. Porphyrins, drugs, and urate crystals may stain the diaper pink and be confused with bleeding. A benzidine test on the diaper can distinguish between hemoglobin and other red hues.[78] Urine that contains old blood, hemosiderin, or myoglobin is characteristically brown.

Specific gravity of neonatal urine is often persistently low (less than 1.004) but may be factitiously elevated by high molecular weight solutes, such as radiographic dye, sugars, or protein. Osmolarity is a more representative measure of the kidney's concentrating abilities. In the absence of extraneous solute, however, there is ordinarily a good correlation between specific gravity and osmolarity. Specific gravity can be measured on as little as two drops of urine, using the small clinical refractometers now available. Maximum concentrating ability of the premature is approximately 750 mOsm (specific gravity 1.018). Occasionally, a full-term infant's urine may reach as high as 1000 mOsm (specific gravity 1.025). This relatively limited concentrating capacity influences the infant's ability to tolerate restricted intake or excessive insensible fluid losses. Under these circumstances, urinary volume then becomes a more useful parameter of hydration than specific gravity. In older children, the specific gravity increases markedly with water deprivation, whereas in young infants it may not.

Persistent proteinuria must be considered pathologic until proved otherwise.[2, 46] Proteinuria may be seen with asphyxia, cardiac failure, massive doses of penicillin, dehydration, or fever or in the presence of x-ray contrast media. Massive proteinuria usually indicates a glomerular injury. Normally 95 per cent of infants have trace or negative tests for protein using qualitative reagent strips; one report found proteinuria in less than 1 per cent of newborns after removal of urates from the urine. Highly alkaline urine may cause a false-positive test for protein when reagent strips are used and a false-negative for protein with sulfosalicylic acid or heat and acetic acid. Quantitative amounts of protein vary with gestational age.[2, 46] Protein excretion averages 0.9 mg/hr/m² in infants at 28 weeks' gestation, rising to 2.5 mg/hr/m² by 34 weeks, then falling to 1.3 mg/hr/m² by 40 weeks. Only 12 per cent of infants excrete more than 96 mg/m²/day of protein. Albumin is the most abundant plasma protein in the urine. Persistent massive proteinuria in a newborn should alert one to consider congenital nephrotic syndrome. Transient intrarenal obstruction has been reported, apparently the result of intratubular obstruction from precipitated Tamm-Horsfall protein; acute renal failure may rarely occur.

Glycosuria is unusual.[2, 13] When the blood glucose is below 100 mg/dl, no infant above 34 gestational weeks and only 13 per cent younger than 34 weeks should have glucose detected by reagent strips. This is because only 93 per cent of the filtered glucose is absorbed in the infants below 34 weeks, while the fraction increases to 99.2 per cent after 34 weeks. Glycosuria can be a manifestation of a proximal tubular defect, often accompanied by phosphaturia and amino aciduria. Initiation of formula feedings might increase both phosphorus and amino acid excretion.

Urinary Sediment

CELLS. Cells in the urine can come from anywhere in the genitourinary tract; their origin may be difficult to determine. Specimens collected in the usual adhesive bag, particularly from females, often have white cell contamination from the perineum or vagina. Very often, when female infants void while supine, the urine contains vaginal washings.

HEMATURIA.[29, 63] Hematuria (> 2–3 red cells per centrifuged HPF) may be seen with blood dyscrasia, infections, neoplasia, stones, trauma, congenital malformations, disseminated intravascular coagulation, nephrotoxic drugs, renal vascular thrombosis, cortical or medullary necrosis, obstructive uropathy, or neonatal asphyxia. Hemoglobinuria has been noted in erythroblastosis fetalis. The presence of red blood cell casts indicates a glomerular irritation. Hematuria occurs at a rate of 0.2/1000 admissions in the first month of life, and its occurrence calls for urgent investigation. Renal vein thrombosis must be particularly considered after traumatic delivery and is more common in infants of diabetic mothers and in those infants with cyanotic congenital heart disease or marked dehydration.

Editorial Comment: Asphyxia remains the most common cause of hematuria in the neonatal period.

PYURIA.[68] Pyuria (> 3–5 white cells per centrifuged HPF) is most commonly associated with urinary tract infection but can come from anywhere in the genitourinary tract as a manifestation of irritation. Pyuria can be seen with glomerular injury, tubular disease, acidosis, interstitial nephritis, dehydration, or following instrumentation. It occurs in only 2 per cent of normal newborn males and 6 per cent of normal newborn females.[27] White blood cell casts are always an indication of renal parenchymal irritation.

CASTS. Casts are the only definitive evidence of upper renal involvement. Red blood cell casts are most commonly seen in glomerular injury. White blood cell casts, however, may be seen with infection, interstitial injury, or renal inflammation. Epithelial cell casts are seen with tubular or interstitial injury. Broad casts are seen with tubular ectasia and destruction. Granular casts are usually partially decomposed cellular casts. They can be seen, however, in dehydration, interstitial injury, or tubular injury.

Urine Collection

Collection of an adequate, uncontaminated urine specimen is extremely difficult in the neonate. The so-called clean voided specimen obtained by cleaning the perineum and applying a sterile adhesive plastic bag may give erroneous results. The technical problems of bladder catheterization in the neonate are real, and the reliability of this specimen is no greater than that of a clean voided specimen, particularly for bacteriologic evaluation. In these circumstances, a suprapubic bladder aspiration may solve many problems and avoid unnecessary instrumentation and study. It is a rapid procedure, subjects the infant to no more distress than a venipuncture, and greatly reduces the chance of contamination of the urine specimen or of the bladder. It is indicated in any infant when urinary tract infection is suspected, particularly when the results of several clean voided specimens are confusing or conflicting. It may also be considered as the initial means of collecting urine for culture in seriously ill infants or in suspected septicemia when delaying the start of antibiotics could be hazardous. When a child is on antibiotics, it is hard to determine whether minimal growth in the urine is due to urethral contamination or represents a persistent low-grade infection; sterile urine by suprapubic aspiration would indicate successful therapy, whereas any growth must be interpreted as persistent infection and so treated. Suprapubic bladder aspiration is also useful in the diagnosis or exclusion of infection in the urinary tract in the presence of vulvovaginitis, urethritis, or balanoposthitis, particularly since catheterization from below is contraindicated because of the increased risk of contamination of the bladder. Suprapubic bladder aspiration is the method of choice whenever contamination appears to be unavoidable, as it often is in the newborn, or when standard techniques have given confusing results.

SUPRAPUBIC BLADDER ASPIRATION.[67, 68] The procedure we use is as follows: In neonates, the bladder is already an abdominal organ easily palpated or percussed. The infant is placed supine and held in a frog-leg position (Figure 14–1). We make no attempt to resist outflow by compressing the penis in the male or the urethra via a rectal digit in the female, although some feel this is important. The lower abdomen is prepared with alcohol sponge or other suitable antiseptic, as for a venipuncture. The symphysis pubis is located with the index finger of the free hand. We use a 5–10 ml syringe with a No. 22 1-inch disposable needle to puncture the abdomen in the midline, about 1.5–2 cm above the symphysis. In many newborns, a transverse lower abdominal skin crease just above the symphysis provides an excellent landmark. The needle is angled about 30° from the perpendicular, toward the fundus, and advanced into the bladder. Minimal negative pressure will aspirate the required volume of urine, and the needle is withdrawn. Pressure until skin bleeding stops is the only dressing required.

In reports now numbering in the thousands, suprapubic bladder aspiration has proved a safe, easy procedure with fewer complications than catheterization. One can anticipate success in over 90 per cent of attempts, with practice. There are only two contraindications to the procedure: (1) an empty bladder, as evidenced by a wet diaper or a reliable history of voiding within 30 minutes; and (2) dilated loops of bowel, from obstruction, ileus, or inflammation. There are very few complications. Transient gross hematuria lasting less than 24 hours (often present on only one void) occurs in about 0.5 per cent of infants. We have had no patients require transfusion or surgical intervention.

RADIOLOGIC EVALUATION[12, 28, 34, 36, 51, 62, 96, 100]

Radiologic evaluation of the genitourinary tract in the newborn can be more difficult than in the older child but is clearly of value. Given the poor ability of a newborn to concentrate the urine and the relatively low glomerular filtration rate, visualization is not always adequate when standard intravenous pyelography (IVP) is performed. However, pyelography can be successful in any infant who can attain a creatinine urine/plasma ratio in excess of 15. Poor visualization can often be overcome by using 3 ml/kg of 25 per cent diatrizoate as a single injection or by utilizing the infusion pyelography technique with 6 ml/kg of diatrizoate. Contrast agents are not totally benign and have been implicated in episodes of renal insufficiency, tubular obstruction, and parenchymal necrosis. It is probably best to perform these studies in a well-hydrated infant.

The time sequence is prolonged in the normal neonate, with the nephrogram phase more persistent and the pyelogram phase

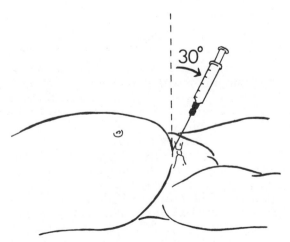

Figure 14–1. Suprapubic bladder aspiration.

more delayed than in the older child. The pyelogram provides information both by excretion and by total body opacification. Since over 75 per cent of neonatal abdominal masses are avascular or cystic lesions, the negative shadow during total body opacification is helpful in alerting us to hydronephrosis, multicystic renal dysplasia, polycystic kidneys, ovarian cysts, and renal vein thrombosis. A unilateral nonfunctioning kidney by pyelography usually means multicystic dysplasia or renal vein thrombosis. Delayed films or ultrasonography is essential, however, to distinguish hydronephrosis from these other lesions. A thin crescent of renal parenchyma during the nephrogram phase is the image of hydronephrosis even before the calyces and pelvis become visualized. Radially arranged, nonopacified shadows early in the IVP that later fill as dilated tubules suggest infantile polycystic kidney disease. An intravenous urogram or ultrasonogram together with a voiding cystourethrogram is indicated in any infant, boy or girl, with the first documented urinary tract infection.

Because reflux is common in obstructive disease, a cystogram probably should be done before the pyelogram in newborn infants.   **W. Weil, Jr.**

Radionuclide scanning provides both anatomic and functional data. Information about size, shape, location, vascular integrity, blood flow, parenchymal function, and obstruction can be obtained even when conventional urography is contraindicated or unsuccessful. Assessment of each kidney's individual contribution to renal function can also be made by radionuclide techniques.[44, 74] Most experience has been with technetium-labeled materials.

Ultrasonography[12, 96] has the advantage of being noninvasive, not requiring radioactive materials, and not requiring either blood flow or renal function. It has been increasingly successful in the differentiation of cystic, solid and complex masses, evaluation of the "nonfunctioning" kidney, delineation of free fluid from loculated fluid, measurement of size, confirmation of position or absence of organs, percutaneous renal biopsy, and evaluation of the bladder and genital tract. Ultrasonography is particularly useful for distinguishing between hydronephrosis, multicystic renal dysplasia, and renal vein thrombosis. It may be the only procedure necessary for the diagnosis of multicystic dysplasia and the most reliable way to differentiate ureteropelvic obstruction from ureterovesical obstruction. Antenatal ultrasonography is discovering urinary tract abnormalities with increasing frequency.[62]

EVALUATION OF RENAL FUNCTION[2, 13, 17, 20, 31, 38, 39, 50, 66, 70, 91-93]

The accurate estimation of the glomerular filtration rate by standard creatinine clearance in neonates and infants is difficult and often virtually impossible, owing largely to incomplete or inaccurate urine collections. When properly done, however, the results are reliable. Investigations have shown that a clearance can be calculated from the plasma disappearance curve of a substance handled such as inulin, if the data are calculated according to a multicompartmental analysis. Such methods have been developed, using sodium iothalamate, Cr-EDTA, and Tc-DTPA.[44, 74] A constant infusion technique with inulin has been adapted to infants as young as 25 weeks' gestation.[50] Because of unequal distribution in the small infant, all of these methods tend to overestimate the glomerular filtration rate. However, since they require no urine collection, their usefulness in the standard nursery more than offsets their minor differences with the classic inulin technique. These methods should be considered when inconsistent results are obtained with standard creatinine clearances.

Although these tests have clinical usefulness, in our experience the only completely reliable measure of glomerular filtration rate is the standard inulin clearance. Single injection techniques with sodium iothalamate, Cr-EDTA, or inulin may overestimate GFR in the first week of life. Creatinine clearance accuracy can be improved if blood creatinine is determined before and at the end of the urine collection period.

Extraction of PAH may not be complete in the first week of life, tending to lead to underestimation of renal plasma flow.   **E. Gautier**

Any collection for creatinine clearance in which the infant excretes creatinine at a rate less than 15 mg/kg/24 hours should be considered erroneous. The serum creatinine in cord blood approximates that of the mother. It usually falls over the first week of life to 0.3–0.4 mg/dl. In this light, a serum creatinine of 0.6–0.8 mg/dl, although normal for a given laboratory, may reflect a reduction of glomerular filtration to half normal for a given infant. Diatrizoate has been reported to interfere with the laboratory measurement of creatinine, leading to a falsely elevated level.

Studies have shown that the pattern of glomerular filtration varies directly with the time since conception, with an apparent abrupt change in the rate of increase at 34 weeks.[2] Accordingly, a premature infant, after 1 or 2 days adjustment, will follow a pattern after delivery that is similar to that of a fetus of the same conceptional age in utero, even though the extrauterine child will increase the filtration rate faster than his intrauterine counterpart after 32–34 weeks.[2] Now standards can be based on gestational age at birth rather than weight and postnatal increases more precisely predicted. In term infants, the average inulin clearance is 20 ml/min/1.73 m² in the first 12 hours of life and 33 ml/min/1.73 m² 2–5 days later. Guignard et al[39] found that the inulin clearance of a group of infants of 35–39 weeks' gestational age was 19 ml/min/1.73 m² at 2–5 days and 33 ml/min/1.73 m² at 6–14 days. Infants whose gestational age at birth was ≤ 34 weeks averaged 33 ml/min/1.73 m² when studied by Leake et al at 1–2 weeks of age.[50]

Renal plasma flow, as measured by PAH, is low at birth and increases with postnatal age also to a mature level by 6 months of age. Guignard et al[39] noted that PAH clearances averaged 75 ml/min/1.73 m² in the first month of life but increased from 53 ml/min/1.73 m² in the first postnatal week to 110 ml/min/1.73 m² by the second week. It is felt by many that this increase in renal plasma flow, secondary to a decrease in the resistance of the renal microvasculature, is a prime contributor to the increase in the glomerular filtration rate postnatally.[42]

Tubular function improves proportional to the increase in glomerular function with glomerulotubular balance generally maintained.[13, 47] The tubular reabsorption of glucose, phosphorus, amino acids, and sodium is significantly less in infants <34 weeks than in more mature newborns.[2]

Clinical methods for evaluation of the various renal functions in infants are listed in order of decreasing accuracy in Table 14–1. Table 14–2 lists values for various renal functions at birth according to gestational ages.

CASE PROBLEMS

Case One

G. R., a 3600 gm male, is transferred to your service at 18 hours of age because of a mass in the left flank. He was born at the termination of a 38 week normal pregnancy and 12 hour spontaneous labor by a nondifficult breech extraction to a 26 year old gravida II mother. Although there was a small amount of meconium in the amniotic fluid, the child had a prompt, good cry and appeared quite well. Initial examination by the nurse in the delivery room was reported as normal, and the child was transferred to the newborn nursery in good condition. An examination at 12 hours of age by the pediatrician disclosed a large left flank mass but was otherwise within normal limits.

Your examination concurs that the infant has a large, firm, superficial, somewhat lobulated mass filling the left flank, extending from the costal margin almost to the iliac crest. He is pale with a poor suck. Temperature is 37°C, hemoglobin is 16.5 mg/dl, hematocrit is 43 per cent, WBC is 8500 per mm³, platelets are normal, and red cell morphology is normal on peripheral blood smear.

What are your diagnostic considerations at this point?

At least 70 per cent of all abdominal masses in the newborn are renal in origin; in some series

TABLE 14–1 RENAL FUNCTION TESTS

Function	Useful Clinical Tests
Glomerular filtration rate	Sodium iothalamate clearance Creatinine clearance Cr-EDTA clearance Blood creatinine
Renal plasma flow	Paraaminohippurate clearance

Proximal tubular transport
  Reabsorption
  Excretion
	
	Tubular maxima glucose
	Tubular maxima paraaminohippurate
	Phenolsulfonphthalein excretion
	Glycosuria
	Aminoaciduria

Distal tubular transport	Concentration and dilution (urine osmolarity) Maximal and minimal urine specific gravity

TABLE 14–2 AVERAGE RENAL FUNCTION AT BIRTH*

	Gestational Age (weeks)					
	28	30	32	34	36	40
Glomerular filtration rate (ml/min)	0.35	0.45	0.50	0.46	1.2	2.2
Tubular reabsorption of glucose (%)	78	97	98	99	99	99
Tubular reabsorption of phosphate (%)	85	89	86	93	93	98
Fractional reabsorption of sodium (%)	92	98	98	98	99	99

*Adapted from Arant.[2]

the percentage is even higher.[65, 73] About 50 per cent of all abdominal tumors are renal. Although the size of the mass is of little diagnostic significance, the location is significant. Flank masses are usually renal or adrenal in origin; bilateral masses usually represent hydronephrosis or polycystic kidneys; unilateral masses often mean multicystic kidney, tumor, hydronephrosis, or vascular accident. Lower abdominal masses more frequently involve the bladder or ovaries or are due to hydrometrocolpos, while a more anterior midline mass is probably an ovarian cyst or intestinal duplication. Renal masses tend to feel smooth and firm.

Thus, the percentages, as well as the location and feel of this mass, strongly suggest it is kidney. The superficiality of the mass might suggest splenic enlargement, but its extension deep into the flank is more supportive of a renal lesion. The breech delivery, although not difficult, coupled with the mass being easily felt anteriorly, might suggest a retrorenal hematoma, but other causes of renal enlargement should be considered. Hydronephrosis and multicystic dysplasia account for 70 per cent of renal masses and 40 per cent of all abdominal masses in the newborn.[24, 51] Other renal lesions to be considered include polycystic kidneys, renal ectopia, duplication of the collecting system, renal vascular thrombosis, horseshoe kidney, malrotation, abscess, leiomyoma, multilocular cysts, or a solitary cyst.[24, 37, 45, 51, 65, 73] Likewise, neoplasia, such as Wilms' tumor, neuroblastoma, or adrenal tumors, cannot be excluded.

What is your next move?

With these considerations in mind, it would be appropriate to evaluate the infant's renal function by BUN, creatinine, electrolytes, and blood gases. Techniques that define anatomically the status of both kidneys are also indicated. Of prime importance, however, would be a careful examination of the urine.

At 22 hours of age, the infant passes the first recorded urine. It is grossly bloody with 1 + protein, no clots, and no casts. The infant has become less active and less responsive, with shallow, rapid respiration. He refuses to suck and has vomited a small amount of yellowish fluid once. Temperature is 35.4°C, electrolytes are normal, BUN is 45 mg/dl, pH is 7.24, and bicarbonate is 15 mEq/l.

Does this change your thinking? What course should be followed now?

The infant is clearly ill and has gross hematuria. The initial nurse's examination now assumes historical importance; the mass not palpable at birth but so easily palpable now would suggest sudden enlargement of one kidney. In general, only renal vascular thrombosis or acute adrenal hemorrhage would produce such rapid change and such a degree of clinical illness. A congenital malformation with secondary infection might, also. The gross hematuria and the size of the mass would suggest renal vein thrombosis as the more likely of the two, as do the azotemia and hypothermia. A coagulation disorder, such as disseminated intravascular coagulation, might be considered. Evaluation of the anatomic status of the kidneys and coagulation studies are clearly indicated.

Would this occur with unilateral disease? No. One good kidney is enough to sustain renal function adequately so that azotemia will not occur. Thus, if the BUN is elevated, there is almost certainly some problem with the other kidney.   **W. Weil, Jr.**

An IVP shows a normal nephrogram on the right with calyces faintly visualized but normal. The bladder fills with radiopaque dye. Although the mass can be seen as a negative shadow during total body opacification, there is no excretion of dye detectable on the left, even on delayed films. A renal scan shows no function on the left. Ultrasonography shows the left kidney to be large with a disordered central collection of echoes. Coagulation studies are normal.

Should surgery be contemplated, or are further studies indicated?

The diagnosis appears quite clear now. The sudden enlargement of one kidney, marked clinical illness, azotemia, metabolic acidosis, gross hematuria, nonvisualization of the kidney on the involved side by IVP, nonfunctioning scan, and typical ultrasonographic findings are quite characteristic of renal vein thrombosis. A unilaterally nonfunctioning kidney by IVP or radionuclide scan implies multicystic dysplasia or vascular thrombosis; however, late films or ultrasonography is essential to exclude hydronephrosis with either ureteropelvic or ureterovesical obstruction. Occasionally a late film will outline the septa of cysts in multicystic dysplasia. Ultrasonography is particularly adept in the delineation of the nonfunctioning kidney, the separation of solid from cystic structures, and the outlining of the collecting system. Since a large kidney usually suggests hydronephrosis, multicystic dysplasia, or renal vein thrombosis, ultrasound, as in this case, often distinguishes between these lesions.[96] Transillumination of abdominal masses such as large cysts and hydronephrotic kidneys can be helpful but is nowhere near as accurate or sensitive as ultrasonography. Venography has also been helpful in showing a lack of renal filling on the affected side and occasionally of the vena cava but is invasive and would not improve either diagnostic or therapeutic accuracy in this instance.

The etiology in this case is not really clear; noncomplicated breech delivery has not been implicated in this disorder, although traumatic deliveries have been suspect. Factors associated with renal vein thrombosis have included dehydration, hyperosmolality, maternal diabetes, anoxia, altered renal plasma flow, polycythemia, gastroenteritis, cyanotic congenital heart disease, pyelonephritis, structural abnormalities of the kidney, and septicemia. Although thrombocytopenia has been reported, this has been thought to be the result of the thrombosis rather than part of a disseminated intravascular coagulation syndrome. Normal platelets, normal red cell morphology, normal coagulation studies, and the absence of systemic bleeding would eliminate this consideration in the present case.

Therapy requires vigorous supportive care.[9, 26] Since the outcome depends largely on the severity of the underlying primary medical conditions, aggressive management directed to associated medical problems may be more important than specific management of the renal vasculature. There is no evidence that nephrectomy improves outcome. In fact, those who appear at higher risk are males with congenital heart defects and those subjected to early nephrectomy. Since the venous thrombosis is primary, originating in the smaller intrarenal vessels, surgical thrombectomy is of little consequence to the kidney. Although anticoagulation has been used, its necessity or effectiveness has not been established. The results with supportive therapy alone, avoiding anticoagulation, are just as encouraging.

Recovery of renal function in the affected kidney is a familiar occurrence. Some degree of renal atrophy is to be expected, and occasionally tubular dysfunctions have appeared as a late sequela.[91] Pyelography after recovery may show calyceal clubbing and reticulated renal calcification.[95] It is exceedingly unusual, however, for subsequent nephrectomy to be necessary.

Case Two

H. Y., a 2680 gm female, was born to a 29 year old gravida I, STS negative, A+ mother, after a 38-week normal pregnancy and a 2½ hour spontaneous labor with vaginal delivery under spinal anesthesia. The infant did well until 3 days of age, when grunting respirations with intermittent cyanosis were noted. The chest is clear on examination; abdominal palpation discloses no organ enlargement. Chest films show no abnormality of the heart or lungs. On the morning of the fifth day, periorbital edema is noted, which becomes less marked as the day progresses. A urinalysis shows 3+ protein, 5–10 RBC per HPF, 4–8 WBC per HPF, and occasional granular casts. Serum electrolytes are normal, pH is 7.38, bicarbonate is 25.6 mEq/l, and P_{CO_2} is 44 mm Hg.

Are the symptoms and signs compatible with cardiac failure? With respiratory distress syndrome? With renal disease?

The clinical picture is not that of cardiac failure or respiratory distress. There is no cardiomegaly, pulmonary vascular changes by x-ray, murmur, hepatomegaly, or tachypnea. Edema is a late finding in infants with cardiac failure, is characteristically not facial, and is usually worse late in the day. Although grunting and cyanosis could be from respiratory distress syndrome, it is unlikely, because they took 3 days to appear, chest x-ray is clear, and blood gases are normal. Other causes of edema in the first few days of life, such as erythroblastosis, maternal toxemia, or excessive exogenous sodium and water loading, do not appear to be operating here either.

Periorbital edema, worse in the morning and improving as the day progresses, is characteristic of hypoproteinemia or renal disease. In this instance, the presence of marked proteinuria and cylindruria is quite compatible with a renal lesion, probably glomerular.

How would you proceed at this point?

Investigation of renal function and anatomic status would be in order. Because of the edema, components of the nephrotic syndrome (proteinuria, hypoproteinemia, and hyperlipemia) should be investigated.

The following laboratory results are obtained: BUN = 11.5 mg/dl, creatinine = 0.6 mg/dl, and total serum protein = 2.4 gm/dl with albumin 27.5

per cent, alpha 2 globulin 39.0 per cent, and gamma globulin 5.5 per cent; cholesterol = 273 mg/dl, and total lipids = 709 mg/dl; Kline is nonreactive; urinary protein = 0.576 gm/dl with 0.288 gm excreted in 24 hours; creatinine clearance is 23 ml/min/1.73 m²; renal ultrasound shows normal anatomic structures with some increase in renal parenchymal echogenicity; and clean voided urine culture shows 10³ col/ml *E. coli* and 10² col/ml diphtheroids.

What are the diagnostic possibilities? What is your diagnosis?

The laboratory data are consistent with some form of nephropathy. Acute pyelonephritis is probably unlikely, since the proteinuria is too high, the renal anatomy normal, and the urine culture not definitive. However, 10³ col/ml *E. coli* on a single culture could be significant in the dilute urine of a newborn, so either a repeat clean voided specimen culture or a suprapubic bladder aspiration would be useful. Acute tubular injury or renal cortical necrosis is not supported by the clinical course or the laboratory findings. A nephrotic syndrome is present. There is hypoalbuminemia with an elevation of alpha 2 globulin; cholesterol and total lipids are elevated for a newborn; and the proteinuria of 0.576 gm/dl is likewise quite massive for a newborn. The diagnosis would be congenital nephrosis.

Should a renal biopsy be performed on such a young infant? Would it help, if it could be done?

Congenital nephrotic syndrome is a heterogeneous group of diseases from which microcystic disease (Finnish type), focal glomerulosclerosis, diffuse mesangial sclerosis, membranous glomerulonephropathy, interstitial nephritis, nail-patella syndrome, and congenital glomerulosclerosis have been separated as histologic entities. The syndrome has been reported in association with congenital syphilis, renal vein thrombosis, nephroblastoma, toxoplasmosis, and cytomegalic inclusion disease. The steroid-responsive minimal lesion form has been described in less than 10 per cent of infants. That the spectrum of histologic alterations cannot be defined clinically suggests that renal biopsy can be useful in the diagnosis and management of these children. It can be performed on such young infants either by open surgical biopsy or by percutaneous needle biopsy under fluoroscopic or ultrasound guidance. In this child, needle biopsy showed the changes of microcystic disease, a form of congenital nephrosis that does not respond to any known type of therapy.

Infants with congenital nephrotic syndrome are often born prematurely, with a large, edematous placenta. Signs of fetal asphyxia are common. They will soon develop edema and ascites. They show the usual serum alterations of the nephrotic

syndrome, including low albumin and an elevation of alpha 2 globulin. The level of hypercholesterolemia and hyperlipidemia is less than that seen in the older child but is persistently above normal for newborns. In general, these children fail to do well and, other than those with the minimal lesion form, do not respond to corticosteroid therapy. The outcome is often death in the first year, though not usually from renal failure. Practically all of these infants fail to thrive and often succumb to infection before renal insufficiency develops. One approach, using constant rate, low flow nasogastric feedings, has successfully prolonged life in several infants and allowed good growth, normal development, and improved outcome. Successful renal transplantation has been reported, without recurrence of the nephrotic syndrome. When due to congenital syphilis, congenital nephrotic syndrome can be successfully treated with penicillin. There is also a report of successful treatment of toxoplasmosis-associated nephrosis with steroids, pyrimethamine, and sulfadiazine.

Most of these infants have an abnormal thyroid screen with low T₄ (thyroxine) secondary to the low protein concentration. Occasionally this may be the first abnormality noted in infants with the congenital nephrotic syndrome. **W. Weil, Jr.**

Case Three

F. D., a 3800 gm newborn male, has a routine urine specimen obtained at 4 days of age prior to circumcision. This urine shows 1+ protein, 25–30 WBC per HPF, no casts, but many motile bacteria in the spun sediment. Pregnancy, labor, and delivery were uncomplicated. Physical examination is normal. He is vigorous, with a good cry, and is afebrile. Feeding has been no problem, and his weight is only 250 gm below birth weight.

Does this child have a urinary tract infection?[10, 52, 53, 55]

Certainly pyuria must raise the suspicion as does the presence of bacteria on smear. Several questions need to be answered first, however. It is not clear how this urine was obtained. Was the prepuce cleaned in any way? Was the foreskin retracted in the cleaning? The problem does not exist here, as it does in a female, of determining if the cells came from vaginal secretions washed out by vaginal reflux in the process of micturition, and one would hope that balanoposthitis has been excluded by examination as a source of pyuria.

The presence of bacteria in the spun sediment is of little value if the urine has been in the bag at room temperature for any length of time. Other than the patient being a male, clinical indications of a urinary tract infection are not present. Some type of infection or pyrexia is present in the mother during labor in 45 per cent of cases. Clinical signs appear more commonly between 5 and 8 days of age, with pyrexia, poor weight gain, palpable kidneys, and diarrhea being the most common reasons for investigation. Pyuria is more often associated with clinical illness. At best, one can only suspect urinary tract infection. Other studies are necessary before a diagnosis can be made.

What other studies should be performed?

The next study would seem to be a reexamination of the urine with culture included. The outlook for a male infant with a urinary tract infection must be viewed with caution. The chance of developing renal insufficiency in the male is four times that of the female, and obstructive uropathy is three times more common than in the female. In the newborn, hematogenous spread of bacteria is a more common route of colonization of renal parenchyma; blood cultures are positive in 33 per cent of males and 14 per cent of females with proven urinary tract infections. Therefore blood cultures and radiologic evaluation of the urinary tract are important when an infant, particularly a male, has a urinary tract infection.

A second urine specimen is obtained the same day by cleaning the prepuce with pHisoHex and applying a sterile adhesive plastic bag. The specimen is removed from the bag as soon as possible. This urine shows no protein, 2–5 WBC per HPF, and no casts. A stained smear of uncentrifuged urine shows no organisms, but the culture shows 10^5 col/ml E. coli.

Can we now document the presence of a urinary tract infection?[27, 55]

No. A single culture, even though a pure growth of more than 10^5 col/ml of a single organism, is insufficient evidence for urinary tract infection in the newborn. As many as 60 per cent of normal newborns will have greater than 10^5 col/ml in a standard clean voided urine, about one quarter of which will yield a pure growth of one type of organism. In the uncircumcised male, as many as 35 per cent will show "significant growth," even with very careful cleansing. Thus, in the newborn, the usual criteria for infection must be even more stringent than in the older child.

What do you do now?

Without a reliable diagnosis, it would not seem wise to start therapy. Since the prognosis must be guarded and the urologic evaluation more extensive in a young male, undue concern and unnecessary study might follow definitive therapy for what may prove to be an erroneous diagnosis.

The second urine is of little help. It is in exactly this sort of confusing situation that the suprapubic bladder aspiration of urine has proved so helpful.[67, 68] When performed in this child, a sterile urine was obtained. The child continued to do well with no medication.

Should urine cultures be part of the nursery routine?

Routine nursery cultures by the usual clean voided technique often create more difficulties than they solve. The incidence of urinary tract infection in the newborn nursery varies between 0.5 and 3 per cent.[27, 55] It is clear that the diagnosis of infection without a suprapubic aspirate is virtually impossible in the usual nursery situation; yet one cannot justify a suprapubic bladder aspiration on 60 per cent of newborns for only a 1 per cent yield. Therefore we do not recommend a routine urine culture. When the clinical situation suggests infection in the child, we recommend culture of a single clean voided urine. In any child with greater than 10^3 col/ml organisms in that specimen, a suprapubic bladder aspiration for culture should be obtained. We do recommend that urinalysis be routine, particularly in the high-risk nursery.

Case Four

A 2300 gm male infant was delivered after a 36 week normal pregnancy. The labor was normal until 30 minutes prior to delivery, when fetal heart rate was noted to be 80. At delivery, the cord was tight about the neck. Apgar at 1 minute = 2; at 5 minutes = 8. Resuscitation included intermittent positive pressure breathing plus intravenous sodium bicarbonate. Blood gases at 15 minutes: pH = 7.11, Pao_2 = 93 mm Hg, and $Paco_2$ = 54 mm Hg. Examination of the first urine passed, at age 36 hours, shows 1+ protein, positive benzidine, and many granular casts.

Is this acute tubular necrosis or glomerulonephritis?

At this point it may not be either. Oliguria or a delay in urination for up to 48 hours is quite common in both perinatal asphyxia and severe respiratory distress syndrome.[20, 22, 38, 39, 86, 89] Proteinuria, hematuria, and cylindruria also are a part of this symptom complex. Fetal lambs with anoxia may show a decrease of 50 per cent in renal blood flow, with a decrease of urine output to one sixth of control and a decrease in glomerular filtration rate to one fourth of control.[21, 81] Mild hypoxia in both the fetal lamb and the human can produce a rise in renal blood flow and increased urine output with increased electrolyte excretion. Severe hypoxia causes a reduction in both glomerular filtration rate and effective renal blood flow.[40] Evidence of intrarenal shunting of blood exists, possibly related to prostaglandins, vasopressin, or the renin-angiotensin system. Persistent anuria should raise concern over bilateral agenesis, dysgenesis, complete obstruction, or renal cortical necrosis.

What therapeutic steps should be taken?

There can be a prerenal component to the altered function.[56] In these circumstances, intravenous infusions of fluids and electrolytes can be cautiously attempted and successful, after positive evidence of hypovolemia is obtained. In most instances, however, vigorous attention to ventilation is the treatment of choice. When oxygenation improves, in most instances urine volume increases, glomerular filtration and renal blood flow improve, and the positive urinary findings clear. Should there be little change in urine output, many will respond to either mannitol, 0.5 mg/kg, or furosemide, 1–1.5 mg/kg, given intravenously. Although furosemide may produce a fourfold increase in urine volume and a tenfold increase in urinary sodium, there is no clear evidence that it alters plasma parameters or improves blood gases; this must be balanced against reports of insidious and progressive nerve deafness appearing in children who received furosemide during a period of impaired renal function.

One has to question the validity of producing a diuresis for its sake alone. There is little to be gained by having more urine, and there is little to suggest that the diuresis is actually therapeutic.   **W. Weil, Jr.**

The infant develops gross hematuria. Laboratory studies now show: serum sodium 128 mEq/l; BUN 29 mg/dl; creatinine 1.1 mg/dl.

What is the significance of these findings?

Hematuria occurs in about 75 per cent of infants with perinatal anoxia; in about half of these it will be gross. This usually represents the more severely asphyxiated infants. Its presence, however, should alert one to the possibility of renal vascular thrombosis (See Case One).

The newborn kidney is particularly at risk for thrombosis because the vessels are small, the renal plasma flow low, and the vascular resistance high. Hypoxia, particularly if associated with hypercapnia, reduces plasma flow still further. Arterial thrombosis was unusual until umbilical artery catheterization became prevalent, particularly with the use of hypertonic solutions. The signs of arterial thrombosis are secondary to renal infarction and include decreased or absent urine output, hematuria, proteinuria, variable degrees of altered function, hypertension, and renal enlargement. Evidence of thrombotic phenomena in other organs is frequently present. Treatment consists of aggressive support of the infant, including dialysis if necessary. The value of anticoagulation has not been adequately determined, and early nephrectomy is rarely required. Hypertension may be particularly difficult to control, requiring dosages of antihypertensive drugs that are proportionately higher than those used in older children.

Renal cortical or medullary necrosis must also be considered.[1] Both have been described in association with umbilical artery catheters (even in the absence of asphyxia), particularly if hypertonic solutions have been administered. Characteristically, there is anuria. The kidneys are often palpable. Edema may not appear, but hypertension, resistant to therapy, can appear very rapidly. With medullary necrosis, polyuria and salt wasting may follow a brief period of oliguria. Thrombocytopenia, as evidence of intravascular coagulation, may be present. Serum potassium levels may rise rapidly. A prolonged nephrogram with dense opacification of the renal pyramids has been said to be more diagnostic of medullary necrosis than cortical necrosis. With cortical necrosis, the renal parenchyma calcifies quite rapidly. Again, treatment is vigorous medical support. Pyelocalyceal abnormalities and renal atrophy are not unusual sequelae in survivors.

Hyponatremia occurs in about one third of asphyxiated infants. It behaves very much like the syndrome of inappropriate secretion of antidiuretic hormone (ADH)[72, 99] with low serum osmolality—low serum potassium, chloride, and calcium; high urinary sodium in the face of severe hyponatremia; and decreased free water clearance. It has been reported in both term and preterm infants. Although reported in the nursery associated with meningitis, pneumonia, hypoplasia of the anterior pituitary, and idiopathic vasopressin secretion, and following surgical repair of a patent ductus arteriosus, the most frequent cause of inappropriate ADH secretion is still asphyxia. The hyponatremia may be compounded by the initial vigorous administration of fluids and electrolytes given these infants in the control of acidosis or in the hope of reversing a presumed hypovolemic state. This is why careful attention to fluid administration and monitoring of weight gain are so important in the management of asphyxiated infants. If initial attempts to increase urine output are not successful, further attempts to provoke urine with parenteral fluids and electrolytes court disaster. The circumstance of inappropriate ADH secretion demands fluid restriction; only unusual occasions require administration of 3 per cent NaCl. However, like the hematuria, it may resolve quickly with improved ventilation and oxygenation.

Unless the hyponatremia is extremely severe (a serum sodium less than 120 mEq/l), we would prefer to manage this situation simply by fluid restriction.   **L. Stern**

It is worth noting that acute adrenal cortical insufficiency, with hyperkalemia and hyponatremia, may mimic this condition. However, in adrenal insufficiency, there is no weight gain, and the hyponatremia does not respond to fluid restriction. Hydrocortisone administration should decrease urinary sodium and elevate urinary potassium.

Questions

A newborn is noted to have a single umbilical artery at the time the cord is clamped and cut. How serious is this anatomic curiosity? Should further investigation be attempted?[14, 15, 32]

This anomaly occurs in 0.7–0.9 per cent of newborns, of whom 10–17 per cent have major malformations. Moreover, a single umbilical artery is associated with a perinatal mortality approximately four times that of the general newborn population; 80 per cent of infants who die will be stillborn or will die in the first week of life. It appears that the reported high incidence of congenital anomalies has been true in those who die but not in those who survive. In addition, the frequency of genitourinary anomalies (27 per cent), although this is the most frequent anomaly seen, is no higher in these infants than in any other infant dying with multiple congenital anomalies. This implies that: (1) those with significant problems die early, and (2) the genitourinary anomalies are a function of the multiple congenital anomalies rather than specifically related to the single umbilical artery. Of importance is that the survivors do as well as other children of comparable weight and socioeconomic status. Defects not present at birth do not develop later; those that are detected later are not detrimental to the infant. We no longer routinely evaluate the genitourinary tract of these infants.

What are the extraurinary findings that would prompt an early radiologic evaluation of the urinary tract?

Certain defects outside the urinary tract are associated with a greater than expected incidence of urinary tract anomalies. The controversy over single umbilical arteries has already been discussed. Other defects include (1) absence of abdominal musculature;[71, 82] (2) congenital heart lesions, especially ventricular septal defect; (3) Turner's syndrome; (4) gastrointestinal abnormalities, especially anorectal anomalies, esophageal atresia, or tracheoesophageal fistula,[4, 8] (5) severe hypospadias;[54] (6) hydrometrocolpos; (7) dysplasia or absence of the radius;[16] (8) vertebral defects; (9) ear anomalies existing with facial bone anomalies; (10) hypoplasia of the pelvis;[5] (11) myelodysplasia; and (12) unexplained pneumothorax or pneumomediastinum.[6] A grouping of defects, indicating a need for further investigation, has been designated by the mnemonic of VATER anomalies (Vertebral defects, Anal atresia, Tracheo-Esophageal fistula with esophageal atresia; Radial and Renal dysplasia).[77] From these associations, it would appear that the fetus is most susceptible to developing anomalies of the genitourinary tract at about 33 days' gestation.

Urography does not seem as indicated in simple cryptorchidism, isolated coronal or penile hypospadias, or uncomplicated imperforate hymen.[43, 58]

How might a BUN of 17 mg/dl be compatible with severe renal disease? How might a BUN of 43 mg/dl be compatible with normal renal function?

The level of blood urea is the difference between production and excretion. Production is influenced by nitrogen intake, tissue nitrogen catabolized, and the nitrogen incorporated into new tissues (anabolism). Excretion is a function of glomerular filtration rate and tubular reabsorption.

Without any change in renal function, the level may rise with excessive catabolism. It may also rise during periods of decreased renal plasma flow, such as is seen in hypovolemia, often accompanied by decreased urine flow, which allows increased tubular reabsorption of urea (so-called prerenal azotemia). If protein intake is allowed to continue unchanged during these periods or if caloric intake is insufficient, the level of urea will rise still higher.

A markedly decreased protein intake, however, may allow the BUN to be 17 mg/dl in the face of severe renal disease, merely because the nitrogen load presented to the kidneys does not exceed their limited capacity to excrete, particularly if sufficient calories are available from carbohydrates and fats so that tissue catabolism is reduced to a minimum. With a normal protein intake, the BUN does not rise above normal until the glomerular filtration rate is below 40 per cent of normal. By reducing the protein intake, the BUN may not rise until the glomerular filtration rate is below 20 per cent of normal.

It is for these reasons that most nephrologists have come to rely more on the serum creatinine level as a more sensitive screening test for general renal function. The serum creatinine concentration can be expected to double for each 50 per cent fall in glomerular filtration rate.

A 1400 gm infant is found to have a serum sodium of 128 mEq/l. Should free water intake be restricted or sodium intake increased?[23, 30, 70, 84, 85]

Hyponatremia in the immature infant has become a common finding during the neonatal period. Whether one adds sodium or restricts fluid is dependent on a careful evaluation of the etiology of the low serum sodium. The timing of this finding can be helpful. Early hyponatremia, often in the first day of life, can be related to events surrounding labor and delivery and should prompt the physician to inquire about a maternal history of diuretics, oxytocin, or hypotonic fluid infusions. When the mother has received diuretics, usually for eclampsia, the total body sodium depletion can involve the fetus as well. Repletion of body water in the infant can then result in hyponatremia. Oxytocin, on the other hand, is antidiuretic, leading to an endogenous water load that can involve the fetus, with dilutional hyponatremia resulting. Large volumes of hypotonic fluid administered to the mother during labor can have the same effect.

The infant with severe respiratory distress is also prone to developing hyponatremia[70, 72, 81, 99] usually as a result of cerebral anoxia leading to inappropriate secretion of antidiuretic hormones (see Case Four). The aim here is to restrict fluids and improve ventilation. Altered renal function, likewise related to asphyxia, may compound the problem. Other causes of hyponatremia during this period include acute adrenal insufficiency (secondary to adrenal hemorrhage, sepsis, or intravascular coagulation), salt-losing adrenogenital syndrome, water intoxication from nebulization with nasal CPAP,[84] and the use of loop diuretics, such as furosemide,[86, 94] with inappropriate free water replacement.

Late hyponatremia is usually seen in the rapidly growing premature taking standard prepared formulae patterned after human breast milk.[3, 49, 85, 97] The infant is usually of < 30 weeks' gestation at birth; the hyponatremia will usually occur between 2 and 8 weeks of age. The electrolyte content of these formulae is not sufficient, in the quantities taken by most prematures, to replace the losses and accommodate the rapidly enlarging body mass. The usual preterm infant needs 2–3 mEq of Na/kg/day; these infants may require as much as 4–8 mEq/kg/day for repair of the hyponatremia (see Chapter 6).

There is generally not a significant dilutional component contributing to the low plasma levels; the major factors appear to be inadequate intake coupled with the immature kidney's high urinary loss of sodium relative to the plasma levels. There is some speculation that additional available sodium is lost to coprecipitation with calcium in bone formation. Improvement is a function of postnatal age rather than gestational age; once the kidney matures enough to retain sodium, supplementation is no longer required.

A 7 day old, 2100 gm male infant has fully recovered from mild respiratory distress and is taking formula well. However, he is not gaining weight, and a blood sample shows pH = 7.25 and TCO_2 = 17 mEq/l. Why?

Late metabolic acidosis[87] is a common problem. It generally appears after the first 3 days of life at a time when feedings are well tolerated. Its prevalence seems inversely related to both gesta-tional and postnatal age and directly related to caloric intake. It usually responds spontaneously in 3–10 days, although some children may require the addition of bicarbonate or a reduction in the amount of protein in the diet for a temporary period. It is possible that late metabolic acidosis in the preterm infant may be prevented by early sodium supplementation. Of interest is a report that net acid excretion in these infants is appropriate for age and that late metabolic acidosis does not result in an increased capacity to excrete hydrogen ion. The low TCO_2 may reflect the infant's low renal bicarbonate threshold.

Anatomic lesions or lesions of disordered nephrogenesis can produce a limited ability to excrete hydrogen ion. Examples include hydronephrosis, renal dysplasia, obstructive uropathy, nephronophthisis, polycystic kidneys, and oligomeganephronia. A reduction of functioning renal mass from any cause sufficient to produce nitrogen retention can also produce metabolic acidosis. An insufficient delivery of phosphate to the distal nephron is a rare cause of limited ability to excrete titratable acid.

Renal tubular acidosis must also be considered; however, it is a much rarer phenomenon in the nursery. Proximal renal tubular acidosis, as an isolated defect, occurs predominantly in males. It is a bicarbonate-resistant, hyperchloremic metabolic acidosis in which the infants do not elaborate an acid urine until the serum bicarbonate falls below the renal threshold, which may be as low as 14 mEq/l. The diagnosis rests on the ability to demonstrate the low renal threshold as well as the infant's ability to acidify the urine eventually at low bicarbonate levels. It is usually self-limiting but does not respond to dietary manipulation, as late metabolic acidosis does. Distal tubular acidosis occurs predominantly in females, is usually diagnosed after the neonatal period, is associated with impaired excretion of an ammonium chloride load, and is usually permanent. These infants fail to produce an acid urine, even with severe systemic acidosis.

On several occasions we have seen persistent acidosis of this kind in full-term infants as the only presenting sign for what subsequently on pyelography turned out to be severe forms of renal dysplasia. The occurrence of this so-called late metabolic acidosis in a full-term infant should always raise the suspicion of either a physiologic or an anatomic defect that is more than just transient in nature. **L. Stern**

REFERENCES

1. Anand, S. K., Northway, J. D., and Smith, J. A.: Neonatal renal papillary and cortical necrosis. Am J Dis Child *131*:773, 1977.
2. Arant, B. S.: Developmental patterns of renal functional maturation compared in the human neonate. J Pediatr *92*:705, 1978.
3. Atkinson, S. A., Radde, I. C., and Anderson, G.

H.: Macromineral balances in premature infants fed their own mothers' milk or formula. J Pediatr *102*:99, 1983.
4. Atwell, J., and Beard, R.: Congenital anomalies of the upper urinary tract associated with esophageal atresia and tracheoesophageal fistula. J Pediatr Surg *9*:825, 1974.

5. Baden, M., Ortiz, A., Goyette, R. E., et al: Hypoplastic pelvis in association with multiple anomalies. Pediatrics 53:270, 1974.

6. Bashour, B. N., and Balfe, W.: Urinary tract abnormalities in neonates with spontaneous pneumothorax and/or pneumomediastinum. Pediatrics 59:S1048, 1977.

7. Beale, M. G., Strayer, D. S., Kissane, J. M., et al: Congenital glomerulosclerosis and nephrotic syndrome in two infants: speculations and pathogenesis. Am J Dis Child 133:842, 1979.

8. Belman, A. B., and King, L. R.: Urinary tract abnormalities associated with imperforate anus. J Urol 108:823, 1972.

9. Belman, A. B., Susmand, D., Burden, J., et al: Nonoperative treatment of unilateral renal vein thrombosis in the newborn. J Am Med Assoc 211:1165, 1970.

10. Bergstrom, T., Larson, H., Lincoln, K., et al: Studies on urinary tract infections in infancy and childhood. J Pediatr 80:858, 1972.

11. Betkerur, M. V., Yeh, T. F., Miller, K., et al: Indomethacin and its effect on renal function and urinary kallikrein excretion in premature infants with patent ductus arteriosus. Pediatrics 68:99, 1981.

12. Boineau, F., Rothman, J., and Lewy, J. E.: Nephrosonography in the evaluation of renal failure and masses in infants. J Pediatr 87:195, 1971.

13. Brodehl, J., Franken, A., and Gellissen, K.: Maximal tubular reabsorption of glucose in infants and children. Acta Paediatr Scand 6:413, 1972.

14. Bryan, E., and Kohler, H.: The missing umbilical artery. I. Prospective study based on a maternity unit. Arch Dis Child 49:844, 1974.

15. Bryan, E., and Kohler, H.: The missing umbilical artery. II. Paediatric follow-up. Arch Dis Child 50:714, 1975.

16. Carroll, R., and Louis, D.: Anomalies associated with radial dysplasia. J Pediatr 84:409, 1974.

17. Catterton, Z., Sellers, B., and Gray, B.: Inulin clearance in the premature infant receiving indomethacin. J Pediatr 96:737, 1980.

18. Clark, D. A.: Times of first void and stool in 500 newborns. Pediatrics 60:457, 1977.

19. Crocker, J., Brown, D., and Vernier, R.: Developmental defects of the kidney. Pediatr Clin North Am 18:355, 1971.

20. Daniel, S., and James, L.: Abnormal renal function in the newborn infant. J Pediatr 88:856, 1976.

21. Daniel, S., Yeh, M., Bowe, E., et al: Renal response of the lamb fetus to partial occlusion of the umbilical cord. J Pediatr 87:788, 1975.

22. Dauber, I., Krauss, A., Symchych, P., et al: Renal failure following perinatal anoxia. J Pediatr 88:851, 1976.

23. Day, C., Radde, I., Balfe, J., et al: Electrolyte abnormalities in very low birth weight infants. Pediatr Res 10:522, 1976.

24. DeKlerk, D. P., Marshall, F. F., and Jeffs, R. D.: Multicystic dysplastic kidney. J Urol 118:306, 1977.

25. Dillon, M. J., Gillin, M. E. A., Ryness, J. M., et al: Plasma renin activity and aldosterone concentration in the human newborn. Arch Dis Child 51:537, 1976.

26. Duncan, R. E., Evans, A. T., and Martin, L. W.: Natural history and treatment of renal vein thrombosis in children. J Pediatr Surg 12:639, 1977.

27. Edelman, C. M., Ogwo, J. E., Fine, B. P., et al: Prevalence of bacteriuria in full term and premature infants. J Pediatr 82:125, 1973.

28. Effmann, E., Ablow, R., and Siegel, N.: Renal growth. Radiol Clin North Am 15:3, 1977.

29. Emmanuel, B., and Aronson, N.: Neonatal hematuria. Am J Dis Child 128:204, 1974.

30. Engelke, S. C., Sham, B. L., Vasan, U., et al: Sodium balance in very low-birth-weight infants. J Pediatr 93:837, 1978.

31. Feldman, H., and Guignard, J.-P.: Plasma creatinine in the first month of life. Arch Dis Child 57:123, 1982.

32. Froehlich, L., and Fujikura, T.: Follow-up of infants with single umbilical artery. Pediatrics 52:6, 1973.

33. Garrett, R., and Franken, E.: Neonatal ascites: perirenal urinary extravasation with bladder outlet obstruction. J Urol 102:627, 1969.

34. Gatewood, O. M. B., Glasser, R. J., and Van Houtte, J. J.: Roentgen evaluation of renal size in pediatric age groups. Am J Dis Child 110:162, 1965.

35. Godard, C., Geering, J. M., Geering, K., et al: Plasma renin activity related to sodium balance, renal function and urinary vasopressin in the newborn infant. Pediatr Res 13:742, 1979.

36. Goldberg, B., Pollack, H., Capitanio, M., et al: Ultrasonography: an aid in the diagnosis of masses in pediatric patients. Pediatrics 56:421, 1975.

37. Greene, L. F., Feinzhig, W., and Dahlin, D. C.: Multicystic dysplasia of the kidney: with special reference to the contralateral kidney. J Urol 105:482, 1971.

38. Guignard, J.-P.: Renal function in the newborn infant. Pediatr Clin North Am 29:777, 1982.

39. Guignard, J.-P., Torrado, A., DaCunha, O., et al: Glomerular filtration rate in the first three weeks of life. J Pediatr 87:268, 1975.

40. Guignard, J.-P., Torrado, A., Mazouni, S. M., et al: Renal function in respiratory distress syndrome. J Pediatr 88:845, 1976.

41. Hiner, L. B., Gruskin, A. B., Baluarte, H. J., et al: Plasma renin activity in normal children. J Pediatr 89:258, 1976.

42. Ichikawa, I., Maddox, D. A., and Brenner, B. M.: Maturational development of glomerular ultrafiltration in the rat. J Physiol 236:F465, 1979.

43. Kahn, R., Duncan, B., and Bowes, W.: Spontaneous opening of congenital imperforate hymen. J Pediatr 87:768, 1975.

44. Kainer, G., McIlveen, B., Höschl, R., et al: Assessment of individual renal function in children using ^{99m}Tc-DTPA. Arch Dis Child 54:931, 1979.

45. Kaplan, B. S., Rabin, I., Nogrady, M. B., et al: Autosomal dominant polycystic renal disease in children. J Pediatr 90:782, 1977.

46. Karlsson, F. A., and Hellsing, K.: Urinary protein excretion in early infancy. J Pediatr 89:89, 1976.

47. Kon, V., and Ichikawa, I.: Glomerulo-tubular balance in the immature kidney. Pediatr Res 16:324, 1982.

48. Kotchen, T., Strickland, A., Rice, M., et al: A study of the renin-angiotensin system in newborn infants. J Pediatr 80:938, 1972.

49. Kumar, S. P., and Sacks, L. M.: Hyponatremia in very low-birth-weight infants and human milk feedings. J Pediatr 93:1026, 1978.

50. Leake, R. D., Trygstad, C. W., and Oh, W.: Inulin clearance in the newborn infant: relationship to

gestational age and postnatal age. Pediatr Res *10*:759, 1976.

51. Lebowitz, R., and Griscom, N.: Neonatal hydronephrosis: 146 cases. Radiol Clin North Am *15*:49, 1977.
52. Lincoln, K., and Winberg, J.: Studies of urinary tract infections in first month of life. Acta Paediatr Scand *53*:307, 1964.
53. Littlewood, J.: Sixty-six infants with urinary tract infection in first month of life. Arch Dis Child *47*:218, 1972.
54. Lutzker, L. G., Kogan, S. J., and Levitt, S. B.: Is routine intravenous urography indicated in patients with hypospadias? Pediatrics *59*:630, 1977.
55. Maherzi, M., Guignard, J.-P., and Torrado, A.: Urinary tract infection in high-risk newborn infants. Pediatrics *62*:521, 1978.
56. Mathew, O. P., Jones, A. S., James, E., et al: Neonatal renal failure: usefulness of diagnostic indices. Pediatrics *65*:57, 1980.
57. Mauer, S., Dobrin, R., and Vernier, R.: Unilateral and bilateral renal agenesis in monoamniotic twins. J Pediatr *84*:236, 1974.
58. McArdle, R., and Lebowitz, R.: Uncomplicated hypospadias and anomalies of the upper urinary tract. Need for screening? Urology *5*:712, 1975.
59. McCracken, G., Jr.: Pharmacological basis for antimicrobial therapy in newborn infants. Am J Dis Child *128*:407, 1974.
60. McCracken, G., Ginsberg, C., Chrane, D. F., et al: Clinical pharmacology of penicillin in newborn infants. J Pediatr *82*:692, 1973.
61. Mendelsohn, H. B., Krauss, M., Berant, M., et al: Familial early onset nephrotic syndrome: diffuse mesangial sclerosis. Acta Paediatr Scand *71*:753, 1982.
62. Mendoza, S. A., Griswold, W. R., Leopold, G. R., et al: Intrauterine diagnosis of renal anomalies by ultrasonography. Am J Dis Child *133*:1042, 1979.
63. Miltényi, M., Bóka, G., and Kun, E.: Haemoglobinuria in erythroblastosis fetalis. Acta Paediatr Scand *71*:231, 1982.
64. Moore, E., and Galvez, M.: Delayed micturition in the newborn period. J Pediatr *80*:867, 1972.
65. Museles, M., Gundry, C. L., and Bason, M. W.: Renal anomalies in the newborn found by deep palpation. Pediatrics *47*:97, 1971.
66. Nash, M. A., and Edelmann, C. M., Jr.: The developing kidney. Immature function or inappropriate standard? Nephron *11*:71, 1973.
67. Nelson, J., and Peters, P.: Suprapubic aspiration of urine in premature and term infants. Pediatrics *36*:132, 1965.
68. Newman, C., O'Neill, P., and Parker, A.: Pyuria in infancy and the role of suprapubic aspiration of urine in diagnosis of infection of urinary tract. Br Med J *2*:277, 1967.
69. Norman, M. E., and Assadi, F. K.: A prospective study of acute renal failure in the newborn infant. Pediatrics *63*:475, 1979.
70. Oh, W.: Disorders of fluid and electrolytes in newborn infants. Pediatr Clin North Am *23*:601, 1976.
71. Pagon, R. A., Smith, D. W., and Shepard, T. H.: Urethral obstruction malformation complex: a cause of abdominal muscle deficiency and the "prune belly." J Pediatr *94*:900, 1979.
72. Paxson, C. L., Stoerner, J. W., Denson, S. E., et al:

Syndrome of inappropriate antidiuretic hormone secretion in neonates with pneumothorax or atelectasis. J Pediatr *91*:459, 1977.
73. Perlman, M., and Williams, J.: Detection of renal anomalies by abdominal palpation in newborn infants. Br Med J *2*:347, 1976.
74. Piepiz, A., Denis, R., Ham, H. R., et al: A simple method for measuring separate glomerular filtration rate using a single injection of ^{99m}Tc-DTPA and the scintillation camera. J Pediatr *93*:769, 1978.
75. Pinto, W., Jr., and Gardner, L.: Abnormal genitalia as a presenting sign in two male infants with hydantoin embryopathy syndrome. Am J Dis Child *131*:452, 1977.
76. Potter, E., and Craig, J.: *Pathology of the Fetus and the Infant.* 3rd Ed. Chicago, Year Book Medical Publishers, 1975.
77. Quan, L., and Smith, D.: The VATER association: *V*ertebral defects, *A*nal atresia, *T-E* fistula with esophageal atresia, *R*adial and *R*enal dysplasia: a spectrum of associated defects. J Pediatr *82*:104, 1973.
78. Rasoulpour, M., McLean, R. H., and Raye, J.: Pseudohematuria in neonates. J Pediatr *92*:852, 1978.
79. Reimold, E. W., Don, T. D., and Woorthen, H. G.: Renal failure during the first year of life. Pediatrics *59*(Suppl):987, 1977.
80. Robillard, J. E., Weismann, D. N., and Herin, P.: Ontogeny of single glomerular perfusion rate in fetal and newborn lambs. Pediatr Res *15*:1248, 1981.
81. Robillard, J. E., Weitzman, R. E., Burmeister, L., et al: Developmental aspects of the renal response to hypoxemia in the lamb fetus. Circ Res *48*:128, 1981.
82. Rogers, L., and Ostrow, P.: The prune belly syndrome: report of 20 cases and description of a lethal variant. J Pediatr *83*:786, 1973.
83. Roodhooft, A. M., and Holmes, L. B.: Family studies: Potter's syndrome of renal agenesis and dysgenesis. Am J Hum Genetics *33*:91A, 1981.
84. Rosenfeld, W., Linshaw, M., and Fox, H.: Water intoxication: a complication of nebulization with nasal CPAP. J Pediatr *89*:113, 1976.
85. Roy, R., Chance, G., Radde, I., et al: Late hyponatremia in very low birth weight infants (<1.3 kilograms). Pediatr Res *10*:526, 1976.
86. Savage, M., Wilkinson, A., Baum, J., et al: Furosemide in respiratory distress syndrome. Arch Dis Child *50*:709, 1975.
87. Schwartz, G. J., Haycock, G. B., Edelmann, C. M., et al: Late metabolic acidosis: A reassessment of the definition. J Pediatr *95*:102, 1979.
88. Siegel, S., and Oh, W.: Renal function as a marker of human fetal maturation. Acta Paediatr Scand *65*:481, 1976.
89. Siegel, S., Fisher, D., and Oh, W.: Renal function and serum aldosterone levels in infants with respiratory distress syndrome. J Pediatr *83*:854, 1973.
90. Springer, C., Eyal, F., and Michel, J.: Pharmacology of trimethoprim-sulfamethoxazole in newborn infants. J Pediatr *100*:647, 1982.
91. Stark, H., and Geiger, R.: Renal tubular dysfunction following vascular accidents of the kidneys in the newborn period. J Pediatr *83*:933, 1973.
92. Stonestreet, B. S., and Oh, W.: Plasma creatinine

levels in low-birth-weight infants during the first three months of life. Pediatrics *61*:788, 1978.

93. Stonestreet, B. S., Bell, E. F., and Oh, W.: Validity of endogenous creatinine clearance in the low birthweight infants. Pediatr Res *13*:1012, 1979.

94. Sulyok, E., Erh, T., Varga, F., et al: Furosemide induced alterations in the electrolyte status, the function of renin angiotensin-aldosterone system and the urinary excretion of prostaglandins in newborn infants. Pediatr Res *14*:765, 1980.

95. Sutton, T. J., Leblanc, A., Gauthier, N., et al: Radiologic manifestations of neonatal renal vein thrombosis on follow-up examinations. Radiology *122*:435, 1977.

96. Teele, R. L.: Ultrasonography of the genitourinary tract in children. Radiol Clin North Am *15*:109, 1977.

97. Tomarelli, R. M.: Osmolality, osmolarity and renal solute level of infant formulas. J Pediatr *88*:454, 1976.

98. Trompeter, R. S., Chantler, C., and Haycock, G. B.: Tolazoline and acute renal failure in the newborn. Lancet *1*:1219, 1981.

99. Weinberg, J., Weitzman, R., Zakauddin, S., et al: Inappropriate secretion of antidiuretic hormone in a premature infant. J Pediatr *90*:111, 1977.

100. Nogrady, M. B., and Outerbridge, E. W.: Roentgenologic sequelae of neonatal septicemia and UTI. Am J Roentgenol Radium Ther Nucl Med *118*:28, 1973.

15

Hematologic Problems

SAMUEL GROSS

The great questions of the day are not decided by speeches and majority votes but by blood and iron.

BISMARCK
SEPTEMBER 30, 1862

This chapter, describing the nature and management of hematologic problems common to the neonate (with the exception of erythroblastosis, discussed in Chapter 11), is organized in a different fashion. Case problems will serve as a basis upon which discussion will be developed, and the sections on Basic Considerations, Clinical Management, and Practical Hints previously seen are incorporated into the cases. For quick reference, the following cases will be discussed in this chapter: (1) accidental blood loss, (2) vitamin K deficiency, (3) low platelets, (4) consumption coagulopathy, (5) iron deficiency, (6) vitamin E deficiency, and (7) a complicated case.

This chapter is not intended to serve as an introduction to basic neonatal hematology, for which the reader is referred to the text of Oski and Naiman.[30]

DISORDERS IN HEMOSTASIS

Blood Volume and Accidental Blood Loss

Case One

Male infant A was the second child born to a healthy, blood type O, Rh-positive mother, whose medications during pregnancy consisted solely of

336

calcium, iron, and vitamins. Labor began spontaneously but was then precipitously hastened following manual rupture of the membranes. The infant's birth weight (2.6 kg) was consistent with the estimated gestational age of 39 weeks. Examination of the placenta revealed a small 1 cm tear at the base of the cord adjacent to its insertion. No bleeding was noted from this site. Although the baby breathed and cried spontaneously, he appeared to be moderately lethargic and accordingly was placed in the observation nursery where he received vitamin K_1 (0.5 mg IM). One hour later, lethargy was more pronounced and accompanied by pallor, tachypnea, and tachycardia (respiratory rate 70/minute; pulse rate 165/minute). Apart from these changes there were no other abnormal physical findings, nor was there evidence of active bleeding. Rectal temperature at that time was 34.7° C. The umbilical vessels were catheterized, and the following studies, including type and cross-match, were obtained.

Hemoglobin	10.2 gm/dl
Hematocrit	29.5 per cent
Arterial pressure (mean)	20 mm Hg
Arterial pH	7.15
Pa_{O_2}	50 mm Hg
Blood type	O, Rh-positive
Coombs' test (direct)	Negative
Platelets	230,000/mm³
Prothrombin time	13 seconds
Partial thromboplastin time	30 seconds
Fibrinogen	200 mg/dl
Erythrocyte morphology	Normochromic, normocytic; 12 nucleated RBCs per 100 WBCs.

As shown, the major abnormalities included low hemoglobin and hematocrit values and low arterial pressure and oxygen tension. The presumptive diagnosis was accidental blood loss with impending shock, presumed to be the result of the tear in the cord at the time of delivery. Twenty minutes later, the infant received 50 ml (20 ml/kg) of whole blood, cross-matched against both mother and infant. There followed an immediate, albeit modest, clinical improvement (mean arterial pressure rose to 28 mm Hg, and the hematocrit rose to 32 per cent). Two hours later, an additional 50 ml of whole blood was transfused, following which the hematocrit rose to 41 per cent and the mean arterial pressure stabilized at 43 mm Hg.

Commentary

The presence of a tear in the umbilical cord and the clinical findings of pallor, tachycardia, and tachypnea, with failure to identify either hemolytic or coagulation abnormalities, are strong presumptive evidence of accidental hemorrhage. This diagnosis was further supported by the lack of any evidence of active internal bleeding (e.g., abdominal distension, shifting dullness, periumbilical ecchymoses) or hemorrhage into the central nervous system (e.g., apnea or convulsions). The association of tachypnea and tachycardia with arterial hypotension further distinguishes blood loss with impending shock from the symptoms of primary pulmonary dysfunction.

Once a hemorrhagic event is identified as a life-threatening process, the hallmarks of which are shock and hypotension, efforts to ameliorate this disorder must be carried out with deliberate haste. Ideally in such situations the measurement of choice is a blood volume determination by radioactive assay. However, in the absence of this technique, dependable estimations can be made on the basis of the studies of Usher et al,[36] who showed that term infants, after immediate cord clamping, had a mean blood volume of 78 ml/kg (red cell volume 52 ml/kg), as compared with 101 ml/kg (red cell volume 51 ml/kg) following a 5 minute delay in clamping. In premature infants,[35] following immediate clamping only, the mean blood volume was 89 ml/kg (red cell volume 51 ml/kg). Insofar as identifying volume losses, reliable estimations may be applied from studies on term infants by Walgren et al,[37] who showed that a 25 per cent reduction in circulating volume halved the initial pulmonary and systemic arterial pressures and that, conversely, a corresponding increase in volume doubled the pressures. Thus, in the absence of specific information, one may estimate volume as 90

ml/kg and losses in accord with arterial pressures (i.e., 50 per cent decline in arterial pressure approximates at least a 25 per cent reduction in volume). Earlier correction of the hypovolemia would have improved the care of the infant.

Equally important is the knowledge of the blood-processing measures characteristic of each institution. For example, in this center, 450 ml of donor blood is collected into a plastic bag containing 67.5 ml of anticoagulant (citrate-phosphate-dextrose), resulting thereby in an average hemoglobin content of 64 gm, or 12.4 gm/dl. When "routinely packed" cells are requested (i.e., a single centrifugation followed by removal of 90 per cent of the plasma volume, the resultant hemoglobin range is 19–22 gm/dl. A double centrifugation of saline-washed cells, followed by removal of both supernatant and the upper 5 per cent cell mass, will increase the hemoglobin range to 27–31 gm/dl.

Another significant factor is the basis upon which cell measurements are made. Capillary blood should not be used for such determinations.[25] During the first 5 days of life in term infants and for as many as 14 days in small premature infants, peripheral stasis may result in a differential of as many as 20 percentage points between central and peripheral determinations. (The peripheral determinations are higher than the central measurements.) In addition, cord blood obtained at the time of delivery is also unsuitable for estimation of red cell mass because of difficulties in collection. Blood from the umbilical or other free-flowing veins is preferred.[3b, 30a]

Earlier application of this information in the treatment of baby A, in whom blood loss was acute and treatment not completed until slightly over 3½ hours had elapsed, would have provided a logical basis of therapy and a more immediate response. The following is our approach to treatment in such cases.

1. Assume an intermediate value for blood volume (i.e., 90 ml/kg). In the case of baby A, 2.6 kg × 90 ml = 234 ml.

2. In slightly more than 90 per cent of term infants, the normal range in hemoglobin and hematocrit values is 16–20 gm/dl and 48–60 per cent, respectively (Appendix C–5). In this infant, who was symptomatic by 1 hour of life, these values were 10.2 gm/dl and 29 per cent, respectively, which would indicate an estimated volume loss between 35 and 45 per cent.

3. A judgment must then be made as to the type of volume replacement. The clinical picture was one of acute blood loss and hypotension (hypovolemia). The pressing goal of therapy in such circumstances is the repair of the "effective" circulating volume. In any situation of profound hemorrhage and vascular collapse, the rapid infusion of 20 ml/kg of saline (or 5 per cent albumin if available) will provide a temporary restoration of volume.

A most effective plasma expander is plasma itself. Arrangements should be made with the blood bank to have an available source of fresh-frozen AB plasma for just such acute emergencies.

However, without restoration of red cell mass, the alleviation of hypoxia will be marginal at best, especially in the infant compromised by hemoglobin that contains low levels of 2,3-DPG (2,3-diphosphoglycerate). The treatment of choice is whole blood, cross-matched against both mother and infant. Since this procedure may not be practical in emergency situations, the initial transfusion may follow a "partial"* match or be provided from a "walking" donor of known blood type.

During this period, appropriate cross-matching must be carried out prior to completing the total calculated transfusion. This should return the hemoglobin level to at least 80 per cent of the estimated loss. This case clearly underlines the need to anticipate therapy. Had a single "routinely packed" cell transfusion (hematocrit 55–65 per cent) been used, a 75 ml infusion (equal in volume and cell mass to the estimated loss) would have corrected the deficit in a relatively brief period of time.

4. The arterial pressure must be monitored in all situations of neonatal hypovolemia. It is the most sensitive early index of volume repair, since the return to a normotensive state precedes restoration of normal hematocrit values. Examination of baby A's therapy demonstrates this point. The initial infusion of whole blood, although it provided transient clinical benefit, did not result in a normotensive state, nor did it correct the loss of red cell volume. The modest rise in arterial pressure indicated that further replacement therapy was necessary. Monitoring of arterial blood pressure also prevents overly vigorous attempts at volume repair with the attendant risks of overexpansion of the intravascular space.

5. Supportive efforts must include the maintenance of an unobstructed airway, adequate oxygenation, and appropriate correction of acid-base balance. In situations in which lengthy laboratory studies are needed to identify possible coagulation abnormalities or internal hemorrhage secondary to trauma, the transfusion procedures must be maintained as long as evidence of continued bleeding persists, especially if surgical intervention is anticipated. Every possible attempt should be made to ensure proper temperature control during manipulation and transfusion procedures.

6. Examination of the placenta and umbilical cord must also be included as an integral part of the initial evaluation. In this instance, identification of the tear in the umbilical cord should have immediately alerted the physician to the possibility of blood loss.

In cases of suspected fetal-maternal hemorrhage or twin-to-twin bleeding of similar clinical severity, the same procedures must be employed. In the former instance, the acid elution technique may confirm the presence of fetal cells in the maternal circulation.[39] If differences in maternal and infant blood typing exist, differential agglutination studies will also be helpful. Although fetal-maternal hemorrhage usually occurs during labor, one may, on occasion, observe pallor after delivery without signs and symptoms of acute blood loss (presumably the result of bleeding into the maternal circulation before labor). It is reasonable to treat such infants solely with iron (see section on the red cell, pp. 346–354). On occasion, blood is identified in the vomitus or stool of the infants suspected of a bleeding disorder. In such situations, the use of the hemoglobin identification test of Abt and Downey[2] will help to distinguish adult from fetal hemoglobin. Because the alkali resistance of fetal hemoglobin is time dependent, the test should be done within 1–2 hours of its procurement.

Editorial Comment: Recent studies indicate that prompt determination of the maternal serum alpha-fetoprotein level is the most accurate measure of fetal-maternal hemorrhage. Bear in mind that maternal-fetal hemorrhage may also produce significant problems, including hydrops fetalis.

---

*In this sense, "partial" indicates a rapid cross-match.

Bowman, J. M., Lewis, M., DeSa, D. J.: Hydrops fetalis caused by massive materno-fetal transplacental hemorrhage. J Pediatr *104*:769, 1984.

Bickers, R. G., and Wennberg, R. P.: Fetomaternal transfusion following trauma. Obstet Gynecol *61*:258, 1983.

Fay, F. A.: Feto-maternal hemorrhage as a cause of fetal morbidity and mortality. Br J Obstet Gynecol *90*:443, 1983.

It is important to anticipate evidence of recent acute blood loss in many high-risk newborn infants. It should be mandatory, therefore, to monitor central venous hemoglobin/hematocrit determinations, along with arterial pressure levels, on all such patients admitted to the high-risk nursery to identify the less apparent cases of acute blood loss, which, without supportive intervention, may progress to delayed, albeit sudden, cardiovascular collapse and death. Utilizing such careful assessment, Faxelius et al[6] noted that almost 25 per cent of high-risk infants, many of whom initially were not severely clinically distressed, had red cell volumes less than 25 ml/kg and an attendant death rate of almost 60 per cent. The sine qua non, in effect, is a high index of suspicion, which should prompt the physician to reassess all pertinent perinatal data, including a review of possible vaginal spotting, placental abnormalities, emergency cesarean sections, or umbilical cord abnormalities. Clinical signs that should alert the physician to the possibility of impending cardiovascular collapse secondary to acute blood loss include asphyxiation, respiratory distress, peripheral vasoconstriction, and low arterial pressure. By scrupulously attending to all of the above details, it should be possible to further diminish the extent of fetal wastage in the high-risk nursery.

Polycythemia

Neonatal polycythemia, by definition, is a hematocrit value in excess of 70 per cent. It occurs most commonly as a result of maternal-to-fetal transfusions but also may occur in twin-to-twin transfusions, infants of diabetic mothers, congenital adrenal hyperplasia, infants born to thyrotoxic mothers, and infants who are small for gestational age. The occurrence of neonatal polycythemia requires appropriate diagnostic studies, including the maternal history, examination of the placenta, fetal and adult hemoglobin levels, IgA and IgM levels, differential erythrocyte agglutination, and, if indicated, glucose, cortisol, and thyroxin levels. In dizygotic twins, a hemoglobin differential greater than 4.0 gm/dl should suggest twin-to-twin transfusion.

The risks of neonatal polycythemia include arterial and venous thromboses, pulmonary hemorrhage, hyperbilirubinemia, apnea, radiographic evidence of interlobar fluid, lethargy, jitteriness, hypoglycemia, signs of impending congestive heart failure, priapism, and necrotizing enterocolitis. Infants with central hematocrits in excess of 65 per cent who display the foregoing findings should receive partial exchange transfusions with whole blood (Hct 36%). It is generally agreed that partial exchange transfusions are not indicated for polycythemic infants who are asymptomatic or have normal blood glucose levels.[6]

Since most infants with polycythemia have normal or even slightly reduced blood volumes and all show some evidence of circulatory insufficiency as a result of the associated hyperviscosity, I don't feel that any of these infants should be treated by simple phlebotomy. All polycythemic infants who require treatment should have partial exchange transfusions. The real problem at present is the identification of the infant who can benefit from the procedure. At the present time we do not routinely perform partial exchange transfusions on polycythemic infants who are asymptomatic and have normal blood glucose levels. Partial exchange transfusions are reserved for those infants with a central hematocrit in excess of 65 per cent who display dyspnea, interlobar fluid on chest film, lethargy or excessive jitteriness, hypoglycemia, signs of impending congestive heart failure, priapism, or possible necrotizing enterocolitis. **F. Oski**

Although diagnostic and management procedures employed in the care of the anemic or polycythemic infant usually require catheterization of the umbilical vessels, it should be emphasized that these manipulations are not without risks (i.e., infection, perforation, thrombosis) (see Chapter 2).

Editorial Comment: Black et al published another randomized study of the effects of partial plasma exchange transfusion on long-term outcome. Ninety-three infants with polycythemia and hyperviscosity were randomly assigned to receive either a partial exchange transfusion or symptomatic treatment. Polycythemic infants demonstrated more neurologic problems than the nonpolycythemic controls. Furthermore, at 2 years the polycythemic infants who had undergone partial exchange transfusions had fewer diagnoses of neurologic problems and fine motor abnormalities than those receiving symptomatic treatment only. Nonetheless, gastrointestinal injury was more prevalent among those receiving partial plasma exchange transfusions. One must conclude that polycythemia with hyperviscosity results in a major incidence of short- and long-term morbidity.

Black, V. D., Lubchenco, L. A., Koops, B. L., et al: Neonatal hyperviscosity: randomized study of effect of partial plasma exchange transfusion on long-term outcome. Pediatrics 75:1048, 1985.

Black, V. D., Rumack, C. M., Lubchenco, L. A., et al:

Gastrointestinal injury in polycythemic term infants. Pediatrics 76:225, 1985.

Vitamin K Deficiency

Case Two

While driving home from the market, Mrs. Y., a 33 year old gravida VI mother of five healthy children, entered spontaneous labor and within a few minutes, in the midst of heavy downtown traffic, delivered a male infant. Further assistance was provided by the rescue squad, who subsequently transported both mother and infant to a nearby hospital. Physical examination in the nursery revealed a normal term male (weight 3.0 kg). Because of the circumstances of the delivery, the baby received prophylactic penicillin and kanamycin. On the second hospital day, breast feeding was begun. On the third day, excessive oozing from a heel site following routine capillary puncture was observed. No further studies were obtained at that time. On the fourth hospital day, the infant was circumcised, and within a short time the surgical dressing and diaper were thoroughly saturated with blood. Venous blood was then obtained for screening hematologic and clotting studies.

Hematocrit	46 per cent
Platelets	205,000/mm³
Partial thromboplastin time	68 seconds (Nl* 35 seconds)
Prothrombin time	28 seconds (Nl 12 seconds)
Fibrinogen	255 mg/dl

On questioning the nursery personnel, it was revealed that the infant did not receive vitamin K, an apparent result of the confusing and unusual circumstances of his birth. At this point, the presumptive diagnosis of hemorrhagic disease secondary to vitamin K deficiency was made.

Commentary

In the absence of vitamin K, the liver is unable to synthesize factors II (prothrombin), VII (proconvertin), IX (plasma thromboplastin component), and X (Stuart-Prower). In the small premature infant, hepatic synthesis of these factors is often minimal, even in the presence of large amounts of vitamin K. Furthermore, the only factors that remain within the range of normal adult values in the immediate newborn period, irrespective of gestational maturity, are factors I, V, VIII,

and with rare exception, platelets (Appendix C–6).[26–28]

A reliable index of vitamin K deficiency is the one-stage prothrombin time determination, which, however, does not measure solely prothrombin levels. It measures the activity of factors II, V, VII, and X, but in situations of vitamin K deficiency, the prothrombin time becomes prolonged because of the progressive deficiencies of factors II, VII, and X. Factor IX is not identified in the prothrombin time determination, and factor V is not vitamin K dependent (Figure 15–1).

The ability of the newborn infant to synthesize and utilize vitamin K is a function of both gestational and chronologic age. In term infants, prothrombin time is most prolonged at 3–4 days and remains increased for an additional 2–3 days. In the small premature infant, the prolonged time may persist for 10–14 days.

The initial diet of the newborn also plays a significant role in the production of vitamin K deficiency.[8] For example, cow's milk contains approximately 6 μg/dl of vitamin K, or four times the amount present in human milk. Furthermore, the frequency of a marked prolongation of prothrombin time in infants fed cow's milk preparations before 12 hours of age is approximately half that of infants whose feedings are delayed during this period.

The prolonged administration of antibiotics, which eliminate intestinal bacterial flora, may contribute to vitamin K deficiency. The combination of antibiotic therapy and formulae low in vitamin K has been related to the occurrence of serious hemorrhagic problems in infants well beyond the newborn period.

In the case of baby Y, failure to administer vitamin K was compounded by the subsequent administration of a diet low in vitamin K (breast milk). It is a moot point, however, whether the antibiotics administered during the first 3 days of life added to this problem.

Editorial Comment: It should be noted that at birth 5 per cent of normal full-term infants are dangerously deficient in vitamin K. This must not be overlooked, particularly in neonates with any hemorrhagic disorder.

Alpan, G., Avital, A., Peleg, O., et al: Late presentation of hemorrhagic disease of the newborn. Arch Dis Child 59:482, 1984.

Payne, N. R., and Hasegawa, D. K.: Vitamin K deficiency in newborns: a case report in alpha-antitrypsin deficiency and a review of factors predisposing to hemorrhage. Pediatrics 73:712, 1984.

*Normal.

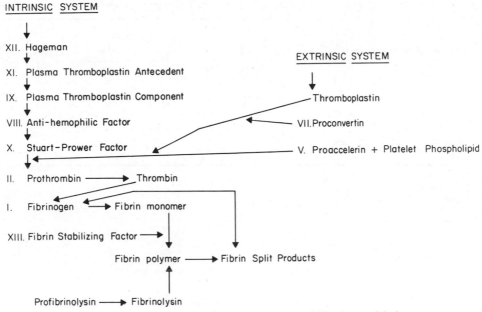

Figure 15–1. The system of clot promotion, stabilization, and lysis.

Although as little as 25 μg/dl of vitamin K$_1$ is sufficient to protect against the prolongation of prothrombin time in term infants, the recommended dose is 0.5–1.0 mg IM, administered immediately after birth. There is no advantage gained by the administration of vitamin K to the mother immediately prior to delivery. In cases of obvious bleeding, it is advisable to use the intravenous route to avoid the occurrence of hematoma formation. In the small premature infant, as much as 2–3 mg may be necessary to effect a favorable response in prothrombin time. However, prolonged bleeding may still persist in such infants, and although administration of fresh plasma may help in replacing some of the deficient factors and aid in shortening the prothrombin time, in no instance should synthetic vitamin K analogues be used. Such agents not only are slow in effecting a response, but in large doses they have the attendant risk of producing hyperbilirubinemia and kernicterus when administered to premature infants. The data relative to a similar response in full-term infants are not clearly established.

Certain of the milk substitute formulae contain less than 25 μg of vitamin K/liter. Infants receiving such preparations should have additional vitamin K in the dietary regimen to raise the daily intake to the level of around 100 μg/l. The same holds true for infants with malabsorption disorders, such as cystic fibrosis or biliary atresia, or infants requiring prolonged parenteral nutritional supplementation. The water-soluble preparation is to be preferred and need not be administered parenterally unless there is unequivocal evidence that vitamin K absorption is impaired.

It should be noted that a prolongation of prothrombin time may reflect primary abnormalities in liver function rather than lack of dietary vitamin K. Table 15–1 contains a summation of the screening tests useful in characterizing the clotting abnormalities in vitamin K deficiency, liver disease, primary clotting factor deficiencies, and consumptive coagulopathies.

Platelets

Case Three

Baby boy Z was born at term to a healthy, gravida II, blood type AB, Rh-positive mother, whose pregnancy was uncomplicated and who received no drugs other than vitamins. A previous sibling, born at another hospital, had a history of chronic umbilical bleeding during the first 3 days of life, which allegedly did not respond to the administration of vitamin K. However, no clotting studies were performed on that infant, and only after a transfusion of fresh whole blood did the bleeding apparently cease. Immediately following delivery of baby Z, scattered petechiae were visible over the entire

TABLE 15–1 CLOTTING DISORDERS AND RELATED SCREENING STUDIES IN THE NEWBORN*

Deficiencies/Disorders	PTT	PT	TT	Fibrin-ogen	FSP	Platelets	Urea Clot Lysis
Vitamin K	↑	↑	NI	NI	NI	NI	NI
Factors VIII, IX, and XI	↑	NI	NI	NI	NI	NI	NI
Factor X	↑	↑	NI	NI	NI	NI	NI
Factor V or VII	NI	↑	NI	NI	NI	NI	NI
Factor XIII	NI	NI	NI	NI	NI	NI	↑
Platelets	NI	NI	NI	NI	NI	↓	NI
Disseminated intravascular coagulation	↑	↑	↑	↓	NI or ↑	↓	NI
Liver disease	↑	↑	↑	NI	NI or ↑	NI or ↑	NI

PTT = Partial thromboplastin time
PT = Prothrombin time
TT = Thrombin time
FSP = Fibrin-split products
↑   = Increased
↓   = Decreased
NI = Normal
Note: Factors V and VII are decreased in DIC.
*Ratnoff, O.: The blood clotting mechanism and its disorders. Disease-A-Month, pp. 1–49, 1965.

body, and during the ensuing 3 hours the subcutaneous bleeding increased and became confluent.

Save for petechiae and ecchymoses, no other abnormalities were noted. Venous blood obtained from readily visible and palpable vasculature revealed:

Hemoglobin	16.0 gm/dl
Hematocrit	49.0 per cent
Blood type	A, Rh-positive
Coombs' test (direct)	Negative
Platelets	18,000/mm³
Partial thromboplastin time	40 seconds (control 33 seconds)
Prothrombin time	14 seconds (control 13 seconds)
Fibrinogen	205 mg/dl
IgG	650 mg/dl
IgA	10 mg/dl
IgM	10 mg/dl

These studies revealed that the only identifiable abnormality was the marked reduction in platelets (18,000/mm³). X-rays of the skull and long bones were normal, and bacterial and viral cultures were negative. A bone marrow examination and stain for morphology revealed a slight increase in erythroid precursors, with normal myeloid activity and a modest decrease in the number of megakaryocytes, some of which were immature. The platelet count on the mother was 253,000/mm³. The presumptive diagnosis was isoimmune thrombocytopenia, and treatment with prednisone (1 mg/kg daily) was initiated. Therapy was discontinued after 4 weeks because the platelet count failed to improve. However, no further bleeding problems were noted. Eight weeks later, the platelet count was 75,000/mm³, and by 3 months of age, the count had stabilized in a range of 170,000–225,000/mm³.

Commentary

The absence of any blood group incompatibilities, coupled with normal bone marrow and x-ray examinations in an infant whose sole clinical abnormality was purpura, effectively excluded the possibilities of erythroblastosis, infection, or tumor (including congenital leukemia). The negative maternal history of drug ingestion (specifically thiazides), as well as her normal platelet count, made unlikely the possibility of an autoimmune, drug-induced thrombocytopenia. With the suggestion of a similar disorder in the previous sibling, the presumptive diagnosis of isoimmune thrombocytopenia was considered likely. Although the diagnosis was made solely by exclusion, the course of the disease was consistent with isoimmune thrombocytopenia. It should be noted that serologic tests for platelet antibodies are both difficult to perform and frequently inconclusive.[33]

The differences between isoimmune and autoimmune thrombocytopenia are usually quite distinct. Isoimmune purpura should be suspected in any otherwise healthy thrombocytopenic infant whose mother has a normal platelet count and a negative history of drug therapy. In this disorder, as in erythroblastosis fetalis, the antibody will attack both the infant's and the father's platelets, and successive pregnancies usually result in thrombocytopenic infants. In both disorders, it is not unusual to observe an amegakaryocytic marrow, presumably the result of a direct antibody attack on the antigenic sites of the megakaryocytes.

Corticosteroid therapy rarely is effective in the treatment of the autoimmune type, but for unknown reasons such therapy may occasionally have an ameliorating effect on the isoimmune variety. Exchange transfusion with fresh, platelet-rich whole blood may also be beneficial, possibly by providing extra sites for antibody absorption.

Unusually severe bleeding can be controlled readily using the mother's washed platelets (which are not agglutinated by antibody). However, her condition may preclude such a procedure, or the facilities in a given institution may not include a cell separator, in which case exchange transfusion with fresh whole blood is acceptable. In anticipation of an isoimmune thrombocytopenic birth, it is suggested that delivery be carried out by cesarean section. However, it may be possible to predict the need for such a delivery by sampling scalp vein blood for platelet count at the time of scalp presentation. A platelet count in excess of 30,000/mm^3 mitigates against the necessity for section. It is appropriate that any mother with an anticipated isoimmune thrombocytopenic birth be admitted in advance of delivery to obtain platelets by pheresis so as to have available a nonimmunized platelet source for transfusion into the affected infant, should the need arise. Also recommended by some is the administration to the mother of prednisone (1 mg/kg) 4–6 hours prior to delivery in an attempt to stabilize the infant's capillary bed. This procedure probably will not increase the infant's platelet level. In the infant with thrombocytopenia of unknown cause, repeat platelet determination at 1 hour and 24 hours following an infusion of 1 unit/5 kg of body weight will help distinguish between productive failure and increased lysis. A rapid decline supports the latter. Failure to produce the expected rise (60,000–75,000/mm^3) with platelets from a random donor followed by successful response to maternal platelets is strongly indicative of isoimmune thrombocytopenia.

Editorial Comment: To avoid intracerebral hemorrhage, cesarean section has been recommended for neonates with low platelet counts, the result of isoimmune thrombocytopenia. A recent report documents ultrasonographic demonstration of intracranial hemorrhage occurring in utero in a family with prior evidence of isoimmune neonatal thrombocytopenia. Nonetheless the recommendation of cesarean section still appears justified when the platelet count is low in the fetus. It would, however, appear to be prudent to perform ultrasound prior to delivery to ascertain whether any CNS catastrophe has already taken place.

There are many causes of thrombocytopenia in the newborn. The investigative approach as outlined by Andrew and Kelton should prove extremely valuable (Table 15–2).

Andrew, M., and Kelton, J.: Neonatal thrombocytopenia. Clin Perinatol 11:359, 1984.

Sia, C. G., Concepcion, A., Chan, N., et al: Cesarean section delivery fails to prevent intracranial hemorrhage in isoimmune neonatal thrombocytopenia. Am J Obstet Gynecol 153:79, 1985.

A platelet transfusion from a random donor, although usually not required for therapeutic purposes, provides diagnostic information as to the cause of the thrombocytopenia. The administration of 1 unit of platelets/5 kg of body weight can be anticipated to increase the platelet count by approximately 75,000/mm^3. Failure to achieve such a rise or failure to maintain it for a period of approximately 24 hours indicates that a destructive process is responsible for the observed thrombocytopenia. When a platelet transfusion from a random donor does not produce the expected rise and platelets from the mother do, then the diagnosis of isoimmune neonatal thrombocytopenia is established even in the absence of supporting serologic data. For guidance in the use of this procedure the reader should consult the report of McIntosh and associates (1973).

I strongly support the suggestion of Dr. Gross that once a mother has given birth to an infant with isoimmune thrombocytopenia, efforts should be directed toward having all subsequent deliveries accomplished by cesarean section. The mother should be admitted the day before surgery so that a platelet-pheresis can be performed, thus ensuring the availability of platelets for transfusion should the need arise.

McIntosh, S., O'Brien, R. T., Schwartz, A. D., et al: Neonatal isoimmune purpura: response to platelet infusions. J Pediatr 82:1020, 1973.

F. Oski

TABLE 15–2 INVESTIGATIONS FOR CLASSIFYING THROMBOCYTOPENIA BY MECHANISM

Laboratory Parameter	Increased Platelet Destruction	Decreased Platelet Production
Platelet size	Increased	Normal
Platelet survival	Decreased	Normal
Platelet associated IgG	Often very increased	Usually normal, or slightly increased
Bleeding time	Usually prolonged	Prolonged
Other cell lines	Usually normal	Often abnormal
Megakaryocytes	Normal or increased	Decreased
Other bone marrow cell lines	Normal	Often decreased or abnormal

Other causes of neonatal thrombocytopenia include erythroblastosis fetalis (although thrombocytopenia may develop following repeated and prolonged exchange transfusions) and congenital absence of megakaryocytes as an isolated phenomenon or in association with phocomelia; it may appear as part of a pancytopenia syndrome (which may on rare occasions respond to the administration of corticosteroids and/or testosterone). Thrombocytopenia may be present in a wide variety of infectious diseases, including bacterial septicemia, herpes simplex, toxoplasmosis, cytomegalic inclusion disease, congenital syphilis, and the rubella syndrome. It is usually a feature of congenital leukemia, Down's syndrome, Wiskott-Aldrich syndrome, Letterer-Siwe disease, and disseminated intravascular coagulation. Although rare before 2 months of life, it may be associated with giant hemangiomata as a result of platelet trapping.

The clinical expression of thrombocytopenia in the immediate newborn period is usually quite dramatic. Unlike the occasional scattered petechiae on the head and shoulders of an otherwise normal infant, subcutaneous bleeding sites are usually profuse and scattered over the entire body. Fortunately, bleeding is rarely of sufficient degree to impair vital function. In such instances, immediate exchange transfusion with fresh whole blood or platelet packs should be administered and followed by splenectomy (but only if megakaryocytes are clearly identified in the marrow).

Platelet counts vary in accordance with both the method of determination and, to a lesser extent, the degree of gestational maturity. In general, platelet levels enumerated by phase microscopy are 25,000–50,000/mm³ lower than those performed under direct microscopy. In small premature infants, occasional platelet values as low as 25,000–50,000/mm³ have been noted in the absence of any clinical disorder. However, this information is not intended to deter the physician from seeking an etiologic agent.

The Consumption of Clotting Factors

Case Four

Baby girl W was born at term (birth weight 3.9 kg) following an uncomplicated pregnancy and delivery. On the first postpartum day it was noted that the mother had a streptococcal breast abscess,

and, as a consequence, breast feeding was not allowed, although rooming-in was permitted. Capillary blood studies, obtained on the third day of life because of the presence of icterus, revealed the following: hematocrit 43 per cent; blood type O, Rh-positive; direct Coombs' test negative; bilirubin D/T 0.7/9.4 mg/dl. The infant appeared to be sluggish during the blood-drawing process. Twelve hours later, she suddenly became pale and voided a small quantity of burgundy-colored urine. The umbilical artery was catheterized and revealed a pressure of 25 mm Hg. Additional blood studies performed at this point included a hematocrit of 31 per cent and a peripheral blood film that contained polychromatophilic and fragmented erythrocytes, increased numbers of normoblasts, and a marked reduction in platelets. Detailed studies are included below.

Hemoglobin	11.1 gm/dl
Hematocrit	31.0 per cent
Reticulocyte count	17.1 per cent
Normoblasts	15/100 WBC
Peripheral smear	Fragmented erythrocytes, decreased platelets
Coombs' test (direct)	Negative
Platelet count	35,000/mm³
Partial thromboplastin time	> 160 seconds
Prothrombin time	> 120 seconds
Thrombin time	> 60 seconds
Fibrinogen	10 mg/dl
Urinalysis	Free hemoglobin, red cells, protein 60 mg/dl*
Fibrin split products	10 per cent*
Factor VIII	10 per cent*
Factor V	10 per cent

The infant's clinical status rapidly deteriorated. She immediately received an infusion of 30 ml of 5 per cent albumin, which was followed in rapid sequence by an exchange transfusion of 24 hour old, type-specific, citrated whole blood. Bleeding from the umbilical vessels, which had been profuse prior to the exchange transfusion, ceased midway through the procedure, and the arterial pressure rose to a normal level. Following the exchange transfusion, the infant was markedly improved and had normal clotting studies, which remained normal throughout the hospital stay. Blood cultures obtained from the umbilical vein prior to the exchange grew β-hemolytic streptococcus, group A, for which the infant accordingly received 10 days of penicillin (initiated after completion of the exchange transfusion). On the eighteenth hospital day, the infant was sent home in good health with

---

*These results were obtained 7 hours later on preexchange plasma stored at −20° C.

a discharge diagnosis of consumptive coagulopathy (disseminated intravascular coagulation) secondary to β-hemolytic streptococcal septicemia, presumably contracted from the mother.

Commentary

In 1962, Abelli and DeLamerans[1] applied the term "secondary hemorrhagic disease" to a group of immature newborn infants with alterations in capillary permeability and abnormally low clotting factors, including fibrinogen (I), factor V, and platelets. In most of these infants, hypoxia and/or sepsis was a major clinical finding, and the response to vitamin K was generally poor, although the administration of fresh whole blood occasionally effected transient improvement. In retrospect, it appears likely that many of these patients did indeed have disseminated intravascular coagulation. It is now well established that a variety of factors can either initiate or worsen disseminated intravascular coagulation. Table 15–3 lists known triggering events.

The diagnosis of disseminated intravascular coagulation (DIC) must be strongly suspected in any newborn infant (particularly the susceptible infant of a high-risk pregnancy) with a bleeding disorder secondary to a deficiency of all factors (including factors I, V, VIII, and platelets) in association with increased levels of fibrin-split products and a peripheral smear characterized by fragmented erythrocytes. The erythrocyte abnormality is presumed to be the result of a shearing effect on the membrane following flow through an angiopathic or semioccluded blood vessel. Such cells rapidly undergo lysis within the vascular space. The newborn has limited capacity to synthesize haptoglobin, with the result that there can be free hemoglobin with brisk hemolysis and free hemoglobin is released into the renal collecting system, imposing a risk for development of tubular damage. Additional albumin and fluid administration will effectively diminish the chances for bilirubin release and the onset of a hemoglobin-induced nephropathy. The elevation of fibrin-split products reflects the response of the fibrinolytic system to the initial increase in clot formation. However, in cases of overwhelming disease, such elevations may not be present or even found on postmortem examination. Furthermore, the clotting abnormalities may not always occur in temporal association. As a consequence, fluctuations in these laboratory determinations are commonly seen during the course of the illness.

The present case illustrates the rapidity with which clinical manifestations of DIC may appear and underlines the urgency of providing rapid diagnostic studies and appropriate therapy. Procedures that are readily accomplished within minutes include: (1) estimation of platelet numbers and erythrocyte morphology by examination of routine blood films, and (2) estimation of fibrinogen content by observing the degree of flocculation of plasma heated at 56° C (no precipitate or only a fine flocculus is strong presumptive evidence of decreased fibrinogen levels). Reliable determinations of partial thromboplastin and prothrombin times, as well as fibrinogen content, can be made within 5 minutes on as little as 3 ml of whole blood. However, because assays for factors VI, VIII, and fibrin-split products are time consuming, such determinations may be held in abeyance until time permits by storage of citrated plasma in plastic tubes at −20° C.

Therapy should be directed against both the inciting cause, if identifiable, and the hemorrhagic event. Heparin in a dose of 100 units/kg, administered every 4–6 hours and continued until sustained improvement is established, has been recommended as the treatment of choice. This is not our experience. Heparin, if it is used at all, should be used in infants with obvious thrombotic events. In the absence of any data to the contrary, the most effective therapy (in addition to identification of the inciting cause) is a two-volume exchange transfusion with citrate-phosphate-dextrose whole blood less than 48 hours old. Repeat exchange transfusions may be performed as indicated. For

TABLE 15–3 ETIOLOGIC FACTORS IN DISSEMINATED INTRAVASCULAR COAGULATION IN THE NEWBORN

Septicemia: bacterial, viral, parasitic, rickettsial, mycotic
Tissue release:
 Antigen-antibody complexes
 Abruptio placentae
 Intravascular hemolysis
 Malignancy
 Idiopathic respiratory distress syndrome
  (asphyxia, hypoxia)
 Burns
Giant hemangioma (platelet trapping)
Purpura fulminans (? septicemia)
Hepatitis and cirrhosis (? tissue release)

more extensive information on problems of hemostasis in the premature infant, the reader is directed to the reviews by Gross and Stuart and Nathan and Oski.[15, 24a]

For the patient actively bleeding the best results in our series have been obtained with citrated whole blood exchange transfusion, repeated if necessary until a favorable response is obtained.[11] For the term infant, blood less than 48 hours old is satisfactory; for the premature infant, fresh blood is preferred. In patients in whom bleeding and hemolysis are not severe (i.e., in the absence of a shocklike state), supportive therapy with platelets suspended in fresh plasma or fresh whole blood will suffice. In the absence of fresh whole blood, platelets suspended in fresh frozen plasma—to which erythrocytes are added to a hematocrit of 50 per cent—is an acceptable alternative.

Several investigators have identified a marked increase in fibrinogen turnover and fibrinolytic activity in infants with respiratory distress syndrome (RDS), while the relationship between hypoxia and DIC has generated much discussion.[5, 18, 21] It has further been postulated that failure to effect optimal perfusion of the pulmonary vasculature in premature infants, as a result of either perinatal hemorrhage or sequestered placental blood, may potentiate or actually initiate the RDS,[7] which may in turn trigger a local bleeding diathesis and the consumption of coagulation factors. However, in the absence of adequate confirmatory findings, one should at least be aware of the potential risks in such patients and obtain appropriate studies in anticipation of such events as intracerebral (or intraventricular) hemorrhage, pulmonary hemorrhage, or severe gastro-intestinal bleeding—all of which may be life-threatening.

Other causes of hemorrhagic disease in the newborn may be related to iatrogenic effects, namely, overzealous flushing of an indwelling umbilical catheter with heparin or thrombus formation secondary to an inappropriately positioned catheter.

The initial presentation of hemorrhagic disease secondary to inherited coagulation abnormalities may, on occasion, occur in the newborn period. As in all clotting disorders, appropriate studies should be obtained and treatment directed to replacement of deficient factors. A variety of differential laboratory examinations relative to various clotting disorders are presented in Table 15–1.

THE ERYTHROCYTE

Iron

Case Five

Baby girl S was born at term (birth weight 2.9 kg) to a healthy, blood type B, Rh-positive primigravida mother following an uneventful pregnancy. However, labor was complicated by vaginal bleeding, which was apparently the result of marginal sinus rupture of the placenta. For this reason, delivery was accomplished by cesarean section. Initial physical examination revealed a vigorous, active infant in no distress. The placenta was not examined. Laboratory data obtained on blood from the umbilical vein included:

Hemoglobin	13.9 gm/dl
Hematocrit	40 per cent
Peripheral smear	Normocytic erythrocytes with 5 nucleated RBC/WBC
Reticulocyte count	8.7 per cent
Platelet count	425,000/mm³

A stain of maternal peripheral blood revealed 3.5 per cent fetal cells. The infant's blood type was B, Rh-positive, and differential agglutination was therefore not attempted. After an uneventful 4 day hospital course, the infant was discharged without further therapy. The mother was instructed to use a milk formula that was not iron supplemented, and the infant was scheduled for a follow-up return visit 1 month after discharge. However, the infant did not return for 6 months, at which time examination revealed an irritable, pale infant whose only other pertinent physical finding was a spleen tip palpable 1 cm below the left costal margin. Laboratory data at this time included:

Hemoglobin	7.0 gm/dl
Hematocrit	24 per cent
Peripheral smear	Marked hypochromia
Reticulocyte count	3.2 per cent
Platelet count	450,000/mm³
Bound serum iron	35 mg/dl
Total iron binding capacity	490 mg/dl

On further questioning of the parents, it was learned that the sole dietary intake during the first 6 months of life was a milk preparation, which averaged approximately 36 ounces/24 hours. Later during this examination the infant passed a stool that was normal in color and consistency but that was found to be 2 + for guaiac.

Commentary

The clinical and laboratory findings were consistent with a diagnosis of iron deficiency anemia. In most normal full-term infants the most common etiologic factor in the production of iron deficiency is inadequate iron intake. This was obviously the situation in this baby. Infrequently, iron deficiency may occur as a result of chronic occult blood loss secondary to the ingestion of large amounts of unmodified cow's milk preparations. In such infants, a reduction in the total milk intake reduces the red cell losses. Bleeding as a result of vascular abnormalities of the gut will also lead to iron deficiency. Tissue desquamation losses (i.e., nails, hair, gut, etc.) account for somewhere between 0.1 and 0.3 mg of elemental iron per day, but this loss is not sufficient to explain iron deficiency per se. Most cases of nutritional iron deficiency in term infants are rarely apparent before 6 months of age; in fact, they usually do not present until some time late in the first year of life. On the other hand, premature infants not supplied with medicinal or dietary iron will present with signs of iron deficiency before 6 months of age, because of the excessive demands secondary to rapid weight increases. Thus, in the case of baby S, dietary deprivation was only one factor in the causation of the iron deficiency anemia, which was present at least by 6 months of age. The following facets of her newborn course are relevant:

1. A history of blood loss from the placenta before delivery.

2. An initial hematocrit of 40 per cent, which is abnormally low for a full-term infant.

3. Delivery by cesarean section. The manipulation of the infant during this type of extraction often results in "trapping" of a significant amount of the infant's blood volume in the placenta prior to clamping of the cord.

Unlike infants who are symptomatic as a result of profound, acute blood loss in the neonatal period, baby S appeared deceptively normal in the newborn period, presumably because she was able to maintain adequate vascular perfusion. However, it is reasonable to implicate blood loss in the neonatal period as the major reason for part of the clinical and laboratory expression of severe iron deficiency 6 months following delivery.

Certain of the clinical and laboratory data noted in this infant at 6 months of age are worthy of comment. The findings of splenomegaly, moderate thrombocytosis, and positive stool guaiac are not unusual phenomena in iron-deficient infants. Approximately one fourth to one third of all such infants have readily palpable spleens (the etiology of which is obscure), which recede to normal following appropriate therapy. The increase in platelets probably represents the overall increase in marrow response early in the course of iron deficiency. In fact, thrombocytopenia may occur later on, related solely to the deficiency of iron or, on occasion, as part of a concomitant folate deficiency. The presence of occult blood in the stool occurs as a result of profound changes within the mucosal structures caused by deficiencies in tissue iron enzymes, which thereby result in loss of cellular integrity and increased exfoliation.

Had the hematologic data on baby S been viewed with greater scrutiny in the immediate newborn period, appropriate preventive measures could have been initiated. The administration of iron-enriched (8–10 mg of elemental iron/l) formula offered at the time of discharge from the hospital, with the addition of iron-rich foodstuffs beginning at 5–6 months of age, would have in part supplied the iron necessary to allow for restoration of losses as well as maintain the needs imposed by growth. For example, the average daily intake of such a formula during the first 6 months of life is approximately 400–500 ml (4–5 mg of elemental iron) per day. With approximately 10 per cent absorption of the iron, during this interval a total iron intake of somewhere between 75 and 100 mg would have resulted. Examination of the iron balance sheet in Table 15–4 (a retrospective study of baby S and her hypothetical normal term counterpart) suggests that an iron-fortified, low-protein formula per se is not sufficient in such an instance. For example, the hemoglobin in the normal baby was 17.5 gm/100 dl, with an estimated total body iron of 200–220 mg at birth. At 6 months of age (a time when birth weight is doubled), the ideal hemoglobin is 12 gm/dl, with a total body hemoglobin iron of around 200 mg (representing two thirds to three fourths of the total body iron, or approximately 270–300 mg/dl). For baby S, the total body hemoglobin iron measured approximately 130 mg, and probably no more than 150 mg; the amount of available iron even in an iron-rich formula would not have been entirely sufficient to provide both maintenance and correction.

Effective treatment would consist of the

TABLE 15—4 IRON BALANCE

	Normal Term Infant	Baby S
Birth weight	2.9 kg	2.9 kg
Mean hemoglobin (gm/dl)	17.5	13.9
Blood volume (90 ml/kg)	261 ml	261 ml
Total body hemoglobin (gm/dl)	$17.5 \times 2.61 = 45.7$	$2.61 \times 13.9 = 36.3$
Total body hemoglobin iron (mg)	$45.7 \times 3.4^* = 155$	$3.4 \times 36.3 = 129$
Storage iron (8 mg/kg)†	$8 \times 2.9 = 23$	$2.9 \times ? = ?$
Tissue iron (12 mg/kg)†	$12 \times 2.9 = 35$	$2.9 \times ? = ?$
Total body iron (mg)	213	129 plus
Total iron deficit at least: 213–129		

*Approximately 3.4 mg of iron/gm of hemoglobin.
†Depleted in iron deficiency anemia when total body iron stores are not maintained.

administration of oral medicinal iron in a dosage of 10 mg of elemental iron/kg of body weight/day for 2–3 months. Deleterious effects are essentially nonexistent—only on rare occasions do oral iron preparations produce either diarrhea or constipation. It is advisable to avoid the use of unmodified cow's milk preparations because of their greater iron binding effects than the low-protein preparations as well as the rare chance, as noted, of initiating gastrointestinal occult red cell losses.

Under circumstances in which medical follow-up of such patients as baby S is uncertain, more rapid replacement of iron losses is desirable. Total replacement of the iron deficit in the immediate neonatal period is easily accomplished with the use of parenteral iron preparations, calculating the deficit as outlined in Table 15–4. The usual parenteral (iron dextran) preparation contains 50 mg of elemental iron/ml. Although it is advised to administer no more than 1 ml/day, 2–3 ml/day has been administered without untoward effect (namely, febrile response). On rare occasions, an anaphylaxis-like response is known to occur, which readily responds to treatment with oxygen and epinephrine.

Once therapy for the iron-deficient state is completed, there is no further need for the use of iron supplements, provided such infants are maintained on a well-balanced dietary regimen. The authors are aware of the recommendations for supplemental iron during the entire first year of life for all infants (Committee on Nutrition, American Academy of Pediatrics).[34, 34a, 34b] However, while this is appropriate for premature infants (whose requirements for hemoglobin synthesis may exceed iron intake during the rapid growth period of the first year), the normal term infant provided with appropriate medical care and dietary instructions (which in-

clude either breast milk or low-protein formula) does not benefit from additional iron supplementation. In a carefully controlled study of formula and solid feeding practices, only those term infants fed cow's milk with the higher protein content had lower hemoglobin values. Iron supplementation for the infants fed lower protein formula did not improve any hematologic parameter (Table 15–5). The ideal formula in this regard is human milk. Although both contain only trace quantities of iron, on a volume-for-volume basis, more iron is absorbed from human milk than from cow's milk. Human milk contains antibacterial properties (lactoferrin), which lose potency when saturated with iron. For breast-fed infants born at term, normal iron stores are maintained for the first 6 months of life, following which iron-rich solid foods should be added to the diet. Whether or not this is applicable to premature infants is a moot point. In the absence of large-scale studies of solely breast-fed pre-

TABLE 15—5 MEAN HEMOGLOBIN (AND % TERM INFANTS) WITH HEMOGLOBIN LEVELS < 10 gm*/dl IN RELATIONSHIP TO PROTEIN AND IRON CONTENT OF FORMULAE†

Months	LP-I	LP	HP	HP-I
2	11.4 (1)	11.8 (1)	11.6 (1)	11.5 (2)
3	11.5 (0)	11.7 (2)	11.9 (1)	11.6 (2)
4	12.4 (0)	12.2 (0)	11.7 (1)	12.5 (0)
5	12.4 (0)	12.6 (0)	11.8 (1)	12.5 (0)
6	12.6 (0)	12.5 (0)	11.8 (1)	12.2 (1)
8	12.5 (0)	12.2 (0)	11.9 (2)	12.4 (0)
10	12.8 (0)	12.4 (0)	12.1 (1)	12.8 (0)
12	12.7 (0)	12.6 (0)	12.1 (0)	12.6 (0)

*Lowest hemoglobin was 9.0 gm/dl.
LP-I: Protein, 1.5 gm/dl; elemental iron, 0.8 mg/dl
LP: Protein, 1.5 gm/dl; trace iron.
HP: Protein, 2.4 gm/dl; trace iron.
HP-I: Protein, 2.4 gm/dl; elemental iron, 0.85 mg/dl.
†Adapted from data of Gross.[10]

mature infants, iron supplementation is clearly mandated to prevent early onset iron deficiency. For all infants, unmodified cow's milk should be avoided. It is inadequate as a source of iron and is also a potential inducer of gastrointestinal bleeding. A further example of complex interrelationships is the paradoxic response to iron administration in tocopherol "deficient" infants.

I do not agree that the exclusively breast-fed infant requires solid foods that are rich in iron at 3–4 months of age. Carefully controlled studies (Saarinen, 1978) demonstrate that the exclusively breast-fed infant maintains normal iron stores for at least the first 6 months of life. After 6 months an additional source of iron may be required. Whole cow's milk should certainly be avoided during this period of life. Not only is it an inadequate source of iron, but it may in fact contribute to the production of iron deficiency anemia by inducing occult gastrointestinal bleeding.

Saarinen, U.: Need for iron supplementation in infants on prolonged breast feeding. J Pediatr *93*:177, 1978.

F. Oski

In the United States, nutritional iron deficiency is most often a reflection of broader dietary inadequacies and the lack of optimal medical care among educationally and socioeconomically deprived families.

Vitamin E

Case Six

Baby boy E was born prematurely to a healthy, 20 year old mother whose pregnancy history, apart from the premature birth, was normal. Birth weight was 1.45 kg, and the physical characteristics of the infant were consistent with an estimated gestational age of 32 weeks. A central hematocrit obtained shortly after birth was 48 per cent. At 3 days of age, icterus was noted (bilirubin D/T 0.5/9.0 mg/dl). The hematocrit remained stable, and there was no evidence of blood group incompatibility. Peripheral blood film obtained shortly after birth revealed normal erythrocyte morphology. Treatment consisted of phototherapy, which was discontinued 4 days later following a bilirubin decline to D/T 0.5/3.1 mg/dl. At 4 weeks of age, the hematocrit and reticulocyte counts were 36 per cent and 7.8 per cent, respectively. Three weeks later, the hematocrit had fallen to 24 per cent, and the reticulocyte count had risen to 14.2 per cent. The platelet count was 425,000/mm³, and a peripheral blood smear revealed approximately 10 per cent pyknotic red cells.

Blood was obtained for evaluation of red cell selenium, red cell enzymes, serum tocopherol, iron, and folic acid. Laboratory results were as follows:

Hemoglobin	8.4 gm/dl
Hematocrit	25 per cent
Reticulocytes	14.2 per cent
WBC	8 × 10³/mm³, normal age-related differential
Platelets	425 × 10³/mm³
Serum folate (total)	3.4 ng/dl (Nl >4.5 ng/ml)
Serum tocopherol	0.23 ng/dl
Serum iron	80 ng/dl
RBC selenium	3.0 × 10⁻¹⁰ ng/cell (Nl >4.0)
RBC G6PD	Nl
RBC pyruvate	Nl
RBC glutathione peroxidase	3.6 × 10⁻¹⁰ ng/cell (Nl 6.4 ± 1.0)

As noted, the infant was deficient in tocopherol and folic acid. However, it was concluded that neither the reticulocytosis nor the thrombocytosis was consistent with folate deficiency, and accordingly the infant was treated solely with a daily oral tocopherol dose of 25 units/kg. Repeat blood counts obtained 1 week later failed to reveal changes in any of the above parameters. Therapy was continued for an additional 14 days, at the end of which time the hematocrit had risen to 28 per cent in association with a decline in reticulocyte count to 4.5 per cent and a rise in the level of vitamin E to 0.85 mg/dl. The intramuscular injectable form of vitamin E is an even more efficacious way of treating the infant.

Commentary

The erythrocyte of the newborn infant, as with many aspects of the clotting mechanism, is not especially suited for extrauterine life. Its hemoglobin has a reduced potential for effective oxygen release owing to a lowered 2,3-DPG content,[29] and although the activity of the glycolytic enzymes (except phosphofructokinase) is increased, glutathione peroxidase and catalase activity is diminished.[26] This results in lessened antiperoxidant protection for the red cell membrane, which in less mature infants has a lipid content 1.5 times greater than that of adult red cells. The instability of the "redox" system is further intensified by lowered levels of reduced glutathione, apparently the result of an unstable nicotinamide-adenine dinucleotide phosphate (NADP) system. The lack of antioxidant protection afforded the red cell of the premature infant is further compounded by vitamin E deficiency[22] (due essentially to inadequate absorption of fatty compounds), which persists in varying degrees until the infant approaches gestational maturity[23] (7 weeks of age in baby E). In the term infant, the instability of the glutathione system is rarely apparent beyond the first week of life, while in very small premature infants, low levels of glutathione peroxidase and an unstable, reduced glutathione system may persist for 4–5 weeks.

The combination of increased red cell lipids and decreased levels of vitamin E renders the red cell particularly susceptible to the adverse effects of peroxidant activity. The administration of agents known to enhance peroxidation, such as iron and oxygen, may further increase lipid peroxidation, resulting in cell leakage and ultimately hemolysis.

In addition to the hemolytic aspects, thrombocytosis and occasional peripheral edema have been noted. The thrombocytosis probably reflects nonspecific heightened marrow response to hemolysis, and the edema is the result of vascular damage to the capillary bed.

Baby E exhibited the essential characteristics of a vitamin E dependent, hemolytic anemia, which responded to appropriate therapy only after he reached gestational maturity of sufficient degree to absorb the fat-soluble preparation of the vitamin (at approximately 36–38 weeks' gestational age). Although the administration of a biologically active water-soluble vitamin E preparation (i.e., D-alpha-tocopherol polyethylene glycol succinate [TPGS]) provides "normal" tocopherol levels early in the postgestational life of the smallest premature infants,[14] this so-called "sufficiency" (serum tocopherol levels >0.5 mg/dl) does not prevent hemolysis in the presence of a high PUFA (polyunsaturated fatty acid) level and/or supplemental iron challenge. Selenium deficiency, brought about by ingestion of only cow's milk (which generally is 50–75 per cent lower in selenium than most human milk),[16] leads to glutathione peroxidase deficiency, which in turn further

reduces antioxidant protection in infants so nourished.[10] In veterinary medicine, certain combined selenium and tocopherol deficiency states have been corrected by the administration of high doses of either tocopherol or selenium,[24] and there is evidence to support a similar occurrence in the human.[38] Moreover, infants fed high PUFA diets do not experience increased hemolysis when stressed with parenteral iron, provided prior (4 days to 1 week) therapy with parenteral tocopherol is given to maintain serum levels in excess of 1.0 mg/dl.[9]

Although the serum folate was low in this infant, a finding common in many premature infants,[32] folate deficiency does not appear to play a role in the development of the early anemia of prematurity. Moreover, the administration of folate to such infants, even in the absence of vitamin E deficiency, apparently does nothing more than raise the level of folic acid in the circulation. The entire story on "folate deficiency," however, is not complete and awaits carefully controlled studies wherein all other known hematologic events are stabilized prior to examining folate responsiveness. Even less is known regarding vitamin B_{12} requirements (or possible deficiency) in the small neonate. It is generally agreed that both B_{12} and folate should be supplemented during the first 3–4 months (or until solid intake is initiated) because of increased demands during rapid growth.

The administration of iron during this early period, as noted, relates not only to vitamin E but to antimicrobial protection as well. It interferes with the intestinal absorption of tocopherol,[23] intensifies the hemolytic process due to vitamin E deficiency, and probably interferes with the antibacterial properties of certain (iron binding) proteins when such proteins become iron saturated. It is advisable therefore to defer the practice of administering large amounts of oral or parenteral iron early in the life of a small premature infant for at least 3–4 weeks or until the risk of major infections diminishes. The early administration of intramuscular tocopherol (for dose, see Appendix A–3, p. 405) will permit subsequent administration of prophylactic iron without the attendant risk of oxidant-induced hemolytic anemia.

TABLE 15–6 TOCOPHEROL VALUES IN PREMATURE INFANTS <1700 gm BIRTH WEIGHT (mg/dl)

Weeks	Unsupplemented	Supplemented*
1	0.30	0.30
2	0.32	0.45
4	0.29	0.55
6	0.25	0.50
8	0.30	0.49
10	0.45	0.75
12	0.75	0.85

*Tocopherol polyethylene glycol succinate.

Editorial Comment: The precise role of vitamin E in the newborn remains undefined. In addition to its role in preventing hemolysis of red cells, reports indicate a protective effect against retinopathy of prematurity, bronchopulmonary dysplasia, and even intraventricular hemorrhage. On the other hand, there have been concerns that sepsis, necrotizing enterocolitis, and hemorrhage may be more prevalent with vitamin E therapy. Furthermore, the risks of introducing untested products into the nursery are exemplified by the reports first emanating from the Centers for Disease Control of the disastrous consequences of the use of a new intravenous form of vitamin E (intravenous E-Ferol). An unusual symptom complex of pulmonary deterioration, thrombocytopenia, liver failure, ascites, renal failure, and even death was noted in some infants.

An equally disastrous outcome was noted as a result of the use of benzyl alcohol as a preservative for intravenous preparations. A gasping syndrome was reported first by Gershanik et al (1982). The infants manifested neurologic deterioration, severe metabolic acidosis, gasping respiration, hematologic abnormalities, skin breakdown, and hepatic and renal failure. Cardiac output diminished, and seizures with EEG abnormalities were common. These infants received multiple injections of heparinized bacteriostatic sodium chloride to flush indwelling catheters, and Gershanik et al estimated that they received far in excess of the lethal dose of benzyl alcohol. Again, this agent was inadvertently introduced into the arena of neonatal care.

Brown, W. J.: Fatal benzyl alcohol poisoning in a neonatal intensive care unit. Lancet 1:1250, 1982.

Centers for Disease Control: Unusual syndrome with fatalities among premature infants. Association with a new intravenous vitamin E product. MMWR 33:198, 1984.

Gershanik, J. J., Boecler, B., Ensley, H., et al: The gasping syndrome and benzyl alcohol poisoning. N Eng J Med 307:1384, 1982.

Lorch, V., Murphy, D., Hoersten, L., et al: Unusual syndrome among premature infants: association with a new intravenous vitamin E product. Pediatrics 75:598, 1985.

Other causes of hemolytic anemia in the newborn include ABO and, to a lesser extent, Rh erythroblastosis. Less frequently occurring are the inherited disorders in the glycolytic mechanism (e.g., deficiencies of glucose-6-phosphate dehydrogenase, pyruvate kinase, etc.) or defects in structure (e.g., hereditary spherocytosis, elliptocytosis, and congenital pyknocytosis), all of which may produce significant anemia and hyperbilirubinemia (the latter of sufficient degree to require treatment with exchange transfusion). The disorders of hemoglobin synthesis, with the exception of Bart's, rarely are apparent before the middle of the first year of life.

Among the aregenerative or megaloblastic anemias, juvenile pernicious anemia usually is not apparent before 3 months of age. In addition, only rare cases of folic acid deficiency anemias are identified during the same interval. Equally uncommon during this period of time are any of the varieties of pancytopenia or erythroid hypoplasia. Included among the anemias of underproduction is congenital hypoplastic anemia (CHA), which occurs with slow onset during the first few months of life. The mechanism of erythrocyte suppression is unknown. Less common is the anemia of lack, which is adequately treated by correcting the underlying deficiency. Osteopetrosis is yet another example of early onset marrow failure, the result of defective osteoclast function. Transient erythroblastopenia of childhood is rarely seen in the neonatal period. It usually presents between 6 months and 4 years of age and rarely persists for longer than 3–4 months.

In approaching the diagnosis of anemia in the newborn, the outline of Blanchette and Zipursky[3a] is most helpful (Figure 15–2). It becomes apparent that it is important to document the volume of blood withdrawn for testing each day, since it is easy to render a preterm infant anemic from excessive blood sampling.

A Complicated Case

The history and clinical course of the next newborn infant provided the physicians who cared for her with almost the entire gamut of the currently reviewed acute hematologic problems as well as many related difficulties that are considered in other sections of this book. Since diagnostic efforts and the clinical management did not necessarily represent optimal care, questions are also provided for the reader's consideration.

Baby girl H, who was transferred from another hospital 2 hours after birth because of suspected Rh incompatibility, was a term product of an uncomplicated pregnancy. One previous pregnancy resulted in a full-term, living child who had no difficulties in the newborn period, although the mother stated that labor was long and painful. The mother was type O, Rh-negative, and antibody titers on two occasions early in pregnancy were reported as 1:64 and 1:128, respectively.

Under these circumstances, what further maternal history should be sought, and what further investigation should have been appropriate during the pregnancy?

Detailed knowledge of the first pregnancy and delivery, including maternal antibody titers.

Once an anti-D titer (anti-Rh) is identified, amniocenteses should be carried out to obtain chromogen levels, which are far more reliable than anti-D titers in estimating the degree of anemia in utero.

Actually, chromogen levels were obtained during this pregnancy and were reported as being in the low zone.

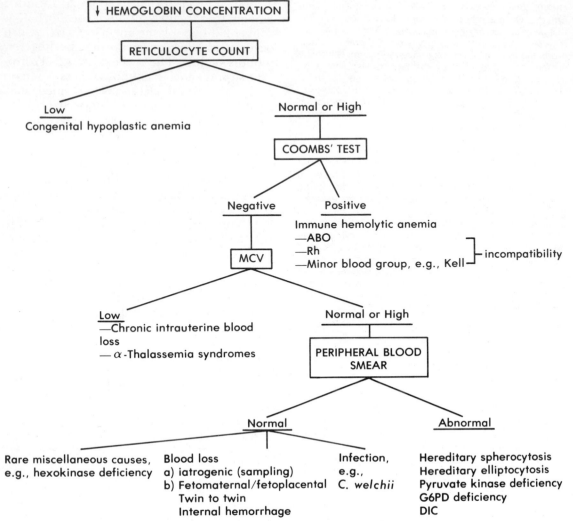

Figure 15-2. Diagnostic approach to anemia in the newborn infant. (From Blanchette, V. S., and Zipursky, A.: Assessment of anemia in newborn infants. Clin Perinatol *11*:489, 1984.)

How should the physician interpret the results of the amniocentesis, and how might this information have affected the course of the pregnancy?

Chromogen levels in the low zone indicate well-compensated hemolysis, or more likely, minimal hemolysis. For this reason, the decision to allow the pregnancy to go to full-term was proper. High-zone chromogen levels obtained before 34 weeks' gestation may indicate the need for intrauterine transfusion of Rh-negative cells. If mid- or high-zone levels occur after 34 weeks, a decision regarding induction of labor or early delivery should be made.

Labor was said to be long and difficult, and the obstetrician reported that considerable effort was necessary to deliver the infant vaginally. Initial physical examination revealed an infant who was pale, cold, and cyanotic. Deep gasping respirations were noted, although auscultation indicated satisfactory pulmonary air exchange. Additional physical findings included a partial left brachial palsy and a slightly distended abdomen. The liver and spleen were not palpable. The laboratory values included a cord bilirubin D/T of 0.5/5.2 mg/dl; central venous hematocrit 30 per cent; blood type O, Rh-positive; and direct Coombs' test 4+.

Given the historical, clinical, and laboratory findings at this point, how would one evaluate the infant's condition?

The difficulties in labor and delivery should cause suspicion that the infant's poor clinical condition immediately after birth was in some way related to these events. In retrospect, the partial brachial palsy was indicative of the vigorous extraction efforts. The condition of the infant at birth suggested that a catastrophic event had occurred in the immediate perinatal period. Although the blood type and positive direct Coombs' test in association with a moderate elevation in cord bilirubin confirmed the presence of Rh incompatibility, the shocklike clinical condition in the absence of hydrops fetalis and the lack of demonstrable hepatosplenomegaly are more consistent with either acute hemorrhage or hemolysis rather than a chronic hemolytic process. Furthermore, the low-zone chromogen studies are in keeping with this impression.

What other laboratory information should be obtained as soon as possible?

The critical nature of her condition required the following essential information:
- Arterial blood gases, pH, and blood pressure determinations.
- Radiologic and ultrasonographic examination of both chest and abdomen in search of internal hemorrhage (and also to provide identification of the site of catheter placement).
- Initiation of cross-matching procedures against fresh donor blood (less than 3 days old).

The mean arterial blood pressure was 24 mm Hg; pH was 7.2; Pao$_2$ was 28 mm Hg; Paco$_2$ was 40 mm Hg; and HCO$_3$ was 18 mEq/l. A stained film of peripheral blood showed increased numbers of immature red cells and adequate numbers of platelets. Following catheterization and blood drawing, several bandage changes were necessary in a short period of time to control oozing.

What is the significance of these blood gas and pressure values?

The patient had a metabolic acidosis without CO$_2$ retention and respiratory insufficiency. The low arterial blood pressure is indicative of hypovolemia or at least peripheral pooling.

What therapeutic approach should be carried out at this point?

Prompt treatment should be directed to the maintenance of optimal body temperature, correction of the metabolic acidosis, improvement of the arterial Pao$_2$, and correction of the presumed hypovolemia (hypotension). In the last instance, this may be provided by an infusion of normal saline, plasma, or plasma expanders.

What is the next course of action?

The transfusion of appropriately cross-matched O, Rh-negative, "routinely packed" cells, if time permits. Otherwise, use the freshest available whole blood.

This infant received 20 ml/kg of O, Rh-negative whole blood, following which the mean arterial pressure rose to 38 mm Hg in association with moderate improvement in the respiratory status. Laboratory values for clotting studies performed prior to the transfusion became available and revealed markedly prolonged prothrombin and partial thromboplastin times, as well as decreased levels of fibrinogen and platelets. At this point, an exchange transfusion was carried out, following which the infant's clinical condition further improved with coincident repair of blood gases and pH. However, at 5 hours of age, the abdomen was noted to be distended and firm, and respirations became labored.

What was the role of the exchange transfusion?

Exchange transfusion is an effective way to treat DIC. In this infant it was performed on the assumption that the fundamental problem was anemia secondary to Rh incompatibility. It is therefore probable that this procedure fortuitously helped in the treatment of two separate disorders. Although citrated whole blood exchange transfusion for the treatment of DIC is known to be effective, in DIC with vascular collapse, exchange transfusions with heparinized (200 units/ml) whole blood have been recommended.

Blank, J. P., Sheagren, T. G., Vajaria J., et al: The role of RBC transfusion in the premature infant. Am J Dis Child *138*:831, 1984.

Dear, P.: Blood transfusion in the preterm infant [Editorial]. Arch Dis Child *59*:296, 1984.

Hovi, L., and Siimes, M. A.: Exchange transfusion with fresh heparinized blood is a safe procedure. Experiences from 1069 newborns. Acta Paediatr Scand *74*:360, 1985.

Stockman, J. A.: The anemia of prematurity and the decision when to transfuse. Adv Pediatr *30*:191, 1983.

Given the change in the infant's course, what further studies should be done?

X-ray and ultrasonographic examination of the abdomen, repeat clotting studies, and needle aspiration of the lower abdominal quadrants.

X-ray examination showed a diffuse haziness throughout the abdomen, clotting studies were normal, and a peritoneal aspiration of the left lower quadrant returned fresh blood, which clotted immediately. The hematocrit had fallen from a 37 per cent postexchange level to 29 per cent. The history of a traumatic delivery and the evidence of blood in the abdominal cavity and corrected or normal clotting studies lent strong support to the presumptive diagnosis of an additional cause of the anemia (i.e., posttraumatic bleeding).

What are the two most frequent causes of internal bleeding in a neonate, and what guide can one use in distinguishing between them?

Capsular tears in the liver or spleen. Blood loss from hepatic capsular tears is usually self-limited and hence requires no direct surgical intervention. However, splenic rupture is a life-threatening event that can be corrected only by splenectomy. If the latter procedure is contemplated, arrangements must be made to obtain adequate supplies of fresh whole blood.

French, C. E., and Waldstein, J.: Subcapsular hemorrhage of the liver in the newborn. Pediatrics *69*:204, 1982.

Over the next 12 hours, abdominal girth and distension steadily decreased, and the hematocrit and arterial blood pressure remained stable. At 24 hours of age, the infant developed seizure activity consisting of frequent, short episodes of tonic-clonic movements of the extremities. However, the seizures did not interfere with feeding or vital functions.

What studies should be undertaken to identify the etiology of the seizure activity?

Seizure activity under these circumstances falls into one of three categories:

- Central nervous system bleeding, possibly related to anoxic damage or trauma.
- Metabolic disturbances incurred in the early course of therapy (possibilities include hypoglycemia, hypocalcemia, hypomagnesemia, or hyponatremia—none of which was present in this infant).
- CNS damage secondary to a wide variety of infectious agents.

Bacterial cultures were negative, a lumbar tap revealed xanthochromic fluid with no other abnor-malities, and a serum bilirubin was D/T 0.6/12.4 mg/dl.

Should the bilirubin level at this point be of concern?

The reader should refer to Chapter 11, Neonatal Hyperbilirubinemia, for a more complete exposition of this dilemma. Briefly, however, although the infant was full term, the period of anoxia and acidosis early in life could significantly alter bilirubin kinetics, and the risk of kernicterus would be slightly increased yet extremely low.

The infant's seizure activity gradually ceased during the next 7 days, and she began to gain weight on oral formula feedings. The infant was discharged at 16 days of life, at which time the hematocrit was 32 per cent.

What type of follow-up should be ensured?

In addition to a careful evaluation of this infant's physical and neurologic development, the hematocrit should be closely followed in the first few months of life. Increased red cell destruction due to Rh incompatibility may continue without the production of jaundice and result in a marked anemia. In such instances, it may be necessary to transfuse with packed cells (15–20 ml/kg) should the hematocrit fall below 20 per cent.

Is vitamin E, iron, or folic acid indicated as adjunct therapy?

Neither vitamin E nor folate levels are abnormally low in the term infant, although it is possible that the demand for folic acid could rise in response to the increase in marrow activity. The possibility of iron deficiency, in view of the past history of some external blood loss and frequent blood specimens for laboratory determinations, would indicate the need for supplemental iron, administered in accordance with the suggestions in the section of this chapter devoted to iron metabolism.

REFERENCES

1. Abelli, A., and DeLamerans, S.: Coagulation changes in the neonatal period and in early infancy. Pediatr Clin North Am *9*:785, 1962.
2. Abt, L., and Downey, W., Jr.: Melena neonatorum: the swallowed blood syndrome. J Pediatr *47*:6, 1955.
3. Ambrus, C., Ambrus, J., Niswander, K., et al: Changes in fibrin stabilizing factor levels in relation to maternal hemorrhage and neonatal disease. Pediatr Res *4*:82, 1970.
3a. Blanchette, V. S., and Zipursky, A.: Assessment of anemia in newborn infants. Clin Perinatol *11*:489, 1984.
3b. Brans, Y. W., Shannon, D. L., and Ramamurthy, R. S.: Neonatal polycythemia: II. Plasma, blood and red cell volume estimates in relation to hematocrit levels and quality of intrauterine growth. Pediatrics *68*:175, 1981.
4. Cade, J., Hirsh, J., and Martin, M.: Placental barriers to coagulation factors. Its relevance to the coagulation defect at birth and to hemorrhage in the newborn. Br Med J *2*:281, 1969.
5. Ekelund, H., and Fumstrom, O.: Fibrinolysis in preterm infants and in infants small for gestational age. Acta Paediatr *61*:185, 1972.
6. Faxelius, J., Gutberlet, R., Swanstrom, S., et al: Red cell volume measurements and acute blood loss in high-risk newborn infants. J Pediatr *90*:273, 1977.
7. Flod, N., and Ackerman, B.: Perinatal asphyxia and

residual placental blood volume. Acta Paediatr 60:1, 1971.

8. Gellis, S., and Lyon, R.: The influence of diet of the newborn infant on the prothrombin index. J Pediatr 19:495, 1941.

9. Graeber, J., Williams, M., and Oski, F.: The use of intramuscular vitamin E in the premature infant. Optimum dose and iron interaction. J Pediatr 90:282, 1977.

10. Gross, S.: The relationship between milk protein and iron content on hematologic values in infancy. J Pediatr 73:521, 1968.

11. Gross, S.: Hemolytic anemia in premature infants: relationship to vitamin E, selenium, glutathione peroxidase, and erythrocyte lipids. Semin Hematol 13:187, 1976.

12. Gross, S., and Melhorn, D.: Exchange transfusion with citrated whole blood for disseminated intravascular coagulation. J Pediatr 78:415, 1971.

13. Gross, S., and Melhorn, D.: Vitamin E, red cell lipids and red cell stability in prematurity. Ann NY Acad Sci 203:141, 1972.

14. Gross, S., and Melhorn, D.: Vitamin E–dependent anemia in the premature infant. III. Comparative hemoglobin, vitamin E, and erythrocyte phospholipid responses following absorption of either water-soluble or fat-soluble d-alpha tocopherol. J Pediatr 85:753, 1974.

15. Gross, S., and Stuart, M. J.: Hemostasis in the premature infant. Clin Perinatol 4:259, 1977.

16. Hadjimarkos, D. M.: Selenium content of human milk: possible effect on dental caries. J Pediatr 63:273, 1963.

17. Hjort, P., and Rappaport, S.: The Shwartzman reaction: pathogenic mechanism and clinical manifestation. Ann Rev Med 16:135, 1965.

18. Kartizky, D., Leine, N., Pringsheim, W., et al: Fibrinogen turnover in the premature infant with and without idiopathic respiratory distress syndrome. Acta Paediatr 60:465, 1971.

19. Kartizky, D., Pringsheim, W., and Kumzen, W.: Fibrinogen and fibrinolysis in the respiratory distress syndrome: observations during the first day of life. Acta Paediatr 59:281, 1970.

20. Markarian, M., Githens, J., Jackson, J., et al: Fibrinolytic activity in premature infants: relationship of the enzyme system to the respiratory distress syndrome. Am J Dis Child 113:312, 1967.

21. Markarian, M., Lindley, A., Jackson, J., et al: Coagulation factors in premature infants with and without the respiratory distress syndrome. Thromb Diath Haemorrh 17:587, 1967.

22. Melhorn, D., and Gross, S.: Vitamin E dependent anemia in the premature infant. I. Relationships between iron and vitamin E. J Pediatr 79:569, 1971.

23. Melhorn, D., and Gross, S.: Vitamin E dependent anemia in the premature infant. II. Relationships between gestational age and absorption of vitamin E. J Pediatr 79:581, 1971.

24. Muth, O. H., Oldfield, J. E., Remmert, L. F., et al: Effect of selenium on white muscle disease. Science 128:1090, 1958.

24a. Nathan, D. G., and Oski, F. A.: Hematology of Infancy and Childhood. 2nd ed. Philadelphia, W. B. Saunders, 1981.

25. Newman, A., and Gross, S.: Capillary and venous hematocrits in the newborn. Clin Pediatr 6:6, 1967.

26. Nielsen, C.: Coagulation and fibrinolysis in normal women immediately post partum and in newborn infants. Acta Obstet Gynecol Scand 48:371, 1969.

27. Nielsen, C.: Coagulation and fibrinolysis in prematurely delivered mothers and their premature infants. Acta Obstet Gynecol Scand 48:505, 1969.

28. Nossel, H., Lanzkowski, P., Levy, S., et al: A comparison of coagulation factor levels in women during labor and in their newborn infants. Thromb Diath Haemorrh 16:185, 1966.

29. Oski, F., and Delevoria-Papadopoulos, M.: The red cell, 2,3-diphosphoglycerate and tissue oxygen release. J Pediatr 77:941, 1970.

30. Oski, F., and Naiman, J.: Hematologic Problems in the Newborn. 3rd ed. Philadelphia, W. B. Saunders Company, 1982.

30a. Ramamurthy, R. S., and Brans, Y. W.: Neonatal polycythemia: I. Criteria for diagnosis and treatment. Pediatrics 68:168, 1981.

31. Rotruck, J. A., Pope, A. L., Ganther, H. E., et al: Selenium. biochemical role as a component of glutathione peroxidase. Science 179:588, 1973.

32. Shojania, A., and Gross, S.: Folic acid deficiency and prematurity. J Pediatr 64:323, 1964.

33. Shulman, N., Aster, R., Pearson, H., et al: Immunoreactions involving platelets. V. Immunoreactions of maternal isoantibodies responsible for neonatal purpura. Differentiation of a second platelet antigen system. J Clin Invest 41:1059, 1962.

34. Statement of the Committee on Nutrition, American Academy of Pediatrics: Iron fortified formulas. Newsletter, Vol. 21. (See also Pediatrics 48:152, 158, 1971.).

34a. Statement of the Committee on Nutrition, American Academy of Pediatrics: Vitamin and supplement needs in normal children in the United States. Pediatrics 66:1015, 1980.

34b. Statement of the Committee on Nutrition, American Academy of Pediatrics: The use of whole cows milk in infancy. Pediatrics 72:253, 1983.

35. Usher, R., and Lind, J.: Blood volume of newborn premature infant. Acta Paediatr 54:419, 1965.

36. Usher, R., Shepard, M., and Lind, J.: The blood volume of the newborn infant and placental transfusion. Acta Paediatr 52:497, 1963.

37. Walgren, G., Barr, W., and Rudhe, U.: Haemodynamic studies of induced acute hypo- and hypervolemia in the newborn infant. Acta Paediatr 53:1, 1964.

38. Williams, M., Shott, R., O'Neal, P., et al: Role of dietary iron and fat on vitamin E deficiency anemia of infancy. N Engl J Med 292:887, 1975.

39. Zipursky, A., Hull, A., White, F., et al: Foetal erythrocytes in the maternal circulation. Lancet 1:451, 1959.

16

Neurologic Problems

CLAUDINE AMIEL-TISON
ROWENA KOROBKIN
MARSHALL H. KLAUS

As for intelligence, there is a little friend of mine who three days after birth weighed only 950 grams. She is seven years old and speaks French and German. I think that the allegations regarding the permanent bodily and mental debility of weaklings ... are entirely without foundation.

PIERRE BUDIN
THE NURSLING

The integrity and function of the nervous system are of utmost importance to the physician, nurse, and parents of the high-risk newborn infant. The aim is intact survival. Disease involving the brain of the infant is a source of major anxiety for the parents. The physician must maintain a considerate attitude and avoid gloomy predictions unless absolutely certain that the prognosis is poor. Except in a few cases of very typical and severe lesions, the late outcome will usually be better than the neonatologist initially forecasts. The hope of the parents remains a necessary component for the quality of the outcome.

Primary disorders of the brain, spinal cord, muscles, and nerves account for a relatively small proportion of the acute neurologic problems of the newborn infant. More frequently, the nervous system disorder is secondary to circulatory, metabolic, physical, infectious, or environmental conditions that may transiently impair function or leave permanent sequelae. Recent advances in perinatology have reduced the incidence of neurologic sequelae. In particular, the early and repeated use of the nonstress test to evaluate

the variability of fetal heart rate has allowed anticipation of impending cerebral ischemia or fetal death, making it possible to deliver very low-birth weight infants before any catastrophe occurs. Advances in neonatal care, with stabilization of respiratory and circulatory systems, and reduction of metabolic and thermal stress have lowered the incidence and severity of intraventricular hemorrhage. Improvement in imaging techniques, especially cribside cranial ultrasonography, has improved clinicopathologic diagnosis[54] and has changed some of our views of pathophysiology. This chapter will discuss common problems and remedial conditions and will outline some pathophysiologic correlations to neonatal cerebral damage, with a brief discussion of aspects of clinical assessment and etiologic considerations. Further descriptions of problems in perinatal neurology may be found in several texts.[30, 33, 43, 64]

PATHOPHYSIOLOGIC CONSIDERATIONS

The nervous system of a newborn infant is extremely immature anatomically, and there are considerable chemical and physiologic differences from the adult brain.[33] The cerebral hemispheres show poor differentiation of gray and white matter; the majority of neuronal cells are present at birth but are immature in appearance and function.

Editorial Comment: Creative studies of fetal neurologic development in animals have taught us much that has been valuable. In fetal animals, preventing movement of a single joint results in freezing of the joint space as well

356

as marked atrophy of the bones, muscles, and nerves surrounding that joint. Fetal movement is thus essential for normal intrauterine musculoskeletal development. The major development of brain cells in the human cortex occurs between 12 and 18 weeks of fetal life. Surprisingly, by 19 weeks the fetus is able to step, as shown in Figure 16–1.

In the premature infant, there is little myelination. Polysynaptic connections are in the early stages of formation. The neurologic function is largely, but not exclusively, at brain-stem and spinal cord level; the infantile reflexes such as Moro's reflex and grasping, stepping, and placing reactions represent release of primitive neuronal function, largely uninhibited by higher cerebral control. However, our present understanding of anatomic and physiologic maturation cannot fully explain the previously unappreciated innate abilities of the normal full-term infant in the first hours of life. In the quiet, alert state, the neonate can follow a face, turn his head toward a sound, move his body to the rhythm of languages, and indeed mimic tongue protrusion, mouth opening, and puckering of the lips![12, 34, 36]

A large variety of primary structural nervous system abnormalities, as well as many causes of brain dysfunction secondary to systemic disorders, are described in the literature. An abbreviated list of some of these conditions is seen in Table 16–1. It is most important to realize that permanent structural changes may occur in the brain if sys-

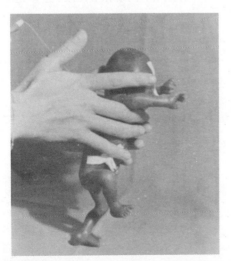

Figure 16–1. Nineteen to twenty week, 420 gm fetus stepping. The baby is receiving additional oxygen. (From Katona, F.: *The Developing Consciousness.* Budapest, Gondolat Ed. Dept. of Developmental Neurology and Rehab., 1979.)

TABLE 16–1 MAIN CAUSES OF CENTRAL NERVOUS SYSTEM MALFUNCTION IN THE NEONATAL PERIOD

Prenatal
Chronic fetal distress:
    Toxemia, maternal diabetes

Chromosomal abnormalities

Congenital malformations

Infections:
    Cytomegalic inclusion disease, rubella, toxoplasmosis, herpes simplex, maternal sepsis

Neurocutaneous syndromes:
    Neurofibromatosis, tuberous sclerosis

Drugs:
    Narcotics, barbiturates, general anesthetic agents, local anesthetics, anticonvulsants, tranquilizers

Vascular:
    Cerebral ischemia, hemorrhage, thrombosis, embolism

During Birth Process
Mechanical birth injury (mainly in full-term), high forceps, cephalopelvic disproportion, breech:
    Tearing of dural sinuses and bridging veins, subdural and subarachnoid hemorrhage, depressed skull fracture, spinal cord injury (breech delivery)

Cerebrovascular compromise:
    Subacute or acute fetal distress with hypoxia and ischemia, in any type of mechanical or functional dystocia or any fetus already compromised; ischemic stress of "normal birth" to a fetus; cerebral embolism

Postnatal
Acute distress (mainly in low-birth-weight infants) with hypoxia and ischemia, apneic spells, bradycardia, cardiac arrest

Infections:
    Bacterial or viral meningoencephalitis

Metabolic:
    Hypoglycemia, hypocalcemia, hypomagnesemia, hyponatremia, hypernatremia, hyperbilirubinemia, hypothyroidism, hyperthyroidism, galactosemia, aminoaciduria, hyperammonemia, hyperviscosity

temic disorders are not recognized and treated promptly and specifically. Therefore, the causes of reversible and treatable abnormalities of function must be considered first in clinical management.

The role of drugs as causes of nervous system malfunction should not be underestimated in terms of drugs administered either to the mother or postnatally to the infant himself. Intoxication with local anesthetic agents, either by direct puncture or from absorption through injudiciously administered paracervical block, can cause serious and, if not recognized early enough, fatal seizures. Depression and hyperexcitability can result from these agents. **L. Stern**

CLINICAL EVALUATION

The basic framework of the neurologic assessment of older infants can be partly adapted to the newborn. The technical aspect of such an examination is described in specialized textbooks.[5, 45, 47, 64] In this chapter we will describe some specific aspects of the neurologic examination of the newborn.

Knowledge of the evolution of signs and symptoms over time is important in understanding etiology and prognosis. Toxic and metabolic derangements cause concurrent neurologic symptoms, even if they are nonspecific. Similarly, sepsis and systemic illness will cause immediate depression of the infant. Hypoxic-ischemic insults, however, cause an evolution of signs and symptoms, depending on the severity of the initial insult. There is progressive depression of the state of consciousness over 24–48 hours, and seizures begin after 12–24 hours, with recovery over the next several days. Central nervous system hemorrhage may be associated with immediate signs, but there will be a progressive worsening if the hemorrhage is associated with cerebral infarction. In any case, the rapidity and completeness of recovery correlate with the severity of cerebral damage and therefore with prognosis.

States of Alertness

The state of quiet alertness is necessary to obtain optimal responses. An important aspect of clinical evaluation of the high-risk neonate is to observe and consider the behavioral state of the infant.

Wolff[68] designed the first descriptive rating scale for the term infant and defined six states. Prechtl and Beintema[45] omitted the drowsy state, regarding it as a transition between states, and defined five states (Table 16–2). Others describe coma as a state. Any of these behavioral classifications can be utilized clinically when describing the infant.

The states can also be differentiated by recordings of physiologic measures, which include respiration, heart rate, eye movements (electrooculogram, or EOG), and the

electromyogram (EMG). Table 16–3 sets forth physiologic parameters in different states of alertness.

It is important to stress that although the states seem like a continuing spectrum, they are qualitatively different, with distinct types of organization and brain center control. They are also relatively stable and, with the exception of short transitional periods, repeat in regular cycles during the day and night.

It is especially important to note sleep state when evaluating muscle tone. During active or REM sleep there is poor tone of the postural muscles (head and neck, intercostal). Tone, posture, and spontaneous movement should be evaluated during state 3 or 4 with the head in the midline (to obviate effects of the tonic neck reflex). **P. Fitzhardinge**

Evaluation of Tone

Appreciation of muscle tone is a fundamental feature of the examination, which includes the study of the resting posture, passive tone, and active tone. One evaluates spontaneous posture by inspection when the infant is lying supine. One evaluates passive tone by manipulating the passive infant and measuring the amplitude of movement of a single joint. Active tone is studied when the infant is in an active situation, with the examiner noting the infant's active reflex movement, such as straightening of the trunk when the infant is placed vertically. There are a few standard maneuvers for evaluating

TABLE 16–2 STATES OF ALERTNESS*

State	Prechtl and Beintema	Wolff
1	Deep sleep: eyes closed, regular respiration, no movements	Same
2	Active sleep (REM): eyes closed, irregular respiration, small movements	Same
3	Quiet alert: eyes open, no movements	Drowsy
4	Active alert: eyes open, gross movements, no crying	Quiet alert: eyes open, no movements
5	Crying (vocalization)	Active alert: eyes open, gross movements, no crying
6	—	Crying (vocalization)

*Adapted from Wolff[68] and Prechtl and Beintema.[45]

TABLE 16–3 PHYSIOLOGIC PARAMETERS IN DIFFERENT STATES OF ALERTNESS*

State of Consciousness	1	2	3	4	5
Rapid eye movements	−	+ +	+ +	+	+
Slow eye movements	−	+ +	−	−	−
Startles	+ +	+	−	−	−
Rhythmic mouthing	+ +	−	−	−	−
Smiles, grimaces	−	+ +	+	+	−
Gross movements	−	+ +	−	+	+ +
Stable heart rate	+	−	+	−	−

− Absent; + and + + present.

*Adapted from Prechtl, H., and O'Brien, M.: Behavioral states of the full-term newborn. The emergence of a concept. *In* Stratton, P. (ed.): *Psychobiology of the Human Newborn.* New York, John Wiley & Sons, 1982, p. 68.

passive and active tone.[3, 7, 47, 58] To detect an abnormal pattern of tone, one must know the gestational age on the day of the evaluation (see Figure 4–4) and the normal pattern of tone for this age. Despite premature birth and/or acute illness in the neonatal period, the time course of maturation is not disturbed unless there has been neurologic damage. Although there are no specific correlates between abnormal signs in the neonatal period and neurologic outcome later in life, a normal pattern of active tone when the former premature infant reaches 40 weeks' gestational age is correlated with a good outcome.

Editorial Comment: An important principle of neurologic development is that a function is usually available and practiced many hours and days before it appears to be obviously required. As an example, it has been beautifully demonstrated by Tison and Grenier (1983) that if the normal tonic neck responses are severely diminished with gentle rubbing for 3–5 minutes while the infant is brought to the quiet alert state, 50 per cent of the infants will reach for objects in the first weeks of life. This is termed liberated motor activity. It is our impression that within the very near future, studies such as these will lead to a more complete neurologic evaluation of the developing premature and full-term infant. Figure 16–2 illustrates how the neck tone is released in a 17 day old full-term infant and demonstrates reaching. Releasing the neck muscle tone prevents the usual slight movements of the infant's head and neck from distorting the arm movements, thereby allowing the infant's inherent capacity for hand-eye coordination and more precise movement to emerge.

Tison, C. A., and Grenier, A.: *Neurologic Evaluation of the Newborn and the Infant.* (Trans. by Steichen, J., Steichen-Asch, P., and Braun, C. P.) New York, Masson Publishers, 1983.

Reflexes

Primary reflexes are normally present in the preterm as well as the full-term newborn. They are not inhibited until the infant reaches several months of age. It is a sign of central nervous system depression when primary reflexes cannot be elicited in the newborn of greater than 28 weeks' gestation. There are many primitive responses, but only a few of them are used for routine evaluation: Moro's reflex, the palmar grasp, automatic walking, and the suck-swallow reflex.

MORO'S REFLEX. Holding both hands of the infant in abduction, the examiner lifts the infant's shoulders a few inches off the bed and then releases the hands briskly. The normal reflex is a brisk active abduction and extension of the arms, followed by complete opening of the hands and then adduction.

PALMAR GRASP. The examiner inserts his index fingers into the hands of the infant to obtain a strong flexion of the infant's fingers. This strong palmar grasp will allow the infant to sustain his whole body weight when the examiner lifts his index fingers. The "response to traction" obtained provides a very good verification of the quality of active tone.

AUTOMATIC WALKING. The examiner holds the infant upright in the standing position to obtain a supporting reaction. The examiner then tilts the infant forward slightly, and the infant should step.

THE SUCK-SWALLOW REFLEX. The examiner places a finger into the infant's mouth and notes the strength and rhythmicity of sucking and the synchrony of swallowing.

DEEP TENDON REFLEXES. Biceps and patellar tendon reflexes should be readily elicited. Ankle clonus in the neonate is of no significance.

Cranial Examination

HEAD CIRCUMFERENCE. This is the largest occipital-frontal circumference. Normal values are well established (see Appendices G–

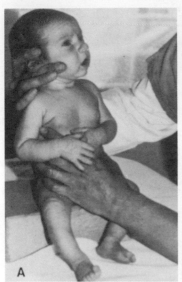
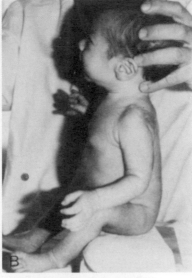
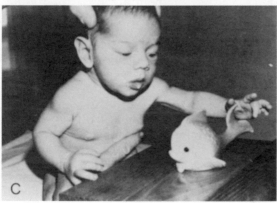

Figure 16–2. *A,* To explore liberated motor activity, manual support and massage are given to the neck while the infant is kept alert and attentive to the examiner. After 3–5 minutes, uncontrolled head movement no longer results in obligatory responses. *B,* Also after 3–5 minutes the infant's back becomes straight. *C,* This 17 day old infant is then able to reach for objects. (From Tison, C. A., and Grenier, A.: *Neurologic Evaluation of the Newborn and the Infant.* Trans. by Steichen, J., Steichen-Asch, P., and Braun, C. P. New York, Masson Publishers, 1983.)

2 and G–3).[42] Daily measurements are sometimes essential. Excessively rapid growth is always to be regarded with suspicion, with hydrocephalus being the most likely pathologic cause. Gestational age and health of the infant are significant factors in determining the pattern of head growth in the premature baby. Difficulty is encountered in separating the rapid growth due to hydrocephalus from that of "catch-up" growth.[28, 52] The size of both anterior and posterior fontanelles is very variable, and except in extreme cases, it is difficult to assess bulging or depression. The palpation of all the sutures is more reliable. The normal range of suture width is a function of both the infant's age and the suture being examined. For the sagittal and parietooccipital sutures, widths of as much as 4–5 mm may be of no significance during the first weeks of life. Such a separation can also be normally observed in the portion of the metopic and coronal sutures close to the angles of the anterior fontanelle. However, separation of 2–3 mm of the parietotemporal sutures (improperly called "squamous sutures") at the level of the helix is a reliable sign of intracranial hypertension (Figure 16–3).

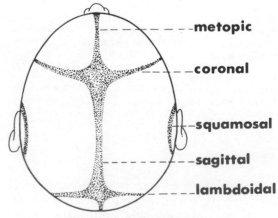

Figure 16–3. Cranial sutures.

TRANSILLUMINATION OF THE HEAD. This simple procedure may provide information about the existence and location of abnormal fluid spaces intracranially. In a darkened room, following a period of adaptation for the examiner's eyes, a cuffed flashlight is held against the skull. Normally, one sees only a small halo (about 1 cm) around the cone, especially prominent in prematures. Asymmetry or extensive transillumination is abnormal. However, the results of transillumination can be difficult to interpret. With the Chun-gun, light is provided by a focus projection lamp that emits a constant bright light, and the results are more reliable.[13]

Editorial Comment: Ultrasound and CT scans have reduced the value of transillumination.

FUNDUSCOPIC EXAMINATION. This is a routine procedure. All quadrants of the retina must be evaluated after dilatation of the pupil. Retinal hemorrhages in the first days of life are very frequent and usually are not indicative of intracranial hemorrhage. Papilledema does not usually appear with cerebral edema because of the separation of the sutures that occurs when intracranial pressure increases. Congenital malformations may be helpful diagnostically, and chorioretinitis may denote underlying congenital infection due to toxoplasmosis, cytomegalovirus, or herpes simplex.

Care must be taken in the use of cycloplegic and mydriatic drugs in the preterm infant. Ocular administration of the sympathomimetic drug phenylephrine (Neo-Synephrine) in solutions of 10 per cent can cause a rise in systemic blood pressure of 12–16 mm Hg within 5 minutes lasting for up to 1 hour. Blood pressure is not affected by instillation of 2.5 per cent phenylephrine, and this dosage produces excellent persistent mydriasis. The cycloplegic parasympatholytic drug cyclopentolate hydrochloride (Cyclogyl) is often used in association with phenylephrine. Atropine-like toxicity has been reported in two premature infants following instillation of 6 drops of 1 per cent Cyclogyl (3 mg cyclopentolate) over a period of 15 minutes. Blood levels 24 hours later were significantly high, especially so in one infant who developed necrotizing enterocolitis. It is recommended that the use of Cyclogyl be limited to a 0.5 per cent solution with a limit of 3 drops per eye (total of 1 mg).

Bauer, C., Trottier, M., and Stern, L.: Systemic cyclopentolate (Cyclogyl) toxicity in the newborn infant. J Pediatr 82:501, 1973.
Borromeo-McGrail, V., Bordiuk, J., and Keitel, H.: Systemic hypertension following ocular administration of 10 per cent phenylephrine in the neonate. Pediatrics 51:1032, 1973.

P. Fitzhardinge

Additional Procedures and Laboratory Investigations

LUMBAR PUNCTURE. Analysis of the CSF should always include culture, cell count, and protein and glucose estimation. The main indications in the neonate are suspicion of intracranial infection or hemorrhage. Normal values in neonates are summarized in Appendices F–1 and F–2.

SUBDURAL TAP. This is now performed only when CT scan or ultrasound has indicated the presence and location of a subdural hemorrhage or fluid collection.

X-RAY OF THE SKULL. This can be extremely valuable, showing the size of the sutures, the digital impressions of increased intracranial pressure, and intracranial calcifications. It remains the procedure of choice for diagnosis of skull fracture.

CRANIAL ULTRASONOGRAPHY. This rapid, noninvasive, cribside imaging technique has become the method of choice for detecting and following the evolution of neonatal intracranial hemorrhage and hydrocephalus (Figure 16–4). It may also detect cysts and

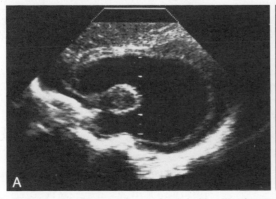
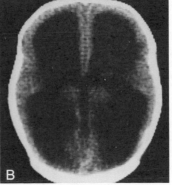

Figure 16–4. *A,* Cranial ultrasound scan, lateral view. Massive congenital hydrocephalus. *B,* CT scan, same case as *A.*

other cerebral malformations, tumors, brain abscesses, and structural damage due to infection and infarction.[8] It is not reliable for detection of subarachnoid hemorrhage or small subdural hemorrhage. The CT brain scan is required for diagnostic confirmation and further structural elucidation of abnormalities detected by ultrasound scan.

COMPUTED TOMOGRAPHIC (CT) BRAIN SCAN. This technique gives the most detailed anatomic imaging of the brain that is currently available for routine clinical use. The main problem is transportation of the sick neonate to and from the scanning room. The CT scan should be reserved to confirm an abnormality suspected by cranial ultrasound or for cases in which clinical suspicion is high, but the ultrasound scan is negative.

MEASUREMENT OF INTRACRANIAL PRESSURE. Several devices can be placed on the anterior fontanelle to allow noninvasive measurement of the intracranial pressure.[37, 44, 60, 68] The normal pressure in the full-term healthy newborn is approximately 100 mm of water and is quite stable. Progressively increasing pressures with values of 150 mm of water or more are definitely abnormal. This very simple measurement has several benefits—detecting preclinical stages of intracranial hypertension, confirming clinical signs, and monitoring the therapeutic efficacy of measures taken to reduce pressure.

ELECTROENCEPHALOGRAPHY (EEG). The EEG is very helpful in the perinatal period in confirming the clinical diagnosis of neonatal seizures and providing valuable information concerning long-term prognosis.[16, 46, 57] Maturation has been studied extensively by this method and may complement clinical assessment.

ELECTROMYOGRAPHY (EMG). This is rarely required in the newborn nursery. When there is suspicion of myopathy or motor neuron disease, muscle biopsy is the procedure of choice.[48] EMG may be helpful in cases of neonatal myasthenia gravis,[67] but one should proceed with the neostigmine or edrophonium test. When there has been damage to a peripheral nerve or nerve root—for example, in facial palsy or brachial plexus palsy—EMG and nerve conduction velocity may indicate the severity of the lesion and may be useful in following recovery.[14]

Standardized Assessments or Scores

One must tailor the neurologic assessment according to the status of the infant, more specifically the respiratory status, the nutritional status, the gestational age, and the hours or weeks of life. There is no single neurologic assessment applicable to all newborn infants, and no simplified scale will suffice to delineate the neurologic status of a sick neonate.

Early Evaluation in a Sick Neonate

Monitoring devices, catheters, respirator, and infusions often make a detailed evaluation impossible during the first days or weeks of life. Thus, much of the evaluation will be dependent upon careful inspection of the infant. It is therefore of the utmost importance to observe the infant for a considerable time before attempting manual examination. One may note spontaneous posture and movement, state of consciousness, and subtle signs of seizure activity. Seizures should be confirmed by EEG. As far as the evaluation of tone is concerned, there is frequently not more than one foot and one hand available for testing. Consequently, it is often impossible to evaluate maturation based on neurologic criteria. Laboratory studies, including lumbar puncture, EEG, and cranial ultrasound scan, confirm the suspicion of neurologic disorder.

Editorial Comment: Recent studies of 183 immature infants by Glass et al (1985) suggest that bright lights in the neonatal intensive care unit may alter the neurologic development of immature infants. Severely reducing light inside the incubator altered the ratio of rapid eye movement sleep to deep sleep and increased the length of time spent with the eyes open from 10 per cent to 47 per cent. They also noted significantly more retrolental fibroplasia in infants living within the present brightly lit intensive care nursery, when compared with the infants raised continuously in reduced light. Graven, in a newly designed unit in Columbia, Missouri, has noted that when small immature infants are moved early in their hospital course (shortly after resolution of acute disease—e.g., respiratory distress) into a quiet, dimly lit room, there is a remarkable change in their behavior. For the first 2–3 days they sleep with little motor activity. Following this period, they begin to have short periods of activity and surprising alertness.

Glass, P., Avery, G. B., Subramanian, K. N. S., et al: Effect of bright light in the hospital nursery on the incidence of retinopathy of prematurity. N Engl J Med 313:401, 1985.

Graven, S.: Personal communication, 1985.

The Importance of Repeat Evaluations

Rapid changes are observed from one day to another during the acute stage following birth injury or simply secondary to adjustment difficulties during the transitional period after birth. Thus, it is useful to evaluate the newborn at least daily and to quantify the abnormalities in a systematic manner. The pattern of evolution will help in the final diagnosis and prognosis. Repeated laboratory evaluations are also important. Cranial ultrasound scan should be repeated at least once a week for the first 3 weeks in low-birth weight infants. The ultrasound scan may show hemorrhage in the first days of life, but later porencephaly, hydrocephalus, and other sequelae will become apparent. Moreover, hemorrhages can occur later in life, even though the highest incidence is within the first 3 days. In some units, the progressive maturation and change in EEG have been followed weekly and appear to provide important prognostic information.

Also with the Brazelton Neonatal Behavior Assessment Scale, serial evaluations seem to have a greater ability to forecast the infant's later developmental outcome.

Lester, B. M.: Meaning and measurement of patterns of change in neonatal behavior. Infant Behav Dev 7:211A, 1984.
Nugent, J. K., Green, S., and Brazelton, T. B.: Predicting three year IQ scores from patterns of change in newborn behavior. Infant Behav Dev 7:269A, 1984.

R. Paludetto

Evaluation of the Convalescent Neonate

The evaluation of the cerebral function of a neonate may be fairly sophisticated in the areas of cognitive function, behavior, and adaptability to the environment. Several types of scales or scores have been described, among which the Brazelton Neonatal Behavior Assessment Scale is the first and the most commonly used.[11]

The Brazelton Behavior Assessment Scale is useful in testing the whole spectrum of state and state control as well as infants' individual characteristics. In the exam there is a graded series of procedures starting with a sleeping infant and slowly arousing him; 20 reflexes and 26 behavioral responses are tested over 30–40 minutes and rated on a 9-point scale. The infant is always rated on his best performance. This assessment scale is utilized clinically not only to assess the infant's cognitive and neurologic status but to demonstrate his marvelous sensory abilities to his parents.

Although we do not evaluate every infant with the full Brazelton Assessment Scale, we have selected certain items as clinically useful when examining the baby—his wakefulness, his visual and auditory response, and the way he responds when we awaken him or soothe him. Normal infants can also fixate on patterns and select between two pictures, preferring those with greater contrast and contour over plainer patterns. This is possible only at a visual distance of 18 cm, since the infant's eyes cannot accommodate greater distances. Using this visual preference technique, we reported a pilot study[38] in which 33 high-risk infants were tested before discharge from the nursery and followed for up to 3 years of age. The neonatal visual preference rating was found to be accurate in 27 infants, whereas the standard newborn exam was correct in only 22 infants. Two infants who were hypotonic and thought to be neurologically abnormal but who had normal visual preferences were normal on follow-up. This test may be useful in the future together with a standard neurologic examination.

M. Hack

Sequential data with the Brazelton Neonatal Behavior Assessment Scale on 30 healthy preterm infants from 35–44 weeks' postconceptional age revealed that the behavior of preterm infants does not progress smoothly in each area toward term. Some features develop faster than others. Motor and orientation performances showed more rapid behavioral evolution than other clusters.

Visual responses to a moving ball or face scored in the median range of healthy term infants at 40–44 weeks' postconceptional age. On the contrary, orientation to a rattle or a voice was in the same range as term infants from 35 weeks onward, which suggests that this behavior is well established early in life.

In our preterm infants from 35–44 weeks' postconceptional age, we also found a decreased ability to bring the hands to the mouth compared with term infants. We need to understand how and why different brain functions do not mature simultaneously in these young infants and if some of our care procedures are influencing these behaviors.

Paludetto, R., Mansi, G., Rinaldi, P., et al: Behavior of preterm newborns reaching term without any serious disorder. Early Hum Dev 6:354, 1982.
Paludetto, R., Rinaldi, P., Mansi, G., et al: Early behavioral development of preterm infants. Dev Med Child Neurol 26:347, 1984.

R. Paludetto

Evaluation in the Delivery Room

Severe neonatal depression or injury is readily apparent and easily detected by standard neurologic examination. However, mild depression or injury is not so readily observable in the newborn. Infants having high Apgar scores may have subtle neurologic signs of drug depression (e.g., mild hypotonia, mediocre primary reflexes, absent or poor habituation to repeated stimuli). Perinatal asphyxia or mild birth trauma may result in subtle imbalances of extensor and flexor tone of the neck muscles or in hypotonia in the upper extremities. There is a progression of neurologic signs dependent on the development of intracellular edema following hypoxic-ischemic cell injury. Immediately after the injury, there may be a state of hyperalertness and hyperactive reflexes. From 12–24 hours after the initial insult, a period associated with intracellular edema and cell death, the infant develops depression of consciousness, seizures, hypotonia, and other neurologic signs. Over the next few days, as the edema clears, the seizures come under control, and the recovery phase begins.

There are several scales for early evaluation of the neonate. The Brazelton scale,[11] described above, has been used for this purpose, but it is too time-consuming and requires a great deal of expertise. The test most commonly used to detect the effects of obstetric medication is the Early Neonatal Neurobehavioral Scale, described by Scanlon and coworkers.[50] We recently described a neurologic and adaptive capacity score for full-term newborns that is easily applied to routine clinical use.[6] By placing more emphasis on muscle tone, this test should identify not only babies having drug depression but also those with birth asphyxia or trauma.

MAJOR PATHOLOGIC CONDITIONS

Hypoxic-Ischemic Encephalopathy

Under the term *perinatal hypoxic-ischemic brain injury*, all varieties of cellular damage are included.[2, 59, 64] The most severe degree (Grade III) in full-term newborns is cerebral necrosis involving all cortical areas, basal ganglia, brain stem, and cerebellum. These changes may be associated with severe brain edema.[32, 64] When cerebral necrosis is massive, status epilepticus is the frequent clinical expression. The seizures generally begin 12–24 hours after the initial insult. Neonatal death or severe sequelae are a frequent outcome. However, the improvement in neonatal care allows a partial or even complete recovery in more and more cases. Recovery depends on the severity of the initial insult, and this frequently cannot be ascertained during the acute phase, when the intracellular edema is responsible for the neurologic signs. As the edema clears over the first week of life, the extent of damage will be more apparent. Even then, because of the immaturity of the neonatal brain, final outcome cannot be predicted with complete accuracy.

With regard to the mechanism of CNS dysfunction, it remains clinically difficult to separate hypoxia from ischemia.[61, 64] In acute fetal distress, both factors are usually present. In subacute distress, when these two factors

are more readily separated, neonatal death is less frequent. Experimental studies, particularly those of partial asphyxia in monkeys, have yielded considerable data and have helped to emphasize the role of brain edema.[39–41] In the last 10 years, the increasing knowledge of the probable pathophysiology of perinatal brain damage and, in some cases, the possibility of prevention or cure have necessitated a more analytic approach. Since it appears possible to separate the clinical pictures that correspond to particular pathologic damage states, schematic guidelines to establish diagnoses with reasonable accuracy follow.

Controversy has arisen as to whether edema plays a significant role in human neonatal asphyxia. Prolonged partial asphyxia in newborn monkeys produces generalized swelling of the brain and a shift of fluid from the extracellular into the intracellular compartments, resulting in ballooning and distortion of the mitochondria (Bondareff et al, 1970). In the asphyxiated human infant, although there is often clinical evidence of increased intracranial pressure, precise pathologic demonstration of increased fluid content is hampered by the fluid and electrolyte shifts that occur postmortem. Controlling for these postmortem changes, Anderson et al (1974) showed increased brain water concentration only in infants surviving more than 48 hours. Electrolyte disturbances (increased sodium, depleted potassium concentrations) were present irrespective of the age at death. In our own preliminary studies of full-term asphyxia, computed tomography (CT) of the brain frequently shows generalized increased water content (i.e., low-density reading) at 12–24 hours of life persisting for 5–7 days. It is debatable whether this increased fluid content plays a cause or effect role in symptomatology and morbidity, but it is usually associated with severe seizure activity.

Anderson, J., and Belton, N.: Water and electrolyte abnormalities in the human brain after severe intrapartum asphyxia. J Neurol Neurosurg Psychiatry 37:514, 1974.

Bondareff, W., Meyers, R., and Brann, A.: Brain extracellular space in monkey fetuses subjected to prolonged partial asphyxia. Exp Neurol 28:167, 1970.

P. Fitzhardinge

After prolonged survival, necrotic lesions are transformed into areas of nodulocortical atrophy, white matter sclerosis, and status marmoratus of the basal ganglia. CT scans taken after several months frequently show enlarged ventricles and a prominent sulcal pattern—the characteristic picture of cerebral atrophy (Figure 16–5).

A moderate degree of injury (Grade II) with moderate cell damage and brain edema can be distinguished using clinical data. Signs of cerebral edema occur in 79 per cent of cases:[7] sequelae, if detectable, are usually

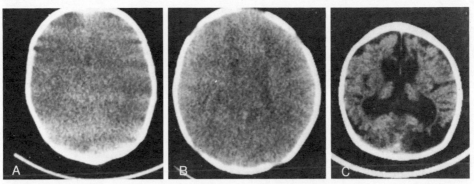

Figure 16–5. CT scans of full-term baby with perinatal asphyxia. *A,* Age 3 days. Cerebral edema. *B,* Age 12 days. Resolving edema. *C,* Age 13 months. Cerebral atrophy with hydrocephalus ex vacuo.

mild to moderate. Mild degrees of injury (Grade I) correlate with animal experiments showing mild edema of the brain without cellular damage.[40] No sequelae are observed in Group I when examination at the end of the first week is normal.[4]

Editorial Comment: A normal neurologic exam at 14 days of age without pathologic reflexes such as increased muscle tone or abnormal reflexes usually signifies an excellent future outcome. It also satisfies our passion to predict the future.[4]

Classification of injury into the three grades of severity was found to be helpful to the clinician, affording some correlation with anatomic data and therefore with prognostic implications.[59] The quantitation of clinical and EEG data, in terms of duration of transient findings within the first week of life, defines the severity of the insult to the brain and increases the accuracy of early prognosis in asphyxiated infants.[49]

The incidence of birth asphyxia has decreased in recent years, owing both to prenatal care and to fetal intrapartum monitoring. The incidence of Grade III cerebral necrosis decreased first and in many obstetric units is now below 1 per cent,[55] so low that it can no longer be used to evaluate the quality of obstetrics. Moreover, the rare cases observed are usually not directly linked with the birth process but with antepartum fetal distress and any of the various in utero causes of cerebral abnormality. These are usually not detected in utero and cannot be detected with present techniques. The process of birth is an asphyxial stress under normal circumstances and is not well tolerated if the brain is already abnormal. A low incidence of Grade II cerebral signs represents the best current index for monitoring the quality of obstetrics.

The site of injury from hypoxic-ischemic insult depends upon the vascular anatomy and relative metabolic activity of the brain. Both of these features change with maturation. Concomitant with neuronal formation, migration, and differentiation, a rich capillary bed with high arterial flow develops in the subependymal germinal matrix. The capillaries empty into major branches of the terminal vein, often at an abrupt right angle. This potential obstruction to flow, together with the fragile walls of the capillary network, makes this area exceptionally vulnerable to changes in arterial blood flow, it is a common site of vascular rupture prior to 33 weeks' gestation. The high metabolic rate of this same area adds to its vulnerability. After 32 weeks the vascularity and metabolic activity subside so that injury to the subependymal area is relatively rare at term.

Toward term, the area of vulnerability shifts to the cortex, which has greatly increased its metabolic rate and blood supply. Although the entire cortex may look edematous in the acute stage, necrosis occurs preferentially in the parasagittal cortex, especially in the posterior portion. This area is the boundary zone between the end-fields of the major cerebral arteries portion. Its vulnerability has been attributed to a watershed effect or local ischemia in the presence of systemic hypotension. However, similar lesions can only be produced in monkeys if they are subjected to hypoxia with or without hypotension. It has been postulated that the ischemic effect is a result of cerebral edema compressing the vulnerable area against rigid portions of the skull.

To summarize, hypoxic-ischemic insults to the immature infant cause hemorrhage in the subependymal area with or without rupture into the ventricles or periventricular white matter. If the infant survives, he is at risk for hydrocephalus and/or cerebral palsy involving the lower extremities. Similar insult to the term infant preferentially causes cortical necrosis, resulting in varying degrees of mental retardation, microcephaly, cortical blindness, and/or cerebral palsy involving primarily the upper extremities. **P. Fitzhardinge**

Periventricular Leukomalacia

The pathologic description of periventricular leukomalacia is distinctive: foci of necrosis are seen grossly as white spots or, when more extensive, as larger areas of brownish softening. The distribution of lesions is in the centrum semiovale, extending from the frontal horn to occipital and temporal horns, adjacent to the bodies of the lateral ventricles. These sites represent border zones between penetrating branches of the middle cerebral artery and the posterior or the anterior cerebral artery. When the lesion is recent, it appears under the microscope as PAS-positive coagulation necrosis. There is early glial infiltration in the first days; a few weeks later, varying degrees of cavitation are observed, and there is a diminution of myelin. The reduction of thickness of white matter will produce hydrocephalus "ex vacuo," the lateral ventricles expanding secondary to cerebral atrophy. When the lesions are very extensive, porencephalic lesions (holes extending from the ventricles) are seen. Historically, these lesions were described first in premature newborns, and the clinical correlation was spastic diplegia as the typical sequela.[9] With the development of neonatal intensive care, it has been shown to be a common lesion in term infants as well in various circumstances, particularly asphyxia or infection.[33, 64] It may also result from a prenatal insult as well as a postnatal one.

From a clinical point of view, it is interesting to summarize some of the certainties as well as the uncertainties regarding periventricular leukomalacia. The pathophysiology is well understood; leukomalacia being a border zone lesion, the main risk circumstance is a decreased cerebral blood flow. This type of border zone ischemia may occur following hypotension, bradycardia, or cardiac arrest. This explains the statistical link between leukomalacia and apneic spells.

Editorial Comment: The marked reduction in cerebral blood flow noted with apnea and bradycardia may explain the association between leukomalacia and apnea.

Perlman, J. M., and Volpe, J. U.: Apnea and bradycardia in the preterm newborn. Pediatrics 76:333, 1985.

The topography of the lesions explains that the major long-term sequela is spastic diplegia, since the region of cerebral white matter mostly affected is traversed by descending fibers from the motor cortex, mainly to lower limbs.[43] Epidemiologic studies amongst newborn infants weighing less than 2500 gm have shown a decreasing incidence of spastic diplegia as neonatal intensive care advances.[24]

From a population-based series of patients with cerebral palsy born during the 20 year period of 1959–1978, Hagberg et al found a significantly decreasing incidence of cerebral palsy from 1959–1970. The incidence increased from 1971–1978. These changing trends in incidence ran parallel to a steadily progressive decline in perinatal mortality through this whole period.

Hagberg, B., Hagberg, G., and Olow, I.: The changing panorama of cerebral palsy in Sweden. IV. Epidemiological trends 1959–78. Acta Paediatr Scand 73(4):433, 1984.

M. Hack

The missing link lies in the clinical and radiologic silence in the neonatal period. There is no specific neurologic symptom during the first months of life, except in severe cases;[29] this explains why it is important to wait at least 3 months to rule out motor problems in a very low-birth-weight infant. There is no definite lesion on ultrasound or CT scan prior to cavitation or definite cerebral atrophy. With current central nervous system imaging techniques, the first weeks of life fail to show any evidence of leukomalacia.

Intracranial Hemorrhage

Intracranial hemorrhage may occur from a variety of causes in the perinatal period, isolated or associated with cellular damage. Until recent years, the localization of the hemorrhage was impossible. Now, with bedside ultrasonography, there is no longer a diagnostic problem. However, the outcome remains uncertain, since ultrasonography does not provide a good evaluation of associated cerebral damage.

Subdural Hemorrhage

This is usually the result of mechanical trauma in full-term newborn infants. When associated with massive tearing of the dural sinuses or of the vein of Galen, the outcome is usually very poor. The symptoms are immediate and severe. Milder forms are associated with tearing of small bridging superficial cerebral veins or bleeding connected with thrombocytopenia or coagulation defects. Development of secondary membranes, liquefaction of the blood clots, and further fluid accumulation take place over a period of days or weeks. Historically, subdural hemorrhage was typically observed in full-term infants after a grossly traumatic delivery. As the proportion of preterm infants surviving the first days of life increases, there is now a similar percentage of such hemorrhages in prematures.[33] Recognition of subdural hemorrhage is important because of the therapeutic implications. Typically the signs begin at birth, with coma and ocular signs, respiratory difficulties, and signs of intracranial hypertension. Rarely, the onset of neurologic deterioration is delayed. Cranial ultrasonography will show the collection of blood, allowing the physician to perform a subdural tap as therapy rather than as a diagnostic exploration for convexity hematomas. Posterior fossa subdural hematomas require surgical evacuation. These produce more severe symptoms because of their location and are associated with apnea and death from brainstem compression. The immediate prognosis for any type of subdural hematoma is poor, considering the severe trauma that causes it and the cellular damage from cerebral asphyxia and cerebral contusion, which are associated in most of the cases. Outcome following evacuation of the hematoma depends on the degree of underlying brain damage.

Primary Subarachnoid Hemorrhage

This is defined by exclusion as not being secondary to the extension of any other type of hemorrhage but having its origin in the subarachnoid space itself.[33, 64] It is a common type of hemorrhage in premature or term infants. It used to be defined by the presence of over 3000 red blood cells/mm^3 in the CSF. The recent definition is the detection by ultrasound or CT scan. It is unnecessary to utilize accessory findings such as xanthochromia, high protein values, or low glucose in the CSF. The source of the bleeding is considered to be venous, from small vessels, with the possibility of asphyxic diapedesis or mild mechanical trauma to the vessels. Hypoxia with secondary capillary rupture is probably the most common mechanism in premature newborns and therefore may occur after a delivery considered mechanically normal. Trauma with increased intravascular pressure and small vessel rupture is often responsible for the hemorrhage in the term infant.

Subarachnoid hemorrhage must be suspected after a somewhat difficult delivery in a neurologically abnormal term infant. Before ultrasonography was available, sub-

arachnoid hemorrhage was divided into two groups based on clinical severity. In the first or mild group—asymptomatic or the only symptoms being irritability, hypertonia, and incessant high-pitched crying—complete recovery is generally observed within the first week of life. In the second, more severe group, recurrent apnea occurs on the second or third day of life with hypotonia, hyporeactivity, and lethargy. These signs signify that blood in the subarachnoid space is likely to be associated with underlying neuronal damage, and the prognosis is obviously dependent on the degree and anatomic extent of the underlying cellular injury and necrosis. Serial ultrasonographic measurements of the size of the ventricles are necessary to detect the preclinical signs of hydrocephalus. In most of the cases, the absorptive defect resolves and rarely ends in hydrocephalus requiring a shunt.

Intraventricular Hemorrhage (IVH)

Anatomic data have clearly shown that this type of hemorrhage is very common in premature newborns, with an incidence decreasing with gestational age.[31, 33] IVH used to be associated with early death. Later studies allowed clinical diagnosis with reasonable accuracy in surviving infants. With progress in neonatal intensive care and increasing survival of very-low-birth-weight infants, there has been an increasing incidence of survivors of IVH showing various sequelae, including hydrocephalus. There is still a considerable mortality rate from massive IVH.

Cranial ultrasonography has changed our understanding of the clinical spectrum of this problem.[53] Recent work has redefined the incidence, epidemiology, evolution, and prognosis of IVH.[1, 10, 63] Oversimplification is necessary here to give the main aspects of past and recent pathogenic concepts. The fragility of brain tissue is one component—more specifically, the huge number of immature cells present in the germinal matrix under 32 weeks' gestation. Arterial vascularization of the germinal matrix is very prominent, feeding a rich capillary network. A rich venous drainage terminates in the great cerebral vein of Galen. The course of venous flow first goes anteriorly to a point of confluence at the level of the foramen of Monro and then posteriorly to join the vein of Galen. The point at which the direction of blood flow changes is the main site of bleeding in the matrix, at the level of the caudate nucleus and the foramen of Monro. This periventricular hemorrhage may rupture into the ventricular system, filling partly or totally one or both lateral ventricles.

Besides the anatomic predisposition to periventricular bleeding secondary to rupture of fragile capillaries, periventricular hemorrhage may actually represent hemorrhagic infarction in many cases.[66] The difficulties in cardiorespiratory adjustments at birth are important in the first hours of life. Hypothermia, hypotension, hypoxic events, hypercapnia, and a pneumothorax have been associated with IVH. Emphasis has since been placed on the lack of vascular autoregulation in the small premature, giving a role to any fluctuations of arterial blood pressure.[35] Therefore monitoring and maintaining blood pressure stability from the first minutes of life seem the most crucial steps in prevention.

The incidence of IVH in very low-birthweight infants, studied first with the help of the CT scan and now with bedside cranial ultrasonography, has been shown to be higher than previously suspected (Figure 16–6). The occurrence in the first two days of life has been confirmed. However, the incidence of delayed bleeding is also high. The ultrasound scan should be repeated systematically during the first weeks of life and not restricted to the first days of life.

The clinical features of IVH have been correlated with ultrasonographic data. There is a complete span of signs, from the abrupt comatose state with seizures and decerebration to more subtle signs, so subtle that they can be overlooked or misinterpreted. Similar to a subarachnoid hemorrhage, the CSF studies are now unimportant compared with imaging techniques.

The immediate outcome is related to the severity of IVH. The majority of newborns with bilateral massive bleeding, usually associated with extensive leukomalacia and intracerebral bleeding, will die in the neonatal period. With less severe lesions, the infant recovers, but the main, immediate concern is the occurrence of hydrocephalus. Careful serial measurements of ventricular size should be made by ultrasonography and should be correlated with the clinical features. Signs of intracranial hypertension in small prematures are distension of sutures (especially the squamous suture), tension of the fontanelle, opisthotonos, the sunset sign, yawning, apnea, and bradycardia. Emesis is a late sign. Progressive hydrocephalus seen on ultrasound scan, especially when associated with apnea and bradycardia, is an indication of significantly increased intracranial pressure. Intracranial pressure may be measured serially by noninvasive pressure measurements across the anterior fontanelle. When the signs are moderate, it seems reasonable to postpone shunting, and to wait for a possible regression of symptoms with the help of medical treatment by acetazolamide,[26] glycerol,[56] or repeated lumbar punctures.[21] When the signs are severe or progressive despite medical measures, shunting is necessary. In some cases, the head circumference does not increase, and there are no clinical signs of intracranial hypertension, but the ultrasound scan shows an increasing size of

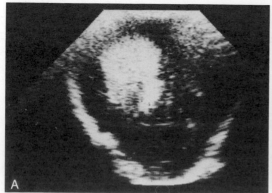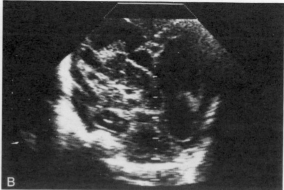

Figure 16–6. *A*, Large intraventricular and intracerebral hemorrhage in a 6 day old premature infant. Cranial ultrasound scans, coronal views. The area of increased density is blood. *B*, Same infant, age 27 days. Hydrocephalus and encephalomalacia. Note the multiple cystlike structures.

the ventricles. This may be interpreted as the result of cerebral atrophy, hydrocephalus ex vacuo linked with white matter sclerosis.

Infants with mild to moderate and uncomplicated IVH may develop absolutely normally.[52] Term infants may develop IVH, particularly as a complication of severe asphyxia.[20] In these cases, there is generally a poor outcome because of the asphyxic neuronal necrosis, despite mild to moderate IVH.

Management of posthemorrhagic hydrocephalus must begin with awareness of the natural history. In nearly all patients the ventricular dilatation initially is slowly progressive and under normal intracranial pressure. In approximately 50 per cent of patients with posthemorrhagic hydrocephalus the progression ceases without intervention, usually within 30 days. In the other 50 per cent, however, progression continues, increased intracranial pressure develops, and intervention is mandatory. Thus, for purposes of devising management, infants with posthemorrhagic hydrocephalus can be divided into two major groups—i.e., those with slowly progressive hydrocephalus with normal intracranial pressure and those who evolve to rapidly progressive hydrocephalus with increased intracranial pressure. The therapeutic approach to these infants differs as discussed next.

The major therapeutic choices in the group of infants with normal pressure hydrocephalus are three—close surveillance, use of serial lumbar punctures, or administration of drugs that decrease CSF production. *Close surveillance* is appropriate initially, since, as discussed above, nearly one half of infants will improve on their own without any specific therapy. This management is particularly appropriate over the first 30 days following the onset of posthemorrhagic hydrocephalus. If the infant does not show spontaneous improvement within that time, then, as discussed above, it is unlikely that spontaneous resolution is likely to occur and more active intervention is necessary.

Serial lumbar punctures are the next most reasonable choice for management of this group of infants. No controlled studies are available to establish that this therapeutic approach is effective. However, two determinations will establish whether at least temporary benefit will result from serial lumbar punctures. These determinations are (1) demonstration of communication between the lateral ventricles and the lumbar subarachnoid space, and (2) definition of the optimal quantity of CSF necessary to be removed to effect a decrease in ventricular size. The communication is established by showing that removal of adequate quantities of CSF causes a decrease in ventricular size, documented by ultrasound scan immediately after the lumbar puncture. Some infants will require removal of as much as 15–20 ml of CSF to effect a decrease in ventricular size. Lumbar punctures are then continued daily over the next 1–3 weeks, with frequency based principally upon the rapidity with which the ventricles return to a dilated state after the puncture and the degree of that dilatation. When progression ceases and improvement ensues, the frequency of the lumbar punctures should be decreased gradually and the punctures discontinued after days to weeks.

Although close surveillance alone over days to weeks is appropriate management for the initial normal pressure hydrocephalus following intraventricular hemorrhage, prompt intervention is mandatory with rapidly progressive ventricular dilatation and increased intracranial pressure. When this phase of rapid progression begins, drastic increases in ventricular size and intracranial pressure often occur over only a few days. The ventriculomegaly may become massive and the intracranial pressure exceed 200 mm of water during this brief interval. Intervention must be prompt and decisive to prevent the deleterious effect on the brain of ventricular enlargement *per se* and of increased intracranial pressure. These deleterious effects are mediated, in part, by mechanical distortion of nerve fibers and, in part, by derangements of cerebral blood flow, the latter documented in the human newborn by the Doppler technique at the anterior fontanelle.

The major therapeutic choices for rapidly progressive posthemorrhagic hydrocephalus with increased intracranial pressure include external ventricular drainage and ventriculoperitoneal shunt. The use of serial lumbar punctures has been advocated by some in this setting. As discussed above, to attain even transient benefit with lumbar punctures, there must be communication between lateral ventricles and lumbar subarachnoid space. Because obstruction at the aqueduct or the outflow of the fourth ventricle is not uncommon in rapidly progressive hydrocephalus, lumbar punctures often are not useful in this setting. Moreover, even in the presence of communication, single daily lumbar punctures may not provide decompression of adequate duration between punctures. Nevertheless, this technique is clearly less invasive than the other two (see below) and thus may be worthy of a trial in selected patients.

External ventriculostomy is the procedure of choice for the infant who is too small or too ill to tolerate placement of a ventriculoperitoneal shunt. When carefully performed, the procedure is safe and highly effective. Ventricular size and configuration are assessed by ultrasound scan, and unless the right lateral ventricle contains a large intraparenchymal lesion or an unusually large intraventricular blood clot, the ventriculostomy is placed on the right side. The procedure is performed rapidly in the neonatal intensive care unit. The catheter is removed after 5–7 days. Experience with ventricular catheters in adult patients suggests that longer duration of placement may increase the risk of infection considerably. Ventricular size usually decreases in association with the ventricular drainage, but several days after removal of the drain the ventricles may begin to increase in size again. A second ventriculostomy may be necessary, although often the infant now is able to tolerate a *ventriculoperitoneal shunt*. In our experience, approximately 10–20 per cent of infants will not redevelop progressive ventriculomegaly and, thus, will not require a ventriculoperitoneal shunt. In those who do subsequently require a shunt, at the least the ventriculostomy has been a safe, decisive, temporizing measure to achieve ventricular decompression and the opportunity for placement of a ventriculoperitoneal shunt under more favorable circumstances.

Hill, A., and Volpe, J. J.: Normal pressure hydrocephalus in the newborn. Pediatrics 68:623, 1981.

Hill, A., and Volpe, J. J.: Decrease in pulsatile flow in the anterior cerebral arteries in infantile hydrocephalus. Pediatrics 69:4, 1982.

Volpe, J. J.: *Neurology of the Newborn*. Philadelphia, W. B. Saunders, 1981, pp. 262–298.

J. Volpe

Seizures

Editorial Comment: Perlman, Volpe, and associates have demonstrated a striking association between a fluctuating pattern of cerebral blood flow velocity in the first day of life in preterm infants requiring mechanical ventilation for the respiratory distress syndrome and the subsequent occurrence of intraventricular hemorrhage. The fluctuating pattern of cerebral blood flow velocity showed good concurrence with a tracing of arterial pressure.

After they determined that the fluctuating pattern could be eliminated by muscle paralysis, they conducted a prospective randomized trial that evaluated the effect of paralysis on both aberrant flow velocity and the incidence and severity of the hemorrhage. IVH developed in all ten control infants (7/10 the most severe) but in only five of the 14 infants subjected to muscle paralysis. In four of these infants, IVH occurred after cessation of paralysis. Although further studies are required, this is a promising observation.

Perlman, J. M., and Volpe, J. J.: Fluctuating cerebral blood flow velocity in respiratory distress syndrome. Relation to the development of intraventricular hemorrhage. N Engl J Med 309:204, 1983.

Perlman, J. M., Goodman, S., Kreusser, K. L., et al: Reduction in intraventricular hemorrhage by elimination of fluctuating cerebral blood flow velocity in preterm infants with respiratory distress syndrome. N Engl J Med 313:1353, 1985.

The physiologically and morphologically immature neonatal cerebral cortex is capable of producing seizure discharges, but the clinical appearance of the seizures is considerably different from that manifested by the mature brain.[46, 62] Classic tonic-clonic seizures are not usually seen in the neonate. Similarly, the typical Jacksonian march of motor seizures and petit mal spells is most uncommon. On the other hand, the relatively advanced maturation of the subcortical structures, such as the limbic system and its descending connections to the diencephalon and brain stem, may explain the high incidence of apnea, chewing, sucking, and abnormal eye movements as manifestations of neonatal seizures. Precise correlation of clinical and EEG findings is still a matter of investigation, so that the identification and classification may vary widely, based on clinical as well as EEG criteria. In the modern intensive care nursery, seriously ill neonates are frequently paralyzed to achieve better ventilation. Such infants are at high risk for seizures or status epilepticus. With no clinical clues to diagnosis, the physician must rely on the EEG.

It is easier, though inappropriate, to ignore the newborn, quietly exhibiting continuous subtle seizures, than the older child, jerking violently in a generalized tonic-clonic seizure. Repeated seizures, even if subtle in type, may

disturb ventilation and cause hypoxemia and hypercapnia. Transcutaneous monitoring of respiratory gases has documented this point clearly. Hypoxemia can cause brain injury directly or, by provoking cardiovascular failure, can lead to ischemic brain injury. In addition, and especially important in the preterm infant, continuous monitoring of blood pressure has shown that abrupt increases regularly accompany subtle seizures. This pressor response, when coupled with certain other accompaniments of seizures—i.e., impaired autoregulation, hypercapnia, and elevated cerebral lactate (secondary to enhanced glycolysis)—may lead to dangerous increases in cerebral blood flow and, perhaps, intraventricular hemorrhage or hemorrhagic infarction. Finally, seizures *per se*, separate from the disturbances of ventilation and perfusion just described, may lead to brain injury, at least in experimental studies of neonatal as well as mature animals.

Perlman, J. M., and Volpe, J. J.: Seizures in the preterm infant: effect on cerebral blood flow velocity, intracranial pressure, and arterial blood pressure. J Pediatr 102:288, 1983.

Volpe, J. J.: *Neurology of the Newborn.* Philadelphia, W. B. Saunders, 1981, pp. 111–137.

Watanabe, K., Kuroyanagi, M., Hara, K., et al: Neonatal seizures and subsequent epilepsy. Brain Dev 4:341, 1982.

J. Volpe

The clinical approach, as described by Volpe,[62] uses a classification based on five types of seizure, noted here in decreasing order of frequency. *Subtle manifestations* may consist of only tonic horizontal deviation of the eyes, tonic posturing of a limb, repetitive blinking of the eyelids, widening of the palpebral fissures, staring episodes, drooling, and clonic movements of the chin. Apnea, when due to a seizure, is usually associated with other subtle manifestations of seizure. Immaturity, metabolic derangement (e.g., hypoglycemia), sepsis, and respiratory distress among other conditions are more frequent causes of apnea than are seizures (Table 16–4).

Tonic seizures may resemble decerebrate or decorticate posturing seen in older patients, with stertorous breathing, eye signs, or occasional clonic movements.

Multifocal clonic seizures are manifested by clonic movements of one or two limbs that migrate to another part of the body in a nonorderly fashion and may sometimes progress to a generalized clonic seizure.

Focal seizures are well localized and not usually accompanied by unconsciousness. Although characteristically produced by discrete lesions, focal seizures do not necessarily mean focal disease and are more commonly due to a generalized cerebral disorder.

Myoclonic seizures are usually synchronous

TABLE 16–4 NEONATAL SEIZURES

Causes Requiring Specific Treatment
Hypoglycemia
Hypocalcemia
Hypomagnesemia
Hyponatremia and hypernatremia
Pyridoxine dependency
Drug withdrawal (barbiturates, narcotics)
Local anesthesia
Septicemia, meningitis
Aminoaciduria—e.g., maple syrup urine
   disease

**Supportive and Symptomatic Treatment
Necessary for Seizure Due to:**
Developmental anomalies
Cerebral birth trauma
Cerebral hemorrhage (intraventricular,
   subarachnoid, subdural), cerebral
   thrombosis
Anoxic encephalopathy
Infection—bacterial meningitis, encephalitis,
   toxoplasmosis, cytomegalic inclusion
   disease, herpes simplex

---

and take the form of single or multiple jerks with flexion of upper or lower limbs. This type of seizure is rare in neonates but may be seen particularly in association with metabolic problems.

Subtle seizures are seen in both premature and full-term infants, generalized tonic seizures more commonly in prematures, and multifocal and focal clonic forms most frequently in full-term infants.[62, 64]

Two pitfalls in the diagnosis of seizures exist for the clinician. First, "jitteriness" has to be distinguished from neonatal seizures. Jitteriness is defined as synchronous tremors or clonic movements not accompanied by other signs and is usually stimulus sensitive. Jitteriness may follow elicitation of Moro's reflex with several very rapid clonic jerks of the extremities, especially of the arms, but may also follow spontaneous movements of the arms and legs without provocative measures. A period of prolonged observation establishing the relationship of jittery movements to spontaneous movements of the limbs or the startle reflex can differentiate these from seizures. Jitteriness is sometimes noted in hypoglycemia or following hypoxia, but more often no cause is found, and this finding may be considered as normal in the first 24–48 hours.

Secondly, subtle manifestations are often overlooked by inexperienced staff, and in addition, small focal myoclonic jerks may be normal manifestations in active sleep. Correlation of clinical and EEG findings is often extremely difficult, and clinical judgment must remain preeminent.[57] Subtle clinical manifestations may be accompanied by minimal, brief, or even no electrical discharges. Multifocal or focal seizures are usually expressed by localized sharp activity or slower rhythmic activity migrating from one area of the cerebral cortex to another. In generalized tonic and myoclonic seizures, the EEG is usually grossly abnormal.

Status epilepticus may be defined as seizures frequently recurring at short intervals without full recovery of consciousness between them. Single seizures lasting beyond 20 minutes may also be regarded as constituting status epilepticus. The EEG patterns associated with status epilepticus have been described extensively. The prognosis is more dependent upon the interictal tracing and, most importantly, upon the etiology of the seizures.[15] Prognostically, normal background activity in the EEG tracing a day or two after seizures is favorable, but this must not be judged immediately following injection of anticonvulsants. In general, a comprehensive approach using the neurologic examination as well as the EEG is most helpful, since seizures can be a nonspecific manifestation of a variety of underlying causes of brain dysfunction. For use in prognosis, the EEG should be performed within 24 hours of the onset of seizures and repeated by the fifth day.[57, 64] However, it is essential that therapy should not be postponed when EEG facilities are not immediately available.

Epilepsia partialis continua is manifested by continuous jerking of one part of the body (for example, a hand or the mouth). This form of seizure is questionably harmful to the infant per se, but its presence usually indicates a significant underlying structural lesion such as infarction, cortical venous thrombosis, or serious infection. These seizures are extraordinarily difficult to stop with medication, and the physician is cautioned against overvigorous therapy. Intravenous drug therapy in large doses should be avoided since respiration may be halted before the seizure stops. Maintenance therapy with phenobarbital and phenytoin should be instituted. A treatment plan for seizures is outlined in Table 16–5.

Phenobarbital is the drug of first choice in neonatal seizures. We administer the drug intravenously in two 10 mg/kg increments, each administered over 5–10 minutes, for a total loading dose of 20 mg/kg, with careful attention to respiration. This dose results in a therapeutic blood level of approximately 20 µg/ml. The response to

TABLE 16–5 TREATMENT OF SEIZURES WITH ANTICONVULSANT DRUGS

Mild or Infrequently Repeated Seizures
Phenobarbital
Loading dose: 20 mg/kg IM or IV; if seizures persist, may repeat once.
Maintenance dose: 5 mg/kg/day IM or PO in 2 divided doses. Maintain blood level 20–40 µg/ml.

Phenytoin (added to phenobarbital in refractory cases):
Loading dose: 10–15 mg/kg IV.
Maintenance dose: 6–10 mg/kg/day IV in 4 divided doses. Maintain blood level 10–20 µg/ml.

Status Epilepticus (be prepared to intubate)
Phenobarbital: intravenously slowly 20 mg/kg; may be repeated once. May push blood level to 50 µg/ml when infant is intubated.

If phenobarbital fails to control seizures:
Phenytoin: 15 mg/kg IV slowly, followed after 8 hours by 6–10 mg/kg/day IV or PO in 4 divided doses. Maintain blood level 10–20 µg/ml.

In refractory cases, paraldehyde may be used but may cause pulmonary damage.
Paraldehyde: (4% solution*) IV over 10–15 minutes (2.5–4.0 ml/kg or 4% solution); repeat as required. Discontinue any single dose as soon as seizures stop or respiratory depression ensues.

*10 ml paraldehyde in 250 ml of 2½% D/W in ½ normal saline or similar solution. Shake often.

this dose depends upon the etiology of the seizure, but in general approximately one half to two thirds of infants will respond. If more anticonvulsant medication is necessary, we recommend additional 5–10 mg/kg increments of phenobarbital, administered over 5–10 minutes, to a maximum dose of 40 mg/kg. With this approach, only approximately 10 per cent of infants will require a second anticonvulsant drug.

Phenytoin is our second choice drug. We administer phenytoin directly into the intravenous line (phenytoin will precipitate if added to the usual intravenous solutions) and follow the injection with a small amount of normal saline (the pH of the parenteral preparation is 12 and is irritating to the vein). A dose of 20 mg/kg will achieve an appropriate blood level of 15–20 µg/ml.

With the regimen just described, the need for a third drug in control of neonatal seizures is rare. Moreover, it is often more dangerous to attempt to stop every remaining remnant of seizure activity by adding more medication. Nevertheless, occasionally we have utilized rectal or intravenous paraldehyde. Others have recommended continuous intravenous infusion of diazepam in the term infant.

Duration of therapy relates principally to the likelihood of recurrence of seizure if the drugs are discontinued. What is the risk of subsequent epilepsy in infants with neonatal seizures? The overall incidence of subsequent epilepsy after neonatal seizures has varied from study to study between approximately 10 and 25 per cent. This incidence can be refined in the individual patient if one considers (1) the cause of the neonatal seizures, (2) the

neonatal neurologic findings, and (3) the neonatal EEG. The first of these is the most critical determinant. Thus, the risk of subsequent epilepsy after neonatal seizures secondary to perinatal asphyxia is approximately 20–30 per cent, whereas neonatal seizures secondary to cortical dysgenesis carry a risk of epilepsy of 81 per cent. However, the risk is 0 per cent with simple, late onset hypocalcemia.

We recommend that these three factors be assessed carefully in each newborn with seizures to determine duration of therapy. In practice, we discontinue phenytoin almost invariably during the neonatal period, usually when intravenous lines are removed. Phenobarbital is discontinued in the neonatal period also if the neurologic examination is normal. In questionable cases, the EEG may be particularly useful. If the infant is discharged on phenobarbital, we reassess the neurologic examination and development at 2–3 months of age and, if the neurologic status is normal, discontinue phenobarbital (over 4 weeks). If the infant is not normal, a sleep EEG is useful, and if not overtly paroxysmal, we believe it reasonable to taper and discontinue the phenobarbital.

J. Volpe

Hypotonia

The evaluation of tone in the newborn infant requires considerable experience, practice, and patience on the part of the physician. Although much has been written about the hypotonic, or floppy, infant, establishing the cause of hypotonia is difficult and often fraught with many pitfalls. The most common cause of neonatal hypotonia is intrauterine asphyxia. For neuromuscular causes, the reader is referred to the monograph by Dubowitz[18] for a detailed account of hypotonic disorders, the diagnostic features of which are summarized in Table 16–6. When a physician is confronted with a hypotonic infant, the history should be carefully reviewed and a detailed physical examination completed prior to the "taken for granted" meticulous neurologic examination. Electrodiagnostic study and/or muscle biopsy is indicated only if the clinical features point clearly to a structural neuromuscular disorder.

Neonatal myasthenia gravis is a life-threatening disorder that requires prompt diagnosis. A history of maternal myasthenia gravis is the diagnostic giveaway. The clinical picture of hypotonia with respiratory weakness should always suggest the possibility of this entity. These infants frequently have difficulty in eye closure, the jaw hangs open, and there is weak sucking and swallowing. The diagnosis is confirmed by intramuscular injection of neostigmine (Prostigmin, 0.1–0.2 mg), which will produce dramatic clinical improvement within 30 minutes. The condi-

TABLE 16–6 APPROACH TO THE DIAGNOSIS OF HYPOTONIA

Anatomic Site	Pathogenesis	Clinical Features						Laboratory Aids			
		Alertness	Cry	Eye Movements	Tongue Fasciculation	Deep Tendon Reflexes	Muscle Bulk	Electromyography	Muscle Biopsy	Muscle Enzyme (CPK)*	Prostigmin Test
Cerebral	Malformation Hemorrhage Hypoxia-ischemia Metabolic Infection Drugs	Poor	Poor	Occasionally abnormal	No	Normal or increased	Normal	Normal	Normal	Normal	Negative
Spinal cord	Injury	Good	Normal	Normal	No	Decreased or increased	Normal	Normal	Normal	Normal	Negative
Anterior horn cell	Spinal muscular atrophy (Werdnig-Hoffmann)	Good	Normal/weak	Normal	Yes	Absent	Decreased	Neurogenic pattern	Neurogenic group atrophy	Normal	Negative
Neuromuscular Junction	Neonatal myasthenia gravis	Good	Weak	Abnormal	No	Normal	Normal	± Normal	Normal	Normal	Positive
Muscle	Congenital myopathy Myotonic dystrophy Glycogen storage	Good	Good	Normal	No	Decreased or normal	Decreased	Myopathic pattern	Myopathic change	Normal or elevated	Negative

*CPK = Creatine phosphokinase. CPK is grossly elevated in Duchenne's dystrophy, which does not usually manifest as hypotonia in neonates.

tion is transient and will usually subside within 6 weeks. During this time, administration of Prostigmin (0.2 mg every 6 hours) will be necessary.

Intracranial Hypertension

Intracranial pressure may be increased in a variety of pathologic states. In most of the cases, there is a combination of cranial and neurologic signs that makes the clinical diagnosis an easy one. The possibility of measuring the pressure by a noninvasive technique has confirmed the clinical evaluation and has shown the high incidence of such cases, as well as the efficacy of treatment.[60]

Cranial signs depend on maturation of cranial bones. They are more prominent in premature than term newborns and may be absent when the skull is very ossified. A moderate disjunction of the sagittal suture (5 mm) and of the initial segment of the coronal and metopic sutures is not uncommon in any normal newborn infant in the first days of life. However, the disjunction of the squamous suture (temporosquamous) is a very reliable sign of high intracranial pressure (just as the overlapping of the squamous suture is a very reliable sign of cerebral atrophy or dehydration). The repeated measurement of head circumference gives a good indication as well, when the curve is clearly crossing percentiles on a standard chart. The enlargement of head circumference, however, may be a late sign of increased intracranial pressure.

Neurologic signs may be observed despite the absence of papilledema in the newborn because of the easy disjunction of the sutures and the compressibility of the brain tissue. The most prominent sign is the sunset sign, permanent or intermittent, although this is nonspecific. Cerebral symptoms include yawning, lethargy and irritability, irregular breathing, apneic spells, bradycardia, and vomiting. There are characteristic abnormalities in passive and active tone.[7] The resting posture is abnormal, with arching of the head to create a free space between the neck and the bed in the supine position. On testing the active tone in the neck muscles, the comparison between extensors and flexors shows an excessive tone in the extensor muscles, keeping the head back when the infant is pulled to the sitting position. With severe hypertonicity of spine extensor muscles, there is permanent opisthotonos.

Measurement of intracranial pressure is possible across the anterior fontanelle.[37, 44, 60, 65] This allows simple monitoring of intracranial hypertension to observe variations of pressure and the efficacy of therapy.

PRACTICAL HINTS

1. In the neonate, the stereotypic clinical response of the infant central nervous system to a variety of pathologic conditions makes differentiation of the underlying cause extremely difficult on the basis of clinical examination alone.

2. The neonate in his early hours of independent life may still have functional abnormalities due to carry-over or dependence on maternal health (e.g., drugs, myasthenia gravis).

3. In assessing neurologic status, especially tone, note time of examination in relation to feeding schedule and state of wakefulness of the infant. The ideal time to evaluate neurologic function is just prior to a feed, when the baby is sometimes in the quiet alert state. Immediately after a seizure, the neurologic examination is not an accurate tool for assessment of the underlying cause or prognosis for disorders of the nervous system. In evaluating the symmetry of movements and tone, the head must be maintained in the midline to avoid changes due to the physiologic tonic neck reflex. The fundi cannot be said to have been examined adequately unless the pupils have been dilated.

4. Be reluctant to make a clinical diagnosis of congenital cerebral defects in the absence of significant abnormalities of the head, facies, extremities, or internal organs.

5. Permanent structural changes can occur in the brain if systemic disorders are not recognized and corrected promptly (e.g., hypoglycemia) (see Table 16–4). Children with asphyxial convulsions are often damaged by failure to attend to supportive measures, such as treatment of hyponatremia, etc. A rare cause of neonatal seizures is direct, accidental needle puncture during caudal anesthesia with injection of local anesthetic into the fetus; exchange transfusion may be life-saving. The treatment of cerebral edema resulting from asphyxia is still open to discussion. Neither the incidence nor the long-term effects of edema are clearly known. Corticosteroids (dexamethasone 0.5 mg/kg/24 hours) and/or mannitol (10 per cent, 1 gm/kg IV) can be utilized. The efficacy and

safety of these measures in preventing further cell damage have not been clearly demonstrated.

Asphyxiated infants often develop generalized and cerebral edema due to water retention secondary to renal insufficiency and/or inappropriate ADH secretion. This may exacerbate convulsions. We monitor urine output of asphyxiated infants very closely and try to minimize brain edema by limiting fluid intake to replacement of insensible fluid loss and urine output. Body weight, serum, and urine sodium and osmolality also need to be monitored, as well as other renal functions. **M. Hack**

6. One third of perfectly normal premature infants under 12–15 days of age and weighing below 2 kg have apnea. Thus, apnea by itself does not signify central nervous system damage.

7. The clinical features of sepsis are so similar to those of anoxia that only the history and confirmation by bacteriologic study can differentiate it from central nervous system dysfunction due to hypoxia.

8. The most critical therapy for seizures is correction of any underlying metabolic cause. Convulsion due to asphyxia or epilepsia partialis continua often cannot be stopped readily with the use of regular doses of anticonvulsants. Avoid excessive dosage, which may be extremely dangerous and depress respiration.

9. The electroencephalogram may be of value in identifying neonatal seizures; however, therapy should not be postponed when EEG facilities are not available. Interpretation of the EEG in the neonate is relatively difficult, with many diagnostic pitfalls.

10. In the treatment of status epilepticus, we recommend phenobarbital (20 mg/kg), given slowly intravenously. In our experience, this has been most effective and relatively safe. Administration should be discontinued immediately if respiratory depression is noted. The latter is always to be recognized as a potential threat with anticonvulsants given via the intravenous route, and the physician must always have facilities available to administer respiratory assistance. Phenobarbital (20 mg/kg) may be repeated once. Phenytoin (Dilantin) (10–20 mg/kg) given slowly intravenously should be used if phenobarbital fails to stop the seizures. Diazepam has been used for treating neonatal seizures, but questions regarding its efficacy and safety have been raised. The drug does not directly cause hyperbilirubinemia, but its constituent, sodium benzoate, will cause uncoupling of protein-bound bilirubin.

11. Maintenance therapy of phenobarbital is continued with a dosage of 5 mg/kg/24 hours in two divided doses. Frequent monitoring of the blood levels is necessary, and an optimal level of around 20–30 µg/l should be aimed for. Phenytoin may be maintained with 8–10 mg/kg/day in divided doses intravenously or orally. The optimal blood level is in the region of 10–20 µg/l. Duration of therapy will be dependent on the cause and course of seizures and should be judged individually.

12. Constant attention to nutrition, temperature regulation, respiratory status, and metabolic balance is essential, no matter how severe the central nervous system disorder may appear. No gloomy prognosis should be given to the parents unless you are 100 per cent sure that permanent damage to the central nervous system has taken place.

QUESTIONS

True or False

Continuous convulsive twitching of the mouth should be terminated with prolonged infusion of paraldehyde.

This continuous twitching (epilepsia partialis continua) may respond transiently to anticonvulsants; however, the seizures almost inevitably recur, and the continued use of large doses of drugs often leads to undesirable effects, especially respiratory depression. Therefore the statement is false.

Jitteriness in the neonate may be an isolated and benign finding.

Careful physical examination is essential to look for an underlying cause, and laboratory tests are sometimes necessary to exclude hypoglycemia, hypocalcemia, or electrolyte disturbance. This statement, however, is true.

Cephalohematomas that transilluminate should be drained by needle aspiration.

These hematomas absorb spontaneously; therefore needle aspiration is unnecessary and could initiate infection in the hematoma. The statement is false.

A CSF protein level of 120 mg/dl is normal in a 2000 gm premature at age 16 days.

Protein levels may be very high in prematures. Therefore the statement is true.

Papilledema is an important sign in the diagnosis of hydrocephalus or cerebral edema in the neonate.

Papilledema is very rarely seen in small infants, because splitting of the cranial sutures and the open fontanelle act as "safety valves," and pressure build-up in the optic nerve is to a large extent prevented. The statement is, therefore, false.

A bulging fontanelle at age 24 hours is an absolute indication for subdural taps.

The fullness of the fontanelle could be due to cerebral edema, subarachnoid or intraventricular hemorrhage, meningitis, or hypercapnia. If these causes were ruled out by appropriate diagnostic measures, subdural taps may be indicated, although CT scans and ultrasound scans have markedly reduced the necessity for needling the subdural space. Therefore the statement is false.

Amyotonia congenita cannot be diagnosed in a floppy newborn infant.

Amyotonia congenita is a meaningless term, denoting no pathologically defined entity. In the hypotonic infant, it is important to determine whether the hypotonia is cerebral in origin, represents a systemic disorder affecting the brain, or is due to a spinal cord injury, muscle, nerve, or anterior horn cell disease, or myasthenia gravis. Specific diagnosis of the hypotonic infant is necessary. There is no justification to continue the use of the term *amyotonia congenita* in pediatric diagnosis. Therefore the statement is true.

A repeatedly isoelectric EEG in a full-term infant denotes brain death.

An isoelectric EEG after 24 hours is evidence of cortical necrosis in term infants and probably also in premature infants. However, this tracing has to be of optimal quality and of sufficient duration. The statement is true.

CASE PROBLEMS

Case One

T. G., a 2680 gm male infant, was born at term to a 26 year old mother, a known epileptic treated throughout pregnancy with phenobarbital (120 mg) and phenytoin (300 mg) daily. The baby appeared normal until 30 hours of age, when he was noted to be lethargic, jaundiced, crying weakly, and hypotonic, and to have a depressed Moro's reflex. The deep tendon reflexes were normal, and the tongue did not fasciculate. The fontanelle was full but not tense, and the neck was supple. Head circumference was 33.5 cm. Transillumination was negative, and the funduscopic examination was normal. Temperature was 35.3°C.

What could be the possible relationship between the anticonvulsant drugs taken by the mother and the hypotonia in the infant?

There is no significant cerebral depression of the infant whose mother is taking the usual therapeutic doses of anticonvulsants. A withdrawal syndrome is possible, though, with agitation, poor sleep, and incessant crying. Anticonvulsants taken during pregnancy can cause coagulation defects in the neonate; thus, cerebral hemorrhage may occur more frequently. (The bleeding disorder associated with maternal anticonvulsant therapy responds to a vitamin K and fresh frozen plasma.) In this infant, all coagulation studies were normal. It is unlikely that drugs taken by the mother will cause depression and hypotonia only at age 30 hours. Drugs affecting the fetus will usually cause problems at birth or soon thereafter.

What diagnostic steps are indicated?

Inspection of Table 16–6 reveals that an infant with hypotonia, lethargy, and a poor cry, with normal deep tendon reflexes, is most likely to have central "cerebral" as opposed to peripheral nervous system disease. The fact that the baby, who was of normal size for a term infant, was perfectly well for the first 30 hours of his life, together with the rapid onset of symptomatology, is strong evidence against anoxic encephalopathy, cerebral birth trauma, or congenital malformation. Infection or a metabolic derangement causing cerebral depression and hypotonia is more likely. With realization of this information, this infant requires a CBC; spinal tap; cultures of blood, urine, skin, and throat; blood sugar, calcium, sodium, potassium, and pH determination; x-ray of the chest; and urinalysis. (With this clinical picture, we do not believe that muscle enzymes, EMG, or biopsy of muscle should even be considered at this time.)

Results of the investigation were: hematocrit 52; WBC 12,000 with 60 per cent segmented polymorphs; urinalysis normal; blood sugar 42 mg; calcium 8.0 mg; sodium 134 mEq; potassium 4.6 mEq; pH 7.37; P_{CO_2} 32; and chest x-ray negative. Spinal fluid was xanthochromic; 96 WBC and 60 polymorphs; sugar 10 mg/dl; protein 279 mg/dl; Gram stain of the spinal fluid was negative for organisms. (Refer to Appendix F–1 for normal values.) There is thus an increase of white cells in the CSF, with low sugar and elevated protein.

In view of the negative Gram stain of CSF, should this baby be treated immediately as having a presumptive case of septicemia and meningitis?

Most definitely. The clinical picture together with the CSF abnormalities is highly suggestive of bacterial meningitis. Absence of a stiff neck and the fact that the fontanelle was flat should not deceive the physician, since it is extremely rare to see neck stiffness in the early phase of bacterial meningitis in the newborn period. Culture of the blood and CSF grew out *E. coli* after 48 hours.

One third of cases of neonatal septicemia will be complicated by meningitis.

The mother was subsequently reported to have a urinary tract infection with *E. coli*. When attention is given to early signs of infection in the mother with immediate notification of the maternal history and maternal laboratory findings to the neonatal unit, diagnosis of potential maternofetal contamination is made at an earlier stage.

Four weeks after the initiation of appropriate antibiotic therapy, the infant began showing a rapid increase in head size on daily head circumference measurements. Does this infant require immediate subdural taps?

No. The most likely cause of rapid head enlargement is hydrocephalus resulting from the infection. Ultrasonography is the most useful diagnostic measure and can demonstrate clearly whether the infant has hydrocephalus and/or subdural effusions (see Figure 16–1).

Case Two

B. D. was delivered at 30 weeks' gestation by cesarean section to a 21 year old gravida IV para 0 mother. Birth weight was 1500 gm, length 40.5 cm, and head circumference 26.5 cm. The mother had systemic lupus erythematosus and was being treated with steroids. She was also hypertensive from the fifteenth week of gestation and was treated with methyldopa. The fetal heart rate was monitored from the twenty-eighth week of gestation. At 30 weeks, the tracing was flat with no variability, the mother noted a decrease of active movements, and the baby was delivered. The Apgar score was 1 at 1 minute. The baby was intubated and resuscitated. The arterial blood pressure was 47/33 mm Hg in the first hour of life. The first blood gas at 30 minutes of age had pH 7.25, Pco_2 19, and base excess (BE) 17. The baby developed respiratory distress syndrome, which was treated by CPAP and oxygen for 3 days, and hyperbilirubinemia (8.0 mg/dl), treated by phototherapy. Feedings were started on the fourth day.

Neurologically, in the first days the infant was active with no abnormal movement and no seizures. The lumbar puncture on the third day was normal. The cranial ultrasound scan was normal on the second day. The EEG repeated over the first 5 days showed positive rolandic sharp waves.

At 3 weeks of age (33 weeks' gestation), the head circumference was 28 cm, the sutures and fontanelle were normal, and the neurologic examination was normal except for excessive hypotonia of neck flexors and hypotonia at the shoulders. The EEG showed left temporal spikes in quiet sleep.

The baby was discharged at 40 weeks' gestation. The parents did not return for follow-up care until the baby was 6 months old (4 months corrected age). At that time he did not use his right hand. At 9 months the right hemiplegia was evident, with the arm affected more than the leg. At 14 months his head circumference was normal, and he was almost walking alone. The CT scan showed a porencephalic area in the territory of the left sylvian artery. The EEG showed decreased activity of the left hemisphere with no seizure activity.

When did the lesion occur?

This is an ischemic lesion in the territory of the left sylvian artery, which could have occurred during the last 2 days of intrauterine gestation when there was poor variability of the fetal heart rate, signifying fetal distress, from an abnormality of placental circulation. It also could have occurred at the time of birth when there was temporary cardiac arrest.

When could it have been seen on cranial ultrasound scan?

Ischemic lesions are not seen on ultrasound or CT scan when they first occur, unless they are accompanied by hemorrhage. There may be focal edema visible on CT scan after 3–5 days, and the cavitation becomes apparent on ultrasound or CT scan after 2–3 weeks. Thus, the ultrasound scan should be repeated weekly for the first 3 weeks of life in small premature infants, even if there are no signs of neurologic abnormality.

What signs lead one to believe that the lesion was already present in the first days of life?

The EEG showed high-voltage positive rolandic sharp waves. These were initially described in infants with IVH and later in infants with other brain damage. The positive rolandic sharp waves are most likely related to cell damage rather than to IVH per se. The prognostic value of the EEG in premature infants as reviewed by Tharp[57] still needs more data and long-term follow-up.

Why did the signs of motor deficit take so long to appear if the lesions was already present?

There is no voluntary cortical control of movement for the first 3 months postterm. The importance of corticospinal pathways does not become apparent clinically until about 4 months of age when the infant starts reaching. In this case, the lesion became apparent clinically at that age.

What hope is there of preventing such deficits?

Regular monitoring of fetal heart rate in very high-risk pregnancies is very important. The infant may be delivered by cesarean section before there are cerebral lesions. The problem is still a difficult one, since abnormalities of fetal heart rate variability may be temporary or difficult to interpret during quiet sleep of the fetus. In very high-risk pregnancies, we have to accept the possibility of saving a neurologically damaged infant by modern technology. Many of these infants would have died in utero if they had not been monitored. We can only hope for a good outcome, or at least acceptable deficits (such as in this case). This is a new population, which demands continuity of care over the first year of life to obtain the best outcome.

The Outcome of Neonatal Intensive Care

MAUREEN HACK
CLAUDINE AMIEL-TISON

Technical advances and improvements in obstetric and neonatal care have been mainly responsible for the improved survival of high-risk neonates and for the accompanying improvement in the quality of the survivors (Figures 16–7 and 16–8). A major concern persists, however, that neonatal intensive care may result in an increase in the pool of permanently handicapped and damaged infants. Since the costs of sustaining the life of such immature infants are enormous, the financial and personnel burden would be difficult to justify if indeed the long-term outcome was less than favorable.

The initial follow-up studies of preterm infants described a decrease in unfavorable neurodevelopmental sequelae as compared with the pre–neonatal intensive care era. However, more recently, despite the continued decrease in mortality, the incidence of neurosensory and developmental handicaps has not continued to decrease but has remained constant.[25, 51] The absolute number of both healthy and neurologically impaired children in the population has thus increased. Furthermore, the increased survival of extremely low-birth-weight infants (< 1 kg), many of whom were previously considered nonviable, has resulted in a high handicap rate (30–40%) in the subpopulation of infants born weighing less than 750 gm. Neonatal intensive care has also resulted in an extended morbidity of various medical complications, which include chronic pulmonary disease, increased susceptibility to infection, sequelae of necrotizing enterocolitis, cholestatic jaundice, multiple rehospitalizations, poor physical growth, and an increase in postneonatal deaths.[23]

When evaluating outcome results there is a considerable difference in the actual figures quoted in different reports. One reason for this variation is the fact that selection of patients by birth weight by no means guarantees a homogeneous group, and such populations studied in

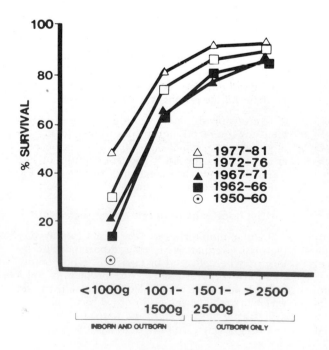

Figure 16–7. Infant survival (Vanderbilt Neonatal Intensive Care Unit), 1950–1981.

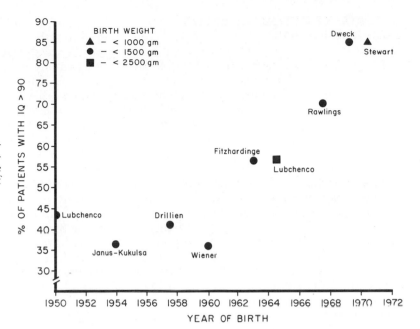

Figure 16–8. A summary of follow-up studies of infants with varying birth weights. Children were assessed between 2 and 10 years of age.

one center may differ considerably from those studied in another center. There are several reasons for these differences. One of the most important factors is the pattern of referral to the neonatal intensive care unit (ICU). An "inborn" unit, which limits admissions to babies born in an adjoining obstetric unit, has a population sample most closely approximating a normal sample. On the other hand, units that receive admissions from numerous outlying hospitals have a selected population that may contain a disproportionate number of the sickest babies or may contain only those infants deemed well enough to transport. In addition, patients treated in the inborn unit have the advantage of consistent and, presumably, good obstetric care coupled with the opportunity for immediate postnatal resuscitation and management. Inadequate resuscitation at birth and prolonged hypoxia and acidemia, together with the cold stress of transport that is seen so frequently in the referred patient, influence not only the immediate neonatal period but also the type and frequency of developmental sequelae. Other factors that may influence the outcome of weight-selected samples are: (1) the socioeconomic profile of the parents; (2) the proportion of infants with intrauterine growth retardation; (3) the incidence of extreme prematurity, i.e., ≤ 28 weeks; (4) a selective admission policy; (5) a selective treatment policy; and (6) changes in therapy during the selection period.   **P. Fitzhardinge**

Regional outcome results reflect a more accurate picture of outcome since they include all infants born in an area.[25, 27, 51] These studies are, however, only rarely undertaken since they are very expensive and time-consuming. In the absence of such regional studies, identification by neonatal disease entities or neonatal complications will yield a more universal method for determining risk that would be applicable to all types of neonatal

units. From studies in Toronto of babies treated in a referral ICU during 1974, Fitzhardinge found that the very low-birth-weight babies at highest risk for subsequent handicap (87%) were those with recurrent neonatal seizures associated with clinical signs of intracranial hemorrhage. Infants with severe intrauterine growth retardation, most of whom had severe perinatal asphyxia, constituted the next highest risk group (53%). The third subgroup at high risk for handicap (36%) consisted of infants with birth weights less than 1001 gm. Handicap in these tiny infants was most closely associated with severe acidemia and/or intracranial hemorrhage. The next group at risk (29%) consisted of those very low-birth-weight infants who required mechanical ventilation. The necessity for ventilation in the neonate reflects serious complications related either to the respiratory tract or to the control of respiration. Such infants sustain periods of hypoxia, acidemia, and frequently sudden changes in cardiac output and cerebral blood supply. It is not, therefore, surprising that, as a group, ventilated very low-birth-weight infants are at higher risk than their nonventilated counterparts. The risk for handicap in the nonventilated babies was 14 per cent, with only 5 per cent presenting with neurologic defects. Children born with multiple major malformations are also a group who, in general, have a poor developmental outcome.

IMPORTANCE OF FOLLOW-UP FOR HIGH-RISK INFANTS

Follow-up clinics should be an integral part of every neonatal intensive care unit. Specialized care of problems of growth, chronic disease, and adaptation are best provided within the setting of such a neonatal follow-up program. This care should initially be provided by the neonatologists themselves and then gradually transferred to a developmental specialist. This initial continuity of care is important to the family, who will find reassurance in the fact that the same people who were responsible for the life-saving decisions are continuing to assume responsibility for the child's adaptation into home life. There is also a moral obligation to maintain this contact. Furthermore, even if the neonatologist does not continue the follow-up for a long period, he/she will benefit greatly by maintaining contact with the nursery graduates and recognizing the sequelae of the early neonatal interventions.

Minor Transient Problems

The first few months after discharge can be considered a period of convalescence for the infant and the parents as well. Many infants have minor problems specifically related to being born preterm, but these may seem major problems to their parents. They include anemia of prematurity, umbilical and inguinal hernias (inguinal hernia is present in at least 50% of males who are born with very low-birth-weight [< 1.5 kg]), relatively large dolichocephalic "premie shaped" heads, and subtle behavioral differences. Most healthy preterm infants are discharged home at 36–37 weeks' gestation (or when they weigh close to 2 kg). At this age they tend still to sleep most of the day, waking only for feeds; to feed slowly and not always demonstrate hunger; to be jittery sometimes; and to have "premie" vocalizations, which include grunts and a relatively high-pitched cry.

Transient Neurologic Abnormality

There is a very high incidence of transient neurologic abnormalities (ranging from 40–80%) in preterm infants.[5, 17, 23] These include abnormalities of muscle tone such as hypotonia or hypertonia. They present as poor head control at 40 weeks' corrected age (the expected term date), poor back support at 4–8 months, and sometimes a slight increase in tone of the upper extremities. Since there is normally some degree of physiologic hypertonia during the first 3 months, it is difficult to diagnose the early developing spasticity related to cerebral palsy. Initially children who will later develop cerebral palsy present with hypotonia (poor head control and back support) and only later with spasticity of the extremities combined with truncal hypotonia. Spasticity during the first 3–4 months is of very poor prognostic significance. Mild hypertonia or hypotonia persisting at 8 months usually resolves by the second year; however it might be indicative of subtle neurologic dysfunction at school age.[17] Persistence of primitive reflexes might also be a sign of early cerebral palsy. Major neurologic handicap will appear obvious during the first 6–8 months post term in about 10 per cent of newborns in the most high-risk categories; however, 90 per cent of high-risk newborns will be or become normal neurologically during the first year (Figure 16–9).

Neurologic Sequelae

Major neurologic handicap can usually be defined during the latter part of the first year of life, or even earlier if very severe. Major neurologic handicap is usually classified as cerebral palsy (spastic diplegia, spastic quadriplegia, or spastic hemiplegia or paresis); hydrocephalus (with or without accompanying cerebral palsy or sensory deficits); blindness (usually due to retrolental fibroplasia); or deafness. The developmental/intellectual outcomes of these children differ according to the neurologic diagnosis. For example, children with spastic quadriplegia and those with microcephaly usually have severe mental retardation, whereas children with spastic diplegia or hemiplegia may have intact mental functioning. Furthermore, this is not always measurable until after 2–3 years of age. Table 16–7 gives the Bayley and the Stanford-Binet test results by neurologic diagnosis of a population of very low-birth-weight children followed at Rainbow Babies and Childrens Hospital, Cleveland, Ohio.

Physical Sequelae and Chronic Disease

Chronic diseases of prematurity, which include chronic lung disease (mainly broncho-

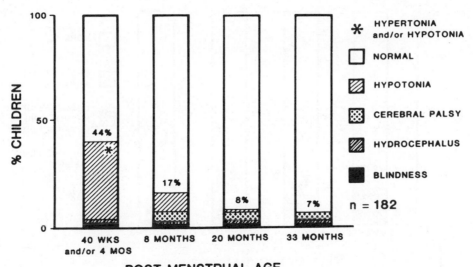

Figure 16–9. Prevalence of neurologic abnormalities among total cohort of very low birth-weight children born in Cleveland, Ohio, in 1977–1978 at 40 weeks' or 4 months' and at 8, 20 and 33 months' postmenstrual (corrected) age.

pulmonary dysplasia), sequelae of necrotizing enterocolitis, and cholestatic jaundice, are present in up to 25 per cent of very low-birth-weight children at 40 weeks' corrected age (for their expected date of delivery) (Figure 16–10). These gradually resolve during infancy. Scars from various neonatal surgery procedures (tracheotomy, thoracocentesis, Broviac lines, shunt procedures) tend also to fade gradually and appear less significant as the children grow. There is, however, a high rate of rehospitalization especially for those children with chronic diseases or neurologic sequelae. Thirty-three per cent of very low-birth-weight children are rehospitalized during the first year of life and up to 10 per cent during the second and third years. Children with neurologic sequelae such as cerebral palsy or hydrocephalus have an even higher rate of rehospitalization for shunt complications, orthopedic correction of spasticity, and eye surgery for strabismus.

TABLE 16–7 NEURODEVELOPMENTAL OUTCOME OF VERY LOW-BIRTH-WEIGHT CHILDREN 1975–1979 (n = 463)

| | N(%) | Bayley (20 months) (mean ± SD) | | | Stanford-Binet (33 months) (mean ± SD) |
		Motor	Mental	DQ*	
Normal outcome	373 (80.6)	97 (±10)	101 (±13)	99 (±11)	99 (±14)
Major congenital malformations	8 (1.7)	55 (±18)	63 (±17)	59 (±16)	64 (±17)
Neurosensory abnormality	47 (10.1)				
Microcephaly	3 (0.6)	81 (±27)	58 (±18)	69 (±18)	64 (±13)
Cerebral palsy					
Spastic quadriplegia 8		46 (±10)	51 (±1)	48 (±4)	50 (±7)
Spastic diplegia 15	25 (5.4)	54 (±12)	94 (±24)	72 (±15)	89 (±15)
Spastic hemiplegia 2				85 (±26)†	97
Hydrocephalus	8 (1.7)‡	66 (±13)	65 (±13)	66 (±10)	78 (±14)
Hypotonia	3 (0.6)	64 (±18)	75 (±12)	70 (±14)	87 (±13)
Severe visual impairment	4 (0.9)	82 (±22)	61 (±11)	71 (±16)	79 (±12)
Deafness	4 (0.9)	88 (±16)	73 (±6)	80 (±5)	72 (±11)
Isolated low DQ (<80)	35 (7.6)	77 (±11)	68 (±8)	72 (±5)	76 (±10)
Total Population	463 (100)	91 (±16)	94 (±18)	93 (±16)	92 (±18)

*DQ = development quotient.
†Stanford-Binet only.
‡One also deaf, two spastic diplegia, and one spastic hemiplegia.

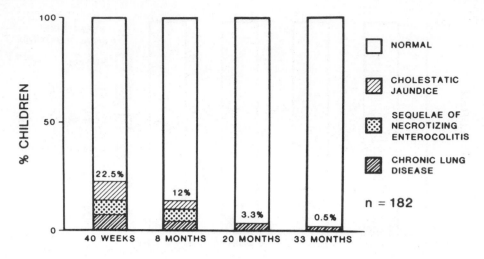

Figure 16–10. Prevalence of chronic disease among total cohort of very low-birth-weight children born in Cleveland, Ohio, in 1977–1978 at 40 weeks', and at 8, 20, and 33 months' postmenstrual (corrected) age.[22]

Physical Growth

Intrauterine and/or neonatal growth retardation is present in up to 50 per cent of high-risk neonates who receive intensive care and require prolonged hospitalizations. For children born appropriate for gestational age, poor neonatal growth is related to inadequate nutrition during the acute phase of neonatal disease; to increased caloric requirements related to breathing in chronic lung disease; to malabsorption related to liver disease following parenteral alimentation; to poor feeding in neurologically impaired children; and to the lack of parental care and/or an optimal environment for growth in the nursery. As these conditions gradually resolve and when an optimal home environment is provided, catch-up of body growth may occur during the first 2–3 years of life. However, up to 20 per cent of these infants still remain subnormal in weight and height by their third year.[22]

The prognosis for catch-up growth is not as good in children born small for gestational age. This is due to the fact that their initial period of growth failure occurred earlier in gestation and extended for a longer time during the critical perinatal period of growth. As many as 50 per cent of SGA very low-birth-weight children remain subnormal in weight by their third year of life.[22]

Growth attainment after discharge is a very good measure of physical, neurologic and environmental well-being. To promote optimal catch-up growth of high-risk infants, neonatal nutrition needs to be maximized and sufficient calories provided during the recovery phase (up to 160 calories/kg/day). This is especially important since catch-up of head circumference in both AGA and SGA children only occurs during the first 6–12 months postterm.

Editorial Comment: There is a rapid spurt in growth when a healthy premature is discharged home. Weight gain per day may jump from 20–30 gm in the hospital to as much as 60–90 gm per day. A check-up at 7–14 days postdischarge with measurement of weight gain is useful in the early detection of environmental (nonorganic failure to thrive) or physical problems.

It is thus evident that most neurologic or physical problems either resolve or become permanent during the first year of life. Clinical follow-up is essential for all high-risk infants during this period. After the first year new problems that become evident are usually subtle motor, visuomotor, and behavioral difficulties, which are best diagnosed and treated in an educational rather than a medical setting. Furthermore, during the second year of life, the environmental effects of parental education and social class begin to influence the outcome measures.

FOLLOW-UP—WHO, WHAT, HOW, AND WHEN

Infants at highest risk should be followed. These include children who had severe asphyxia complicated by seizures and/or signs of brain edema, intraventricular or other cranial hemorrhage, meningitis, and multisystem congenital malformations; those who required assisted ventilation, and those born with very low-birth-weights (especially those weighing < 1 kg).

Growth (weight, height, and head circumference), neurologic development, psychomotor development, ophthalmologic status and vision, and hearing should all be examined.

Timing of Follow-up Visit

The initial follow-up visit should be 7–10 days after discharge. This is essential to evaluate how the child is adapting to the home environment. This visit usually occurs around the time of the expected date of delivery.

A clinic visit at 4 months' corrected age is important to document problems of inadequate catch-up growth and severe neurologic abnormality that might require intervention or physical therapy.

Eight months' corrected age is a good time to confirm the presence of cerebral palsy or other neurologic abnormality. It is also an excellent time for the first developmental assessment (preferably the Bayley Scales of Infant Development) to be performed since the children show very little outward or combative stranger-anxiety at this age and are most cooperative. (Some physicians, however, prefer 12 months of age for the first developmental assessment.)

By 18–24 months of age, most transient neurologic findings will have resolved, and the neurologically abnormal child will be showing some adaptation to neurologic sequelae. Furthermore, most of the potential catch-up growth will have been achieved, and some prediction can be made of the child's ultimate growth attainment. The mental scale of the Bayley Scales will provide at this age some assessment of the child's ultimate mental performance. Prior to 1 year of age this is not easily measured, since most of the test is based on motor function.

The Bayley score attained at 8–12 months' corrected age tends to drop about 10 points by the second year (partly a function of the test and partly due to the increased effect of the environment) and is not of great prognostic significance. However, low scores, of less than 80, are predictive of poor later functioning.

At 3 years of age, a Stanford-Binet IQ test can be performed. This test further validates the child's mental abilities. Language is easily measurable at this age.

From 4 years of age, more subtle neurologic, visuomotor, and behavioral difficulties are measurable. These difficulties will affect school performance even in those children who have normal intelligence.[27a]

NEUROSENSORY AND DEVELOPMENTAL ASSESSMENT

Neurodevelopmental handicap is usually defined in children suffering from a neurologic abnormality and/or a developmental quotient or IQ of less than 80. However, some researchers include only a subnormal IQ (< 70), while others include all children with IQ less 1 SD from the norm (IQ < 84). Neurologic abnormality is usually classified by neurologic diagnosis, which can include hypotonia or hypertonia, cerebral palsy (spastic diplegia or quadriplegia), hydrocephalus, blindness, deafness, etc.

The neurologic examination during infancy is best based on changes in muscle tone that occur during the first year of life. We use the scale developed by Amiel-Tison.[5] This measures the progressive increase in active muscle tone (head control, back support, sitting, standing, and walking) together with the concomitant decrease in passive muscle tone. It furthermore documents visual and auditory responses and some primitive reflexes. This method gives a qualitative assessment of neurologic integrity, which is defined as normal, suspect, or abnormal during the first year. Since the Amiel-Tison method of evaluation extends only to the end of the first year, a conventional neurologic examination should be performed thereafter.

Psychomotor Developmental Tests

BAYLEY SCALES OF INFANT DEVELOPMENT. These are performed prior to 2 years of age. They include a mental and a motor subscale, which together give a Developmental Quotient, or DQ. This test is standardized with a mean of 100. Prior to 1 year of age, these scales are heavily weighted by motor function. It is only during the second year that mental function can be more reliably tested. For example, children with spastic diplegia will have low Bayley scores prior to 12 months of age, but by 2 years they might have a normal mental but low motor score.

STANFORD-BINET TEST OF INTELLIGENCE. Performed between 2 and 6 years of age, this test gives a measure of mental function or IQ.

McCARTHY SCALES OF INFANT DEVELOPMENT. Used mainly between 3 and 5 years of age, these scales have recently become popular. In contrast to the Stanford-Binet test, they have five subscales that measure different functions: verbal, perceptual performance, quantitative, memory, and motor. In addition there is a general cognitive index, which is equivalent to the IQ on the Stanford-Binet test.

DENVER TEST OF DEVELOPMENT. This test is good for clinical use; however, it does not give a quantitative assessment and thus cannot be used to document outcome in specific high-risk populations.

VISUAL TESTING. An ophthalmologic examination should be performed on all high-risk children prior to discharge. If abnormal, repeat examinations should be performed at the discretion of the ophthalmologist. All children should have a repeat eye examination between 12 and 24 months of age.

HEARING. Hearing should be screened prior to discharge from the neonatal intensive care nursery. A behavioral response to sound can be utilized; however, most nurseries now utilize the cribogram or base of brain evoked responses. Hearing should be reexamined between 12 and 24 months since the most common cause of hearing loss is related to middle ear infections, which occur after the neonatal period and during the first 2 years of life.

Editorial Comment: It is important to note that long-term follow-up studies from two large counties in Sweden reveal that 70 per cent of children with severe mental retardation had prenatal causes such as Down's syndrome (32%) while perinatal causes such as birth asphyxia accounted for only 9 per cent of the severely retarded children.[24]

POINTS TO REMEMBER

1. Correct for gestational age (preterm birth) until at least 3 years of age.

2. Do not emphasize to the parents the many abnormalities observed during the 3 month postdischarge period of convalescence since most are transient and have little prognostic significance.

3. Be available, be honest, be optimistic. After the initial abnormal diagnosis is made, most children show improvement, restitution, and growth.

4. The majority of high-risk children do well.

5. In some cases, the diagnosis of cerebral palsy, hydrocephalus, blindness, or cortical atrophy has to be accepted during the first year of life. Early intervention with the child and supportive psychologic help that can be facilitated by the follow-up clinic are crucial.

6. Except when a severe organic disorder persists, ultimate development is dependent on parental education, social class, and environment.

7. The functional capacity attained is more important than the medical diagnosis of abnormality.

REFERENCES

1. Ahmann, P., Lazzara, A., Dykes, F., et al: Intraventricular hemorrhage in the high-risk preterm infant: incidence and outcome. Ann Neurol 7:118, 1980.
2. Amiel-Tison, C.: Cerebral damage in the full-term newborn. Aetiological factors, neonatal status and long term follow-up. Biol Neonate 14:234, 1969.
3. Amiel-Tison, C.: Neurological evaluation of the small neonate: the importance of the head straightening reactions. In Gluck, L. (ed.): Modern Perinatal Medicine. Chicago, Year Book Medical Publishers, 1974.
4. Amiel-Tison, C.: A method for neurological evaluation within the first year of life: experience with full term newborn infants with birth injury. In Major Fetal Handicap: Methods and Costs of Prevention. Ciba Foundation Symposium 59, 1978.
5. Amiel-Tison, C., and Grenier, A.: Neurologic Examination of the Infant and Newborn. New York, Masson Publishers, 1983.
6. Amiel-Tison, C., Barrier, G., Shnider, S. M., et al: A new neurologic and adaptive capacity scoring system for evaluating obstetric medications in full-term newborns. Anesthesiology 56:340, 1982.
7. Amiel-Tison, C., Korobkin, R., and Esque-Vaucouloux, M.: Neck extensor hypertonia: a clinical sign of insult to the central nervous system of the newborn. Early Hum Dev 1/2:181, 1977.
8. Babcock, D., and Han, B.: Cranial Ultrasonography of Infants. Baltimore, Williams & Wilkins, 1981.
9. Banker, B., and Larroche, J.: Periventricular leukomalacia of infancy. Arch Neurol Psychiatry 7:386, 1962.

10. Bejar, R., Cubelo, V., Coen, R., et al: Diagnosis and followup of intraventricular and intracerebral hemorrhages by ultrasound studies of infant's brain through the fontanelles and sutures. Pediatrics 66:661, 1980.

11. Brazelton, B.: Neonatal Behavior Assessment Scale. Clinics in Developmental Medicine, No. 50. London, Spastics Society with Heinemann Medical Books, 1973.

12. Brazelton, T. B.: Behavioral competence of the newborn infant. Semin Perinatol 3:35, 1979.

13. Cheldelin, L., Davis, P., and Grant, W.: Normal values for transillumination of skull using a new light source. J Pediatr 87:937, 1975.

14. Cohen, H., and Brumlik, J.: Manual of Electroneuromyography. Hagerstown, Maryland, Harper & Row, 1976.

15. Dreyfus-Brisac, C., and Monod, N.: Neonatal status epilepticus. In: Handbook of EEG and Clinical Neurophysiology. XVB, 38, Amsterdam, Elsevier, 1972.

16. Dreyfus-Brisac, C., and Monod, N.: Prognostic value of the neonatal EEG in full term newborns. In: Handbook of EEG and Clinical Neurophysiology. XVB, Amsterdam, Elsevier, 1972.

17. Drillien, C. M., Thomson, A. J. M., and Burgoyne, K.: Low birthweight children at early school age: a longitudinal study. Dev Med Child Neurol 22:26, 1980.

18. Dubowitz, V.: Muscle Disorders in Childhood. Major Problems in Clinical Pediatrics, Vol. XVI. London, W. B. Saunders Co., 1978.

19. Fantz, R.: Pattern vision in newborn infants. Science 140:296, 1963.

20. Fitzhardinge, P. M., Flodmark, O., Fitz, C. R., et al: The prognostic value of computed tomography as an adjunct to assessment of the term infant with postasphyxial encephalopathy. Pediatrics 99:777, 1981.

21. Goldstein, G., Chaplin, E., and Maitland, J.: Transient hydrocephalus in premature infants: treatment by lumbar punctures. Lancet 1:512, 1976.

22. Hack, M., and Fanaroff, A. A.: Outcome of growth failure associated with preterm birth. Clin Obstet Gynecol 27:647, 1984.

23. Hack, M., Caron, B., Rivers, A., et al: The very low birthweight infant: the broader spectrum of morbidity during infancy and early childhood. JDBP 4:243, 1983.

24. Hagberg, B., Hagberg, G., and Olow, I.: Gains and hazards of intensive neonatal care: an analysis from Swedish cerebral palsy epidemiology. Dev Med Child Neurol 24:13, 1982.

25. Horwood, S. P., Boyle, M. H., Torrance, G. W., et al: Mortality and morbidity of 500–1499 gram birthweight infants live-born to residents of a defined geographic region before and after neonatal intensive care. Pediatrics 69:613, 1982.

26. Huttenlocher, P.: Treatment of hydrocephalus with acetazolamide. J Pediatr 66:1023, 1965.

27. Kiely, J., Paneth, N., and Stanley, F.: Monitoring the morbidity outcomes of perinatal health services. In Stanley, F., and Alberman, E. (eds.): The Epidemiology of the Cerebral Palsies. Clinics in Developmental Medicine, No. 87, SIMP. Philadelphia, J. B. Lippincott Co., 1984.

27a. Klein, N., Hack, M., Gallagher, J., et al: School performance of the normal intelligence very low birthweight infant. Pediatrics 75:531, 1985.

28. Korobkin, R.: The relationship between head circumference and development of communicating hydrocephalus following intraventricular hemorrhage. Pediatrics 56:74, 1975.

29. Korobkin, R.: Congenital hemiplegia. In Korobkin, R., and Guilleminault, G. (eds.): Progress in Perinatal Neurology. Baltimore, Williams & Wilkins, 1981, pp. 183–196.

30. Korobkin, R., and Guilleminault, G. (eds.): Progress in Perinatal Neurology. Baltimore, Williams & Wilkins, 1981.

31. Larroche, J.: Hemorragies cérébrales intraventriculaires chez le prématuré. I. Anatomie et physiologie. Biol Neonate 7:26, 1964.

32. Larroche, J.: Nécrose cérébrale massive chez le nouveau-né. Biol Neonate 13:340, 1968.

33. Larroche, J.: Developmental Pathology of the Neonate. North Holland, Elsevier Excerpta Medica, 1976.

34. Lipsitt, L. P.: The study of sensory and learning processes of the newborn. Clin Perinatol 4:163, 1977.

35. Lou, N. C., Lassen, N. A., and Friis-Hansen, B.: Impaired autoregulation of cerebral blood flow in the distressed newborn. J Pediatr 96:119, 1979.

36. Meltzoff, A., and Moore, M.: Imitation of facial and manual gestures by human neonates. Science 198:75, 1977.

37. Menkes, J. A., Miles, R., McIlhany, M., et al. The fontanelle tonometer: a noninvasive method for measurement of intracranial pressure. J Pediatr 6:960, 1982.

38. Miranda, S., Hack, M., Fantz, R., et al: Neonatal pattern vision: a predictor of future mental performance. J Pediatr 91:642, 1977.

39. Myers, R.: Two patterns of perinatal brain damage and their conditions of occurrence. Am J Obstet Gynecol 112:246, 1972.

40. Myers, R.: Four patterns of perinatal brain damage and their conditions of occurrence in primates. Adv Neurol 10:223, 1975.

41. Myers, R., Beard, R., and Adamson, K.: Brain swelling in the newborn rhesus monkey following prolonged partial asphyxia. Neurology 19:1012, 1969.

42. Nellhaus, G.: Composite international and interracial graphs. Pediatrics 41:106, 1968.

43. Pape, K. E., and Wigglesworth, J. S.: Haemorrhage, Ischaemia and the Perinatal Brain. Clinics in Developmental Medicine, 69/79. Philadelphia, J. B. Lippincott Co., 1979.

44. Philip, A. G. S.: Noninvasive monitoring of intracranial pressure. Clin Perinatol 6:123, 1978.

45. Prechtl, H., and Beintema, D.: The neurological examination of the full term newborn infant. Clinics in Developmental Medicine, No. 12. London, Spastics Society with Heinemann Medical Books, 1964.

46. Rose, A., and Lombroso, C.: Neonatal seizure states: a study of clinical, pathological and electroencephalographic features in 137 full-term babies with a long-term follow-up. Pediatrics 45:404 1970.

47. Saint-Anne Dargassies, S.: Neurological Development in the Full Term and Premature Neonate. Amsterdam, Excerpta Medica, 1977.

48. Sarnat, H.: Diagnostic value of the muscle biopsy in the neonatal period. Am J Dis Child 132:782, 1978.

49. Sarnat, H., and Sarnat, M.: Neonatal encephalopathy following fetal distress. Arch Neurol 33:696, 1976.

50. Scanlon, J. W., Brown, W. V., Weiss, J. B., et al: Neurobehavioral responses of newborn infants after maternal epidural anesthesia. Anesthesiology, 40:121, 1974.

51. Shapiro, S., McCormick, M. C., Starfield, B. H., et al: Changes in infant morbidity associated with decreases in neonatal mortality. Pediatrics 72:408, 1983.

52. Sher, P., and Brown, S.: A longitudinal study of head-growth in pre-term infants. II. Differentiation between "catch-up" head growth and early infantile hydrocephalus. Dev Med Child Neurol 17:711, 1975.

53. Silverboard, G., Horder, M., Ahmann, P., et al: Reliability of ultrasound in diagnosis of intracerebral hemorrhage and post hemorrhagic hydrocephalus: comparison with computed tomography. Pediatrics 66:507, 1980.

54. Stewart, A. L., Thorburn, R. J., Hope, P. L., et al: Relation between ultrasound appearance of the brain in very preterm infants and neurodevelopmental outcome at 18 months of age. Arch Dis Child 8:598, 1983.

55. Sureau, C., LeBrun, F., and Amiel-Tison, C.: Cesarean birth rate and neurological morbidity in the full term newborn, at the Baudeleuque Maternity Hospital in 1981. Submitted to Am J Clin Perinatol.

56. Taylor, D., Hill, A., Fishman, M., et al: Treatment of post hemorrhagic hydrocephalus with glycerol. Presented at the Meeting of the Child Neurology Society, Minneapolis, Minn., October, 1981.

57. Tharp, B. R.: Neonatal electroencephalography. In Korobkin, R., and Guilleminault, G. (eds.): Progress in Perinatal Neurology. Baltimore, Williams & Wilkins, 1981, pp. 31–64.

58. Thomas, A., Chesni, Y., and Saint-Anne Dargassies, S.: The neurological examination of the infant. Clinics in Developmental Medicine, 1, London, National Spastics Society, 1960.

59. Varangot, J., Henrion, R., Amiel-Tison, C., et al: La souffrance cérébrale du nouveau-né a terme. Nouv Presse Méd 4:1257, 1975.

60. Vidyasagar, D., Raju, T. N. K., and Chiang, J.: Clinical significance of monitoring anterior fontanel pressure in sick neonates and infants. Pediatrics 62:996, 1978.

61. Volpe, J.: Perinatal hypoxic-ischemic brain injury. Pediatr Clin North Am 23:383, 1976.

62. Volpe, J.: Neonatal seizures. Clin Perinatol 4:43, 1977.

63. Volpe, J.: Current concepts in neonatal medicine. Neonatal intraventricular hemorrhage. N Engl J Med 304:886, 1981.

64. Volpe, J.: Neurology of the Newborn. Major Problems in Clinical Pediatrics, Vol. XXII. Philadelphia, W. B. Saunders Co., 1981.

65. Weathall, D., and Smallwood, R.: Methods of measuring intracranial pressure via the fontanelle without puncture. J Neurol Neurosurg Psychiatry 37:88, 1974.

66. Wigglesworth, J., and Page, K.: An integrated model for hemorrhagic and ischaemic lesions in the newborn brain. Early Hum Dev 2:179, 1978.

67. Wise, G., and McQuillen, M.: Transient neonatal myasthenia. Clinical and electromyographic studies. Arch Neurol 22:556, 1970.

68. Wolff, P.: Observations on newborn infants. Psychosom Med 21:110, 1959.

17

Transportation of the High-Risk Infant

AVROY A. FANAROFF
MARSHALL H. KLAUS

The development of neonatal intensive care units in the industrialized nations of the world has precipitated the growth of transportation systems for conveying the sick infant from his place of birth to specialized care centers. As early as the 1900s, Budin used warm water bottles for maintaining the baby's temperature during transport. This was followed in the early part of the century both in England and in the United States by the development of containers for transport of the infants with simple but inadequate heating devices and in some cases a method for administering oxygen. With the advent of modern neonatal intensive care, major refinements in the construction of the transport vehicles and incubators permit the infant to be kept warm and well oxygenated while allowing the physician or nurse transporting the infant to render necessary care during transit.

Each year, an increasing number of neonates are transported at an earlier stage in the course of their illness. Transport equipment has become more specialized and is usually adapted to meet local geographic and climatic conditions. Helicopters and fixed wing aircraft supplement ground transportation when appropriate. Recent technologic advances now permit the transport team to render sophisticated care during transfer in specially designed vehicles. This includes mechanical ventilation and continuous transcutaneous monitoring of blood gases,[2, 4, 10] permitting early recognition and amelioration of hyperoxia, hypoxia, or hypercarbia. Maintenance of communication with the base hospital during transport has enabled prompt and appropriate consultation and intervention, particularly for unique problems. Through extensive educational programs for health care workers, babies are receiving care prior to transfer and are better prepared for transfer. As a result, the effectiveness of these transport systems has improved markedly.

Most encouraging has been the observation that the outcome for transported infants now closely parallels that for inborn infants, with notable exceptions such as a greater incidence of intraventricular hemorrhage among transported infants. This improved outcome for outborn infants contrasts with the previous data (Figure 17–1, Table 17–1) clearly documenting a less favorable outcome at all birth weights for outborn infants as compared with those delivered adjacent to the neonatal intensive care unit (NICU).

It must be emphasized that transportation of the high-risk infant following delivery is probably not the ideal health care delivery system for the high-risk mother or infant.

Most experts in perinatal health care would agree that when risk factors can be predicted, maternal transport is far preferable to neonatal transport and that delivery of a known high-risk infant should occur adjacent to the

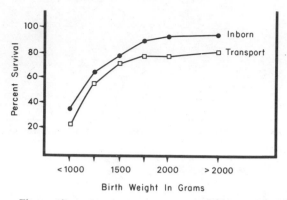

Figure 17–1. Comparison of outcome related to birth weight, Neonatal Intensive Care Unit (NICU), University Hospitals of Cleveland, 1973–1976.[9]

NICU. Programs of maternal transport are currently on the increase in many areas of the United States. Early fears that obstetricians would be less amenable to this new concept than were the pediatricians are proving unfounded. When the staff of the perinatal center works closely with the community physicians in program planning and when the center maintains an open staff and admissions policy for high-risk maternity patients, the obstetrician has demonstrated eagerness to participate.

Nonetheless, despite a measurable increase in the number of maternal transports, medicopolitical and economic pressures have curtailed the growth of these programs. During the past 5 years, coincident with consolidation of the tertiary perinatal centers, we have observed the development and emergence of the level II perinatal teams and units offering care for a wide range of neonatal problems and almost all pregnancy complications and competition with the tertiary units for high-risk patients. Hospital administrators and boards of trustees responding to the economic pressure of keeping the beds full have forced obstetricians and pediatricians to offer more complicated care, transfer fewer patients, and be available to accept reverse transports earlier.

The current uncertain and changing climate of health care delivery and reimbursement with the emergence of organizations dictating the flow that patients are forced to follow to avoid financial penalties has already resulted in significant organizational changes for regional transport programs. More contractual arrangements are being established, with the patients as passive pawns trapped in the system. There is fierce competition to attract the patients into the various systems. We hope that level heads will prevail so that decisions will be based on the best interests of all patients.

Historically, studies in Quebec Province and Arizona first suggested that when the infant is delivered in a hospital with an infant intensive care unit, mortality and morbidity rates are lower. Subsequently, this has been confirmed by many tertiary centers.

TABLE 17–1 NEONATAL INTENSIVE CARE AND PERINATAL MORTALITY*
(PROVINCE OF QUEBEC, 1967, 1968)[17]

Neonatal Intensive Care Facility†	No. Hospitals	No. Births > 1000 gm	Incidence of LBW‡ (1001–2500 gm) *(0/1000 Live Births)*	LBW Neonatal Mortality *(0/1000 LBW Live Births)*	Full-Size (> 2500 gm) Neonatal Mortality *(0/1000 F-S Live Births)*	Stillbirth Rate *(0/1000 Live Births)*	Perinatal Mortality Rate *(0/1000 Live Births)*
Intramural facility	6	12,532	69	62	2.2	8.7	15.0
Referral facility utilized	13	20,962	75	74	2.0	9.8	17.2
Neither intramural nor referral facility utilized	43	73,974	75	86	3.6	10.2	19.9

*For all infants of birth weights more than 1000 gm.

†Including only metropolitan region (Montreal and Quebec City) hospitals delivering more than 1000 infants per year.

‡Low birth weight.

No one would dispute the fact that the possession of an intensive care unit contiguous with the place of birth of the infant represents the ideally superior situation. However, considerations of personnel, economics, and the absolute impossibility of repeating this kind of organization in every hospital in which infants are born require that the statement be analyzed much more carefully. Reference to Table 17–1 will show that, with respect to low-birth-weight infants, the mortality rate is best (i.e., lowest) in those institutions with an intramural intensive care facility, closely followed by those institutions that utilize a referral intensive care facility; institutions that neither have a facility of their own nor refer their patients are at the bottom of the list. The differences between intramural facilities and the utilization of a referral facility, however, should be analyzed a little more carefully. To begin with, in Table 17–1 the incidence of low birth weight is lower in the intramural group and some of the difference (62/1000 as opposed to 74/1000) would be accounted for by this difference in the incidence of low birth weight. Of much greater importance, however, is the difference in the time at which therapy can be undertaken. This difference depends not upon the referral facility but upon the willingness and speed with which the referring institutions transfer their infants. It is generally agreed that earlier transfer, and not just a desperation move when inept attempts at therapy in an unqualified institution have been carried out, would bring the mortality statistics for low-birth-weight infants in institutions using a referral unit even closer to that of the intramural facility itself. (This, in fact, is now happening.) It should also be noted from Table 17–1 that, with respect to mortality rates for full-term infants, there are no differences between intramural and referral utilization of facilities, but the ability to place the child either intramurally or through a referral facility in an intensive care unit results in a full-term neonatal mortality almost half that of infants for whom neither facility is utilized.

L. Stern

A transport system must be considered as only one component of the larger organization required for optimal care of the fetus and newborn. It is our opinion that the uterus is the ideal "transport incubator," and the development of combined maternal and neonatal intensive care units, with the referral to and delivery of high-risk mothers in these special centers, is the ideal arrangement. This will not obviate the need for a transport system, for even though the majority of neonatal problems occur with high-risk pregnancies (including maternal hypertension, antepartum hemorrhage, erythroblastosis, premature ruptured membranes, and premature labor), some infants develop difficulties following a seemingly normal pregnancy and uncomplicated labor and will require transport after delivery.

Although this chapter will discuss the transportation of the infant, this system must not stand alone but must be combined with the development of high-risk maternity-infant centers.

PRINCIPLES AND PRACTICAL ASPECTS OF TRANSPORTATION

All hospitals require some transportation facilities for which the same principles apply, whether the baby is being transported from one city to another or simply within the hospital to the operating room, x-ray department, etc. The transportation of a sick, small infant is a complex act requiring the coordinated action of a number of personnel and institutions. Although in most cases each act is simple, a single omission in the intricate chain may be detrimental to the infant's health. *Communication* and *teamwork* are the keynotes to a successful transport system.

The following discussion and outline consider ground transportation using an ambulance for trips less than 50–60 miles. A slight alteration in the details can be made for longer trips using planes, helicopters, or trucks. In any transport system, plans must be made for the entire 24 hours, and alternative hospitals must be available for accepting infants when the referral center is over crowded or closed for any reason. We have found it useful in Northern Ohio to link two large referral centers together; thus, when one unit is filled or overwhelmed, the other unit can accept all of the other infants. Our working plan is outlined in Table 17–2. The act of transporting a baby, as noted in Table 17–2, is a collaborative effort, and as in any medical endeavor, differences of opinion will arise; however, these must be submerged and reasonable harmony maintained, for otherwise chaos may occur. The individual duties in a transportation system require that all referring hospitals, physicians, and ambulance drivers, as well as the accepting hospitals with their physicians and nurses, have a clear understanding of the local organization and ground rules. In one successful center this was quickly achieved by the director having a discussion with each referring physician over a glass of wine. The responsibilities of every individual and the unit responsibilities must be clearly defined. In our system, this has been helped by having the duties of all physicians and referring hospitals clearly outlined on forms kept in their nurseries.

The transport is *initiated* by a physician requesting transfer to a regional center. His request is influenced by his experience, training, local facilities, personnel, and the overall ability to cope with the problem. (It has continued to be our policy to accept all in-

TABLE 17–2 PLANS FOR TRANSPORTATION

1. Physician controller on call receives incoming referrals and makes the decision as to which nursery can accept an infant after checking on space available.
2. The controller will require that the following essential material and information be available at time of pickup of the infant:
   - Photocopy or duplication of mother's and infant's charts.
   - 5 ml of mother's blood (clotted).
   - Any x-rays of the infant.
   - Infant's name, M.D.'s name, parents' names, address, and phone number.
   - The father should be instructed to follow in his own car (so that he can furnish pertinent information and remain with the infant for 2–3 hours and report back to the mother).
   - With great diplomacy, request that referring physician maintain infant's temperature and color. Tactfully give specific instructions for interim treatment.
3. The controller will delegate a transport team to pick up the infant. This call takes top priority, and the team must be ready to travel in 10 minutes. All team members must receive special training.
   - The intensive care nursery is informed to prepare for infant's arrival.
   - The controller calls driver or ambulance service or special van and relays time of its arrival to the team.
4. The team members collect the transport incubator and emergency bag with drugs and equipment. (Check battery and O_2 cylinder.)
5. Plug incubator into ambulance during trips and use battery operation when moving in and out of hospitals. Plug in at referring hospital.
6. Prepare infant for trip, correcting acute conditions (asphyxia, metabolic acidosis, hypoglycemia, etc.) before transport. Explain plan of action to the parents.
7. No matter how healthy the infant looks, he must be transferred.
8. Record procedures carried out, including drugs, problems, or complications, on the information form.
9. Oxygen tank will last 80 minutes at 7 liters. Battery will last for 45 minutes of constant use.

fants referred from outlying hospitals, even though the physician controller may have the impression that the infant is not seriously ill or is even possibly completely normal. The fact that the referring physician believes that the patient requires further specialized facilities reflects a call for help and is justification for accepting the infant. Rarely have we collected an infant not requiring any special care.) The referring physician communicates the nature of the infant's problem and his condition to the *physician controlling* the transport system, who in turn notifies the transport team and the *nurses on the intensive care unit* of the specific nature of the problem, so that a plan of action may be formulated and any special equipment prepared before setting out.

The *timing* of transport is, of course, particularly important in the premature infant. Approximately one third of all infant deaths occur within the first 24 hours following birth, and early treatment of many conditions appears to alter outcome favorably. Therefore, for whatever reason the physician considers referring an infant, be it an illness that cannot be handled properly at his own hospital or inadequate equipment, we recommend early transportation. While on the subject of timing, it is most helpful to inform the staff of the referring hospital of the anticipated arrival time of the transport team. This allays much anxiety.

After initiating the transport, the referring physician is requested to make the following arrangements:

1. Obtain a sample of blood from the mother, copy the mother's and infant's charts, and have x-rays available. (These data are invaluable in the management of the patient.)

2. The physician controller may often make helpful suggestions to the referring physician so that the infant is prepared for the trip. These include:

- Increasing the environmental oxygen (if this is indicated on clinical grounds — see Chapter 8, Respiratory Problems).
- Administering small doses of bicarbonate if indicated.
- Checking the infant's hematocrit and blood sugar by means of a Dextrostix.
- Placing the infant in the neutral thermal environment.
- Correcting hypotension and hypovolemia.
- Suctioning and decompressing the abdomen when indicated.

(The referring physician may thus warm, oxygenate, and check the blood sugar of the infant before the ambulance arrives and have the patient's records prepared.)

3. The referring physician informs the parents of the reasons for transport and requests that the father be ready to accompany the ambulance in his own car.

Calling before leaving the referring hospital and checking the plan of management as well as preparing the NICU for the anticipated problems constitute time well invested and are mandatory in our system.

It is mandatory that the transportation be carried out by a team from the receiving institution and not just by haphazard selection of a local ambulance company with unqualified personnel.   **L. Stern**

When the ambulance arrives at the referring hospital, the team remains only long enough to stabilize the infant's condition so that the trip back can be accomplished without catastrophe. They must be satisfied that the infant is in reasonable condition and fit to be transported. In order for the transportation to be accomplished without damage to the infant, conditions such as asphyxia, metabolic acidosis, hypoglycemia, and hypovolemia should be promptly treated before transport. A quick clinical appraisal together with several simple laboratory tests (if necessary), such as a Dextrostix, a hematocrit on a pale infant, and a review of the x-rays, is carried out. If there is a history of asphyxia or the presence of respiratory distress and blood gases are not readily available, we make an arbitrary correction of the probable metabolic acidosis by using 1–2 mEq/kg of sodium bicarbonate IV. If the infant is gasping and pale, he may require O_2, bicarbonate, and colloid or crystalloid, preferably cross-matched blood, before the trip commences. Some type of assisted ventilation may have to be started in the referring hospital. The use of transcutaneous monitoring permits adjustment of the fractional inspired oxygen during transport. As a result, fewer infants are arriving at the tertiary centers with either hypoxemia or hyperoxemia.[4] When there is any doubt about controlling ventilation during the trip, it is preferable to intubate the infant prior to departure (infants with severe apnea or respiratory failure).

Transportation should be carried out in an optimally controlled environment. The interior of the transport vehicle should be warm and well-lit so that the infant can be *closely observed* at all times. Difficulties should be anticipated and provisions made for emergency treatment. The team must be in a position to relieve airway obstruction promptly, oxygenate, assist ventilation, correct acidosis, support circulation, control seizures, and maintain temperature during the trip. Table 17–3 outlines the drugs and equipment that we use in our transport system. This checklist stays in the bag, which is replenished after each trip. The major aim is to improve the condition of the infant, and certainly the infant should arrive in no worse condition than when he started.

TABLE 17–3 CHECKLIST OF DRUGS AND EQUIPMENT

Quantity	Item
1	Laryngoscope handle with premature infant blade
	Clear endotracheal tubes, sizes 2.5, 3.0, 3.5, and 4.0 mm
1	Universal endotracheal tube adaptor
1	Breathing bag
1	Set of small Bennett masks
2	Infant airways
2	10 or 12.5 ml syringes, sterile, with # 20 needle
5	3 or 2.5 ml syringes, sterile, with # 22 needle
4	Medicut 18–21
2	T-connectors
5	Three-way stopcocks, sterile
1	Umbilical catheterization set and extra catheters
2	# 5 F single-hole catheters
2	# 5 and 8 F feeding tubes
3	Stopcock plugs (needle caps)
2	Tuberculin syringes with # 26 needle
2	30 ml amp. sterile distilled water
2	30 ml amp. sterile saline
1	10 ml heparin, sterile, 1000 units/ml
1	Amp. phenobarbital, 130 mg
2	50 ml vials sodium bicarbonate
1	50 ml vial 50% glucose
1	Amp. calcium gluconate
1	Amp. 25% albumin
1	1:1000 aqueous adrenalin
2	Amp. (200 mg/ml) naloxone (Narcan)
	6 feet of latex tubing
1	de Lee mucus trap
1	Scissors, nonsterile
2	Hemostats, nonsterile
1	Scotch tape or equivalent
3	Vial files—sharp
	Forms
	Dextrostix
1	Suction catheter with rubber tubing
1	Tape measure
	Disposable gloves
	Specimen tubes
8	Alcohol sponges
2	Urine bags
	Preparation tray with cleansing solution
	Intensive care record sheet
2	Glass 3 ml syringes for artery sticks
2	# 23 scalp needles
1	# 21 scalp needle
	Rubber bands
	Lancets
2	Receiving blankets
1	Stethoscope

Editorial Comment: It is helpful for the transport team to distribute brochures and maps containing key telephone numbers together with information describing the intensive care unit's location and operation.

Detailed notes and recordings of observations made during the transport are essential for the physicians who will ultimately be caring for the infant.

The physician must have a brief discussion with the mother if at all possible and show her the infant before leaving the referring hospital. Although it is obviously impossible to allay all her fears, a short discussion of the reasons for the transportation and the nature of the care the infant will receive in the intensive care unit is helpful. We explain that the mother can receive information on her infant's condition by calling the ICU directly 24 hours a day and that she may visit as soon as she is discharged. We have observed that most mothers believe that their baby probably will not survive following transfer, and they need much reassurance to the contrary. Their initial comment on seeing the infant in the ICU is often: "I never thought I'd see him again." For these reasons, we have found it helpful to work closely with the father, who accompanies the ambulance in his own car. He remains in the intensive care unit for several hours, learning about the condition of the infant, becoming acquainted with the physicians and nurses, and getting a better understanding of his infant's problems. (A cup of coffee and a quiet chat are most useful.) We take a photograph of the infant so that the mother can see how her baby looks. We depend upon him for communicating the infant's condition and progress to his wife. She also receives a report of progress directly from her pediatrician, together with a call from the physician in the ICU.

Problems of transportation are often related mainly to the mechanical equipment. These may be minimized by careful maintenance. In our system, a specific transport team including inhalation therapists cleans and maintains the transport equipment. We have used a battery-operated incubator, which is adapted so it can be plugged into the ambulance during the trip out to reduce the heat loss from the incubator and conserve the battery. To maintain adequate oxygen concentrations, we carry a small plastic hood to fit over the infant's head, connected to the oxygen source. The chief difficulty during transport has been to maintain temperature. To overcome this, it is worth waiting at the referring hospital until the baby has started to warm up before undertaking a journey.

The transportation of ill neonates by inadequately trained staff with inadequate facilities results in increased mortality following the arrival of cold hypoxic infants, particularly those who weigh less than 1500 gm. In a controlled study of skilled assistance, Chance and associates demonstrated not only reduced mortality and morbidity but also a one third reduction in duration of hospitalization for infants less than 1500 gm when transported by a skilled team.[3]

Over the years, selection of the transport team has engendered much discussion. An increasing number of transports are now accomplished by nonphysicians. In analyzing the effectiveness of a highly motivated and specially trained transport team of nurses from their intensive care unit, Thompson in Minnesota documented their ability to assess, manage, stabilize, and transport sick neonates in a manner resulting in comparable outcome to a group transported by physicians.[17] (Physician supervision and consultation were always available.) In Alabama, a "community-based" transport program was organized. Decisions regarding allocation of resources to individual transports reflected distance and the capability of the staff at the referring hospital as well as the nature and severity of the neonates' problems. Physician participation in transports was reduced from 95 per cent to 15 per cent of the trips without adversely affecting neonatal survival.[15] It is the responsibility of the director of the transport program to ensure that all transporters are comprehensively trained and continually supervised so that they will return with an infant in optimal condition. A flexible and diverse staff enhances the capability of the transport program.

On arrival at the intensive care nursery, a short information form is completed by the transport team (Table 17–4). This form is helpful in the care of the infant and in the organization and maintenance of the transportation system.

Once the infant's condition has been evaluated and the diagnosis established, the referring doctor should be called and informed of the infant's condition, provisional diagnosis, etc., so that the mother can be kept up to date. When dealing with neonates, it must be remembered that there are two patients — the mother and the infant.

The ideal vehicle and equipment for transporting infants over different distances are at present unknown. There have been major improvements in the transport vehicles, so that in effect they represent mobile intensive care units. Nonetheless, Shenai et al documented significant mechanical vibration lev-

TABLE 17–4 INFORMATION FORM

Date _____

Time of call _____

Time of departure _____

Time of return _____

Referring person _____ Specialty _____

Hospital _____

Referring diagnosis _____

Name of infant _____ Sex _____ Gest. _____

Date and time of birth _____ Place of birth _____

Category of patient after transfer: Staff _____ Private attending _____

Parents' names _____ Address _____

_____ Phone (home) _____

Your diagnosis _____

What was done before leaving hospital? _____

Bicarb _____ O₂ _____ Bag _____ IV _____ Other _____

What, if any, Rx was given en route? _____

Baby's condition upon arrival _____

Rectal temp. _____ Blood gases _____ Transport temp. _____

Statement of mechanical difficulties, including transport _____

_____

Statement of problems at or with ref. hospital _____

General course of Rx and baby's response in overall transport _____

Suggestions: _____

_____

_____

els, higher than adult tolerance levels, which they suggested may jeopardize the safety of transported infants, particularly when long distances are involved.[12] Many physicians have found the helicopter difficult to work in because of noise, shaking, and inadequate temperature control.

Unless under circumstances in which no other form of transport is available, we are not at all inclined toward the use of helicopters. The question of temperature loss because of the outside cold environmental temperature at such heights is critical, and relatively few helicopters are of the double-walled variety that would prevent such loss. In addition, the choice of a landing site is crucial. In most northern portions of North America, helicopter landing pads that are not low down on the ground generally present conditions too windy to permit the helicopter to land, and although a pad on the roof may look very impressive, it is rarely utilized because of adverse weather conditions. If a helicopter must be used, then an adjacent schoolyard or parking lot would appear to offer the best possibility for its regular operating capacities.   **L. Stern**

The transportation of the infant away from the mother has a profound effect on the mother's relationship with her infant. Procedures for preventing the depression and anticipatory grief that occur in the mother at the time of transportation continue to be studied. Should the mother always accompany the infant? Should she be housed with the infant 2–3 days later when she is discharged? See Chapter 7.

Neonatal back or reverse transfer is defined as the return of previously ill neonates from level III NICU to level II and level I hospitals for intermediate and/or convalescent care. The criteria delineating the levels of care have in general been defined individually in different states, with level II hospitals able to render more complicated care than level I hospitals and hence to accept back sicker and smaller babies.

The initial impetus for reverse transports was a combination of pressure from the need for-intensive care beds and an attempt to reunite mother and infant in the same hospital. Reverse transports now account for a significant proportion of the activity of a transport system and because of their financial impact are highly sought after by the primary hospitals. In Utah, Jung and Bose documented a 44 per cent reduction in the need for services in their neonatal intensive care unit with implementation of the reverse transport program, equivalent to 10 beds per day.[6]

It is imperative that the lines of communication be wide open regarding reverse transports, so that all the health professionals involved in the past and future care of the neonate will relay the appropriate information concerning the course of the infant in a timely and comprehensive manner. We have designated a special nurse to perform the function of reverse transports, and the time at the community hospital is spent on education as well as public relations. The summary forms used to supplement the discharge notes and a copy of the chart are included (Table 17–4). Reverse transports appear to have been very successful, with few infants relapsing or developing new complications requiring a second trip to the NICU.

PRACTICAL HINTS IN TRANSPORTATION OF INFANTS WITH SPECIFIC CASE PROBLEMS

1. Gastrointestinal obstruction—infants with this condition should have indwelling nasogastric tubes and be suctioned prior to and during transportation if necessary.

2. Myelomeningocele—these should be kept covered with moist sterile gauze.

3. Gastroschisis or omphalocele—the intestines should be kept covered, preferably with moist, warm, sterile saline packs.

4. Respiratory obstruction—the infants' airways are to be maintained patent, either with an indwelling endotracheal tube or with an oropharyngeal airway (whichever method is best suited to the individual).

5. Pneumothorax, but no evidence of tension—place the infant in an enriched oxygen environment; be prepared to aspirate and decompress. A tension pneumothorax should be treated before leaving the referring hospital.

6. Severe heart failure—commence therapy before leaving referring hospital (see Chapter 13, The Heart).

7. Seizures—maintain airway and control seizures before leaving the referring hospital (see Chapter 16, Neurologic Problems).

There is a large variety of other technical and operational details that need to be fully understood before effective transport systems can be organized and specifically operated. For example, it is not well known but it is of critical importance that there are striking differences in amperage when AC current—operated equipment (as used in hospitals) needs to be run from DC battery conversion in ambulances. Failure to appreciate this difference generally results in complete breakdown of the ambulance, usually somewhere en route between the two hospitals. This and a large number of other mechanical and administrative considerations are dealt with in a manual on infant transportation published under the aegis of the Canadian Pediatric Society.[11] **L. Stern**

REFERENCES

1. American Academy of Pediatrics, Committee on the Fetus and Newborn: *Hospital Care of Newborn Infants.* 6th ed. Evanston, Ill. 1977.
2. Bose, C. L., Kochenour, N. K., and Brimhall, D. C.: Current Concepts in Transport . . . Neonatal, Maternal, Administrative. Columbus, Ohio, Ross Laboratories, 1982.
3. Chance, G. W., Matthew, J. D., Gash, J., et al: Neonatal transport: a controlled study of skilled assistance. J Pediatr 93:662, 1978.
4. Clarke, T, A., Zmora, E., Chen, J. H., et al: Transcutaneous oxygen monitoring during neonatal transport. Pediatrics 65:884, 1980.
5. Dobrin, R. S., Block, B., Gilman, J. I., et al: The development of a pediatric emergency transport system. Pediatr Clin North Am 27:633, 1980.

6. Jung, A. L., and Bose, C. L.: Back transport of neonates: improved efficiency of tertiary nursery bed utilization. Pediatrics 71:918, 1983.
7. Marks, K. H., Maisels, M. J., and Lee, C. A.: Temperature control during computerized tomography and in-hospital transport of low-birth-weight infants. Clinical memorandum. Am J Dis Child 134:1176, 1980.
8. Merenstein, G. B., Pettet, G., Woodall, J., et al: An analysis of air transport results in the sick newborn. II. Antenatal and neonatal referrals. Am J Obstet Gynecol 128:520, 1977.
9. Merkatz, I., and Fanaroff, A.: The regional perinatal network. In Caplan, R., and Sweeney, W., III (eds.): Advances in Obstetrics and Gynecology. Baltimore, Williams & Wilkins, 1978.
10. Miller, C., Clyman, R. I., Roth, R. S., et al: Control of oxygenation during the transport of sick neonates. Pediatrics 66:117, 1980.
11. Segal, S. (ed.): Manual for the Transport of High-Risk Newborn Infants: Principles, Policies, Equipment, Techniques. Vancouver, Canadian Pediatric Society, 1972.
12. Shenai, J. P., Johnson, G. E., Varney, R. V.: Mechanical vibration in neonatal transport. Pediatrics 68:55, 1981.
13. Shepard, K.: Air transportation of high-risk infants utilizing a flying intensive care nursery. J Pediatr 77:148, 1970.
14. Simon, J. E., Smookler, S., and Guy, B.: A regionalized approach to pediatric emergency care. Pediatr Clin North Am 28:677, 1981.
15. Sumners, J., Harris, H. B., Jones, B., et al: Regional neonatal transport: impact of an integrated community/center system. Pediatrics 65:910, 1980.
16. Sunshine, P. (ed.): Regionalization of perinatal care. Report of the 66th Ross Conference on Pediatric Research. Columbus, Ohio, Ross Laboratories, 1974.
17. Thompson, T. R.: Neonatal transport nurses: an analysis of their role in the transport of newborn infants. Pediatrics 65:887, 1980.
18. Usher, R.: Clinical implications of perinatal mortality statistics. Clin Obstet Gynecol 14:855, 1971.

Appendices

Appendix A–1 Drugs Used for Emergency and Cardiac Indications in Newborns

Compiled with the assistance of Celeste Martin Marx, Pharm.D.

Agent	Dosage	Comments
Atropine	IV (rapid push) or SC: 0.01–0.03 mg/kg. Maximum of 0.04 mg/kg.	
Calcium gluconate 10% (9 mg Ca^{++}/ml)	Emergency dose IV (over 10 min): 1–4 ml/kg/dose; up to 5 ml in prematures and 10 ml in term babies. Maintenance PO or in IV fluids: 30–80 mg/kg/day of elemental calcium (3.3–9 ml/kg/day), diluted and divided q 4 h.	Extravasation may lead to necrosis.
Digoxin	*Total digitalizing dose* (TDD)—divided into three doses, given q 8 h or q 6 h. IV (over 15 min): Premature (1000–1499 gm): 15–23 μg/kg Premature (1500–2500 gm): 23–30 μg/kg Term newborns: 45 μg/kg Term infants (over 1 month): 60 μg/kg PO or IM: TDD is increased by 1/3. *Daily maintenance dose*—PO, IM, or IV: 1/4 of TDD, divided q 12 h.	Serum levels by radioimmunoassay are not useful in neonates (interference by endogenous substances).
Dobutamine	IV (constant infusion): 2.5–7.5 μg/kg/min. Higher doses may be required; maximum rate of 40 μg/kg/min.	
Dopamine	IV (constant infusion): 2–20 μg/kg/min.	Extravasation may lead to necrosis; phentolamine (Regitine) infiltration is an antidote.
Epinephrine	IV or endotracheally: 0.1–0.2 ml/kg of 1:10,000 solution. IV (constant infusion): 0.5–1.5 μg/kg/min.	
Hydralazine	IV or IM: 0.15 mg/kg every 6 hours; increased by 0.1 mg/kg every 6 hours prn. Maximum dose is 4 mg/kg/day. PO: 0.7 mg/kg/day in divided doses.	
Indomethacin (Indocin)	IV: 0.1–0.25 mg/kg/dose given q 12 h for 3 doses IV: 0.2 mg/kg is followed in 12 hours (if needed) by 1 to 2 doses of 0.1 mg/kg (less than 48 hours old), 0.2 mg/kg (2–7 days of age), or 0.25 mg/kg (over 7 days)	

Agent	Dosage	Comments
Isoproterenol (Isuprel)	IV (constant infusion): 0.1–1.0 μg/kg/min. Standard dilution is 1–4 mg in 200 ml D5W, to equal 5–20 μg/ml.	
Lidocaine	IV (over 5–10 min): 1–2 mg/kg, given as a 1% injection. May repeat in 10 min; maximum dosage of 5 mg/kg. IV (constant infusion): 10–50 μg/kg/min.	Watch for hypotension.
Naloxone (Narcan)	IV, IM, or SC: 0.01 mg/kg/dose (equals 0.5 ml/kg/dose of neonatal injection 0.02 mg/ml), repeated prn.	Effect lasts approximately 4 hours.
Neostigmine (Prostigmin)	IM: 0.04 mg/kg.	
Nitroprusside, sodium	IV (constant infusion): 1 μg/kg/min increased prn.	Must have continuous intraarterial blood pressure monitoring. May produce severe hypotension and thiocyanate intoxication.
Procainamide (Pronestyl)	IV (over 10–30 min): 1.5–2 mg/kg, repeated in 30 min if needed.	Watch for hypotension.
Propranolol (Inderal)	IV (over 10 min): 0.01–0.15 mg/kg. May be repeated in 10 min, then q 8 h. PO: 0.5–1 mg/kg/day in 3 or 4 divided doses.	
Prostaglandin E_2 (Prostin VR, Alprostadil)	IV: Begin infusion at 0.1 μg/kg/min. Increase as needed to 0.4 μg/kg/min. Once response established, halve infusion rate serially to lowest tolerated dose. Usual dosage range, 0.01–0.4 μg/kg/min.	
Quinidine	IM: 2–10 mg/kg every 2–6 hours. Total dosage—10–30 mg/kg/day.	IV use not recommended.
Sodium bicarbonate	IV (slow push): 1–3 mEq/kg/dose (equals 2–6 ml/kg/dose 0.5 mEq/ml $NaHCO_3$).	
Tolazoline (Priscoline)	IV (over 10 min): 1–2 mg/kg, followed by 1–2 mg/kg/hour, through a scalp vein.	Monitor blood pressure.
Verapamil	IV (over 1–2 min): 0.1–0.2 mg/kg; may be repeated in 30 min.	Monitor ECG continuously for bradycardia, AV blockade, or asystole. Hypotension may occur, especially with prolonged injection.

Appendix A—2 Antibiotic Therapy in the Newborn

Compiled with the assistance of Celeste Martin Marx, Pharm.D.

Where range is given, newborns less than 1 week of age should receive lowest dose and longest interval; after 1 week use higher dose and shorter interval. For meningitis therapy use highest dose, shortest interval, and IV route.

Antibiotic	Premature	Term	Comments
Penicillins			Penicillins may adversely affect clotting, particularly at high doses and for those agents noted.
Ampicillin	50–100 mg/kg/day IV q 8–12 h	150–200 mg/kg/day IV q 8–12 h	
Carbenicillin	200–300 mg/kg/day IV, IM q 8–12 h	200–400 mg/kg/day IV, IM q 6–8 h	Contains 7.5 mEq Na$^+$/gm. Inhibits platelet function.
Oxacillin/Nafcillin	50–150 mg/kg/day IV q 8–12 h	100–200 mg/kg/day IV q 6–8 h	Monitor liver enzymes and white blood cell count with prolonged treatment.
Penicillin G	50,000–150,000 U/kg/day IV q 6–12 h	150,000–200,000 U/kg/day IV q 6–12 h	Group B streptococcal infections require 200,000–250,000 U/kg/day. Contains approximately 2 mEq Na$^+$ or K$^+$ per million units.
Piperacillin	100–200 mg/kg/day IV q 12 h	150–300 mg/kg/day IV q 6–8 h	Contains 1.9 mEq Na$^+$ per gm. May inhibit platelet function.
Ticarcillin	150–200 mg/kg/day IV q 12 h	200–300 mg/kg/day IV q 6–8 h	Contains 5.2 mEq Na$^+$ per gm. May inhibit platelet function.
Cephalosporins			
Cefazolin (Kefzol)/ Cephalothin (Keflin)	40–50 mg/kg/day IV q 12 h	50–60 mg/kg/day IV q 8 h	Poor CSF penetration.
Cefotaxime (Claforan)	50–100 mg/kg/day IV q 8–12 h	75–150 mg/kg/day IV q 6–8 h	Good CSF penetration.
Cefoxitin	90 mg/kg/day IV, IM q 8 h	90 mg/kg/day IV, IM q 8 h	Poor CSF penetration.

Antibiotic	Premature	Term	Comments
Moxalactam	100 mg/kg/day IV q 8–12 h	100–200 mg/kg/day IV q 6–12 h	Good CSF penetration.
Aminoglycosides Amikacin	15 mg/kg/day IV, IM q 12 h	15–30 mg/kg/day IV, IM q 8–12 h	Monitor serum levels (peak <40 μg/ml, trough <10 μg/ml)
Gentamicin/ Tobramycin	5 mg/kg/day IV, IM q 12 h	5–7.5 mg/kg/day IV, IM q 8–12 h	Monitor serum levels (peak $\leq$10 μg/ml, trough <2 μg/ml)
Others Amphotericin B	0.25–0.5 mg/kg/day IV single dose	0.25 mg/kg/day IV single dose	Monitor renal function and serum K^+; doses up to 1 mg/kg/day or 1.5 mg/kg every other day may be gradually reached.
Chloramphenicol	25 mg/kg/day IV single dose	25 mg/kg/day IV single dose if less than 14 days old; 50 mg/kg/day IV q 12 h if older.	Monitor free (unmetabolized) drug levels (peak 3 hour postdose 10–25 μg/ml).
Flucytosine	100 mg/kg/day PO q 6 h	100 mg/kg/day PO q 6 h	Tentative dose. If serum levels available, maintain below adult toxic level of 100 μg/ml.
Vancomycin	30 mg/kg/day IV q 6–12 h	30–60 mg/kg/day IV q 6–12 h	Monitor serum levels (peak 20–30 μg/ml). Potentially ototoxic; rarely nephrotoxic except when used with aminoglycosides.
Vidarabine	15 mg/kg/day IV q 12 h	15 mg/kg/day IV q 12 h	Poorly soluble; requires high fluid load.

Appendix A–3 Other Drugs Used in the Newborn

Compiled with the assistance of Celeste Martin Marx, Pharm.D.

Agent	Dosage	Comments
Acetaminophen	PO or PR: 5 mg/kg/dose every 4 hours.	
Acetazolamide (Diamox)	IV or PO: 5 mg/kg/day in one or more doses.	
Albumin, human serum, 25%	IV (over 10 min): 1 gm/kg/dose.	
Aminophylline (see theophylline)		
Caffeine citrate	PO: Loading dose—10 mg/kg caffeine base (20 mg/kg caffeine citrate). Maintenance—2.5 mg/kg caffeine base as a single daily dose.	Caffeine serum levels are 5–20 µg/ml.
Calcium glubionate (Neo-Calglucon) (syrup, 23 mg Ca^{++}/ml)	PO: Supplement premature infant to a total intake of 150 mg/kg/day, including feedings.	Gradually increase supplement to avoid osmotic diarrhea.
Chloral hydrate	PO or PR: 10–30 mg/kg/dose every 6 hours prn; maximum daily dose is 50 mg/kg/day.	May irritate mucous membranes.
Chlorothiazide (Diuril)	PO: 10–40 mg/kg/day, divided every 12 hours.	Hyperglycemia, hypercalcemia, and hypokalemia may occur.
Cholestyramine	PO: 240 mg/kg/day in 3 divided doses.	Do not give other oral medications within 1 hour before and 6 hours after cholestyramine.
Cimetidine (Tagamet)	PO or IV (over 15–20 min): Premature: 2–10 mg/kg/day in 3 divided doses. Term: 15–20 mg/kg/day in 3 divided doses.	Reduce dose in renal failure.
Corticotropin (ACTH)	IM, SC: 3–5 U/kg/day in 4 divided doses.	
Cortisone acetate	PO: Physiologic replacement: 15–25 mg/m² (or 1 mg/kg) daily in 3 equal doses, doubled in times of stress. Pharmacologic therapy: 10 mg/kg/day.	
Dexamethasone (Decadron)	IM or IV: Loading dose: 0.5–1.0 mg/kg. Maintenance: 0.05–0.1 mg/kg q 6 h.	

Agent	Dosage	Comments
Diazepam (Valium)	As anticonvulsant—IV (over 3 min): 0.1 mg/kg, repeated as needed, up to a total dose of 0.25 mg/kg. As sedative—PO or IM: 0.02–0.3 mg/kg every 6–8 hours.	May displace bilirubin. Do not dilute injection.
Edrophonium chloride (Tensilon)	IV (slow push): 0.04 mg test dose, followed by 0.16 mg/kg after 1 minute, as diagnostic test.	Keep atropine available for reactions.
Fludrocortisone (9-alpha-fluorohydrocortisone) (Florinef)	PO: 0.025–0.1 mg/day.	Drug of choice for chronic mineralocorticoid deficiency.
Folic Acid	IM: 5 mg, repeated in 7–14 days. PO: 1 mg weekly for premature; 50 μg daily for term infant.	
Furosemide (Lasix)	IV or IM: 1 mg/kg/dose up to a maximum of 2 mg/kg/day. PO: 1–4 mg/kg/day divided into 2–3 doses.	Potentially ototoxic. Increases urinary calcium, chloride, and potassium loss.
Glucagon	IM or IV: 30 μg/kg/dose. May be repeated after 6–12 hours. Dose is increased (300 μg/kg) for infants of diabetic mothers.	
Heparin	IA or IV: 0.5–1 U/ml of flushing and parenteral solutions. IV (for anticoagulation): Loading dose—50 U/kg. Maintenance—16–35 U/kg/hour.	Maintain clotting time of 2–3 times baseline.
Hepatitis B immune globulin (HBIG)	IM: 0.5 ml in delivery room (or within 1 hour of birth); repeated twice at 3 month intervals.	
Hepatitis B vaccine	IM: 0.5 ml at birth, repeated at 1 and 6 months of age.	
Hydrochlorothiazide	PO: 4–5 mg/kg/day, usually divided in 2 doses.	Hypercalcemia, hyperglycemia, and hypokalemia may occur.

Table continued on following page.

Agent	Dosage	Comments
Hydrocortisone	IM or IV: Adrenal crisis—3–10 mg/kg/day as hydrocortisone sodium succinate, in 3 or 4 doses. Physiologic replacement—1 mg/kg/day or 15–25 mg/m²/day.	
Insulin (crystalline zinc, regular)	IV: 0.01–0.1 U/kg/hour.	
Iron	PO: Treatment of iron deficiency—6 mg/kg/day elemental iron. Prevention of iron deficiency—2 mg/kg/day elemental iron.	
Isoniazid	PO: 10 mg/kg/day in a single dose.	
Magnesium sulfate	25–50 mg/kg at 4–8 hour intervals; prepare injection as follows. IM: 0.05–0.1 ml/kg of 50% solution—dilute with 1½ times volume of saline to make 20% injection. IV: Dilute injection to 1% and give 2.5–5 ml/kg over 1 hour.	
Meperidine (Demerol)	IV, IM, SC, or PO: 1–1.5 mg/kg/dose every 4 hours prn.	
Methylene blue	IV (for methemoglobinemia): 0.1–0.2 mg/kg as a 1% solution; infused slowly.	
Morphine sulfate	IV, SC, or IM: 0.05–0.2 mg/kg every 2–4 hours.	
Pancuronium bromide (Pavulon)	IV: Initial dose—0.02–0.3 mg/kg, repeated twice as needed. Maintenance—0.03–0.1 mg/kg every 1½–4 hours as needed.	
Paraldehyde	IV, PO, or PR: 0.15–0.2 ml/kg.	Highly irritating; dilute for IV or PR use, avoid IM injection. IV use risks pulmonary hemorrhage and circulatory collapse.
Phenobarbital	Loading dose—IV (over 10 min) or IM: 10 mg/kg; may be repeated 2 times at 20 min intervals. Maintenance—IV, IM, or PO: 2.5–4 mg/kg/day or more.	Therapeutic serum levels: 15–30 μg/ml.
Phenytoin (Dilantin)	IV (over 5–15 min): Loading dose—10 mg/kg; may be repeated once in 20 min. Maintenance—5–8 mg/kg/day or more.	IM or PO forms unreliably absorbed. Therapeutic neonatal serum levels: 5–15 μg/ml. To increase level, give small loading doses and increase maintenance dose slightly; steady state not reached for weeks without loading.
Phosphate supplement (Neutra-Phos) (3.3 mg phosphorus/ml)	PO: Supplement premature infant to a phosphorus intake of 75 mg/kg/day, including content of feedings.	Gradually increase supplement to prevent diarrhea.
Prednisone	PO: 2 mg/kg/day.	

Agent	Dosage	Comments
Protamine sulfate:	IV: 1 mg for each 100 U of heparin given in preceding 4 hours.	
Pyridoxine (see also vitamin B₆)	IV: 50 mg as single diagnostic dose.	
Sodium polystyrene sulfonate (Kayexalate)	PO: 1 gm/kg every 6 hours. PR: 1–1.5 gm/kg every 6 hours.	Give as solution with 20% sorbitol to prevent intestinal obstruction. May cause electrolyte disturbances.
Spironolactone (Aldactone)	PO: 1–3 mg/kg/day, divided every 6–8 hours.	Hyponatremia and hyperkalemia may be seen.
Theophylline	Loading dose—IV (over 15–20 min): aminophylline 6.9–7.8 mg/kg (= theophylline 5.5–6.8 mg/kg) Maintenance—IV: aminophylline 2.5–8 mg/kg/day; PO: theophylline 2–6.5 mg/kg/day, in divided doses.	Therapeutic serum levels: 4–15 µg/ml. Steady state not reached for days when loading doses not given. Use small boluses to reach desired level; maintain by raising maintenance dose by 25% or less. Tachycardia, seizures, jitteriness, or feeding intolerance may indicate toxicity.
Vitamin A	PO: 250–750 U daily.	Intramuscular forms in oil poorly absorbed.
Vitamin B₁ (thiamine)	PO: 0.5–1 mg/day for prematures; 5–10 mg every 6 hours is therapeutic dose for deficiency.	
Vitamin B₆ (pyridoxine)	PO: 0.3 mg/day for normal term infant; 2–5 mg/day is therapeutic dose for deficiency; 50 mg IV is test dose for dependency.	
Vitamin C	PO or IM: 25–50 mg/day for term baby; 50 mg daily for premature. Therapy for deficiency is 100 mg q 4 hours.	
Vitamin D	PO: 400–1000 IU daily for premature; 40–100 IU daily for term baby.	
Vitamin E	PO (for prevention of hemolysis): 25 IU daily. PO (for prevention of retrolental fibroplasia): 100 IU/kg/day. IM: (for prevention of intraventricular hemorrhage): 15 mg/kg on day 1, followed by 10 mg/kg on days 2, 4, and 6 and every third day thereafter until fed.	Serum tocopherol levels should not exceed 3.5 mg/dl (desired 1.1–3.1 mg/dl).
Vitamin K₁ oxide (AquaMEPHYTON)	IM, SC, or IV (slow push): Preventative dose—0.5 mg for baby less than 2500 gm; 1 mg for heavier newborn. Therapeutic dose: 1 mg IV.	Severe reactions resembling anaphylaxis have occurred with excessively fast intravenous injection.

Appendix A—4 Use of Drugs by Nursing Mothers

Compiled with the assistance of Celeste Martin Marx, Pharm.D.

I. *Agents that are contraindicated: these drugs are known to have produced adverse effects on nursing infants or have a high potential for adverse effects and are known to be excreted in human milk.*

Androgens
Antimetabolites (amethopterin, cyclophosphamide, methotrexate)
Bromides (at high maternal dosage: 5.4 gm/day)
Bromocriptine
Chloramphenicol
Cimetidine
Clemastine
^{69}Gallium: may resume nursing after 2 wks
Gold salts
Heroin
Iodides
^{125}Iodine: may resume nursing after 12 days
^{131}Iodine: may resume nursing after 2 wks
Marijuana

Methimazole
Metronidazole
Nalidixic acid, nitrofurantoin
(if baby is G6PD-deficient)
Phenelzine
Phenindione
Radioactive sodium: may resume nursing after 4 days
Radiopharmaceuticals: in absence of more specific information from radiologist
Sulfonamides (in initial 6–8 wks of infant life)
^{99m}Technetium: may resume nursing after 3 days
Tetracycline
Thiouracil
Valproic acid

II. *Agents about which controversy exists regarding use by nursing mothers.*

Alcohol*	Occasional drinks do not result in the transfer of significant amounts of alcohol to the nursing baby. In mothers who are chronic alcohol abusers, tolerance to very high blood alcohol levels may increase infant exposure and preclude nursing.
Amantadine	Few indications exist for the use of this drug in the lactating population; it is generally possible to avoid its use.
Chloroquine*	Because of potential toxicity to the eyes, exposure is best avoided.
Clindamycin	There is a single report of bloody stools in a nursed infant during maternal clindamycin therapy. The expected infant dose is small.
Diazepam*	An occasional dose is unlikely to produce adverse effects on the infant; because accumulation in milk may occur and infant elimination is slow, chronic therapy should be discouraged.
Ergot alkaloids*	(ergotamine, methylergonovine [Methergine]) Early, crude preparations of ergot were associated with infant ergotism (cardiovascular instability, vomiting, diarrhea, and convulsions). Although chronic use of ergots is best avoided, a short course of methylergonovine for control of postpartum bleeding does not preclude nursing. The purported adverse effect on lactation does not appear to be clinically significant.
Isoniazid (INH)*	Although the infant might not be exposed to toxic amounts of INH via milk and may have been exposed in utero, the potential toxicity of INH to liver and eyes usually results in nursing being discouraged.
Indomethacin	Reports of an infant who developed convulsions during maternal indomethacin therapy have led to relative prohibition of this agent for nursing mothers. Alternative nonsteroidal antiinflammatory agents have been measured in milk and are present in extremely small amounts; those considered compatible with nursing are ibuprofen (Motrin), naproxen (Naprosyn), piroxicam (Feldene).*
Lithium	Although lithium transfer in milk is low, neonatal toxicity has been observed; this may be an artifact of fetal exposure. Because babies are very susceptible to fluid and electrolyte disturbances that may increase the risk of lithium toxicity, it remains best for mothers requiring lithium therapy to avoid nursing.

Methadone	Methadone therapy with less than 20 mg daily has not been associated with adverse effects, but a death has been reported with a higher dose, and the time course of withdrawal may be prolonged.
Oral contraceptives*	Human milk normally contains small amounts of hormones, and the American Academy of Pediatrics Committee on Drugs does not consider oral contraceptive use incompatible with nursing.
Reserpine	Nasal congestion from the pharmacologic action of the drug may impair the infant's ability to nurse.

III. *Agents that have previously been prohibited but that are now considered compatible with nursing.*

Anticonvulsants* (carbamazepine, ethosuximide, phenobarbital, phenytoin, primidone)
Antithyroid drug* (propylthiouracil only)
Atropine
Diuretics* (chlorothiazide, hydrochlorothiazide, spironolactone)
Narcotic analgesics* (butorphanol, codeine, meperidine, morphine)
Psychotherapeutic agents* (antipsychotics: chlorpromazine, haloperidol, mesoridazine, piperacetazine, prochlorperazine, thioridazine, trifluoperazine; tricyclic antidepressants: amitriptyline, amoxapine, desipramine, dothiepin, imipramine)

---

*Although the doses of these agents received by the nursing infant are unlikely to produce toxic or therapeutic effects, the long-term effects of nursing during maternal therapy with these drugs have not been studied. Therefore, their use should be discussed with the parents and the child carefully monitored, if breast feeding is chosen.

REFERENCES

American Academy of Pediatrics, Committee on Drugs: The transfer of drugs and other chemicals into human breast milk. Pediatrics 72:375, 1983.

Lawrence, R. A.: *Breastfeeding: A Guide for the Medical Profession.* St. Louis, C V Mosby, 1980.

Riordan, J., and Riordan, M.: Drugs in breast milk. Am J Nurs. 84(3):328, 1984.

White, G. J., and White, M. K.: Breastfeeding and drugs in human milk. Vet Hum Toxicol 22 (Suppl):1, 1980.

Wilson, J. T.: *Drugs in Breast Milk.* New York, ADIS Press, Australasia Pty Ltd, 1981.

Appendix B–1   Pediatric Hyperalimentation Form—Central Line

UNIVERSITY HOSPITALS OF CLEVELAND
DEPARTMENT OF PHARMACY SERVICES

PEDIATRIC HYPERALIMENTATION REQUEST

PHYSICIAN SIGNATURE: _____

PRINT NAME: _____ DATE: __

PEDIATRIC HYPERALIMENTATION (For Central Line)
EACH 1000 ml CONTAINS:

CRYSTALLINE AMINO ACIDS	27.5 gm	VITAMIN A	10,000 U
NITROGEN	4.6 gm	VITAMIN D	1000 U
PROTEIN EQUIVALENT	27.5 gm	THIAMINE	50 mg
DEXTROSE (FINAL CONC. = 25%)	250 gm	RIBOFLAVIN	10 mg
NONPROTEIN CALORIES	850 kcal	PYRIDOXINE	15 mg
SODIUM	35 mEq	NIACINAMIDE	100 mg
POTASSIUM	40 mEq	DEXPANTHENOL	25 mg
MAGNESIUM	5 mEq	VITAMIN E	5 U
CALCIUM	10 mEq	VITAMIN C	500 mg
CHLORIDE	35 mEq	PHYTONADIONE	2 mg
PHOSPHATE	30 mEq	VITAMIN B_{12}	1 µg
ACETATE	50 mEq	FOLIC ACID	1 mg
GLUCONATE	10 mEq	HEPARIN	1000 U

TOTAL CALORIES (DEXTROSE & AMINO ACIDS) = .95 kcal/ml

PLEASE NOTE: 1. Any change in the above formula, except for additional requirements, must have the prior approval of the Pediatric Hyperalimentation Committee.
2. The concentration of iron is less than one (1) part per million. Supplemental iron, if required, must be given by another route.

ADDITIONAL REQUIREMENTS

ADD SODIUM (as chloride) TO EQUAL A TOTAL CONCENTRATION OF _____ mEq/1000 ml

ADD SODIUM (as acetate) TO EQUAL A TOTAL CONCENTRATION OF _____ mEq/1000 ml

ADD POTASSIUM (as chloride) TO EQUAL A TOTAL CONCENTRATION OF _____ mEq/1000 ml

ADD POTASSIUM (as acetate) TO EQUAL A TOTAL CONCENTRATION OF _____ mEq/1000 ml

OTHER _____

RATE OF ADMINISTRATION_____ ml/hour   PATIENT BODY WEIGHT _____ kg

A 24 HOUR SUPPLY WILL BE SENT IN NO LESS THAN TWO CONTAINERS

PLEASE NOTE: The above formula will be supplied each day unless a revised formula is received in the Department of Pharmacy Services by 8 P.M. for delivery at 10 A.M. the next day.

SEND COPY TO PHARMACY SERVICES   RETAIN ORIGINAL ON NURSING DIVISION

P

FC8236

Appendix B—2   Pediatric Hyperalimentation Form—Peripheral Line

UNIVERSITY HOSPITALS OF CLEVELAND
DEPARTMENT OF PHARMACY SERVICES

PEDIATRIC PERIPHERAL HYPERALIMENTATION
REQUEST

PHYSICIAN SIGNATURE: _____

PRINT NAME: _____ DATE: __

PEDIATRIC PERIPHERAL HYPERALIMENTATION
EACH 1000 ml CONTAINS:

CRYSTALLINE AMINO ACIDS	11.0 gm	VITAMIN A	5000 U
NITROGEN	1.84 gm	VITAMIN D	500 U
PROTEIN EQUIVALENT	11.0 gm	THIAMINE	25 mg
DEXTROSE (FINAL CONC. = 10%)	100 gm	RIBOFLAVIN	5 mg
NONPROTEIN CALORIES	340 kcal	PYRIDOXINE	7.5 mg
SODIUM	38 mEq	NIACINAMIDE	50 mg
POTASSIUM	20 mEq	DEXPANTHENOL	12.5 mg
MAGNESIUM	2 mEq	VITAMIN E	2.5 U
CALCIUM	7 mEq	VITAMIN C	250 mg
CHLORIDE	14 mEq	PHYTONADIONE	1 mg
PHOSPHATE	12 mEq	VITAMIN B_{12}	5 µg
ACETATE	52 mEq	FOLIC ACID	0.5 mg
GLUCONATE	7 mEq	HEPARIN	500 U

TOTAL CALORIES (DEXTROSE & AMINO ACIDS) = .4 kcal/ml

PLEASE NOTE: 1. Any change in the above formula, except for additional requirements, must have the prior approval of the Pediatric Hyperalimentation Committee.
2. The concentration of iron is less than one (1) part per million. Supplemental iron, if required, must be given by another route.

ADDITIONAL REQUIREMENTS

ADD SODIUM (as chloride) TO EQUAL A TOTAL CONCENTRATION OF _____ mEq/1000 ml

ADD SODIUM (as acetate) TO EQUAL A TOTAL CONCENTRATION OF _____ mEq/1000 ml

ADD POTASSIUM (as chloride) TO EQUAL A TOTAL CONCENTRATION OF _____ mEq/1000 ml

ADD POTASSIUM (as acetate) TO EQUAL A TOTAL CONCENTRATION OF _____ mEq/1000 ml

OTHER _____

_____

RATE OF ADMINISTRATION _____ ml/hour   PATIENT BODY WEIGHT _____ kg

A 24 HOUR SUPPLY WILL BE SENT IN NO LESS THAN TWO CONTAINERS

PLEASE NOTE: The above formula will be supplied each day unless a revised formula is received in the Department of Pharmacy Services by 8 P.M. for delivery at 10 A.M. the next day.

SEND COPY TO PHARMACY SERVICES   **PP**   RETAIN ORIGINAL ON NURSING DIVISION

SP1495

Appendix C–1   Blood Chemistry Values in Premature Infants During the First 7 Weeks of Life* (Birth Weight 1500–1750 gm)

Constituent	Age 1 Week			Age 3 Weeks			Age 5 Weeks			Age 7 Weeks		
	Mean	SD	Range	Mean	SD	Range	Mean	SD	Range	Mean	SD	Range
Na (mEq/liter)	139.6	±3.2	133–146	136.3	±2.9	129–142	136.8	±2.5	133–148	137.2	±1.8	133–142
K (mEq/liter)	5.6	±0.5	4.6–6.7	5.8	±0.6	4.5–7.1	5.5	±0.6	4.5–6.6	5.7	±0.5	4.6–7.1
Cl (mEq/liter)	108.2	±3.7	100–117	108.3	±3.9	102–116	107.0	±3.5	100–115	107.0	±3.3	101–115
CO_2 (mM/liter)	20.3	±2.8	13.8–27.1	18.4	±3.5	12.4–26.2	20.4	±3.4	12.5–26.1	20.6	±3.1	13.7–26.9
Ca (mg/dl)	9.2	±1.1	6.1–11.6	9.6	±0.5	8.1–11.0	9.4	±0.5	8.6–10.5	9.5	±0.7	8.6–10.8
P (mg/dl)	7.6	±1.1	5.4–10.9	7.5	±0.7	6.2–8.7	7.0	±0.6	5.6–7.9	6.8	±0.8	4.2–8.2
BUN (mg/dl)	9.3	±5.2	3.1–25.5	13.3	±7.8	2.1–31.4	13.3	±7.1	2.0–26.5	13.4	±6.7	2.5–30.5
Total protein (gm/dl)	5.49	±0.42	4.40–6.26	5.38	±0.48	4.28–6.70	4.98	±0.50	4.14–6.90	4.93	±0.61	4.02–5.86
Albumin (gm/dl)	3.85	±0.30	3.28–4.50	3.92	±0.42	3.16–5.26	3.73	±0.34	3.20–4.34	3.89	±0.53	3.40–4.60
Globulin (gm/dl)	1.58	±0.33	0.88–2.20	1.44	±0.63	0.62–2.90	1.17	±0.49	0.48–1.48	1.12	±0.33	0.5–2.60
Hb (gm/dl)	17.8	±2.7	11.4–24.8	14.7	±2.1	9.0–19.4	11.5	±2.0	7.2–18.6	10.0	±1.3	7.5–13.9

*Adapted from Thomas, J., and Reichelderfer, T.: Premature infants: analysis of serum during the first seven weeks. Clin Chem 14:272, 1968.

Appendix C–2   Other Serum Values

Ammonia (ng/dl)	Newborn	90–150
	0–2 weeks	70–129
Cholesterol (ng/dl)	Full term	50–120
	1–2 years	70–190
Fatty acids, "free" (mEq/L)	Newborn	0–1845
Phenylalanine (ng/dl)	Newborn	Up to 4
Serum Enzymes		
Creatine kinase (CPK) (U/l)	Premature	37.0–106.9
	3–12 weeks	30.1–70.2
Lactate hydrogenase (U/l)	Birth	290–501
	1 day–1 month	185–404
Aspartate aminotransferase (SGOT) (U/l)	Birth–10 days	6–25

See Meites, S. (ed.): *Pediatric Clinical Chemistry; A Survey of Normals, Methods and Instruments.* Washington, D.C., American Association for Clinical Chemistry, 1977.

Appendix C–3 Plasma-Serum Amino Acids in Premature and Term Newborns (μmol/liter)

Amino Acid	Premature (First Day)	Newborn (Before First Feeding)	16 Days–4 Months
Taurine	105–255	101–181	
OH-proline	0–80	0	
Aspartic acid	0–20	4–12	17–21
Threonine	155–275	196–238	141–213
Serine	195–345	129–197	104–158
Asp + Glut	655–1155	623–895	
Proline	155–305	155–305	141–245
Glutamic acid	30–100	27–77	
Glycine	185–735	274–412	178–248
Alanine	325–425	274–384	239–345
Valine	80–180	97–175	123–199
Cystine	55–75	49–75	33–51
Methionine	30–40	21–37	15–21
Isoleucine	20–60	31–47	31–47
Leucine	45–95	55–89	56–98
Tyrosine	20–220	53–85	33–75
Phenylalanine	70–110	64–92	45–65
Ornithine	70–110	66–116	37–61
Lysine	130–250	154–246	117–163
Histidine	30–70	61–93	64–92
Arginine	30–70	37–71	53–71
Tryptophan	15–45	15–45	
Citrulline	8.5–23.7	10.8–21.1	
Ethanolamine	13.4–105	32.7–72	
α-Amino-n-butyric acid	0–29	8.7–20.4	
Methylhistidine			

Data from Dickinson, J. C., Rosenblum, H., and Hamilton, P. B.: Ion exchange chromatography of the free amino acids in the plasma of the newborn Infant. Pediatrics 36:2, 1965. Dickinson, J. C., Rosenblum, H., and Hamilton, P. B.: Ion exchange chromatography of the free amino acids in the plasma of infants under 2,500 gm at birth. Pediatrics 45:606, 1970.

Source: Behrman, R. E.: *Neonatal-Perinatal Medicine: Disease of the Fetus and Infant.* 2nd ed. Table 20, Appendix. St. Louis, C. V. Mosby, 1977.

Appendix C–4   Normal Hematologic Values

Value	Gestational Age (wks)		Full-Term Cord Blood	Day 1	Day 3	Day 7	Day 14
	28	34					
Hb (gm/dl)	14.5	15.0	16.8	18.4	17.8	17.0	16.8
Hematocrit (%)	45	47	53	58	55	54	52
Red cells (mm³)	4.0	4.4	5.25	5.8	5.6	5.2	5.1
MCV (μ³)	120	118	107	108	99	98	96
MCH (pg)	40	38	34	35	33	32.5	31.5
MCHC (%)	31	32	31.7	32.5	33	33	33
Reticulocytes (%)	5–10	3–10	3–7	3–7	1–3	0–1	0–1
Platelets (1000s/mm³)			290	192	213	248	252

MCV—mean corpuscular volume.
MCH—mean corpuscular hemoglobin.
MCHC—mean corpuscular hemoglobin concentration.

Appendix C–5   Hematologic Values in the First Weeks of Life Related to Gestational Maturity

MEAN CORPUSCULAR HEMOGLOBIN CONCENTRATION (PER CENT)*

Weeks	3 Days	1	2	3	4	6	8	10
<1500 gm								
28–32 weeks	32	32	32	33	33	33	33	32
1500–2000 gm								
32–36 weeks	32	32	32	33	33	33	33	32
2000–2500 gm								
36–40 weeks	32	32	33	33	33	33	33	33
>2500 gm								
Term	32	33	33	33	33	33	33	33

*MCV and MCH, the mean corpuscular volume and mean corpuscular hemoglobin in μ³ and pg, respectively, depend upon red cell counts that are not generally reliable.

HEMOGLOBIN (gm/dl)—MEAN ± [1 SD]

Weeks	3 Days	1	2	3	4	6	8	10
<1500 gm	17.5	15.5	13.5	11.5	10.0	8.5	8.5	9.0
28–32 weeks	[1.5]	[1.5]	[1.1]	[1.0]	[0.9]	[0.5]	[0.5]	[0.5]
1500–2000 gm	19.0	16.5	14.5	13.0	12.0	9.5	9.5	9.5
32–36 weeks	[2.0]	[1.5]	[1.1]	[1.1]	[1.0]	[0.8]	[0.5]	[0.5]
2000–2500 gm	19.0	16.5	15.0	14.0	12.5	10.5	10.5	11.0
36–40 weeks	[2.0]	[1.5]	[1.5]	[1.1]	[1.0]	[0.9]	[0.9]	[1.0]
>2500 gm	19.0	17.0	15.5	14.0	12.5	11.0	11.5	12.0
Term	[2.0]	[1.5]	[1.5]	[1.1]	[1.0]	[1.0]	[1.0]	[1.0]

HEMATOCRIT (PER CENT)—MEAN ± [1 SD]

Weeks	3 Days	1	2	3	4	6	8	10
<1500 gm	54	48	42	35	30	25	25	28
28–32 weeks	[5]	[5]	[4]	[4]	[3]	[2]	[2]	[3]
1500–2000 gm	59	51	44	39	36	28	28	29
32–36 weeks	[6]	[5]	[5]	[4]	[4]	[3]	[3]	[3]
2000–2500 gm	59	51	45	43	37	31	31	33
36–40 weeks	[6]	[5]	[5]	[4]	[4]	[3]	[3]	[3]
>2500 gm	59	51	46	43	37	33	34	36
Term	[6]	[5]	[5]	[4]	[4]	[3]	[3]	[3]

RETICULOCYTE COUNT (PER CENT)—MEAN ± [1 SD]

Weeks	3 Days	1	2	4	6	8	10
<1500 gm	8.0	3.0	3.0	6.0	11.0	8.5	7.0
28–32 weeks	[3.5]	[1.0]	[1.0]	[2.0]	[3.5]	[3.5]	[3.0]
1500–2000 gm	6.0	3.0	2.5	3.0	6.0	5.0	4.5
32–36 weeks	[2.0]	[1.0]	[1.0]	[1.0]	[2.0]	[1.5]	[1.5]
2000–2500 gm	4.0	3.0	2.5	2.0	3.0	3.0	3.0
36–40 weeks	[1.0]	[1.0]	[1.0]	[1.0]	[1.0]	[1.0]	[1.0]
>2500 gm	4.0	3.0	2.0	2.0	2.0	2.0	2.0
Term	[1.5]	[1.0]	[1.0]	[1.0]	[0.5]	[0.5]	[0.5]

Appendix C–6   Coagulation Factor Levels, Screening Studies, and Fibrinolysis Times in Relation to Gestational Maturity

Factors	I	II	V	VII & X	VIII	IX	XI	XIII	Platelets	PTT	PT	TT	FT
	mg/dl	Per Cent of Normal			Mean			Titer × $10^3/mm^3$ (+ SD)		Seconds			
<1500 gm 28–32 weeks	215	21	64	42	50	—	—	—	300 (70)	117	21	—	326
1500–2000 gm 32–36 weeks	220	25	67	37	44	—	—	1/8	260 (60)	113	18	14	214
2000–2500 gm 36–40 weeks	240	35	66	48	67	—	—	1/8	325 (75)	77	17	10	214
>2500 gm Term	210	60	92	56	67	26	42	1/8	325 (70)	71	16	9	95
Mothers of premature infants	520	92	110	178	—	—	—	—	225 (45)	73	14	7	—
Mothers of term infants	500	92	110	206	196	130	69	1/16	215 (41)	75	14	8	278

PTT—Partial thromboplastin time
PT—Prothrombin time
TT—Thrombin time
FT—Fibrinolysis time
See Chapter 15, reference 30.

Appendix C–7 Coagulation Factors in the Fetus and Neonate

FETAL COAGULATION FACTORS*

Authors	Gestational Age (wks)	Fibrinogen (mg/dl)	Prothrombin coag. act. (U/ml)	Factor V coag. act. (U/ml)	Factor VII coag. act. (U/ml)	Factor VIII: C (U/ml)	Factor VIIIR: Ag (U/ml)	Factor IX coag. act. (U/ml)	Source of Material
Vahlquist et al	15–20	50–290							H
Heikinheimo	12–60	<290	0–38	0–81	0–18				H
Fortune and Cox	11–22					<0.01		<0.01	H
Holmberg et al	12–24	60–180		0.4–1.12	0.23–1.12	0.23–1.34		0.14–0.40	H
Mahoney et al	18–20					0.36–1.17	0.17–0.60		F
Firshein et al	18–21					0.5 –1.55	0.17–0.65		F
Mibashan et al	16–22				0.32–0.73		0.1 –0.23	0.08–0.18	F
Peake et al	18–22					0.53–2.72			F

*Oski, F., and Naiman, J.: Hematologic Problems in the Newborn. Philadelphia, W. B. Saunders Co., 1982.

COAGULATION FACTOR ASSAYS (MEAN ± 1 SD) AND SCREENING TESTS IN THE FETUS AND NEONATE*

Assays of Coagulation Factors	Normal Adult Values	28–31 Weeks' Gestation	32–36 Weeks' Gestation	Term	Time at Which Values Attain Adult Norms
Fibrinogen (mg/dl)	150–400	215 ± 28 (SE) / 270 ± 85	226 ± 23 (SE) / 244 ± 55	246 ± 18 (SE) / 246 ± 55	
II (%)	100	30 ± 10	35 ± 12	45 ± 15	2–12 months
V (%)	100	76 ± 7 (SE) / 90 ± 26	84 ± 9 (SE) / 72 ± 23	100 ± 5 (SE) / 98 ± 40	
VII and X (%)	100	38 ± 14	40 ± 15	56 ± 16	2–12 months
VIII (%)	100	90 ± 15 (SE) / 70 ± 30	140 ± 10 (SE) / 98 ± 40	168 ± 12 (SE) / 105 ± 34	
IX (%)	100	27 ± 10	NA	28 ± 8	3–9 months
XI (%)	100	5–18	NA	29–70	1–2 months
XII (%)	100	NA	30 ±	51 (25–70)	9–14 days
XIII					
Bioassay (%)	100	100	100	100	
Quantitative (U/ml)	21 ± 5.6	5 ± 3.5	NA	11 ± 3.4	3 weeks
Prothrombin time (sec)	12–14	23 ±	17 (12–21)	16 (13–20)	1 week
Activated partial thromboplastin time (sec)	44	NA	70 ±	55 ± 10	2–9 months
Thrombin time (sec)	10	16–28	14 (11–17)	12 (10–16)	few days
Prekallikrein	100	27	NA	33 ± 6	unknown
HMW kininogen	100	28	NA	56 ± 12	unknown

*Oski, F., and Naiman, J.: Hematologic Problems in the Newborn. Philadelphia, W. B. Saunders Co., 1982.

Appendix C–8   Serum Vitamin E (mg/dl)— Mean ± [1 SD]

Weeks	1	2	3	4	5	6	7	8	9	10
<1500 gm	0.40	0.30	0.25	0.25	0.25	0.25	0.25	0.25	0.35	0.45
28–32 weeks	[0.05]	[0.04]	[0.03]	[0.03]	[0.03]	[0.03]	[0.03]	[0.03]	[0.04]	[0.05]
1500–2000 gm	0.45	0.40	0.40	0.45	0.45	0.45	0.50	0.50	0.60	0.70
32–36 weeks	[0.05]	[0.05]	[0.05]	[0.05]	[0.05]	[0.05]	[0.05]	[0.05]	[0.06]	[0.06]
2000–2500 gm	0.50	0.45	0.50	0.60	0.70	0.75	0.75	0.75	0.75	0.80
36–40 weeks	[0.05]	[0.05]	[0.05]	[0.06]	[0.06]	[0.06]	[0.60]	[0.60]	[0.60]	[0.70]
>2500 gm	0.55	0.55	0.55	0.60	0.75	0.80	0.85	0.85	0.85	0.85
Term	[0.60]	[0.60]	[0.60]	[0.60]	[0.70]	[0.70]	[0.80]	[0.80]	[0.80]	[0.80]

Appendix C–9   White Cell and Differential Counts in Premature Infants

Birth Weight	<1500 gm			1500–2500 gm		
Age in Weeks	1	2	4	1	2	4
Total Count (× 10³/mm³)						
Mean	16.8	15.4	12.1	13.0	10.0	8.4
Range	6.1–32.8	10.4–21.3	8.7–17.2	6.7–14.7	7.0–14.1	5.8–12.4
Per Cent of Total						
Polymorphs						
Segmented	54	45	40	55	43	41
Unsegmented	7	6	5	8	8	6
Eosinophils	2	3	3	2	3	3
Basophils	1	1	1	1	1	1
Monocytes	6	10	10	5	9	11
Lymphocytes	30	35	41	9	36	38

Appendix C–10 Leukocyte Values and Neutrophil Counts in Term and Premature Infants

LEUKOCYTE VALUES IN TERM AND PREMATURE INFANTS (10^3 cells/μl)*

Age (hrs)	Total White Cell Count	Neutrophils	Bands/Metas	Lymphocytes	Monocytes	Eosinophils
Term Infants						
0	10.0–26.0	5.0–13.0	0.4–1.8	3.5–8.5	0.7–1.5	0.2–2.0
12	13.5–31.0	9.0–18.0	0.4–2.0	3.0–7.0	1.0–2.0	0.2–2.0
72	5.0–14.5	2.0–7.0	0.2–0.4	2.0–5.0	0.5–1.0	0.2–1.0
144	6.0–14.5	2.0–6.0	0.2–0.5	3.0–6.0	0.7–1.2	0.2–0.8
Premature Infants						
0	5.0–19.0	2.0–9.0	0.2–2.4	2.5–6.0	0.3–1.0	0.1–0.7
12	5.0–21.0	3.0–11.0	0.2–2.4	1.5–5.0	0.3–1.3	0.1–1.1
72	5.0–14.0	3.0–7.0	0.2–0.6	1.5–4.0	0.3–1.2	0.2–1.1
144	5.5–17.5	2.0–7.0	0.2–0.5	2.5–7.5	0.5–1.5	0.3–1.2

*Oski, F., and Naiman, J.: *Hematologic Problems in the Newborn.* Philadelphia, W. B. Saunders Co., 1982.

TOTAL NEUTROPHIL COUNT REFERENCE RANGE IN THE FIRST 60 HOURS OF LIFE*

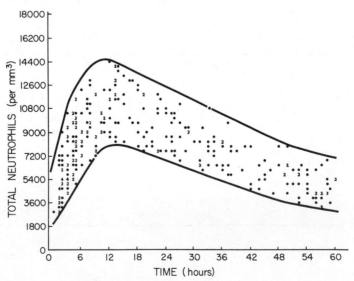

*Manroe, B. L., Weinberg, A. G., Rosenfeld, C. R., et al.: The neonatal blood count in health and disease. I. Reference values for neutrophilic cells. J. Pediatr. 95:91, 1979.

Appendix D–1 Urine Amino Acids in Normal Newborns (μmol/day)

Amino Acid	μmol/day
Cysteic acid	Tr–3.32
Phosphoethanolamine	Tr–8.86
Taurine	7.59–7.72
OH-proline	0–9.81
Aspartic acid	Tr
Threonine	0.176–7.99
Serine	Tr–20.7
Glutamic acid	0–1.78
Proline	0–5.17
Glycine	0.176–65.3
Alanine	Tr–8.03
α-Aminoadipic acid	
α-Amino-n-butyric acid	0–0.47
Valine	0–7.76
Cystine	0–7.96
Methionine	Tr–0.892
Isoleucine	0–6.11
Tyrosine	0–1.11
Phenylalanine	0–1.66
β-Aminoisobutyric acid	0.264–7.34
Ethanolamine	Tr–79.9
Ornithine	Tr–0.554
Lysine	0.33–9.79
1-Methylhistidine	Tr–8.64
3-Methylhistidine	0.11–3.32
Carnosine	0.044–4.01
β-Aminobutyric acid	
Cystathionine	
Homocitrulline	
Arginine	0.088–0.918
Histidine	Tr–7.04
Sarcosine	
Leucine	Tr–0.918

Adapted from Meites, S. (ed.): *Pediatric Clinical Chemistry; A Survey of Normals, Methods and Instruments.* Washington, D.C., American Association for Clinical Chemistry, 1977.

Source: Behrman, R. E.: *Neonatal-Perinatal Medicine: Disease of the Fetus and Infant.* 2nd ed. Table 21, Appendix. St. Louis, C. V. Mosby, 1977.

Appendix E–1 Siggaard-Andersen Alignment Nomogram

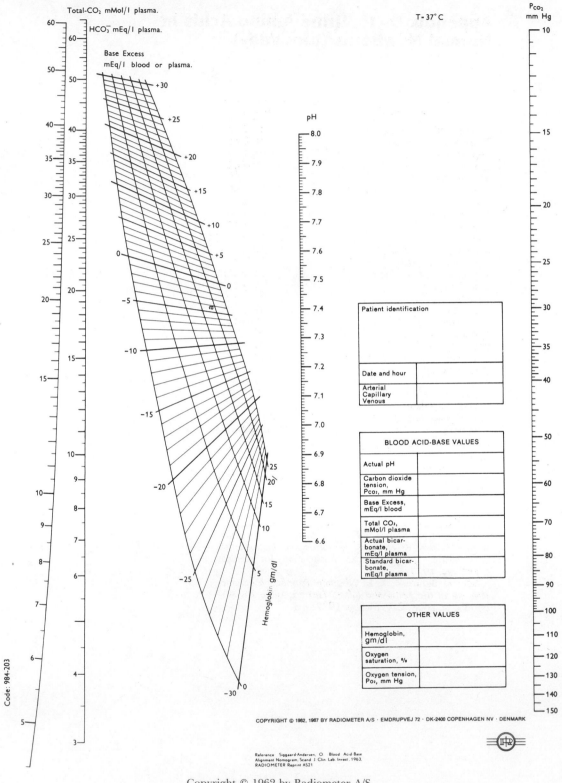

T-37°C

Total-CO₂ mMol/l plasma.

HCO₃⁻ mEq/l plasma.

Base Excess
mEq/l blood or plasma.

pH

Hemoglobin gm/dl

P$_{CO_2}$
mm Hg

Code: 984-203

Reference: Siggaard-Andersen, O. Blood Acid-Base
Alignment Nomogram. Scand J Clin Lab Invest. 1963.
RADIOMETER Reprint AS21.

Patient identification

Date and hour	
Arterial Capillary Venous	

BLOOD ACID-BASE VALUES

Actual pH	
Carbon dioxide tension, Pco₂, mm Hg	
Base Excess, mEq/l blood	
Total CO₂, mMol/l plasma	
Actual bicarbonate, mEq/l plasma	
Standard bicarbonate, mEq/l plasma	

OTHER VALUES

Hemoglobin, gm/dl	
Oxygen saturation, %	
Oxygen tension, Po₂, mm Hg	

418

Appendix F–1 Cerebrospinal Fluid Findings in Term and Premature Infants

CEREBROSPINAL FLUID EXAMINATION IN HIGH-RISK NEONATES WITHOUT MENINGITIS

	Term	Preterm
WBC count (cells/mm³)		
No. of infants	87	30
Mean	8.2	9.0
Median	5	6
SD	7.1	8.2
Range	0–32	0–29
± 2 SD	0–22.4	0–25.4
Percentage PMN*	61.3%	57.2%
Protein (mg/dl)		
No. of infants	35	17
Mean	90	115
Range	20–170	65–150
Glucose (mg/dl)		
No. of infants	51	23
Mean	52	50
Range	34–119	24–63
CSF/blood glucose (%)		
No. of infants	51	23
Mean	81	74
Range	44–248	55–105

*PMN – Polymorphonuclear cells
From: Sarff, L., Platt, L., and McCracken, G.: Cerebrospinal fluid evaluation in neonates: comparison of high risk infants with and without meningitis. J. Pediatr 88:473, 1976.

CEREBROSPINAL FLUID FINDINGS IN FIRST 24 HOURS OF LIFE IN 135 FULL-TERM INFANTS*

	Range	Mean	2 SD
Red blood cells	0–1070	9	0–884
Polymorphs	0–70	3	0–27
Lymphocytes	0–20	2	0–24
Proteins	32–240	63	27–144
Sugar	32–78	51	35–64
Chloride	680–760	720	660–780

*Naidoo, T.: The cerebrospinal fluid in the healthy newborn infant. South Afr. Med J 42:933, 1968.

CEREBROSPINAL FLUID FINDINGS ON FIRST AND SEVENTH DAYS IN FULL-TERM INFANTS*

	Day 1 (n = 135)		Day 7 (n = 20)	
	Range	Mean	Range	Mean
Red blood cells	0–620	23	0–48	3
Polymorphs	0–26	7	0–5	2
Lymphocytes	0–16	5	0–4	1
Protein	40–148	73	27–65	47
Sugar	38–64	48	48–62	55
Chloride	680–760	720	720–760	720

*Naidoo, T.: The cerebrospinal fluid in the healthy newborn infant. South Afr Med J 42:933, 1968.

CEREBROSPINAL FLUID FINDINGS IN PREMATURE INFANTS

Number	Per Cent Xanthrochromic	Per Cent Bloody	Leukocytes (per mm³)	Protein mg/dl	Reference
20	90	10	0–13 mean = 12	50–180 mean = 105	Wolf and Hoepffner*
100	97	1	7–44	1st wk = 100 2nd wk = 128	Otila†

*Wolf, H., and Hoepffner, L.: The cerebrospinal fluid in the newborn and premature infant. World Neurol 2:871, 1961.
†Otila, E.: Studies on the cerebrospinal fluid in premature infants. Acta Paediatr Scand 35 (Suppl. 8):9, 1948.

Appendix F–2   Comparison of WBC Counts in Neonates With and Without Meningitis

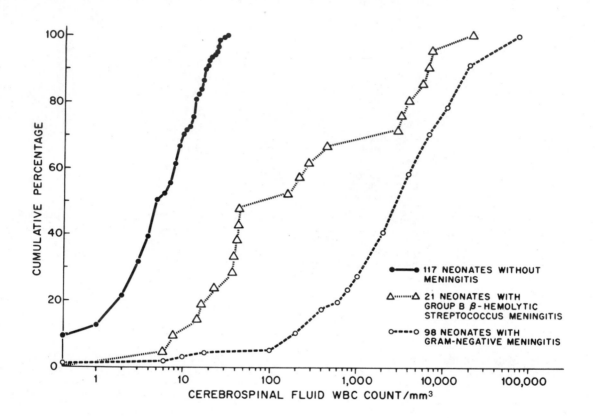

Appendix G–1   Growth Record for Infants

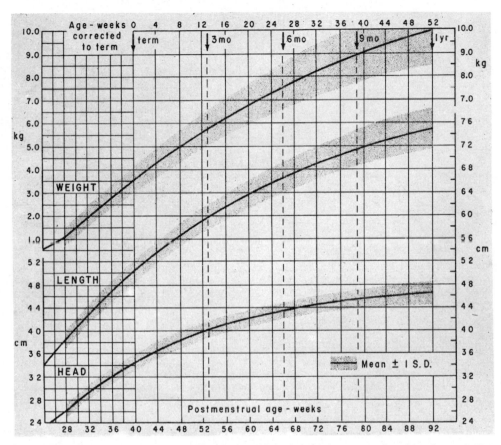

Growth record for infants in relation to gestational age and fetal and infant norms (combined sexes), University of Oregon. (Babson, S.: Growth of low-birthweight infants. J Pediatr 77:11, 1970.)

Appendix G–2   Head Circumference (Boys)

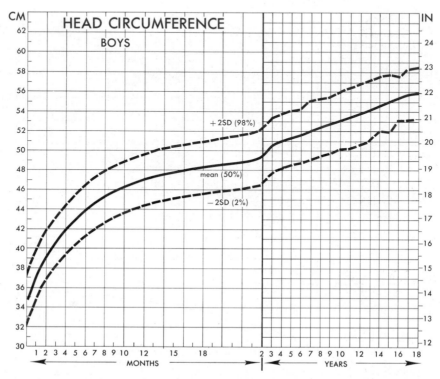

Nellhaus, G.: Composite international and interracial graphs. Pediatrics *41*:106, 1068.

Appendix G—3 Head Circumference (Girls)

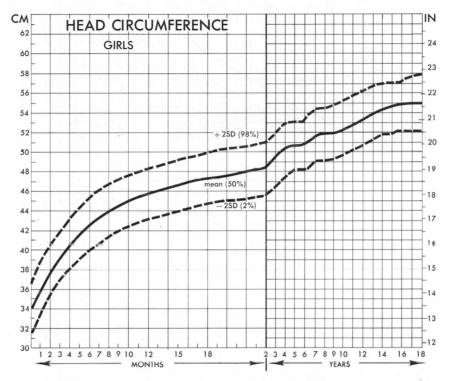

Nellhaus, G.: Composite international and interracial graphs. Pediatrics *41*:106, 1968.

Appendix G—4   Intrauterine Growth Curves

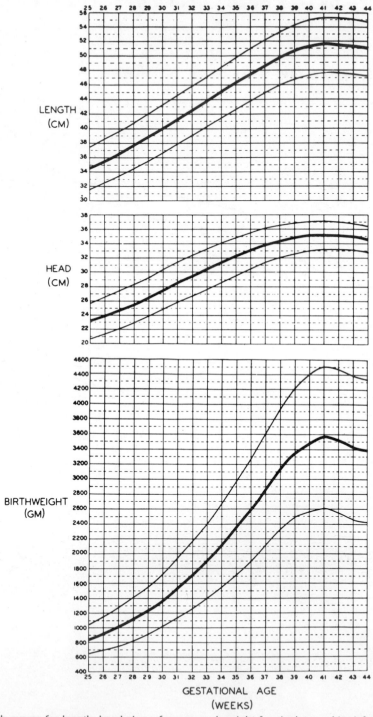

Intrauterine growth curves for length, head circumference, and weight for singleton white infants born at sea level (mean ± 2 standard deviations). (Composite of graphics from Usher, R., and McLean, F.: Intrauterine growth of liveborn Caucasian infants at sea level: standard obtained in 7 dimensions of infants born between 25 and 44 weeks of gestation. J Pediatr 74:901, 1969.)

Appendix G–5 Conversion of Pounds and Ounces to Grams

P O U N D S	Ounces 0	1	2	3	4	5	6	7	8	9	10	11	12	13	Ounces 14	15
0	—	28	57	85	113	142	170	198	227	255	283	312	340	369	397	425
1	454	482	510	539	567	595	624	652	680	709	737	765	794	822	850	879
2	907	936	964	992	1021	1049	1077	1106	1134	1162	1191	1219	1247	1276	1304	1332
3	1361	1389	1417	1446	1474	1503	1531	1559	1588	1616	1644	1673	1701	1729	1758	1786
4	1814	1843	1871	1899	1928	1956	1984	2013	2041	2070	2098	2126	2155	2183	2211	2240
5	2268	2296	2325	2353	2381	2410	2438	2466	2495	2523	2551	2580	2608	2637	2665	2693
6	2722	2750	2778	2807	2835	2863	2892	2920	2948	2977	3005	3033	3062	3090	3118	3147
7	3175	3203	3232	3260	3289	3317	3345	3374	3402	3430	3459	3487	3515	3544	3572	3600
8	3629	3657	3685	3714	3742	3770	3799	3827	3856	3884	3912	3941	3969	3997	4026	4054
9	4082	4111	4139	4167	4196	4224	4252	4281	4309	4337	4366	4394	4423	4451	4479	4508
10	4536	4564	4593	4621	4649	4678	4706	4734	4763	4791	4819	4848	4876	4904	4933	4961
11	4990	5018	5046	5075	5103	5131	5160	5188	5216	5245	5273	5301	5330	5358	5386	5415
12	5443	5471	5500	5528	5557	5585	5613	5642	5670	5698	5727	5755	5783	5812	5840	5868
13	5897	5925	5953	5982	6010	6038	6067	6095	6123	6152	6180	6209	6237	6265	6294	6322
14	6350	6379	6407	6435	6464	6492	6520	6549	6577	6605	6634	6662	6690	6719	6747	6776
15	6804	6832	6860	6889	6917	6945	6973	7002	7030	7059	7087	7115	7144	7172	7201	7228
16	7257	7286	7313	7342	7371	7399	7427	7456	7484	7512	7541	7569	7597	7626	7654	7682
17	7711	7739	7768	7796	7824	7853	7881	7909	7938	7966	7994	8023	8051	8079	8108	8136
18	8165	8192	8221	8249	8278	8306	8335	8363	8391	8420	8448	8476	8504	8533	8561	8590
19	8618	8646	8675	8703	8731	8760	8788	8816	8845	8873	8902	8930	8958	8987	9015	9043
20	9072	9100	9128	9157	9185	9213	9242	9270	9298	9327	9355	9383	9412	9440	9469	9497
21	9525	9554	9582	9610	9639	9667	9695	9724	9752	9780	9809	9837	9865	9894	9922	9950
22	9979	10007	10036	10064	10092	10120	10149	10177	10206	10234	10262	10291	10319	10347	10376	10404

Appendix G—6 The Time of First Void and Stool

Time	Time of 1st Voiding by 920 Full-Term Infants			Time	Time of Passage of 1st Stool by 920 Full-Term Infants		
	No.	Per Cent	Cumulative %		No.	Per Cent	Cumulative %
Delivery room	139	15.1	15.1	Delivery room	210	22.8	22.8
Hours				Hours			
1–24	743	80.8	95.9	1–24	674	73.3	96.1
24–48	35	3.8	99.7	24–48	35	3.8	99.9
Over 48	3	0.3	100.0	Over 48	1	0.1	100.0

Time	Time of Passage of 1st Urine by 280 Premature Infants			Time	Time of Passage of 1st Stool by 280 Premature Infants		
	No.	Per Cent	Cumulative %		No.	Per Cent	Cumulative %
Delivery room	62	22.1	22.1	Delivery room	30	10.7	10.7
Hours				Hours			
1–24	201	71.8	93.9	1–24	191	68.2	78.9
24–48	17	6.1	100.0	24–48	46	16.4	95.3
Over 48	.			Over 48	13	4.7	100.0

Adapted from Sherry, S., and Kramer, I.: The time of passage of the first stool and first urine by the newborn infant. J Pediatr 46:158, 1955.

Kramer, I., Sherry, S.: The time of passage of the first stool and urine by the premature infant. J Pediatr 51:353, 1957.

Clark, D.: Times of first void and stool in 500 newborns. Pediatrics 60:457, 1977.

Appendix H—1 Classification of Newborn Infants and Mortality Risk

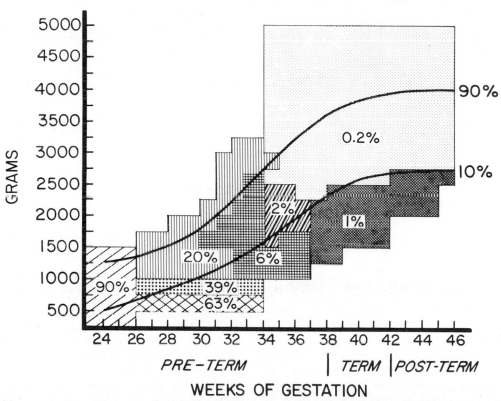

Mortality risk according to birth weight—gestational age relationship. Based on 14,413 live births at University of Colorado Health Sciences Center (1974–1980).

Appendix I–1   Equipment Found on the Umbilical Catheterization Tray, University Hospitals, Cleveland, Ohio

---

2 2 ml Luer-lock syringes
1 Small needle holder
2 Curved mosquito hemostats
1 Straight iris scissors
2 Straight mosquito hemostats
1 Straight suture scissors
1 Smooth straight iris forceps
2 Smooth deep-curved iris forceps
1 Medicine glass
2 Cord ties (10 in long)
2 3-way stopcocks
4 3 × 3 gauze sponges
1 Size 5–0 silk suture set with needle (#682)
1 Eye treatment sheet
2 Needle caps

Appendix I–2   Umbilical Vessel Catheterization

Use of central catheters requires careful consideration of the risks involved, culminating in a decision as to whether the need for the catheter outweighs the risks of the catheterization procedure and the subsequent presence of an indwelling catheter. A central catheter inserted into the aorta via an umbilical artery may be required in the management of the sick neonate for monitoring of blood pressure, intermittent sampling of blood to monitor acid-base status, and, while in place, infusion of parenteral fluids and medications.

Umbilical artery catheters must be precisely located. A major objective is to avoid the origin of the renal arteries, since a catheter may occlude a renal artery and catheters in the area may produce thrombosis.[7] Both situations can result in renal infarction. Our preference is to position the catheter tip between L3 and L4 (low); others prefer a midthoracic location (high).[6, 14, 15] Thrombotic complications are reported with both high[4]

and low[6] placement. Fortunately, resolution of the thrombus or development of collateral circulation generally occurs, even when extensive thrombosis (aorta distal to renal arteries, common iliac) has been documented.[4, 7] Occasionally a neonatal death is considered a direct consequence of complications related to umbilical vessel catheterization. Hypertension in the neonate following use of high umbilical artery catheters has been described.[11] However, in a prospective study the incidence of hypertension was similar with low and high catheters.[12]

Hemorrhage, as a result of loose connections or careless use of the stopcocks or occurring at the time of removal, is a major complication of arterial catheters. Another major complication of catheterization is thrombosis of the vessel around the catheter with subsequent release of microemboli. The catheter tip can traumatize the vessel wall, which may release tissue thromboplastin, and activate intravascular coagulation. Alternatively, the presence of the catheter itself may promote clot formation.

Arterial blood samples may be obtained by multiple arterial punctures (radial, brachial, or temporal) or an indwelling radial artery cannula as the method of choice or when umbilical artery catheterization is unsuccessful.[1, 13] As transcutaneous monitoring of oxygen tension ($tcPO_2$) has become more readily available, the need for indwelling catheters has decreased.

In general, umbilical vein catheterization is technically easier. However, it should be avoided except when immediate access to a vein is needed for an unexpected emergency (delivery room resuscitation), since complications may be serious and difficult to avoid. An umbilical vein catheter tip may locate in a branch of the portal vein and lead to areas of liver necrosis without perforation of the vein wall[5, 9, 10] following infusions of hypertonic solutions such as sodium bicarbonate and hypertonic glucose. Portal vein thrombosis has also occurred with and without infection. In addition, spontaneous perforation of the colon following exchange transfusion via an umbilical vein catheter has been reported. X-ray verification of catheter tip location was not done in any of these cases; most likely the catheter tip was in the portal vein, and the cause of perforation was local necrosis of bowel wall following hemorrhagic infarction secondary to retrograde microemboli or obstructive hemodynamic changes.[3]

In the first hour or so of life in a normal term infant, or for many hours and occasionally for many days in a sick or preterm infant, an umbilical venous catheter may be passed through the ductus venosus into the inferior vena cava.

Depending on the circumstances and preference of the physician, exchange transfusions can be done using either vessel or both, but not infusing into the artery.

The umbilical vessel catheter should be removed as soon as possible and a peripheral IV substituted, if necessary. In the undistressed newborn infant requiring parenteral fluids, under no circumstances should an umbilical vessel catheter be used when a peripheral IV could be started via a scalp vein or an extremity vein. An exception may be made in the infant weighing less than 1000 gm for whom the risks of the umbilical artery catheter are weighed against the stress associated with repeated attempts at peripheral IV placement.

Technique of Catheterization

In the small premature infant, the entire procedure should be done as an operating room procedure in an incubator or under a radiant heater to avoid chilling the infant. In the delivery room, a radiant heater should be used.

When not precluded by an emergency (e.g., acute asphyxia), the following protocol should be followed. The operator carefully scrubs hands and arms to the elbows and puts on sterile gloves. A 3.5–4 (for infants <1500 gm) or 5 French catheter with rounded tip, which has a radiopaque line and end hole (Argyle Umbilical Artery Catheter), or an indwelling arterial oxygen electrode (Orange Medical Instruments) is attached to a syringe by a three-way stopcock, and the system is filled with heparinized saline solution (1 unit heparin/ml of 0.25 N saline). (Appendix I–1 lists the equipment found on the catheterization tray.) Before the procedure is begun, the length of the catheter to be inserted should be marked according to the location desired (Figures I–1 and I–2). After the umbilical stump and surrounding abdominal wall are carefully prepared with an antiseptic solution, sterile towels are placed around the stump and a "circumcision drape" placed with the hole over the stump. The cord stump is then grasped at the base with a gauze sponge, and the stump of cord is cut to within about 1.5 cm of the abdominal wall with a scissors or surgical blade. The exposed vessels are identified—a thin-walled oval vein and two smaller thick-walled round arteries with tightly constricted lumens.

The lumen of the vessel to be used is gently dilated with a curved eye dressing forceps or small obturator (Figure I–3A and B). The catheter is then inserted and gently advanced. Obstruction at the level of the abdominal wall may be relieved by gentle traction on the umbilical cord stump accompanied by steady but gentle pressure for about 30 seconds. During umbilical artery catheterization, obstruction may also occur at the level of the bladder. It may be overcome by gentle, steady pressure for 30 seconds. If this is not successful, 0.1–0.2 ml of 2 per cent lidocaine (without epinephrine) can be injected via the catheter to relieve the vasospasm. (Remove the catheter first to add lidocaine to its tip.) If this procedure is unsuccessful, the other artery should be used. If the leg on the side of the catheterization

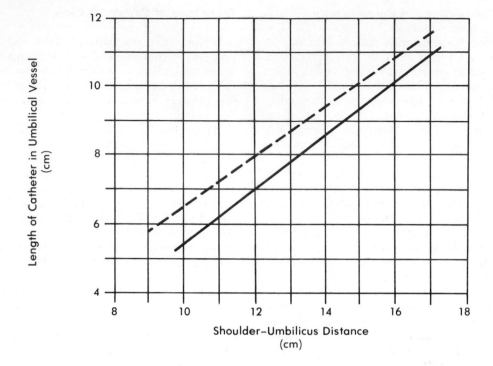

— — — — Umbilical vein—to junction of inferior
vena cava and right atrium

————— Umbilical artery—to bifurcation of aorta

Figure I–1. Determination of length of catheter to be inserted for appropriate arterial or venous placement. The length of the catheter read from the diagram is to the umbilical ring; the length of the umbilical cord stump present must be added. The shoulder-umbilicus distance is the perpendicular distance between parallel lines at the level of the umbilicus and through the distal ends of the clavicles. (Adapted from data of Dunn[2].)

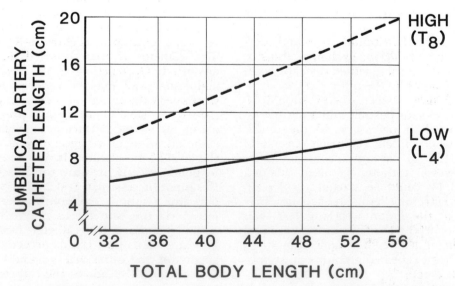

Figure I–2. Catheter position determined from total body length. (Modified from Rosenfeld et al.[8])

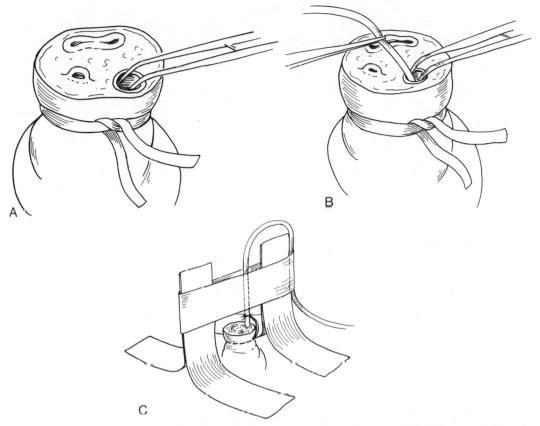

Figure I–3. *A,* Cross-section of umbilical cord. Tie in place. Dilatation of artery with iris forceps. *B,* Insertion of catheter into umbilical artery. *C,* Bridge technique used to secure catheter after suturing. Use purse string suture incorporating all three vessels. Tie square knot at the base of the catheter and a second knot 1 cm above the base. The tape bridge further ensures against the line becoming dislodged.

blanches, the catheter should be removed immediately and the other umbilical artery used. Cyanosis involving toes or part of the foot on the side of the catheter may be relieved by warming the contralateral foot; when this is not successful the catheter should be removed.

If an umbilical vein catheterization is performed, the next site of obstruction after the abdominal wall is the portal system. (The catheter meets resistance several cm before the distance marked on the catheter is reached.) The catheter should be withdrawn several centimeters, gently rotated, and reinserted in an attempt to get the tip through the ductus venosus into the inferior vena cava. Occasionally, it will not be possible to get the catheter into the inferior vena cava for anatomic reasons, and vigorous attempts to advance the catheter are to be avoided.

An umbilical vessel catheter should be tied in place with a silk suture around the vessel and catheter and sutured to the umbilical stump or taped to the abdominal wall (Figure I–3C). Disastrous hemorrhage can occur if the catheter is inadvertently pulled out or the stopcocks are disconnected by the activity of the infant. The position of the catheter must be identified by x-ray immediately after insertion.

If the x-ray following umbilical vessel catheterization indicates that the catheter has been inserted too far, it may be gently withdrawn an estimated amount for appropriate placement. If the catheter is not in far enough, it must be completely withdrawn and a new sterile one inserted after appropriately preparing the area again.

REFERENCES

1. Adams, J., and Rudolph, A.: The use of indwelling radial artery catheters in neonates. Pediatrics 55:261, 1975.
2. Dunn, P.: Localization of the umbilical catheter by post-mortem measurement. Arch Dis Child 41:69, 1966.
3. Friedman, A., Abellera, R., Lidsky, I., et al: Perforation of the colon after exchange transfusion in the newborn. N Engl J Med 282:796, 1970.
4. Goetzman, B., Stadalnik, R., Bogren, H., et al: Thrombotic complications of umbilical artery catheters: a clinical and radiographic study. Pediatrics 56:374, 1975.
5. Larroche, J.: Umbilical catheterization: its complications. Biol Neonate 16:101, 1970.
6. Mokrohisky, S., Levine, R., Blumhagen, J., et al: Low positioning of umbilical-artery catheters increases associated complications in newborn infants. N Engl J Med 299:561, 1978.
7. Oppenheimer, D., Carroll, B., and Garth, K.: Ultrasonic detection of complications following umbilical arterial catheterization in the neonate. Radiology 145:667, 1982.
8. Rosenfeld, W., Biagtan, J., Schaeffer, H., et al: A new graph for insertion of umbilical artery catheters. J Pediatr 96:735, 1980.
9. Sarrut, S., Alain, J., and Alison, F.: Les complications precoces de la perfusion par la veine ombilicale chez le premature. Arch Fr Pediatr 26:651, 1969.
10. Scott, J.: Iatrogenic lesions in babies following umbilical vein catheterization. Arch Dis Child 40:426, 1965.
11. Skalina, M. E. L., Annable, W., Kliegman, R. M., et al: Hypertensive retinopathy in the newborn infant. J Pediatr 103:781, 1983.
12. Stork, E., Carlo, W., Kliegman, R., et al: Neonatal hypertension appears unrelated to aortic catheter position. Pediatr Res 18:321A, 1984.
13. Todres, I., Rogers, M., Shannon, C., et al: Percutaneous catheterization of the radial artery in the critically ill neonate. J Pediatr 87:273, 1975.
14. Uhari, M., Tarkka, M., and Koskinen, M.: Renal blood flow in high and low positions of aortic catheter in rabbits. J Perinatal Med 9:219, 1981.
15. Wesstrom, G., Finnstrom, O., and Stenport, G.: Umbilical artery catheterization in newborns. I. Thrombosis in relation to catheter type and position. Acta Paediatr Scand 68:575, 1979.

Appendix I–3   Endotracheal Tubes

ENDOTRACHEAL TUBE SIZE

Infant Weight (gm)	ET Tube Diameter	
	Inside	Outside
Less than 1000	2.5 mm	12 Fr.
1000–1500	3.0 mm	14 Fr.
1500–2200	3.5 mm	16 Fr.
2200 and over	4.0 mm	18 Fr.

From Avery, G. (ed.): *Neonatology.* Philadelphia, J. B. Lippincott, 1975.

INSERTION DISTANCE, ENDOTRACHEAL TUBE

Infant Weight (gm)	Cord-Carina Distance (cm)	Insertion Past Cords (cm)
1000–1500	4.0	1.5–2.0
1500–2500	4.5	2.0
2500–3500	5.0	2.2
3500–4000	5.5	2.5

From Avery, G. (ed.): *Neonatology.* Philadelphia, J. B. Lippincott, 1975.

Appendix J–1 Intake Range Recommended for Growing Stable 2 Week Old, 29 Week Gestational Age Infant (Cow Milk–Based Formula)

Nutrient	
Vitamin B_{12}	0.15 μg/100 Kcal
Folate	15 μg/kg per day
Vitamin C	30 mg/100 Kcal
Niacin	4 mg preformed niacin/100 Kcal
Thiamine	250 μg/100 Kcal
Riboflavin	335 μg/100 Kcal
Pyridoxine	250 μg/100 Kcal
Vitamin A	1400 IU/day
Vitamin E	25 IU/day[a]
Vitamin K	5 μg/kg per day
Vitamin D	400 IU/day
Fe	2 mg/kg per day by doubled birth weight[b]
Ca	Up to 200 mg/kg per day[c]
P	Up to 113 mg/kg per day[c]
Mg	5–6 mg/kg per day
Na	3–8 mEq/kg per day[d] up to 3 weeks, then 1–3 mEqkg[e] per day[e]
K	1–3 mEq/kg per day
Cl	3–8 mEq/kg per day (can reduce to 1.0 if HCO_3^- given)
Zn	800–1200 μg/kg per day[f]
Cu	100–200 μg/kg per day
Se	1.5–2.5 μg/kg per day
Mn	10–20 μg/kg per day
Cr	2–4 μg/kg per day
Mo	2–3 μg/kg per day
Biotin	0.6–2.3 μg/kg per day
Pantothenic acid	1.0–1.4 mg/kg per day
Choline	5–9 mg/kg per day

[a]25 IU/day is recommended to establish tissue vitamin E stores in the first 2–4 weeks; beyond that, 5 IU/day is satisfactory.

[b]1–2 mg/kg per day prior to this time, if blood loss not replaced.

[c]Low calcium and phosphorus concentrations in human milk fed to preterm infants result in low bone mineral content, which may be prevented by using mineral supplements. Preterm infants receiving exclusively human milk for prolonged periods should be examined, at least at 2 months of age, for rickets and fractures using x-ray, serum phosphorus, and possibly alkaline phosphatase measurements.

[d]Decrease to 2 mEq/kg per day if serum Na is greater than 144 mEq/liter.

[e]Increase again if serum sodium less than 132 mEq/liter.

[f]Infants appear to be generally in negative balance even at these levels of intake.

From Tsang, R. C.: *Vitamin and Mineral Requirements in Preterm Infants.* New York, Marcel Dekker, Inc., 1985.

Index

Numbers in *italics* refer to illustrations; numbers followed by (t) refer to tables; and numbers followed by (c) refer to case problems.